TØ100705

Childhood Asthma

LUNG BIOLOGY IN HEALTH AND DISEASE

Executive Editor

Claude Lenfant

*Former Director, National Heart, Lung, and Blood Institute
National Institutes of Health
Bethesda, Maryland*

The opinions expressed in these volumes do not necessarily represent the views of the National Institutes of Health.

Childhood Asthma

Edited by

Stanley J. Szefler
National Jewish Medical and Research Center
Denver, Colorado, U.S.A.

Søren Pedersen
Kolding Hospital
Kolding, Denmark

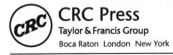

CRC Press
Taylor & Francis Group
Boca Raton London New York

CRC Press is an imprint of the
Taylor & Francis Group, an **informa** business

CRC Press
Taylor & Francis Group
6000 Broken Sound Parkway NW, Suite 300
Boca Raton, FL 33487-2742

First issued in paperback 2019

© 2006 by Taylor & Francis Group, LLC
CRC Press is an imprint of Taylor & Francis Group, an Informa business

No claim to original U.S. Government works

ISBN-13: 978-0-8247-2735-2 (hbk)
ISBN-13: 978-0-367-39206-2 (pbk)

This book contains information obtained from authentic and highly regarded sources. Reasonable efforts have been made to publish reliable data and information, but the author and publisher cannot assume responsibility for the validity of all materials or the consequences of their use. The authors and publishers have attempted to trace the copyright holders of all material reproduced in this publication and apologize to copyright holders if permission to publish in this form has not been obtained. If any copyright material has not been acknowledged please write and let us know so we may rectify in any future reprint.

Except as permitted under U.S. Copyright Law, no part of this book may be reprinted, reproduced, transmitted, or utilized in any form by any electronic, mechanical, or other means, now known or hereafter invented, including photocopying, microfilming, and recording, or in any information storage or retrieval system, without written permission from the publishers.

For permission to photocopy or use material electronically from this work, please access www.copyright.com (http://www.copyright.com/) or contact the Copyright Clearance Center, Inc. (CCC), 222 Rosewood Drive, Danvers, MA 01923, 978-750-8400. CCC is a not-for-profit organization that provides licenses and registration for a variety of users. For organizations that have been granted a photocopy license by the CCC, a separate system of payment has been arranged.

Trademark Notice: Product or corporate names may be trademarks or registered trademarks, and are used only for identification and explanation without intent to infringe.

Library of Congress Cataloging-in-Publication Data

Catalog record is available from the Library of Congress

Visit the Taylor & Francis Web site at
http://www.taylorandfrancis.com

and the CRC Press Web site at
http://www.crcpress.com

Introduction

For small children, if asthma comes from the blockage of the airways, make this proven remedy. In a rough pot enclose a baby hare that has been taken from its mother's womb, cover the pot with clay and put it in the oven long enough until it turns to charcoal; give the powder of this charcoal to the small children, together with *trifera magria* and women's milk.

—Johannes de Santo Paulo, School of Salerno
(Published in the 13th Century)

Surely we all—and especially children with asthma—can be thankful that approaches to asthma care have changed and that other "proven" remedies have been developed.

The quest for better strategies to manage asthma is as old as time. Asthma and its treatment were the subject of considerable interest in ancient Egypt, in early Chinese medicine, and in the teaching of Ayurvedic medicine in India around 500 BC. In a general way, therapies for asthma continued to be based on empirical approaches until the 19th century when anticholinergics, adrenergics, and methylxanthines were introduced, albeit on a limited scale. In the mid–20th century, a better understanding of the pathogenesis of asthma, particularly the role of inflammation, finally gave us a more active and anticipatory approach to treatment.

In children, asthma may be more severe than in adults, and drug dosage, action, and metabolism may be different. It goes without saying, therefore, that children with asthma must be carefully monitored in order to ensure effective control of their disease. This new volume, *Childhood Asthma*, offers a timely and comprehensive exposition of this important issue. Editors Stanley J. Szefler and Søren Pedersen, with their extensive clinical knowledge and well-recognized scientific achievements in asthma, bring unique expertise, and they have enlisted the contributions of many acknowledged experts in the field.

For years, the series of monographs Lung Biology in Health and Disease has presented volumes introducing promising pioneering research on asthma etiology, pathogenesis, and treatment. This latest, *Childhood Asthma*, opens a new window on "the landscape of asthma care." It is certain to provide guidance to practicing pediatricians so that their young patients can lead full lives—and grow and flourish—as they deserve.

As the executive editor of this series of monographs, I want to thank the editors and authors for this important contribution to the series.

Claude Lenfant, MD
Gaithersburg, Maryland, U.S.A.

Preface

With worldwide prevalence of asthma increasing at an alarming rate over the last 20 years, it is timely to maintain frequent updates on the current concepts of asthma epidemiology, natural history, and management, as well as projecting a view for future management. We have gathered together a group of world experts to discuss the current understanding of asthma and to project their views on the major advances that will shape the management of asthma over the next 10 years.

The goals of asthma management have changed from symptom resolution to symptom prevention to early diagnosis and intervention that can effectively alter the natural history of asthma. The first section of this book is devoted to a comprehensive review of the natural history of asthma, including epidemiology, development immunology, airway pathology, and features that differentiate childhood asthma from adult-onset asthma. In addition, the effects of asthma on the growing child are discussed.

Part two reviews those conditions that can significantly alter the course of asthma, including viral infections, the environment, and the effect of early pharmacologic intervention. Part three reviews advances in technology that will impact the diagnosis and monitoring of asthma, including pulmonary function measurement, inflammatory mediators, imaging, and pharmacogenetics.

Part four reviews management principles that include education, application of asthma guidelines, selecting medication delivery devices, assessing the variable response to treatment intervention, and immunotherapy. In addition, the unique features of asthma management in special populations, such as inner-city children, adolescents, the competitive athlete, and the difficult-to-control asthmatic, will be discussed. This section will also address the challenging issues of medication adherence and concomitant medical disorders that impact asthma control.

Finally, we will project what lies in store for the future, with the rapid advances in technology and the introduction of many new medications that will change the landscape of asthma care.

Stanley J. Szefler, M.D.
Søren Pedersen, M.D.

Contributors

David B. Allen   Pediatric Endocrinology and Residency Training, University of Wisconsin Children's Hospital, Madison, Wisconsin, U.S.A.

Talissa A. Altes   Department of Radiology, Children's Hospital of Philadelphia, Philadelphia, Pennsylvania, and University of Virginia Health Sciences Center, Charlottesville, Virginia, U.S.A.

Andrea J. Apter   Division of Pulmonary, Allergy, Critical Care Medicine, Department of Medicine, University of Pennsylvania, Philadelphia, Pennsylvania, U.S.A.

Leonard B. Bacharier   Department of Pediatrics, Washington University School of Medicine, and the Division of Allergy and Pulmonary Medicine, St. Louis Children's Hospital, St. Louis, Missouri, U.S.A.

Peter J. Barnes   Department of Thoracic Medicine, National Heart and Lung Institute, Imperial College, London, U.K.

Allan Becker   Section of Allergy and Clinical Immunology, Department of Pediatrics and Child Health, University of Manitoba, Winnipeg, Manitoba, Canada

Bruce G. Bender Department of Pediatrics, National Jewish Medical and Research Center, Denver, Colorado, U.S.A.

Céline Bergeron Meakins-Christie Laboratories, McGill University, Montréal, Québec, Canada

Gordon R. Bloomberg Department of Pediatrics, Washington University School of Medicine, and the Division of Allergy and Pulmonary Medicine, St. Louis Children's Hospital, St. Louis, Missouri, U.S.A.

Alan S. Brody Department of Radiology, Cincinnati Children's Hospital Medical Center, Cincinnati, Ohio, U.S.A.

Ronina Covar Department of Pediatrics, Divisions of Clinical Pharmacology and Allergy-Clinical Immunology, Ira J. and Jacqueline Neimark Laboratory of Clinical Pharmacology in Pediatrics, National Jewish Medical and Research Center, and University of Colorado Health Sciences Center, Denver, Colorado, U.S.A.

Patrick Daigneault Meakins-Christie Laboratories, McGill University, Montréal, Québec, Canada

Myrna B. Dolovich Department of Medicine, Faculty of Health Sciences, McMaster University, Hamilton, Ontario, Canada

Peyton A. Eggleston Johns Hopkins University School of Medicine, Baltimore, Maryland, U.S.A.

James E. Gern Division of Pediatric Allergy, Departments of Pediatrics and Medicine, Immunology, and Rheumatology, University of Wisconsin Medical School, Madison, Wisconsin, U.S.A.

Peter G. Gibson Respiratory and Sleep Medicine, Hunter Medical Research Institute, John Hunter Hospital, New South Wales, Australia

Theresa Guilbert Arizona Respiratory Center, University of Arizona, Tucson, Arizona, U.S.A.

Qutayba Hamid Meakins-Christie Laboratories, McGill University, Montréal, Québec, Canada

Patrick G. Holt Division of Cell Biology, Telethon Institute for Child Health Research, Centre for Child Health Research, University of Western Australia, Perth, Western Australia, Australia

Meyer Kattan Department of Pediatrics, Mount Sinai School of Medicine, New York, New York, U.S.A.

Stephen Lake Channing Laboratory, Pulmonary and Critical Care Medicine, Brigham and Women's Hospital, Boston, Massachusetts, U.S.A.

Gary L. Larsen National Jewish Medical and Research Center, University of Colorado Health Sciences Center, Denver, Colorado, U.S.A.

Ross Lazarus Channing Laboratory, Pulmonary and Critical Care Medicine, Brigham and Women's Hospital, Boston, Massachusetts, U.S.A.

Robert F. Lemanske Division of Pediatric Allergy, Departments of Pediatrics and Medicine, Immunology, and Rheumatology, University of Wisconsin Medical School, Madison, Wisconsin, U.S.A.

Andrew H. Liu Department of Pediatrics, National Jewish Medical and Research Center, and University of Colorado Health Sciences Center, Denver, Colorado, U.S.A.

Henry Milgrom Department of Pediatrics and Medicine, National Jewish Medical and Research Center, and Department of Pediatrics, University of Colorado Health Sciences Center, Denver, Colorado, U.S.A.

Wayne Morgan Arizona Respiratory Center, University of Arizona, Tucson, Arizona, U.S.A.

Harold S. Nelson Department of Medicine, National Jewish Medical and Research Center, and University of Colorado Health Sciences Center, Denver, Colorado, U.S.A.

James Y. Paton Department of Child Health, University of Glasgow, Glasgow, Scotland, U.K.

Søren Pedersen Department of Pediatrics, University of Southern Denmark, Kolding Hospital, Kolding, Denmark

Susan L. Prescott School of Pediatrics and Child Health, University of Western Australia, and Princess Margaret Hospital, Perth, Western Australia, Australia

John F. Price Guy's, King's and St. Thomas School of Medicine, King's College Hospital, Denmark Hill, London, U.K.

Cynthia Rand Division of Pulmonary and Critical Care Medicine, Johns Hopkins University Medical Center, Baltimore, Maryland, U.S.A.

Brent Richter Channing Laboratory, Pulmonary and Critical Care Medicine, Brigham and Women's Hospital, Boston, Massachusetts, U.S.A.

Gail G. Shapiro Northwest Asthma and Allergy Center, University of Washington Medical School, Seattle, Washington, U.S.A.

Edwin K. Silverman Channing Laboratory, Pulmonary and Critical Care Medicine, Brigham and Women's Hospital, Boston, Massachusetts, U.S.A.

Eric Silverman Channing Laboratory, Pulmonary and Critical Care Medicine, Brigham and Women's Hospital, Boston, Massachusetts, U.S.A.

Jodie L. Simpson Respiratory and Sleep Medicine, Hunter Medical Research Institute, John Hunter Hospital, New South Wales, Australia

Joseph D. Spahn Department of Pediatrics, Divisions of Clinical Pharmacology and Allergy-Clinical Immunology, Ira J. and Jacqueline Neimark Laboratory of Clinical Pharmacology in Pediatrics, National Jewish Medical and Research Center, and University of Colorado Health Sciences Center, Denver, Colorado, U.S.A.

David A. Stempel INFOMED Northwest, Bellevue, and Department of Pediatrics, University of Washington School of Medicine, Seattle, Washington, U.S.A.

Robert C. Strunk Department of Pediatrics, Washington University School of Medicine, and the Division of Allergy and Pulmonary Medicine, St. Louis Children's Hospital, St. Louis, Missouri, U.S.A.

Stanley J. Szefler Department of Pediatrics and Pharmacology, Divisions of Clinical Pharmacology and Allergy and Immunology, Helen Wohlberg and Herman Lambert Chair in Pharmacokinetics, National Jewish Medical and Research Center, University of Colorado Health Sciences Center, Denver, Colorado, U.S.A.

Kelan G. Tantisira Channing Laboratory, Pulmonary and Critical Care Medicine, Brigham and Women's Hospital, Boston, Massachusetts, U.S.A.

Meri K. Tulic Meakins-Christie Laboratories, McGill University, Montréal, Québec, Canada

Frederick S. Wamboldt Department of Medicine, National Jewish Medical and Research Center, Denver, Colorado, U.S.A.

J. O. Warner Southampton General Hospital, Southampton, U.K.

Scott T. Weiss   Channing Laboratory, Pulmonary and Critical Care Medicine, Brigham and Women's Hospital, Boston, Massachusetts, U.S.A.

Glenn Whelan   Department of Pediatrics, Associate Clinical Pharmacologist, Clinical Coordinator, National Jewish Medical and Research Center, Denver, Colorado, U.S.A.

Contents

1

The Epidemiology and Burden of Pediatric Asthma

DAVID A. STEMPEL

INFOMED Northwest, Bellevue, and Department of Pediatrics, University of
 Washington School of Medicine
Seattle, Washington, U.S.A.

I. Introduction

Epidemiology, the science of the prevalence and determinants of disease, provides an assessment of disease frequency and burden of pediatric asthma. In addition it allows researchers to explore associations of risk factors for childhood asthma and the study of disease progression as well as the effect of therapeutic interventions. The data gathered from epidemiological reports permits the calculations of the economic impact of the disease to an individual, family, and society. Disease prevention and reduction in the short-term and long-term consequences of untreated illness are fundamentals of pediatric care. The application of prevalence and cost of illness may be used to determine the resources that should be allocated to effectively limit the morbidity and mortality associated with pediatric asthma.

The past two decades have witnessed significant advances in both the understanding of the pathophysiology of asthma and corresponding breakthroughs in therapeutic approaches with better knowledge of mechanisms of older medications and the development of novel therapeutic agents. National and international expert committees have reviewed the literature and written evidence-based guidelines designed to reduce the morbidity and mortality associated with childhood asthma (1–3). Parallel with these advances has been an epidemic growth during the last two decades in the number of children diagnosed with asthma. In addition, the morbidity and mortality of the disease initially increased rapidly in the 1980s and early 1990s and has recently plateaued (4). The inner city and urbanized areas appear to have experienced a disproportionate burden of severe childhood asthma (5). This chapter will focus on the epidemiology of pediatric asthma and its burden to the child and society.

II. Working Definitions of Asthma

Prior to determining the prevalence of pediatric asthma it is important to establish a working definition of asthma in children. Two longitudinal studies provide complementary data to begin this process. The Tucson Children's Respiratory Study (TCRS) offers an initial classification system for childhood asthma (6). It describes three distinct phenotypes of wheezing illnesses based on duration of symptoms and atopic status: transient wheeze, non-atopic wheeze, and persistent wheeze. The children with transient wheeze have wheezing illnesses noted from infancy that may persist until age six when they appear to be asymptomatic. These children tend to be non-atopic and have diminished lung function at birth that persists but does not progress. The non-atopic wheezers have disease that persists beyond age six, declines in frequency with age, is associated with respiratory synctial virus lower airway disease and have evidence of persistent bronchodilator response observed at the age of 11. The children with persistent wheeze continue to have symptomatic asthma after age six, have normal lung function at birth and reduced lung function at the age of six and are predominantly atopic individuals. This third group of children forms the cohort with persistent disease that warrants persistent treatment and monitoring. This group forms the cohort that we will define for this paper as the children with asthma.

The second longitudinal study is a descriptive population from Melbourne, Australia (7). This study followed children from age seven to 42 years and utilized definitions that correlate closely with those of the TCRS. Mild wheezy bronchitis and transient wheeze both appear to be self-limited diseases of early childhood that do not seem to progress to persistent asthma. Wheezy bronchitis and non-atopic asthma both have limited progression and similar time patterns. The asthma and severe asthma cohorts in Australian studies are similar to the persistent wheeze phenotype from the TCRS.

There is still no direction on how to differentiate the transient, non-atopic wheezers or the wheezy bronchitis infants and toddlers with active wheezing from first symptoms until they enter remission. In the first years of life the transient and non-atopic children may have multiple episodes of recurrent wheeze associated with viral infections. Their disease is persistent during these years and may warrant treatment with asthma controller medications. Their phenotype as infants and toddlers is not fully expressed and may not permit the characterization of this self-limited disease. Furthermore the definition of the atopic potential may be difficult to assess until they reach ages 6 to 11 years. This population remains problematic during the first years of life.

Kurukulaaratchy et al. (8) followed a birth cohort from the Isle of Wight and attempted to establish criteria to identify asthma at the age of four. At birth, family history of atopy, household pets, cigarette smoke exposure, and social class were recorded, and cord IgE levels were measured. The health status of children was assessed by questionnaire at ages 1, 2, 4, and 10 years. At the age of four, 32.5% and by 10, 40.3% of the cohort were recorded as "ever wheezed." Among the cohort of 336 children noted to wheeze by age 4, 37% (12.1% of the entire birth cohort who had complete data) were persistent wheezers. The multivariate analysis revealed that recurrent chest infections at age two, family history of asthma and atopy (defined as skin test positive at age four) were predictive of asthma and that nasal symptoms at age one were protective against persistent asthma. There were seven independent variables for persistent asthma. (Atopy demonstrated by age four, eczema diagnosed at age one, eczema at age four, rhinitis at age four, family history of asthma, maternal smoking at birth, parental smoking at age four, and chest infections at two years.) When each of these variables was given a one-point value, a risk-scoring index was created. A score of four had a positive predictive value of wheezing of 83%. This study suggests that one may be able to categorize a child with persistent asthma by age four using these variables and this scoring system.

The question of who to include in the cohort with persistent asthma may also be complicated by children with persistent asthma that enters a clinical remission. Some patients who meet the Tucson or Melbourne definitions of persistent asthma will have prolonged periods of clinical remission (9). Van den Toorn et al. (10) studied young adults with a history of persistent childhood asthma that had evolved into a clinical remission of at least one and a median of five years. Although these young adults had no symptoms and were off all asthma medications, their FEV_1 predicted was normal and FEV_1 reversibility was intermediate between a group of asthmatics and an age-matched group that had never wheezed. Of interest, the patients in remission had evidence of active inflammation noted on bronchial biopsies with increased major basic protein, mast cells, markers of active T cells, and thickening of the reticular basement membrane. In addition these young adults had positive surrogate markers demonstrating active asthma with increased exhaled nitric oxide and peripheral eosinophils.

These patients have achieved the goals of asthma therapy as established by the National Asthma Education Prevention Program. They no longer meet the clinical criteria of active asthma whether intermittent or persistent in spite of the findings of active inflammation. Although one could make a case for diagnosing active asthma based on laboratory tools demonstrating inflammation on biopsy or less invasive test of bronchial hyperreactivity (BHR) or exhaled nitric oxide, the gold standard for recording prevalence of active asthma is through standardized survey tools that record symptoms, albuterol use, and lung function. Of interest is the finding that standardized questionnaires do correlate with tests of BHR (11). BHR, though, is a sensitive but non-specific test for asthma.

The article by Phalen et al. (7) points out the necessity of validated questions for determining asthma. They are concerned that there was an underestimation of minor wheeze especially associated with exercise when the cohort was 14 years of age. These surveys relied on maternal answers to questions. They raise the issue of how people respond to questions and then offer the following statement: "I no longer get asthma but only wheeze a bit when I play sports or have a cold." The accuracy of the survey tool and need for validation is important in determining the soundness of the results. The International Study of Asthma and Allergies in Childhood (ISAAC) was designed to address this concern when comparing prevalence data from around the world with the use of a standardized survey tool.

III. International Study of Asthma and Allergies in Childhood

ISAAC is a systematic approach to recording the worldwide prevalence of pediatric asthma. It provides the ability to compare data with the use of a universal survey tool overcoming most of the difficulties of differences in methodology and criteria (12). Phase one of the study was designed to determine a baseline prevalence of asthma in 13- to 14-year-olds in multiple countries and at several sites within these countries. The study was performed with a core survey tool that asked eight core questions starting with: "Have you had wheezing or whistling in the chest in the last 12 months?" (Table 1). ISAAC was translated into 39 languages with the recognized inherent difficulty that "wheezing" was not a universal colloquial term in all languages. In 75% of the sites performing this survey a video questionnaire was also employed. The ISAAC results demonstrate over a 20-fold variation in prevalence from the lowest to highest prevalence rates between countries for 13- and 14-year-olds with asthma. The highest rates were noted in the United Kingdom, New Zealand, and Australia, and the lowest rates in Indonesia, Eastern Europe, Greece, China, India, and Ethiopia. The prevalence rates ranged from 1.6% to 36.8%. Rates were

Table 1   Core ISAAC Questionnaire for 13- to 14-Year-Olds

---

1. Have you ever had wheezing or whistling in the chest at any time in the past? Yes [ ] No [ ] IF YOU HAVE ANSWERED "NO" PLEASE SKIP TO QUESTION 6
2. Have you had wheezing or whistling in the chest in the last 12 months? Yes [ ] No [ ] IF YOU HAVE ANSWERED "NO" PLEASE SKIP TO QUESTION 6
3. How many attacks of wheezing have you had in the last 12 months? None [ ] 1–3 [ ] 4–12 [ ] More than 12 [ ]
4. In the last 12 months, how often, on average, has your sleep been disturbed due to wheezing? Never woken with wheezing [ ] Less than one night per week [ ] One or more nights per week [ ]
5. In the last 12 months, has wheezing ever been severe enough to limit your speech to only one or two words at a time between breaths? Yes [ ] No [ ]
6. Have you ever had asthma? Yes [ ] No [ ]
7. In the last 12 months, has your chest sounded wheezy during or after exercise? Yes [ ] No [ ]
8. In the last 12 months, have you had a dry cough at night, apart from a cough associated with a cold or chest infection? Yes [ ] No [ ]

Abbreviation: ISAAC, International Study of Asthma and Allergies in Childhood.

generally lower for the video questions because they were perceived to elicit response for more severe disease. In some of the non-English countries the prevalence of asthma was higher with the video survey tool possibly related to difficulties in translating the written questions. In general there was a concordance between the two survey tools.

The finding of the highest prevalence of asthma in English speaking countries raises several potential questions regarding possible environmental exposures. ISAAC reveals, though, that air pollution does not appear to correlate with the increased prevalence of asthma in adolescents. Areas of the world with high particulate matter and sulfur dioxide, such as China and Eastern Europe, had some of the lowest rates of asthma. Some developing regions of the world, including Indonesia and China, had low prevalence rates of asthma in contrast to Hong Kong and Japan, where the rates were higher. Higher economic status was not universally associated with increased prevalence where it was not a factor in parts of Europe and South America. There was also evidence that within countries with similar ethnic and genetic backgrounds such as China (including Taiwan and Hong Kong), India, Italy, and Spain there was evidence of significant variability in prevalence.

Epidemiological studies such as ISAAC have the ability to generate future questions for research of potential disease associations. Ecological studies employ different databases to perform simple comparisons.

They do not prove cause and effect but rather demonstrate potential associations for further analysis. Ecological studies in phase one of ISAAC demonstrated increased prevalence of asthma in countries with greater prosperity associated with greater consumption of processed foods, the increased use of acetaminophen, a modest increase in the gross domestic product (GDP), and a inverse association with rates of tuberculosis. No associations were observed with increased childhood immunization rates. Asthma prevalence increased with increasing indoor humidity and was inversely associated with increasing altitude. No association with outdoor temperatures and outdoor humidity were found.

The potential association of acetaminophen and asthma is addressed in an analysis by Newson et al. (13). This article explores the strengths and potential limitations of ecological studies. Acetaminophen use has been associated with a higher prevalence of asthma in a dose-dependent fashion. Whether this is a cause and effect is uncertain. The GDP is inversely related to the prevalence of asthma. In this study, when controlling for GDP, there was still an association with asthma and other atopic disorders and the use of acetaminophen. It has been proposed that this medication is not the cause of the increase in the incidence of asthma but rather the substitution of acetaminophen for aspirin that may have a protective effect against the development of asthma (14). ISAAC and other large population surveys allow for study of these central hypotheses, which if confirmed may lead to important interventions.

Diet is another variable that has been considered a potential, if not controversial, variable in the epidemic of asthma noted over the past decades. Farchi et al. (15) studied a group of children aged six and seven participating in ISAAC. They correlated the frequency of wheeze and the consumption of foods high in antioxidants, animal fats, and foods containing omega-3 fatty acids. Increased consumption of cooked vegetables, tomatoes, and fruits conferred a protective effect against wheeze and shortness of breath with wheeze in the last 12 months. Consumption of bread, butter, and margarine were associated with increased asthma symptoms. There were no effects, positive or negative, found with the consumption of omega-3 fatty acids. This study provides some interesting initial data concerning the impact of diet on the changes in asthma prevalence and stimulates thought concerning the potential impact of the robust ISAAC survey.

IV. The Underdiagnosis of Pediatric Asthma

The underdiagnosis of pediatric asthma is an essential clinical issue. Unless diagnosed these children are under-counted, have less resources allocated for their care and do not receive appropriate medical attention. A 1999 North Carolina School Asthma Survey studied over 122,000 12–14-year-olds (16). This study employed the ISAAC questionnaire using both the written and video tools. The children were divided into four cohorts: undiagnosed frequent wheezers (6.2%), diagnosed current asthma (9.9%), asymptomatic (52.6%), and infrequent wheezers (31.3%). Being a member of the undiagnosed first cohort was associated with female gender; active or passive household smoke exposure; low socioeconomic class; African American, Native American, and Mexican American race/ethnicity; and weakly with urban residence. Those children with undiagnosed frequent wheezing were more likely than the diagnosed current asthmatics to report sleep disturbances (OR: 1.9, 95% CI: 1.7–2.1), limited activities (OR: 1.6, 95% CI: 1.4–1.9), and missed school (OR: 1.2, 95% CI: 1.0–1.5) related to wheezing. Significant disease-associated morbidity did not appear to identify these children. Unfortunately the odds of these children having a physician visit for asthma was approximately half that of the cohort with diagnosed current asthma and may, in part, contribute to some of the disease morbidity that these children experience. This study illustrates the importance of community-wide assessment of asthma prevalence as opposed to relying on data from physician contact only. It also illustrates the importance of data that collects prevalence with the use of a standardized and validated tool.

In the assessment of disease prevalence one needs to report patients that have the signs or symptoms of the disease, those that require specific treatment of the illness, and those that experience morbidity. In reporting patients with asthma one needs to assess disease control and severity and from this information attempt to determine the need for treatment with as-needed reliever, daily controller, or a combination. Yeatts et al. (16) illustrate the need for direct survey of patients. Halterman et al. (17) further demonstrate the importance of patient surveys to quantify disease severity. Children, ages four to six, with persistent asthma defined by symptoms three or more days a week or three or more nights a month were enrolled. The providers classified only 40% of the 90 study subjects correctly as having persistent asthma. For those children who were appropriately evaluated, 83% were given controller medications; for those who were not diagnosed by their provider as being persistent, only 28% were on prescribed controller treatment. Acute care visits or hospitalizations were not predictors of appropriate clinician assessment. The only criteria associated with accurate diagnosis was if the child had been seen in the physician's office in the past six months or if the family perceived that the clinician was aware of the patient's symptoms. This study illustrates the need for better patient (family) communication with the provider to appropriately assess disease severity as important in the prescription of appropriate treatment.

In the United States ISAAC has been limited to only a few sites and with somewhat limited enrollment. The one-year prevalence of asthma in these studies has ranged between 19.8% and 24.6%. These results differ significantly from the national health surveys for several important reasons. ISAAC is a specific survey tool assessing the prevalence of asthma, allergic rhinitis, and eczema. In contrast, the U.S. Centers for Disease Control uses the annual National Health Interview Survey (NHIS) that is used to record data on 17 chronic respiratory conditions. ISAAC reports the prevalence of asthma and the limitations imposed by the disease. The NHIS survey is conducted throughout the year to avoid confounders produced by seasonal variation of asthma severity. Each has its own strengths and limitations.

A. National Health Interview Survey

In 1997 the NHIS adjusted its questionnaire to distinguish active asthma and asthma in remission by asking the following two questions. "Has a doctor or other health professional ever told you that you had asthma?" and "During the past 12 months, have you ever had an episode of asthma or an asthma attack?" (4). These two questions attempt to get a broader picture of asthma prevalence. National asthma prevalence data in the United States also includes the National Center for Health Statistics (NCHS) that collects data on office visits, emergency department utilization, and hospitalizations associated with asthma reported in several other survey tools.

The prevalence of asthma is reported in the NHIS database in two pediatric cohorts: 0–4 and 5–14. The older teenage population is blended into the adult population and is therefore excluded from this review. The prevalence of asthma increased significantly from 1980 to 1995 and then appeared to stabilize from 1996 to 1999. For the zero–four age group rates increased from 2.3% to 6.0% and then for the last four years stabilized between 4% and 4.6%. In this age group no differences were noted with the change in survey questions. A similar pattern of increased prevalence was noted in the 5- to 14-year-olds, rising from 4.5% in 1980 to 8.2% in 1995. In 1996 the prevalence declined to 7.0% and declined further for the last three years with the newer survey tool to 5.6–6.0% (Fig. 1).

B. Mortality of Pediatric Asthma

Mortality associated with pediatric asthma is fortunately an infrequent event. When studied in relation to the prevalence of asthma for the zero–four age groups, the risk of an asthma-associated fatality was 7.9×10^{-5} in 1980. For all other time points in the subsequent two decades the rate showed some variability at each measurement period and has been relatively stable from 1985 to 1999 with some possible declines noted in recent years. In the 5- to 14-year-old group the lowest fatality rate was recorded in 1980 and then increased approximately 50% over the next two decades to the present rate of 6.3×10^{-5}. The biggest inflection in this rate appears to have been in 1985 with a more gradual increase in recent years (Fig. 2). Due to the small numbers of events small increases or decreases may be responsible for some of this variation. It should be noted that the overall population has experienced a decline in asthma fatalities in

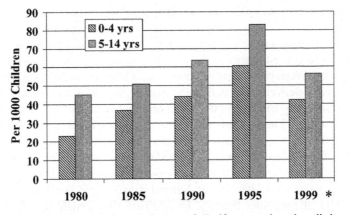

Figure 1 Estimated annual prevalence of "self-reported asthma" in children 0 to 14 years of age (4).
* Change in asthma definition in 1999 from self-reported asthma prevalence during the preceding 12 months (1980–1996) to episode of asthma or asthma attack during the preceding 12 months (1997–1999).

recent years after two decades of increasing mortality (18). Asthma fatalities associated with sports have been reported in children. These events have occurred in competitive as well as non-competitive athletes who were not perceived to have severe asthma (19). This group of children

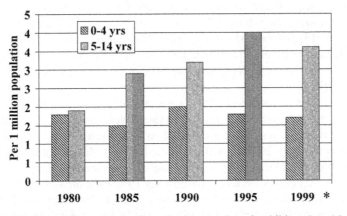

Figure 2 Estimated annual rate of deaths from asthma in children 0 to 14 years of age (4).
* Change in asthma definition in 1999 from self-reported asthma prevalence during the preceding 12 months (1980–1996) to episode of asthma or asthma attack during the preceding 12 months (1997–1999).

was not previously recognized as an at-risk population and deserves further attention.

The increase and relative persistence in the mortality associated with asthma in the United States in the past two decades contrasts with patterns seen in many Western European countries. There are significant differences in health care delivery between these two regions with more universal care available in many of the Western European countries with lower asthma mortality rates. There have also been observational studies that have observed that as the sales of inhaled corticosteroid increased decreases in mortality have been observed. Goldman et al. demonstrated that as the use of inhaled corticosteroids use increased in Israel, mortality from asthma significantly declined (20). In the United States there is a lower utilization of this class of controller therapy. In addition the persistence of this higher rate of mortality may be associated with certain at-risk populations such as the children of the inner city. The disparity in the delivery of health care to this population may partially explain the higher rate of mortality due to asthma in the United States. In addition there is the need for further research in understanding at-risk populations such as the African-American community that appears to be at greater risk.

V. Morbidity of Pediatric Asthma

Hospitalization and emergency department rates show a significant disparity between the two pediatric cohorts in the MMWR data. The number of hospitalizations per 100 identified asthmatics was approximately fourfold greater for the infants and toddlers than the older pediatric cohort. In 1980 there were 16.5 hospitalizations/100 active asthmatics and ranging from 10 to 15/100 over the subsequent two decades. In contrast the older children had rates of 4.1/100 in 1980 to 3.7/100 in the latest data. The higher rates noted in both groups may reflect the change in the survey definition of asthma to include active symptoms in the last year. In the younger cohort the rate was lowest in 1995 when the older definition was employed and then reverted to the 1990 rate when the newer definition was used (Fig. 3).

The rate of emergency department visits was again higher for the younger group ranging from 20/100 to 40/100 and for the older group from 10/100 to 19/100 (Fig. 4). ED rates were not available for the measurement period in the 1980s (1992 ED rates were calculated with 1990 data on asthma prevalence); 1995 had the lowest rates of hospitalizations and emergency department events. It is unclear whether the differences in hospitalization rates are due to variations in the intensity of viral respiratory disease epidemics, allergen exposure, other environmental insults, or differences in treatment.

The failure to see a significant decline in the rate of hospitalization in the United States over the past decade is in contrast to observations

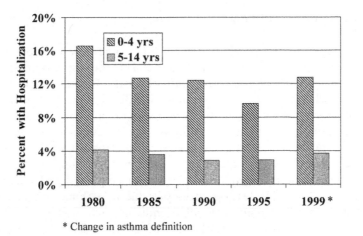

* Change in asthma definition

Figure 3 Percent of asthmatics by age group and year with an asthma-related hospitalization (4).

in Western European countries. Wennergren et al. reported a two-thirds reduction in pediatric hospital days and a 45% decrease in asthma-related admissions concurrent with the large increase in the use of inhaled corti-costeroids for asthma in Göteborg, Sweden (21). The reduction in hospitalizations were found in children older than five years rather than the younger children, where the use of inhaled corticosteroids was less common. Resource utilization records from Harvard Pilgrim Health Care also demonstrated that when inhaled corticosteroids were dispensed the relative risk of an asthma-related hospitalization significantly declined in children by 50% (22). The variables identified in the rates of ED visits, and hospitalization may be related to the changes in the disease frequency, potential differences in disease severity, and the effects of extrinsic triggers that may vary annually and with treatment.

A. Assessment of Asthma Control

Epidemiological reports such as ISAAC and the NHIS present data on the prevalence of disease and the utilization of some of the health care resources. Neither of these reports assesses disease control. Over the past several years there has been the development of several asthma control questionnaires (23–25). Although these tools have not been validated, at present, for pediatric populations they have the potential to explore whether asthma is being adequately controlled. The study by Vollmer et al. (23) has demonstrated the association of poor asthma control and the subsequent risk of acute care for asthma. Surveys, such as this, may in the future better quantify the status of asthma care.

VI. Burden of Pediatric Asthma

Calculating the burden of childhood asthma is complex and open to many different interpretations and formulations. The economic burden may be divided into the direct costs and indirect costs of care. The direct costs correlate with the resources consumed with the treatment of asthma. The indirect costs are more difficult to measure but include the cost of the child's caretaker during the periods of illness, the caretaker's lost wages and expenses related to travel for medical care, and loss of productivity to an employer. How does one calculate the burden of the loss of a night sleep on the child's or parent's productivity on the subsequent day? Even more difficult to quantify is the lost opportunities due to asthma: lost educational experiences, inability to interact with friends in sports, and impaired quality of life. The social or emotional burden of asthma may be quantified with health-related quality of life assessments to assess changes with disease or therapy but do not attempt to place a value on these measurements.

The 2002 MMWR asthma surveillance report (4) documents children with asthma have higher resource utilization than adult patients. In 1997 children 0 to 14 years of age were responsible for 33% of the office visits for asthma as a percent of the total population of asthmatics. This pediatric age group accounted for 44% of the hospitalizations and 37% of the emergency department visits for asthma in the United States. Stanford et al. (26) reported the 1997 cost for an emergency department visit at $234.48 and for an asthma-related hospitalization at $3,102.53. The 1997 estimated cost of pediatric asthma ED events may then be calculated at approximately $157 million and for hospitalizations, $669 million.

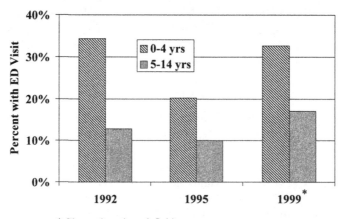

* Change in asthma definition

Figure 4   Percent of asthmatics by age group and year with an asthma-related emergency department visit (4).

Children with asthma have a disproportional greater use of medical expenditures. Using the 1987 National Medical Expenditure Survey children with asthma were compared to a non-asthmatic cohort (27). The period prevalence of asthma in this report was 8.8%. The two important findings in this study are that total medical expenditures for the asthma cohort were greater in all areas including medications, office visits, ED visits, and hospitalizations. Overall expenditures were 2.8-fold greater than non-asthmatic children. The second finding of interest is that the expenses for non-asthma-related medical care was also significantly greater for children with asthma.

School absences for children with asthma per year are 48% greater in 1994–1996 than work absence for adults with asthma. The pediatric survey reported only children 5 to 17 years of age. For those children in this age cohort there were 14 million absences from school. The economic burden of school days lost can be then modeled with certain assumptions. In 2002 the average day's wages and benefits were $171 for an eight-hour day (28). If 25% of caregivers lost a day's work to take care of their asthmatic child who missed school, the cost would be approximately $600 million, and if 50% missed a days work, then there are $1.2 billion of lost wages. These calculations do not take into account the children under age five, the loss of productivity to the employer, the additional dollars lost because of the parent's decreased productivity due to a night with disrupted sleep, the value given to the at-home parent, nor the impact on the child with lost opportunities of education. It may be appropriate to assign this dollar value to all children without regard to the caregiver's employment. The model would then suggest a cost of $2.4 billion. What is clear is that the indirect burden of asthma may be significantly greater than the resource utilization in the ED and hospital.

Children experience significant morbidity as manifested not only with lost school days but also decreased productivity at school due to asthma. It is difficult to give a cost associated with the time missed from school or time with impaired learning due to asthma. It is also difficult to quantify the burden of lost activity for children with asthma. There is no monetary formula that can address the inability to perform physical activity, lost time playing with peers, or a dollar value associated with the missed opportunities of education. Diette et al. (29) have attempted to assess the burden associated with the loss of sleep. They performed a cross-sectional survey utilizing three managed care organizations in the United States. Children were identified if they had two or more medical claims for asthma (ICD-493.XX) or one or more dispensings for asthma. Of the 438 patients completing the survey 40% had been awakening in the previous four weeks due to symptoms of asthma and 66% had asthma symptoms related to exercise. During that same time period 35% of children missed school because of asthma and 36% of parents reported that their children's school performance suffered because of their asthma. The number of nights with asthma correlated with school absences. Sleep disruption and school absences correlated. If the child awakened between one and three nights in the month 44% of parents missed work and it rose to 56% if the child awoke due to wheezing on seven nights.

In a cross-sectional study Lozano et al. (30) assessed the level of asthma control and the use of medications. In this survey of 638 children nearly a third of patients had 5 to 14 symptom-days in the past two weeks. This group of children had an increased burden of disease that is not being adequately managed whether one uses the GINA or NAEPP guidelines. Inadequate control in this study was related to inadequate dosing of controller medications but poor control was found even in the presence of some controller medications. Poverty, non-white ethnicity, and younger children were also risk factors for poor asthma control. Having seen a specialist in the past six months was a protective factor. This study reports the greater burden of asthma in children with lower socioeconomic status. Inadequate control of asthma symptoms increases the burden of disease without an apparent means to calculate a monetary or social value. This study suggests that the more appropriate use of controller medications would result in decreasing the symptom burden of childhood asthma. Greater use of controllers would increase the pharmaceutical costs with some, but probably not complete reduction in other areas of direct resource utilization. The largest gains in implementation of guidelines treatment may be in the reduction of the indirect costs and the social burden of the disease.

VII. Summary

Pediatric asthma is a high prevalence disease. Rates of asthma are higher in children than adults. Resource consumption is greater for children both in the ED and hospital for this disease. The burden of pediatric asthma is significant whether one calculates direct or indirect costs of the disease. Epidemiological reports, such as the one from the MMWR, allow for consideration of where resources should be allocated to reduce the consequences of inadequately or inappropriately treated disease. Are the persistent rates of disease morbidity and mortality associated with the changes in the characteristics of the disease, failure to respond to therapy, a breakdown of the health care delivery system to adequately identify patients that require treatment or the inequality of the system to deliver care to the inner city children who appear to be at greatest risk for asthma exacerbations? The ISAAC study gives us further insight into the growing epidemic of pediatric asthma. Future ecological studies may help determine areas of potential research.

References

1. Guidelines for the Diagnosis and Management of Asthma. U.S. Department of Health and Human Services, National Institutes of Health, NIH publication No. 97–4051, April 1997.

2. National Asthma Education and Prevention Program, Expert Panel Report: Guidelines for the diagnosis and management of asthma update on selected topics-2002. J Allergy Clin Immunol 2002; 110:S141–S219.
3. Global Strategy for Asthma Management and Prevention. National Institutes of Health and National Hearty, Lung and Blood Institute, Revised 2002. Available at www.ginasthma.com.
4. Mannino DM, Homa DM, Akinbami LJ, Moorman JE, Gwynn C, Redd SC. Surveillance for asthma—United States, 1980–1999. MMWR 2002; 51:1–14.
5. Federico MJ, Lui AH. Overcoming childhood asthma disparities of the inner-city poor. Pediatr Clin N Am 2003; 50:655–675.
6. Taussig LM, Wright AL, Holberg CJ, Halonen M, Morgan WJ, Martinez FD. Tucson Children's Respiratory Study: 1980 to present. J Allergy Clin Immunol 2003; 111:661–675.
7. Phaeln PD, Robertson CF, Olinsky A. The Melbourne asthma study; 1964–1999. J Allergy Clin Immunol 2002; 109:189–194.
8. Kurukulaaratchy RJ, Matthews S, Holgate ST, Arshad SH. Predicting persistent disease among children who wheeze during early life. Eur Resp J 2003; 22:767–771.
9. Sears MR, Greene JM, Willan AR, Wiecek EM, Taylor R, Flannery EM, Cowan JO, Herbison P, Silva PA, Poulton R. A longitudinal population-based, cohort study of childhood asthma followed to adulthood. N Engl J Med 2003; 349:1414–1422.
10. van den Toorn LM, Overbeek SE, de Jongste JC, Leman K, Hoogsteden HC, Prins JB. Airway inflammation is present during clinical remission of asthma. Am J Respir Crit Care Med 2001; 164:2107–2113.
11. Lai CKW, Chan JKW, Chan A, Wong G, Ho A, Choy D, Lau J, Leung R. Comparison of ISAAC video questionnaire (AVQ3.0) with ISAAC written questionnaire for estimating asthma associated with bronchial hyperreactivity. Clin Exp Allergy 1997; 27:540–545.
12. Beasley R, Ellwood P, Asher I. International patterns of the prevalence of pediatic asthma: the ISAAC program. Pediatr Clin N Am 2003; 50:539–553.
13. Newson RB, Shaheen SO, Chinn S, Burney PGJ. Paracetamol sales and atopic disease in children and adults: an ecological analysis. Eur Respir J 2000; 16:817–823.
14. Varner AE, Busse WW, Lemanske RF Jr. Hypothesis: decreased use of pediatric aspirin has contributed to the increasing prevalence of childhood asthma. Ann Allergy Asthma Immunol 1998; 81:347–351.
15. Farchi S, Forastiere F, Agabati N, Corbo G, Pistelli R, Fortes C, Dell'Orco C, Perucci CA. Dietary factors associated with wheezing and allergic rhinitis in children. Eur Respir J 2003; 22:772–780.
16. Yeatts K, Johnston Davis K, Peden D, Shy C. Health consequences of frequent wheezing in adolescents without asthma diagnosis. Eur Respir J 2003; 22: 781–786.
17. Halterman JS, Yoos L, Kaczororoski JM, McConnochie K, Holzhaurer RJ, Conn KM, Lauver S, Szilagyi PG. Providers underestimate symptom severity among urban children with asthma. Arch Pediatr Adolesc Med 2002; 156: 141–146.

18. Sly RM. Continuing decrease in asthma mortality in the United States. Ann Allergy Asthma Immunol 2004; 92:313–318.
19. Becker JM, Rogers J, Rossini G, Mirchandani H, D'Alonzo GE. Asthma deaths during sports; report of a 7-year experience. J Allergy Clin Immunol 2004; 113:264–267.
20. Goldman M, Rachmiel M, Gendler L, Katz Y. Decrease in asthma mortality rate in Israel from 1991 to 1995: is it related to increased use of inhaled corticosteroids. J Allergy Clin Immunol 2000; 105:71–74.
21. Wennergren G, Kristjánsson S, Stannegård IL. Decrease in hospitalizations for treatment of childhood asthma with increased use of anti-inflammatory treatment, despite an increase in the prevalence of asthma. J Allergy Clin Immunol 1996; 97:742–748.
22. Donahue JG, Weiss ST, Livingston JM, Goetsch MA, Greineder DK, Platt R. Inhaled corticosteroids and the risk of hospitalization for asthma. JAMA 1997; 227:887–891.
23. Vollmer W, Markson L, O'Connor E, Sanocki L, Fitterman L, Berger M, Buist S. Association of asthma control with health care utilization and quality of life. Am J Respir Crit Care Med 1999; 160:1647–1652.
24. Juniper EF, O'Byrne PM, Guyatt GH, Ferrie PJ, King DR. Development and validation of a questionnaire to measure asthma control. Eur Respir J 1999; 14(4):902–907.
25. Nathan R, Sorkness C, Kosinski M, Schatz M, Li J, Marcus P, Murray J, Pendergraft T. Development of the Asthma Control Test: a survey for assessing asthma control. J Allergy Clin Immunol 2004; 113:59–65.
26. Stanford R, McLaughlin T, Okamoto LJ. The cost of asthma care in the emergency department and hospital. Am J Respir Crit Care Med 1999; 160: 211–215.
27. Lozano P, Sullivan SD, Smith DH, Weiss KB. The economic burden of asthma in US children: estimates from the national medical survey. J Allergy Clin Immunol 1999; 104:957–963.
28. The state of working America: 2002–03, Table 2.3. Accessed 3/26/04 at www.epinet.org/datazone/02/comp_2_3r.pdf.
29. Diette GB, Markson L, Skinner EA, Nguyen TTH, Algatt-Bergstrom P, Wu AW. Nocturnal asthma in children affects school attendance, school performance, and parents' work attendance. Arch Pediatr Adolesc Med 2000; 154:923–928.
30. Lozano P, Finkelstein JA, Hecht J, Shulruff R, Weiss KB. Asthma medication use and disease burden in children in a primary care setting. Arch Pediatr Adolesc Med 2003; 157:81–88.

2

Developmental Regulation of Immune Functions and Risk for Allergy and Asthma

SUSAN L. PRESCOTT

School of Pediatrics and Child Health,
    University of Western Australia, and
    Princess Margaret Hospital
Perth, Western Australia, Australia

PATRICK G. HOLT

Division of Cell Biology, Telethon Institute
    for Child Health Research, Centre for
    Child Health Research, University
    of Western Australia
Perth, Western Australia, Australia

I. Introduction: The Importance of Early Immune Events in the Subsequent Development of Allergic Disease

Although the propensity for allergy can manifest at any age, allergic diseases frequently develop in the first years of life, suggesting that very early events play an important role in initiating these disease processes. A high proportion of infants with early symptoms of atopic dermatitis and food allergy frequently develop more persistent, recurrent airway pathology. The burden of these diseases has been steadily rising in Western countries, with almost 40% of these populations showing evidence of allergic sensitization. There is now mounting concern that billions of people will be affected as developing countries begin to show the same trends (1).

While decades of research have provided a detailed knowledge of the immunological processes that underlie the acute allergic immune response, surprisingly little is known about how or why these inflammatory processes are initiated and why an increasing number of individuals are affected. A better knowledge of early initiating events is critical in both understanding disease pathogenesis and planning prevention strategies.

17

II. Current Concepts of Immune Dysregulation in Allergic Disease

There are clear parallels between human allergic disease and the "Th-1/ Th-2 paradigm" originally described in rodents (2,3). A substantial body of evidence implicates type T helper cell (Th-2) cytokines [interleukin (IL)-4, IL-5, IL-9, IL-13] in the development and expression of allergy and airways inflammation (4–12). However, while it is generally accepted that established immunoglobulin (IgE)-mediated allergic disease is the result of excessive and inappropriate Th-2 responses to allergens, the previous notion that this is the result of a simple "skewing" of immune responses away from "normal" type 1 (Th-1) responses has been called into question. In fact, many recent studies suggest that allergic children are more generally responsive to allergens with increases in both Th-1 and Th-2 responses (13–15), suggesting a breakdown of more fundamental common regulatory processes that affect many aspects of immune function. This also challenges the notion that modern environmental changes are having a simple "Th-2 skewing effect" by specifically promoting Th-2 responses or inhibiting Th-1 responses.

More recently, it has been proposed that environmental changes may be in some way affecting regulatory systems such that they inadequately prevent over-expression of inappropriate Th-1 and Th-2 responses in predisposed individuals (Fig. 1) (16). This new model may also explain the otherwise paradoxical observation that "Th-1 diseases" (such as type 1

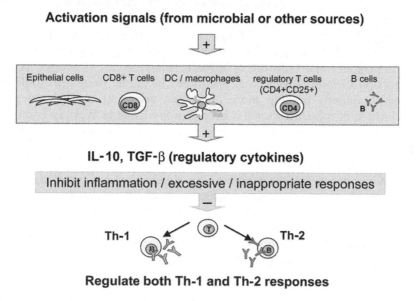

Figure 1   Cells involved in immune regulation.

diabetes, Crohn's disease, and multiple sclerosis) have also increased during the same period of the "Th-2 allergy epidemic" (17). As a result of this perspective, there has been intense interest in aspects of the immune network with known homeostatic and immunomodulatory effects (particularly cells that produce key regulatory cytokines such as IL-10 and transforming growth factor (TGF-β) and how these might be influenced by environmental factors. Many cells produce these regulatory cytokines, but there has been particular interest in the role of antigen-presenting cells (APC) including dendritic cells (DC), and regulatory T (Tr) cells, which can influence both the pattern and magnitude of effector T cell signaling. The DC at mucosal surfaces play a pivotal role during "first contact" with allergens. After local uptake and processing, DC migrate to regional nodes where they receive maturation signals (including granulocyte monocyte lineage colony simulating factor (GM-CSF)) (18), which result in functional changes and increased capacity to present antigen switching (reviewed in Ref. 19). Recent studies suggest that IL-10 derived from myeloid DC appears to be an important factor in controlling the balance between tolerance and sensitization (20). In resting state these cells selectively prime for Th-2 immunity unless Th-1 trophic stimuli are present (18). The production of Th-1-trophic cytokines by DC can be influenced by local factors such as viral infections (21) and is a clear avenue through which environmental factors may influence local immune development (as discussed further below).

III. Evidence of Early Immune Dysregulation in Allergic Infants

Clinical features of atopic disease frequently manifest within two or three months of life, usually as food allergies or atopic dermatitis. Although these conditions generally improve with age, a high proportion of these individuals go on to develop persistent sensitization to aeroallergens and associated respiratory tract disease.

A. Developing Immune Responses to Food Allergens

Most children show early transient lymphoproliferation to food allergens (22), and this is not usually associated with disease. Those who develop clinical reactivity to foods (such as egg) typically show more prolonged and more exaggerated cellular responses, although these are also typically transient (13). As with other forms of allergic disease, the presence of strong Th-2 responses (IL-4, IL-5, and IL-13) is also the defining characteristic of food allergy in infancy (13,23,24). However, these children also secrete high levels of Th-1 cytokines [Interferon gamma (IFN-γ)] and IL-10 in response to egg (13). This generalized mixed cytokine "hyperresponsiveness" in allergic children further suggests abnormal tolerance mechanisms rather than a simple "Th-2 immune skewing." Vaccine studies indicate that this "mixed Th-0 hyperresponsiveness" is not limited to allergens. Infants (18 months of age) at high risk of atopy also show transiently stronger Th-0 (Th-1 and Th-2) responses to vaccine antigens (tetanus toxoid) and allergens [House dust mite (HDM)] compared to low-risk infants (25).

The development of clinical tolerance to food allergens is typically associated with loss of both lymphoproliferation and Th-2 responses to food allergens (13), usually before four to five years of age (with the well-documented exceptions of peanuts, nuts, and shellfish). However, some food-specific cytokine responses appear to persist (IL-10 and IFN-γ) (13) with the development of clinical tolerance (26) suggesting that this may be an active regulatory process rather than due to deletion of allergen-responsive cells. Despite decades of research, oral tolerance is still poorly understood, and remains an important priority for future research. There is currently considerable interest in immunological events in the gastrointestinal mucosa during this early period of life, particularly how other environmental factors (such as intestinal microflora) can influence systemic immune development (discussed further below).

B. The Development of Aeroallergen Responses

Aeroallergen "memory" increases with age to become virtually universal by adulthood according to environmental exposure. Although both atopic and non-atopic individuals show lymphoproliferative responses to common aeroallergens, the presence of Th-2 responses to inhalant allergens is also the defining characteristic of individuals with aeroallergen allergy. Infants destined to develop aeroallergen sensitizations frequently develop hallmark Th-2 responses within the first year of life, even though many remain asymptomatic (22,27). These Th-2 responses to inhalants are frequently seen in children with food allergy (13). As with food allergen responses, Th-1 IFN-γ responses to inhaled allergens are not deficient and may actually be increased compared to non-allergic children (13,14,25,28,29). The origins of these apparently excessive or inappropriate immune responses are unclear. They may be due to a breakdown in regulatory mechanisms that normally control inappropriate responses, or may represent a transiently excessive developmental "rebound" during the phase in which the long-term balance is being established between the Th-1 and Th-2 arms of the adaptive immune response. Other studies (30) have shown that T cells from allergic infants have higher expression of activa tion markers (such as cluster of differentiation marker 25 (CD25) and CD30) suggesting that they are intrinsically more responsive to allergens. The significance of this is unclear and more information is needed about the function of regulatory cells in this period.

C. The Potential Importance of Regulatory Pathways in Early Postnatal Life

Regulatory pathways provide an essential counterbalance to immune defense mechanisms, helping to avert excessive or inappropriate responses. A diverse range of cells have regulatory or suppressive properties (Fig. 1), through direct cell–cell contact or the production of cytokines (such as IL-10 and TGF-β). The current understanding of these pathways is still fairly rudimentary, but it is clear that these cell populations are likely to have a critical role in shaping patterns of response during early immune development.

The gut is believed to be central in the development of regulatory immune function. The gastrointestinal tract and associated mucosal immune system is an IL-10 and TGF-β dominant environment, promoting mucosal immune response and systemic immune tolerance (reviewed in Ref. 16). It is of note that when animals do not achieve normal gut colonization (germ-free conditions) they develop profound disorders of immune tolerance including both autoimmunity and allergy (31).

Although initially classified as a Th-2 cytokine, IL-10 is produced by a much wider range of cell types (DC, monocytes, macrophages, CD4+ and CD8+ T cells, natural killer cells, neutrophils, and epithelial cells) and is now viewed more as a potent immunoregulatory cytokine. It plays an important role modulating and dampening excessive immune responses across the whole immune system. IL-10 is produced by a recently described T cell subset: the CD4+CD25+ Tr cell (reviewed in Ref. 32). IL-10 also inhibits T cell activation, IgE production, eosinophil recruitment and many other aspects of allergic inflammation (as reviewed in Refs. 33 and 34).

There is obviously key interest in the role of IL-10 during early development. A number of IL-10 "knock out" murine models demonstrate increased AHR, and eosinophilia exaggerated Th-2 responses compared with wild-type mice (Ref. 35 and others), although other reports are conflicting (36). IL-10–deficient animals also develop spontaneous inflammatory bowel disease (37). Studies in humans are less conclusive. Lower IL-10 (protein) levels have been measured in Bronchoalveolar Lavage (BAL) from human asthmatics (38), who also show reduced IL-10 responses by their purchase point media corporation (PBMC) (in response to endotoxin) compared with control subjects (38). Allergic patients also demonstrate reduced IL-10 responses after viral infections, with reduced IL-10 detected in nasal lavage fluid (39) and following in vitro PBMC stimulation (40). However, other studies have demonstrated higher expression of IL-10 mRNA in asthmatic airways (41) and gut mucosa (42). Less is known about the role of TGF-β in the development of allergic diseases and asthma in humans. Both IL-10 and TGF-β gene polymorphisms have been noted in association with asthma and atopy (43). Further research is now needed to determine how these and other immunomodulatory pathways regulate evolving patterns of immune response, which can lead to either future health or disease.

IV. The Significance of Perinatal Immune Responses

A. The Significance of Fetal Responses to Allergens

There has been ongoing speculation about whether allergen-responsive fetal T cells have been primed by allergen exposure in vivo or if these reflect some other poorly understood process. Only half of the allergen-responsive T cells in cord blood have recently been shown to have the CD45RO+ "memory" phenotype (44), and it is not clear why the remaining responses are being observed in "naïve" cell populations (44). For many reasons it may be inappropriate to assume that neonatal CD4+CD45RO+ T cells are equivalent to adult T cells with the same "memory" markers (45). Mechanisms of potential in utero allergen exposure are also unconfirmed. Allergens have been measured in amniotic fluid (46), and there is also indirect evidence that allergens can cross the placenta (47). Cells capable of presenting antigens are present in the fetal gut (48) and allergen priming through this route has also been proposed (48). The significance of these observations is unclear. Of note, there are no clear correlations between levels of maternal allergen exposure and the presence, magnitude, or character of fetal immune responses to these allergens (49–51). This suggests that maternal allergen encounter in pregnancy may not have a major influence on infant immune development, although more studies are needed.

More recent studies appear to confirm that cord blood responses to allergens are very different from mature memory responses. Although allergens (and other antigens) induce major histocompatibility complex (MHC) class II dependent cord blood lymphoproliferative responses, this is associated with unusually high levels of apoptosis (51a). Furthermore, the surviving cell populations appear to have "suppressive" or "regulatory" properties in culture. These cells also express markers including CD4, CD25, and cytotoxic lymphocyte antigen 4 (CTLA4) (intracellular), which are common (but not exclusive) to T regulatory cells (51a). The significance of this is still unclear, and further studies are needed. There is obvious interest in the role of these cells in early regulation of immune development.

The current state of knowledge regarding perinatal immune function is summarized in Table 1, including the main areas of controversy or uncertainty, where further research is still needed.

B. Predisposition for Type 2 Immune Responses in the Neonatal Period

During pregnancy, maternal immune responses are normally skewed to favor production of Th-2 cytokines, with similar effects seen in the neonate

Table 1 Perinatal Immune Development: Current Knowledge and Future Directions

	Current knowledge: supported by sound experimental data and/or consistent observations	Future research priorities: issues that are yet to be determined (aims of future research)
APC and regulatory populations	1. APC function is immature in neonates (including Th-1 trophic signals) 2. These functions mature slowly in the postnatal period	1. To determine if infants that go on to develop allergy have intrinsic differences in APC function 2. To determine what factors modify APC maturation 3. To find strategies that can safely modify early immune development to prevent allergic immune responses
T cell responses	1. Allergen-responsive T cell clones are evident in the neonatal period, although the significance of these is unclear 2. Neonatal T cells are more susceptible to postactivation anergy or apoptosis 3. There is a propensity for Th-2 responses in the neonatal period (due to hormonal influences and patterns of APC signaling) 4. Th-1 functions are immature at birth, but can be induced 5. Hypermethylation of the IFN-γ gene promotor is associated with reduced IFN-γ expression in neonatal CD4 T cells 6. There is gradual postnatal maturation of Th-1 function, but this is not apparent until the second year of life	1. To define the mechanism of perinatal T cell "priming", and to determine the role of these populations in subsequent immune development 2. To determine the role (or relevance) of regulatory T cells in the perinatal period, and the factors that can influences this 3. To determine the significance of differential IFN-γ gene regulation (methylation) in CD4 and CD8 populations 4. To define the relationship between perinatal immune function and risk of allergic disease (and strategies to modify this) 5. To determine what factors contribute to the wide variation in rates in immune maturation in a given population
B cell responses	1. Allergen-specific maternal antibodies cross the placenta 2. There is gradual increase in the production of allergen-specific IgE (and IgG) in allergic infants	1. To define the effects (if any) of maternal antibodies on specific cellular immune responses in the neonate 2. To determine whether allergen-speicfic IgG antibodies modulate IgE-mediated effector mechanisms 3. To determine why only a subgroup of infants with elevated allergen-specific IgE develop allergic symptoms

Abbreviations: IFN, interferon; CD, cluster of differentiation marker; APC, antigen presenting cell; IgE, immunoglobulin E.

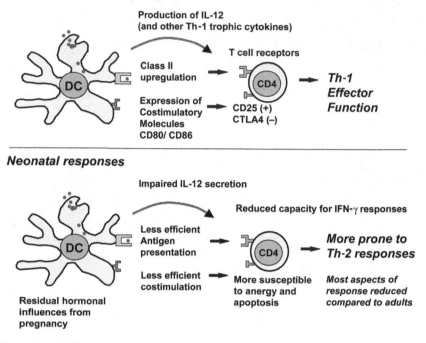

Figure 2   Differences between adult and neonatal responses.

(52) and the placenta (53). This appears to be the result of both pro-Th-2 products from the placenta (progesterone, IL-10, IL-4, and PGE2), and relative immaturity of APC signaling and specific aspects of Th-1 function at birth (Fig. 2). This includes relative inhibition of T cell IFN-γ gene transcription by hypermethylation of IFN-γ promoter region in neonatal CD4+ T cells (54) as discussed further below. The relationship between Th-2 responses at birth and atopic risk or atopic outcomes has been unclear, with a number of studies showing conflicting reports. In a number of recent studies, atopic risk (maternal atopy) has been associated with higher numbers of CD4+IL-13+ cells in cord blood (55) and stronger neonatal IL-13 (type 2) responses to milk allergen (β-lactoglobulin) (56). Atopic disease (at one year) has also been associated with higher neonatal polyclonal IL-13 responses (57) or increased numbers of CD4+IL-13+ cells in cord blood (55). However, other studies suggest an opposite relationship, with weaker Th-2 responses to allergens in high risk (or subsequently atopic infants) (58–60). Another larger cohort study (15) also found that lower cytokine levels (IFN-γ, IL-4, and TNF-α) in cord plasma (*n* = 406) were significantly associated with an increased risk of subsequent doctor-diagnosed asthma, wheeze, and aeroallergen sensitizations at six

years. The authors speculate that this may reflect greater immaturity in infants predisposed to allergy. This is consistent with multiple reports that Th-1 function (discussed below) is also less mature in neonates and infants at high risk of allergic disease (60–64).

C. Impaired Th-1 Immune Function in the Perinatal Period

Neonatal Th-1 IFN-γ responses are significantly attenuated compared to adults (52), and many groups have observed that newborns and infants at high risk of allergy (parental disease) have a greater "relative deficiency" of IFN-γ responses compared to infants at low risk of allergy (27,60–64). This observation has been confirmed in another recent study (65).

We initially speculated that impaired Th-1 immune function might contribute in some way to persistence of the Th-2 responses in allergic individuals (66,67). While this is likely to be an important contributing factor, associated perinatal abnormalities of immune regulatory cells leading to unchecked expansion of allergen-responsive Th-2 and Th-1 clones may also be involved (16,17). There are still no data that clearly describe these early causal pathways. There is suggestive data from both animals and human studies that providing pro-Th-1 stimulation (in the form of a variety of bacterial products and DNA) may improve Th-2 related disease in animals and humans (68–71). Although this lends further support to notions that allergy could be related to suboptimal Th-1 signaling, it remains inconclusive. While there has been speculation that bacterial endotoxin exposure in early life (72,73) may promote Th-1 function and protect from allergy there is no direct evidence to support this. Rather, one recent study showed that higher endotoxin levels at three months of age were associated with a higher risk of subsequent recurrent wheezing and sensitization to inhalant allergens (74). Thus further studies are needed to determine the role and action of early endotoxin exposure (reviewed in Ref. 75).

In addition to effects on Th-1 function, bacteria may also act through enhanced regulatory functions (TGF-β and IL-10) (76) (Fig. 1). Similarly, recent studies also suggest that suppression of Th-2 responses during allergen immunotherapy is also mediated by enhanced regulatory cell function (77) rather than simple Th-1 activation. Thus, the specific contribution of neonatal Th-1 immaturity to the development of Th-2 disease in high-risk infants remains unclear.

Reduced capacity for Th-1 responses during the perinatal period may be related to reduced capacity of neonatal APC to provide adequate pro-Th-1 T cell stimulation during activation, in the form of IL-12 and other cytokines (78,79) (Fig. 2). Although some have suggested that reduced production of IL-12 is a feature of the atopic state (80,81), others dispute this (82). Recent cross-sectional data indicate that the capacity of APC to produce IL-12 is orders of magnitude lower in neonates compared to adults, and may not approach adult levels until late childhood (83). It has been suggested that a relative absence of IL-12 favors the development of a default Th-2 cytokine profile, although other factors are clearly involved. Accordingly, the principal APC involved in activation of naïve T cells (DC) are also less mature in neonates and have been observed to be intrinsically programmed against Th-1 responses (78). However, while reduced neonatal IL-12 capacity is related to the Th-2 skewed allergen-specific responses observed in the neonate (79), there is currently no conclusive evidence that high-risk infants have more immature APC IL-12 signaling to account for relatively weaker type Th-1 responses. Although one recent study (84) suggests that IL-12 responses to allergens are lower in neonates with a family history of allergic disease, other studies show no differences in capacity of high-risk neonates to mount IL-12 responses to bacterial lipopolysaccharide (LPS) (79). Findings in older children have produced conflicting results with atopic children showing weaker IL-12 responses after the age of seven years, but higher levels in early childhood compared to non-allergic children (85).

An observed lack of correlation between IL-12 and IFN-γ responses in the neonate (79) could also indicate that neonatal T cells are less responsive to IL-12. Functional differences in the capacity of T cells to respond to IL-12 and other pro-type 1 signals from APC may occur in atopic or high-risk infants. Although there is one report that neonates at high risk of atopy (86) have reduced T cell expression of IL-12 receptor (IL-12Rβ1) further studies are required to establish if T cells of high-risk infants are less responsive to Th-1-trophic signals.

Differences in IFN-γ gene regulation in the neonate also indicate that neonatal T cells are intrinsically different from mature adult T cells. White et al. (54) have recently reported that neonatal expression of IFN-γ is inhibited by hypermethylation of IFN-γ promotor CpG sites. This finding was restricted to CD4+ T cells and not seen in CD8+ or NK cells. It is not yet clear how variations in perinatal Th-1 gene methylation status relates to the risk of subsequent allergic disease. The regulation of Th-2 cytokine gene transcription has not been investigated in the neonatal period, although there are some preliminary studies in adults (87). It has been recently observed that "Th-2" CD8+ T cells (rather than CD4+ T cells) are the main source of IL-13 in the neonate (52). The possible immuno-regulatory role of these and other cells still remains to be determined.

D. Predictive Value of Perinatal Cytokine Responses

At this stage, perinatal allergen-specific cytokine responses do not appear to have predictive value (88), but support the concept that the processes, which lead to immune dysregulation, are initiated very early in life. With the development of allergy prevention strategies there is a growing need to more accurately predict children at the highest risk for both atopy and related airways disease. However, recent studies from our group (89) (89a) suggest that polyclonal responses of cord blood mononuclear cells (CBMC) to agents such as staphylococcus enterotoxin B (SEB) and phyto-haemagglutinin (PHA) may provide insight into susceptibility to subsequent allergic sensitizations. In particular, high-level IFN-γ production by CD8+ (as opposed to CD4+) T cells of high-risk neonates is strongly associated with sensitizations at outcome age two years (89a).

V. How Perinatal Immaturity Leads to Excessive Postnatal Responses in Atopic Children

The recent observations that allergen-specific Th-1 responses are also stronger in children with established atopy (13,14,29) has led to another challenge: the need to explain the transition from apparently weaker Th-1 responses in the perinatal period. This apparent immunologic immaturity of future atopic individuals may also involve other cell types, as suggested by reduced expression of hemopoietic cytokine receptors on cord blood progenitor cells in neonates at risk for atopy (90). Although we may speculate that parallel immaturity of regulatory immune function during this period could predispose "a child" to the excessive and inappropriate mixed Th-1 and Th-2 responses seen in atopy, there is currently no direct evidence of this and further studies are needed to examine this. Table 2 summarizes the currently recognized differences in immune responses in both symptomatic allergic disease and presymptomatic (high-risk) children. This table distinguishes generally accepted immunological features of allergy as well as more controversial (or more recent) observations.

VI. The Relationship Between Atopy and the Development of Organ-Specific Disease

Despite the clear association with atopy, there is accumulating evidence that local expression of cutaneous or mucosal (airways) allergic disease occurs through independent processes in "Th-2-predisposed" individuals. Local epithelial–mesenchymal interactions are now believed to play a critical role in asthma pathogenesis (91). Epithelial cells, which produce many chemokines, cyokines, and growth factors, have been shown to be essential for Th-2-induced disease expression in animal asthma models (92,93) Th-2 cytokines have also been shown to have direct effects on human epithelial cells (94). Together, these observations suggest that asthma is the culmination of both local epithelial dysfunction and generalized Th-2 propensity (atopic predisposition). The development of atopic dermatitis appears even more complex. At this stage, the exact events leading to tissue-specific

Table 2 Early Immunological Differences in Atopic Children (Relative to Non-atopic Children)

	Generally accepted "facts"	Consistent observations	More recent observations (unconfirmed)
Presymptomatic (neonatal responses)			
Cord blood IgE	No practical predictive value	Higher cord blood IgE associated with later allergic disease, and more severe disease	
Proliferative responses to allergens	No predictive value	Stronger lymphoproliferative responses in high risk neonates	Allergen-specific responses in cord blood do not appear to be true "memory" responses
Perinatal Th-1 responses	No practical predictive value	Weaker Th-1 responses noted in high-risk neonates	
Perinatal Th-2 responses	No predictive value	Th-2 responses develop earlier in high risk +/or subsequently allergic infants	Some studies suggest weaker Th-2 responses in high risk (while others suggest stronger)
Symptomatic allergic disease			
Antibody levels	Elevated IgE to allergens in allergic disease	Higher food-specific IgE associated with persistent inhalant allergy	Increased IgG also seen with allergic disease
Proliferative responses to allergens			Allergy may not necessarily be associated with higher magnitude and frequency of lymphoproliferative responses to allergens
Th-2 responses	Th-2 responses are associated with symptoms		IL-5 appears to be the best cytokine marker for symptomatic disease
Th-1 responses	Th-1 responses to allergens common in both allergic and non-allergic children	Increased Th-1 responses to allergens in allergic children	Recent data does not support the original assumption that Th-1 responses might be impaired in established allergic disease

manifestations of Th-2 propensity are unclear. It is also not clear why only a portion of atopic individuals develop allergic disease, and there is still no clear explanation for the variable and heterogeneous manifestations of disease. A better knowledge of how early tissue-specific events lead to allergic disease may also provide opportunities to target secondary prevention strategies in children who are already showing evidence of allergen sensitizations.

There is a substantial body of evidence implicating most "Th-2" cytokines (IL-4, IL-5, IL-9, and IL-13) in the expression and development of airway inflammation and hyperactivity (AHR). While all of these cytokines appear to have a role, the recent literature indicates that IL-13 is especially critical and may be "sufficient and necessary" for the development of reactive airways disease, at least in animal models (93). Repeated exposure to IL-13 leads to murine airway inflammation, AHR and increased mucous production (95,96). While blocking the effects of other Th-2 cytokines (IL-4, IL-5, and IL-9) results in an incomplete reduction in the asthmatic airways response in mice, blocking the effects of IL-13 completely abolishes asthmatic responses (97). Accordingly, IL-13 "knock out" mice also have reduced airways eosinophilia, inflammation, fibrosis and epithelial, and mucous cell hyperplasia compared with wild-type mice (98). IL-13 appears to act directly on airways epithelial cells to produce the pathological features of asthma (92,93) without the need for an associated inflammatory infiltrate. Kupermann et al. elegantly demonstrated that mice lacking the vital Th-2 "signal transducer and activator of transcription" 6 (STAT6) were protected from all of the IL-13-induced features of airways disease. Reconstitution of STAT6 only in airways epithelial cells was sufficient to lead to all of the features of IL-13-induced AHR and mucus production. In humans, genetic variants of IL-13 (Arg 110 Gln) have been associated with asthma and homozygotes have been noted to have increased serum IL-13 levels (99) suggesting functional differences. However, while IL-13 plays a central role in animal models, the contribution in human is less clear.

Thus it appears that allergic diseases are the result of both local and underlying systemic immune dysregulation. Cytokines appear to play a key role in the initiation and perpetuation of allergic inflammation. However, it is still not clear if this dysfunction is initiated locally in the mucosal surfaces (and related immune networks) where disease is manifest, or if it is due to a more generalized abnormality in host responses. There is growing evidence that both of these processes occur and interact to produce local disease, but significantly more information is still needed.

Local airways APC (DC) populations play a critical role in programming T cell responses, following their migration-induced maturation in regional nodes (100). Although knowledge in this area is still incomplete, these cells appear to have a major role in the late phase response (100,101) and are therefore likely to contribute to the development of airway damage in inflammatory airway disease. Animal studies suggest that resting DC stimulate Th-2 development unless they receive obligatory Th-1-trophic signals during antigen processing (18). These signals may occur under conditions of infection or other local stress (21,102), which evoke protective Th-1 effector T cell responses. Age-related immaturity in DC function (83) may lead to a reduced capacity for these cells to respond to these stimuli. Foreseeably, variations in both local inflammatory factors and DC maturation could have a key role in determining the subsequent pattern of local T cell responses. Animal studies confirm that local airway DC networks are less developed in infant animals, and additionally these DC populations display markedly attenuated responses to inflammatory triggers (103,104). There is also preliminary evidence that this may be true in humans. In the first year of life, infants do not typically show DC in the airways in the absence of inflammation (105). However, despite this apparent immaturity, mature DC do appear in association with severe respiratory infection at this age (105). This suggests that local tissue events in infancy can influence the maturation of DC and modify downstream T cell programming in early life. This has renewed interest in the role of respiratory infection in early life in the etiology of atopic asthma (discussed further below).

To date, relatively few studies have directly investigated possible differences in early DC function in allergic and non-allergic individuals. One recent flow cytometric study found no differences in cord blood DC populations in neonates at high and low risk of atopy although they did not provide data on functional responses (106). However, they did observe that older children with established disease (atopic asthma) had lower levels of circulating plasmacytoid DC (106), possibly indicating increased migration to local tissues. The significance of this is unclear, particularly in view of the observation by other groups that plasmacytoid DC are increased in adults with disease (107). This may represent developmental differences that need to be investigated further.

VII. Factors That May Influence Early Immune Development

Although genetic studies will provide important information about biological pathways and potential mechanisms, it is virtually axiomatic that environmental as opposed to genetic factors must be primarily responsible for the recent epidemic rise in allergic disease with progressive Westernization. There remains a pressing need to identify perinatal exposures that can be readily modified to reduce the risk of subsequent disease (reviewed by Ref. 108). While many potential in utero and perinatal exposures have been associated with allergic disease and asthma (109), the significance of these and potential causal pathways are unclear.

A. Role of Respiratory Tract Infections

The relationship between early respiratory tract infections and allergic airway disease has been confusing. These infectious agents have been clearly identified as asthma triggers in children with established disease, and in addition early respiratory syncytial virus (RSV) infection in infancy has also been long regarded as a risk factor for subsequent asthma, at least in the first six years of life (110). This may be in part because of the Th-2-trophic properties of this and other respiratory viruses (111), but may also be an indirect consequence of the delayed capacity to mount Th-1-IFN-γ responses in the early postnatal period (28). In this context, Oddy et al. (112) have recently demonstrated that predisposition to wheezing lower respiratory infection in the first year of life is a strong risk factor for asthma at six years of age in both non-atopic (OR 4.1, $p < 0.0005$) and atopic (OR 9.0, $p < 0.0005$) children. The findings strongly suggested that significant infection-induced airway inflammation during the early period of postnatal lung growth and development can have profound long-term effects, which appear to be more marked than those resulting from inflammation occurring at later ages (113). Moreover, susceptibility to RSV infection and its subsequent spread to the lower respiratory tract in children at high risk of atopy appears directly related to their diminished capacity to mount Th-1-polarised immune responses during the early postnatal period (28,113). However, the notion that infection can serve only as a priming factor for subsequent allergic inflammation is at odds with other observations that under some circumstances infections appear to protect from allergic disease (114–118). This suggests the possibility that early encounter with infectious agents has the potential to accelerate the maturation of local immune networks (including DC as discussed above) producing Th-1 defense responses which may override the Th-2 default response in immunologically immature infants.

The complexity of these relationships needs to be further dissected. In particular, variations in the consequences of infections on allergic propensity may involve differences in the timing of exposure, the nature of the infectious agent, the location of the infection (upper or lower airway), in addition to genetic factors.

B. Other Factors That May Influence Early Immune Development: Targets for Allergy Prevention?

Many of the targets for prevention such as modifying early allergen exposure and infant feeding practices, may not actually be directly implicated in the increase in disease. In fact, a number of recent findings challenge existing notions that early allergen avoidance and breast-feeding prevent allergic disease (discussed elsewhere, and reviewed in Ref. 119). New approaches for primary allergy prevention include investigation of the role of dietary factors [antioxidants, hydrolyzed infant formulae, prebiotics, and polyunsaturated fatty acids (120,121)], primary (mucosal) allergen immunotherapy, and bacterial products (122,123) as discussed in more detail elsewhere. Strategies that reduce the risk (even slightly) or the severity of disease expression could have enormous impact in this global context.

VIII. Conclusion

Asthma and allergic disease remain the most common diseases in the modern world, making it essential to determine the causal pathways and underlying mechanisms, in the hope that this may lead to more definitive treatment and prevention strategies. A more complete understanding of the processes involved in local and systemic immune development is a crucial part of this process. A number of issues need to be investigated as research priorities, including the specific issues summarized in Tables 1 and 2. However, in more general terms, we need a much more detailed understanding of normal immune tolerance mechanisms, particularly a better understanding of:

    a.   basic cellular interactions and pathways of tolerance during early immune development,

    b.   the environmental and genetic factors that drive this process,

    c.   why this process appears to be failing in an increasing number of individuals, and

    d.   how these pathways can be safely modified to prevent immune mediated diseases.

Abbreviations

APC	Antigen presenting cells
CBMC	Cord blood mononuclear cells
CD-(4, 8, or other)	Cluster of differentiation marker (4, 8, or other)
CTLA4	Cytotoxic lymphocyte antigen 4
DC	Dendritic cells
GMCSF	Granulocyte monocyte lineage colony stimulating factor
HDM	House dust mite
IFN-γ	Interferon gamma
IL-(4, 5, 6, or 13)	Interleukin (4, 5, 6, or 13)
LPS	Lipopolysaccharide
PHA	Phytohaemagglutinin
RSV	Respiratory syncytial virus
SEB	Staphylococcus enterotoxin B
TGF-β	Transforming growth factor beta
Th-1	Type 1 T helper cell
Th-2	Type 2 T helper cell
Tr	Regulatory T cells

References

1. Lewis S. ISAAC—a hypothesis generator for asthma? International Study of Asthma and Allergies in Childhood. Lancet 1998; 351:1220–1221.
2. Romagnani S. Human Th-1 and Th-2 subsets: doubt no more. Immunol Today 1991; 12:256–257.
3. Mosmann T, Sad S. The expanding universe of T-cell subsets: Th-1, Th-2 and more. Immunol Today 1996; 17(3):138–146.
4. Byron K, O'Brien R, Vaigos G, Wooton A. *Dermatophagoides pteronyssinus* ii-induced interleukin-4 interferon-γ expression by freshly isolated lymphocytes of atopic individuals. Clin Exp Allergy 1994; 24:878–883.
5. Imada M, Simons FE, Jay FT, Hayglass KT. Allergen-stimulated interleukin-4 and interferon-gamma production in primary culture: responses of subjects with allergic rhinitis and normal controls. Immunology 1995; 85:373–380.
6. Gabrielsson S, Paulie S, Roquet A, Ihre E, Lagging E, van Hage-Hamsten M, Harfast B, Troye-Blomberg M. Increased allergen-specific Th2 responses in vitro in atopic subjects receiving subclinical allergen challenge. Allergy 1997; 52:860–865.
7. Kimura M, Tsuruta S, Yoshida T. IL-4 production by PBMCs on stimulation with mite allergen is correlated with the level of serum IgE antibody against mite in children with bronchial asthma. J Allergy Clin Immunol 2000; 105: 327–332.
8. Chang JH, Chan H, Quirce S, Green T, Noertjojo K, Lam S, Frew A, Keown P, Chan-Yeung M. In vitro T-lymphocyte response and house dust mite-induced bronchoconstriction. J Allergy Clin Immunol 1996; 98:922–931.
9. Till S, Dickason R, Huston D, Humbert M, Robinson D, Larche M, Durham S, Kay AB, Corrigan C. IL-5 secretion by allergen-stimulated CD4+ T cells in primary culture: relationship to expression of allergic disease. J Allergy Clin Immunol 1997; 99:563–569.
10. Li Y, Simons FE, HayGlass KT. Environmental antigen-induced IL-13 responses are elevated among subjects with allergic rhinitis, are independent of IL-4, and are inhibited by endogenous IFN-gamma synthesis. J Immunol 1998; 161:7007–7014.
11. Macaubas C, Prescott S, Smallacombe T, Yabuhara A, Venaille T, Holt B, Sly P, Holt P. Perinatal and early childhood cytokine responses to environmental allergens. In: Sanderson, C, eds. IL-5: From Molecule to Drug Target. New York: Marcel Dekker Inc., 1999:119–126.
12. Jenmalm MC, van Snick J, Cormont F, Salman B. Allergen-induced Th-1 and Th-2 cytokine secretion in relation to specific allergen sensitization and atopic symptoms in children. Clin Exp Allergy 2001; 31:1528–1535.
13. Ng TW, Holt PG, Prescott SL. Cellular immune responses to ovalbumin and house dust mite in egg—allergic children. Allergy 2002; 57:207–214.
14. Smart JM, Kemp AS. Increased Th-1 and Th-2 allergen-induced cytokine responses in children with atopic disease. Clin Exp Allergy 2002; 32:796–802.
15. Macaubas C, de Klerk NH, Holt BJ, Wee C, Kendall G, Firth M, Sly PD, Holt PG. Association between antenatal cytokine production and the development of atopy and asthma at age six years. Lancet 2003; 362:1192–1197.

16. Wills-Karp M, Santeliz J, Karp CL. The germless theory of allergic disease: revisiting the hygiene hypothesis. Nat Rev Immunol 2001; 1:69–75.
17. Bach JF. The effect of infections on susceptibility to autoimmune and allergic diseases. N Engl J Med 2002; 347:911–920.
18. Stumbles PA, Thomas JA, Pimm CL, Lee PT, Venaille TJ, Proksch S, Holt PG. Resting respiratory tract dendritic cells preferentially stimulate T helper cell type 2 (Th2) responses and require obligatory cytokine signals for induction of Th-1 immunity. J Exp Med 1998; 188:2019–2031.
19. Holt PG, Upham JW. The role of dendritic cells in asthma. Curr Opin Allergy Clin Immunol 2004; 4:39–44.
20. Charbonnier AS, Hammad H, Gosset P, Stewart GA, Alkan S, Tonnel AB, Pestel J. Der p 1-pulsed myeloid and plasmacytoid dendritic cells from house dust mite-sensitized allergic patients dysregulate the T cell response. J Leukoc Biol 2003; 73:91–99.
21. Yamamoto N, Suzuki S, Shirai A, Suzuki M, Nakazawa M, Nagashima Y, Okubo T. Dendritic cells are associated with augmentation of antigen sensitization by influenza A virus infection in mice. Eur J Immunol 2000; 30:316–326.
22. Prescott S, Macaubas C, Smallacombe T, Holt B, Sly P, Loh R, Holt P. Development of allergen-specific T-cell memory in atopic and normal children. Lancet 1999; 353(9148):196–200.
23. Campbell DE, Hill DJ, Kemp AS. Enhanced IL-4 but normal interferon-gamma production in children with isolated IgE mediated food hypersensitivity. Pediatr Allergy Immunol 1998; 9:68–72.
24. Kuwabara N, Kondo N, Fukutomi O, Agata H, Orii T. Relationship between interferon-gamma, interleukin-4 and IgE production of lymphocytes from hen's egg-sensitive patients. J Investig Allergol Clin Immunol 1995; 5:198–204.
25. Holt PG, Rudin A, Macaubas C, Holt BJ, Rowe J, Loh R, Sly PD. Development of immunologic memory against tetanus toxoid and pertactin antigens from the diphtheria-tetanus-pertussis vaccine in atopic versus nonatopic children. J Allergy Clin Immunol 2000; 105:1117–1122.
26. Noma T, Yoshizawa I, Aoki K, Yamaguchi K, Baba M. Cytokine production in children outgrowing hen egg allergy. Clin Exp Allergy 1996; 26:1298–1307.
27. van der Velden VH, Laan MP, Baert MR, de Waal Malefyt R, Neijens HJ, Savelkoul HF. Selective development of a strong Th-2 cytokine profile in high-risk children who develop atopy: risk factors and regulatory role of IFN-gamma, IL-4, and IL-10. Clin Exp Allergy 2001; 31:997–1006.
28. Rowe J, Macaubas C, Monger T, Holt BJ, Harvey J, Poolman JT, Loh R, Sly PD, Holt PG. Heterogeneity in diphtheria-tetanus-acellular pertussis vaccine-specific cellular immunity during infancy: relationship to variations in the kinetics of postnatal maturation of systemic Th-1 function. J Infect Dis 2001; 184:80–88.
29. Kimura M, Yamaide A, Tsuruta S, Okafuji I, Yoshida T. Development of the capacity of peripheral blood mononuclear cells to produce IL-4, IL-5, and IFN-gamma upon stimulation with house dust mite in children with atopic dermatitis. Int Arch Allergy Immunol 2002; 127:191–197.
30. Schade RP, Van Ieperen-Van Dijk AG, Versluis C, Van Reijsen FC, Kimpen JL, Bruijnzeel-Koomen CA, Knol EF, Van Hoffen E. Cell-surface expression

of CD25, CD26, and CD30 by allergen-specific T cells is intrinsically different in cow's milk allergy. J Allergy Clin Immunol 2002; 109:357–362.

31. Sudo N, Sawamura S, Tanaka K, Aiba Y, Kubo C, Koga Y. The requirement of intestinal bacterial flora for the development of an IgE production system fully susceptible to oral tolerance induction. J Immunol 1997; 159:1739–1745.

32. Shevach EM. Certified professionals: CD4(+)CD25(+) suppressor T cells. J Exp Med 2001; 193:F41–F46.

33. Koulis A, Robinson DS. The anti-inflammatory effects of interleukin-10 in allergic disease. Clin Exp Allergy 2000; 30:747–750.

34. Umetsu DT, DeKruyff RH. Interleukin-10: the missing link in asthma regulation? Am J Respir Cell Mol Biol 1999; 21:562–563.

35. Grunig G, Corry DB, Leach MW, Seymour BW, Kurup VP, Rennick DM. Interleukin-10 is a natural suppressor of cytokine production and inflammation in a murine model of allergic bronchopulmonary aspergillosis. J Exp Med 1997; 185:1089–1099.

36. Makela MJ, Kanehiro A, Borish L, Dakhama A, Loader J, Joetham A, Xing Z, Jordana M, Larsen GL, Gelfand EW. IL-10 is necessary for the expression of airway hyperresponsiveness but not pulmonary inflammation after allergic sensitization. Proc Natl Acad Sci USA 2000; 97:6007–6012.

37. Kuhn R, Lohler J, Rennick D, Rajewsky K, Muller W. Interleukin-10-deficient mice develop chronic enterocolitis. Cell 1993; 75:263–274.

38. Borish L. IL-10: evolving concepts. J Allergy Clin Immunol 1998; 101:293–297.

39. Corne JM, Lau L, Scott SJ, Davies R, Johnston SL, Howarth PH. The relationship between atopic status and IL-10 nasal lavage levels in the acute and persistent inflammatory response to upper respiratory tract infection. Am J Respir Crit Care Med 2001; 163:1101–1107.

40. Gentile DA, Patel A, Ollila C, Fireman P, Zeevi A, Doyle WJ, Skoner DP. Diminished IL-10 production in subjects with allergy after infection with influenza A virus. J Allergy Clin Immunol 1999; 103:1045–1048.

41. Robinson DS, Tsicopoulos A, Meng Q, Durham S, Kay AB, Hamid Q. Increased interleukin-10 messenger RNA in atopic allergy and asthma. Am J Respir Cell Mol Biol 1996; 14:113–117.

42. Lamblin C, Desreumaux P, Colombel JF, Tonnel AB, Wallaert B. Overexpression of IL-10 mRNA in gut mucosa of patients with allergic asthma. J Allergy Clin Immunol 2001; 107:739–741.

43. Hobbs K, Negri J, Klinnert M, Rosenwasser LJ, Borish L. Interleukin-10 and transforming growth factor-beta promoter polymorphisms in allergies and asthma. Am J Respir Crit Care Med 1998; 158:1958–1962.

44. Devereux G, Seaton A, Barker RN. In utero priming of allergen-specific helper T cells. Clin Exp Allergy 2001; 31:1686–1695.

45. Prescott SL, Jones CA. Cord blood memory responses: are we being naïve? Clin Exp Allergy 2001; 31:1653–1656.

46. Holloway JA, Warner JO, Vance GH, Diaper ND, Warner JA, Jones CA. Detection of house-dust-mite allergen in amniotic fluid and umbilical- cord blood. Lancet 2000; 356:1900–1902.

47. Szepfalusi Z, Loibichler C, Pichler J, Reisenberger K, Ebner C, Urbanek R. Direct evidence for transplacental allergen transfer. Pediatr Res 2000; 48:404–407.

48. Jones CA, Vance GH, Power LL, Pender SL, Macdonald TT, Warner JO. Costimulatory molecules in the developing human gastrointestinal tract: a pathway for fetal allergen priming. J Allergy Clin Immunol 2001; 108: 235–241.

49. Smillie FI, Elderfield AJ, Patel F, Cain G, Tavenier G, Brutsche M, Craven M, Custovic A, Woodcock A. Lymphoproliferative responses in cord blood and at one year: no evidence for the effect of in utero exposure to dust mite allergens. Clin Exp Allergy 2001; 31:1194–1204.

50. Marks GB, Zhou J, Yang HS, Joshi PA, Bishop GA, Britton WJ. Cord blood mononuclear cell cytokine responses in relation to maternal house dust mite allergen exposure. Clin Exp Allergy 2002; 32:355–360.

51. Chan-Yeung M, Ferguson A, Chan H, Dimich-Ward H, Watson W, Manfreda J, Becker A. Umbilical cord blood mononuclear cell proliferative response to house dust mite does not predict the development of allergic rhinitis and asthma. J Allergy Clin Immunol 1999; 104:317–321.

51a. Thotnyon CA, Upham JW, Wikstrom ME, Holt BJ, White GP, Sharp MJ, Sly PD, Holt PG. Functional maturation of CD4+CD25+CTLA4+CD45RA+ T regulatory cells in human neonatal T cell responses to environmental antigens/allergend. J Immunol 2004; 173:3084–3092.

52. Ribeiro-do-Couto LM, Boeije LC, Kroon JS, Hooibrink B, Breur-Vriesendorp BS, Aarden LA, Boog CJ. High IL-13 production by human neonatal T cells: neonate immune system regulator?. Eur J Immunol 2001; 31:3394–3402.

53. Sverremark Ekstrom E, Nilsson C, Holmlund U, van der Ploeg I, Sandstedt B, Lilja G, Scheynius A. IgE is expressed on, but not produced by, fetal cells in the human placenta irrespective of maternal atopy. Clin Exp Immunol 2002; 127:274–282.

54. White GP, Watt PM, Holt BJ, Holt PG. Differential patterns of methylation of the IFN-gamma promoter at CpG and non-CpG sites underlie differences in IFN-gamma gene expression between human neonatal and adult CD45RO- T cells. J Immunol 2002; 168:2820–2827.

55. Spinozzi F, Agea E, Russano A, Bistoni O, Minelli L, Bologni D, Bertotto A, de Benedictis FM. CD4+IL13+ T lymphocytes at birth and the development of wheezing and/or asthma during the 1st year of life. Int Arch Allergy Immunol 2001; 124:497–501.

56. Kopp MV, Zehle C, Pichler J, Szepfalusi Z, Moseler M, Deichmann K, Forster J, Kuehr J. Allergen-specific T cell reactivity in cord blood: the influence of maternal cytokine production. Clin Exp Allergy 2001; 31:1536–1543.

57. Ohshima Y, Yasutomi M, Omata N, Yamada A, Fujisawa K, Kasuga K, Hiraoka M, Mayumi M. Dysregulation of IL-13 production by cord blood CD4+ T cells is associated with the subsequent development of atopic disease in infants. Pediatr Res 2002; 51:195–200.

58. Williams TJ, Jones CA, Miles EA, Warner JO, Warner JA. Fetal and neonatal IL-13 production during pregnancy and at birth and subsequent development of atopic symptoms. J Allergy Clin Immunol 2000; 105:951–959.

59. Prescott S, Macaubas C, Holt B, Smallacombe T, Loh R, Sly P, Holt P. Transplacental priming of the human immune system to environmental allergens:

universal skewing of initial T-cell responses towards Th-2 cytokine profile. J Immunol 1998; 160:4730–4737.

60. Prescott SL, Macaubas C, Smallacombe T, Holt BJ, Sly PD, Loh R, Holt PG. Reciprocal age-related patterns of allergen-specific T-cell immunity in normal vs. atopic infants. Clin Exp Allergy 1998; 28(Suppl 5):39–44; discussion 50–51.

61. Holt PG, Clough JB, Holt BJ, Baron-Hay MJ, Rose AH, Robinson BWS, Thomas WR. Genetic "risk" for atopy is associated with delayed postnatal maturation of T cell competence. Clin Exp Allergy 1992; 22:1093–1099.

62. Martinez F, Stern D, Wright A, Holberg C, Taussig L, Halonen M. Association of interleukin-2 and interferon-g production by blood mononuclear cells in infancy with parental allergy skin tests and with subsequent development of atopy. J Allergy Clin Immunol 1995; 96:652–660.

63. Liao S, Liao T, Chiang B, Huang M, Chen C, Chou C, Hsieh K. Decreased production of IFNg and decreased production of IL-6 by cord blood mononuclear cells of newborns with a high risk of allergy. Clin Exp Allergy 1996; 26:397–405.

64. Warner JA, Miles EA, Jones AC, Quint DJ, Colwell BM, Warner JO. Is deficiency of interferon gamma production by allergen triggered cord blood cells a predictor of atopic eczema? Clin Exp Allergy 1994; 24:423–430.

65. Lehmann I, Thoelke A, Weiss M, Schlink U, Schulz R, Diez U, Sierig G, Emmrich F, Jacob B, Belcredi P. T cell reactivity in neonates from an East and a West German city—results of the LISA study. Allergy 2002; 57:129–136.

66. Holt PG, Macaubas C. Development of long-term tolerance versus sensitisation to environmental allergens during the perinatal period. Curr Opin Immunol 1997; 9:782–787.

67. Prescott SL, Holt PG. Abnormalities in cord blood mononuclear cytokine production as a predictor of later atopic disease in childhood. Clin Exp Allergy 1998; 28:1313–1316.

68. Cavallo GP, Elia M, Giordano D, Baldi C, Cammarota R. Decrease of specific and total IgE levels in allergic patients after BCG vaccination: preliminary report. Arch Otolaryngol Head Neck Surg 2002; 128:1058–1060.

69. Ota MO, Vekemans J, Schlegel-Haueter SE, Fielding K, Sanneh M, Kidd M, Newport MJ, Aaby P, Whittle H, Lambert PH. Influence of Mycobacterium bovis bacillus Calmette-Guerin on antibody and cytokine responses to human neonatal vaccination. J Immunol 2002; 168:919–925.

70. Barlan IB, Tukenmez F, Bahceciler NN, Basaran MM. The impact of in vivo Calmette-Guerin Bacillus administration on in vitro IgE secretion in atopic children. J Asthma 2002; 39:239–246.

71. Arkwright PD, David TJ. Intradermal administration of a killed Mycobacterium vaccae suspension (SRL 172) is associated with improvement in atopic dermatitis in children with moderate-to-severe disease. J Allergy Clin Immunol 2001; 107:531–534.

72. Roy SR, Schiltz AM, Marotta A, Shen Y, Liu AH. Bacterial DNA in house and farm barn dust. J Allergy Clin Immunol 2003; 112:571–578.

73. von Mutius E, Braun-Fahrlander C, Schierl R, Riedler J, Ehlermann S, Maisch S, Waser M, Nowak D. Exposure to endotoxin or other bacterial components might protect against the development of atopy. Clin Exp Allergy 2000; 30:1230–1234.

74. Bolte G, Bischof W, Borte M, Lehmann I, Wichmann HE, Heinrich J. Early endotoxin exposure and atopy development in infants: results of a birth cohort study. Clin Exp Allergy 2003; 33:770–776.

75. Niven R. The endotoxin paradigm: a note of caution. Clin Exp Allergy 2003; 33:273–276.

76. Zuany-Amorim C, Sawicka E, Manlius C, Le Moine A, Brunet LR, Kemeny DM, Bowen G, Rook G, Walker C. Suppression of airway eosinophilia by killed Mycobacterium vaccae- induced allergen-specific regulatory T-cells. Nat Med 2002; 8:625–629.

77. Francis JN, Till SJ, Durham SR. Induction of IL-10+CD4+CD25+ T cells by grass pollen immunotherapy. J Allergy Clin Immunol 2003; 111: 1255–1261.

78. Langrish CL, Buddle JC, Thrasher AJ, Goldblatt D. Neonatal dendritic cells are intrinsically biased against Th-1 immune responses. Clin Exp Immunol 2002; 128:118–123.

79. Prescott S, Taylor A, King B, Dunstan J, Upham J, Thornton C, Holt P. Neonatal IL-12 capacity is associated with variations in allergen specific immune responses in the neonatal and postnatal periods. Clin Exp Allergy 2003; 33:566–572.

80. Hammad H, Charbonnier AS, Duez C, Jacquet A, Stewart GA, Tonnel AB, Pestel J. Th-2 polarization by Der p 1-pulsed monocyte-derived dendritic cells is due to the allergic status of the donors. Blood 2001; 98:1135–1141.

81. Reider N, Reider D, Ebner S, Holzmann S, Herold M, Fritsch P, Romani N. Dendritic cells contribute to the development of atopy by an insufficiency in IL-12 production. J Allergy Clin Immunol 2002; 109:89–95.

82. Bellinghausen I, Brand U, Knop J, Saloga J. Comparison of allergen-stimulated dendritic cells from atopic and nonatopic donors dissecting their effect on autologous naive and memory T helper cells of such donors. J Allergy Clin Immunol 2000; 105:988–996.

83. Upham JW, Lee PT, Holt BJ, Heaton T, Prescott SL, Sharp MJ, Sly PD, Holt PG. Development of interleukin-12-producing capacity throughout childhood. Infect Immun 2002; 70:6583–6588.

84. Gabrielsson S, Soderlund A, Nilsson C, Lilja G, Nordlund M, Troye-Blomberg M. Influence of atopic heredity on IL-4-, IL-12-, and IFN-gamma-producing cells in in vitro activated cord blood mononuclear cells. Clin Exp Immunol 2001; 126:390–396.

85. Itazawa T, Adachi Y, Okabe Y, Hamamichi M, Adachi YS, Toyoda M, Morohashi M, Miyawaki T. Developmental changes in interleukin-12-producing ability by monocytes and their relevance to allergic diseases. Clin Exp Allergy 2003; 33:525–530.

86. Janefjord CK, Jenmalm MC. PHA-induced IL-12R beta(2) mRNA expression in atopic and non-atopic children. Clin Exp Allergy 2001; 31:1493–1500.

87. Macaubas C, Lee PT, Smallacombe TB, Holt BJ, Wee C, Sly PD, Holt PG. Reciprocal patterns of allergen-induced GATA-3 expression in peripheral blood mononuclear cells from atopics vs. non-atopics. Clin Exp Allergy 2002; 32:97–106.

88. Prescott SL, King B, Strong TL, Holt PG. The value of perinatal immune responses in predicting allergic disease at 6 years of age. Allergy 2003; 58:1187–1194.

89. Sharp MJ, Rowe J, Kusel M, Sly PD, Holt PG. Specific patterns of responsiveness to microbial antigens staphylococcal enterotoxin B and purified protein derivative by cord blood mononuclear cells are predictive of risk for development of atopic dermatitis. Clin Exp Allergy 2003; 33:435–441.

89a. Rowe J, Heaton T, Kusel M, Suriyaarachchi D, Serralha M, Holt BJ, de lerk N, Sly PD, Holt PG. High IFN-gamma production by CD8+ T cells and early sensitization among infants at high risk of atopy. J Allergy Clin Immunol 2004; 113:710–716.

90. Upham JW, Hayes LM, Lundahl J, Sehmi R, Denburg JA. Reduced expression of hemopoietic cytokine receptors on cord blood progenitor cells in neonates at risk for atopy. J Allergy Clin Immunol 1999; 104:370–375.

91. Holgate ST, Davies DE, Lackie PM, Wilson SJ, Puddicombe SM, Lordan JL. Epithelial-mesenchymal interactions in the pathogenesis of asthma. J Allergy Clin Immunol 2000; 105:193–204.

92. Venkayya R, Lam M, Willkom M, Grunig G, Corry DB, Erle DJ. The Th-2 lymphocyte products IL-4 and IL-13 rapidly induce airway hyperresponsiveness through direct effects on resident airway cells. Am J Respir Cell Mol Biol 2002; 26:202–208.

93. Kuperman DA, Huang X, Koth LL, Chang GH, Dolganov GM, Zhu Z, Elias JA, Sheppard D, Erle DJ. Direct effects of interleukin-13 on epithelial cells cause airway hyperreactivity and mucus overproduction in asthma. Nat Med 2002; 8:885–889.

94. Wenzel SE, Trudeau JB, Barnes S, Zhou X, Cundall M, Westcott JY, McCord K, Chu HW. TGF-beta and IL-13 synergistically increase eotaxin-1 production in human airway fibroblasts. J Immunol 2002; 169:4613–4619.

95. Wills-Karp M, Luyimbazi J, Xu X, Schofield B, Neben TY, Karp CL, Donaldson DD. Interleukin-13: central mediator of allergic asthma. Science 1998; 282:2258–2261.

96. Grunig G, Warnock M, Wakil AE, Venkayya R, Brombacher F, Rennick DM, Sheppard D, Mohrs M, Donaldson DD, Locksley RM. Requirement for IL-13 independently of IL-4 in experimental asthma. Science 1998; 282:2261–2263.

97. Temann UA, Ray P, Flavell RA. Pulmonary overexpression of IL-9 induces Th-2 cytokine expression, leading to immune pathology. J Clin Invest 2002; 109:29–39.

98. Kumar RK, Herbert C, Yang M, Koskinen AM, McKenzie AN, Foster PS. Role of interleukin-13 in eosinophil accumulation and airway remodelling in a mouse model of chronic asthma. Clin Exp Allergy 2002; 32:1104–1111.

99. Arima K, Umeshita-Suyama R, Sakata Y, Akaiwa M, Mao XQ, Enomoto T, Dake Y, Shimazu S, Yamashita T, Sugawara N. Upregulation of IL-13 concen-

tration in vivo by the IL-13 variant associated with bronchial asthma. J Allergy Clin Immunol 2002; 109:980–987.

100. Huh JC, Strickland DH, Jahnsen FL, Turner DJ, Thomas JA, Napoli S, Tobagus I, Stumbles PA, Sly PD, Holt PG. Bidirectional interactions between antigen-bearing respiratory tract dendritic cells (DCs) and T cells precede the late phase reaction in experimental asthma: DC activation occurs in the airway mucosa but not in the lung parenchyma. J Exp Med 2003; 198:19–30.

101. Jahnsen FL, Moloney ED, Hogan T, Upham JW, Burke CM, Holt PG. Rapid dendritic cell recruitment to the bronchial mucosa of patients with atopic asthma in response to local allergen challenge. Thorax 2001; 56:823–826.

102. Stampfli MR, Wiley RE, Neigh GS, Gajewska BU, Lei XF, Snider DP, Xing Z, Jordana M. GM-CSF transgene expression in the airway allows aerosolized ovalbumin to induce allergic sensitization in mice. J Clin Invest 1998; 102:1704–1714.

103. Nelson D, McMenamin C, McWilliam A, Brenan M, Holt P. Development of the airway intraepithelial Dendritic Cell network in the rat from class II MHC (Ia) negative precursors: differential regulation of Ia expression at different levels of the respiratory tract. J Exp Med 1994; 179:203–212.

104. Nelson D, Holt P. Defective regional immunity in the respiratory tract of neonates is attributable to hyporesponsiveness of local Dendritic Cells to activation signals. J Immunol 1995; 155:3517–3524.

105. Tschernig T, Debertin AS, Paulsen F, Kleemann WJ, Pabst R. Dendritic cells in the mucosa of the human trachea are not regularly found in the first year of life. Thorax 2001; 56:427–431.

106. Hagendorens MM, Ebo DG, Schuerwegh AJ, Huybrechs A, Van Bever HP, Bridts CH, De Clerck LS, Stevens WJ. Differences in circulating dendritic cell subtypes in cord blood and peripheral blood of healthy and allergic children. Clin Exp Allergy 2003; 33:633–639.

107. Matsuda H, Suda T, Hashizume H, Yokomura K, Asada K, Suzuki K, Chida K, Nakamura H. Alteration of balance between myeloid dendritic cells and plasmacytoid dendritic cells in peripheral blood of patients with asthma. Am J Respir Crit Care Med 2002; 166:1050–1054.

108. Liu AH. Allergy and asthma prevention: the cup half full. Allergy Asthma Proc 2001; 22:333–336.

109. Devereux G, Barker RN, Seaton A. Antenatal determinants of neonatal immune responses to allergens. Clin Exp Allergy 2002; 32:43–50.

110. Stein RT, Sherrill D, Morgan WJ, Holberg CJ, Halonen M, Taussig LM, Wright AL, Martinez FD. Respiratory syncytial virus in early life and risk of wheeze and allergy by age 13 years. Lancet 1999; 354:541–545.

111. Sigurs N, Bjarnason R, Sigurbergsson F, Kjellman B, Bjorksten B. Asthma and immunoglobulin E antibodies after respiratory syncytial virus bronchiolitis: a prospective cohort study with matched controls. Pediatrics 1995; 95: 500–505.

112. Oddy WH, de Klerk NH, Sly PD, Holt PG. The effects of respiratory infections, atopy, and breastfeeding on childhood asthma. Eur Respir J 2002; 19: 899–905.

113. Holt PG, Sly PD. Interactions between respiratory tract infections and atopy in the aetiology of asthma. Eur Respir J 2002; 19:538–545.
114. Gerrard JW, Geddes CA, Reggin PL, Gerrard CD, Horne S. Serum IgE levels in white andmetis communities in Saskatchewan. Ann Allergy 1976; 37: 91–100.
115. Strachan DP. Hay fever, hygiene, and household size. BMJ 1989; 299: 1259–1260.
116. Martinez F. Role of viral infections in the inception of asthma and allergies during childhood: could they be protective? Thorax 1994; 49:1189–1191.
117. Bråbäck L, Breborwiz A, Dreborg S, et al. Atopic sensitisation and respiratory symptoms among Polish and Swedish school children. Clin Exp Allergy 1994; 24:826–835.
118. Martinez FD, Stern DA, Wright AL, Taussig LM, Halonen M. Association of non-wheezing lower respiratory tract illnesses in early life with persistently diminished serum IgE levels. Thorax 1995; 50(10):1067–1072.
119. Sly PD, Holt PG. Breast is best for preventing asthma and allergies—or is it? Lancet 2002; 360:887–888.
120. Dunstan JA, Mori TA, Barden A, Beilin LJ, Taylor AL, Holt PG, Prescott SL. Maternal fish oil supplementation in pregnancy reduces IL-13 levels in cord blood of infants at high risk of atopy. Clin Exp Allergy 2003; 33:442–448.
121. Dunstan J, Mori TA, Barden A, Beilin LJ, Taylor A, Holt PG, Prescott SL. Fish oil supplementation in pregnancy modifies neonatal allergen-specific immune responses and clinical outcomes in infants at high risk of atopy: a randomised controlled trial. J Allergy Clin Immunol 2003; 112:1178–1184.
122. Kalliomaki M, Salminen S, Arvilommi H, Kero P, Koskinen P, Isolauri E. Probiotics in primary prevention of atopic disease: a randomised placebo-controlled trial. Lancet 2001; 357:1076–1079.
123. Kalliomaki M, Salminen S, Poussa T, Arvilommi H, Isolauri E. Probiotics and prevention of atopic disease: 4-year follow-up of a randomised placebo-controlled trial. Lancet 2003; 361:1869–1871.

3

Origins of Asthma

J. O. WARNER

Southampton General Hospital, Southampton, U.K.

I. Introduction

Asthma is a disorder affecting conducting airways in which inflammation interacts with structural changes to cause variable airflow limitation (1). Conventional treatment of established asthma is highly effective in controlling symptoms and improving quality of life. With the possible exception of immunotherapy, however, no treatment has been shown to modify long-term outcomes and no cure has been identified (2–4). Most asthma has its origins in early life and the best predictors of continuation into adulthood are: early age of onset, sensitization to house dust mites (in environments where this is a prevalent allergen), reduced lung function, and increased bronchial hyper-responsiveness (BHR) in childhood (5). Under such circumstances attention must focus on an understanding of the early life origins of the disease in order to identify targets for primary prevention.

While there is a strong genetic predisposition to asthma, the increased prevalence of the disease that has occurred over the last 30 years is too rapid to be accounted for by genetic change in the population. It is likely that the increase is due to a change in environmental influences acting on pre-existing genetic susceptibilities. There are two basic components that contribute to airflow limitation in asthma, namely, airway inflammation and a structural alteration in the airway wall, which has been termed "remodeling." Both features contribute to the induction of BHR. Most studies hitherto have concentrated on the genetic and early life origins of allergy and the way it induces airway inflammation (6). It has been assumed that inflammation is the main cause of remodeling and BHR. However, it is now clear that genetic and environmental factors can affect BHR independent of allergic sensitization (7). Indeed BHR can be detected as early as four weeks of age and its presence is a predictor of asthma at six years of age, independent of allergic sensitization (8). Much less attention has focused on the early life factors influencing airway form and function.

II. Atopy and Asthma

Successive studies have demonstrated that both the prevalence and severity of asthma is increasing in the developed world (9). In the United Kingdom, prevalence surveys among 12- to 14-year-olds have shown an increase in point prevalence from 1973 to 1988, and finally to 1996 from 4% to 9% to 20.9%, respectively (10,11). Other atopic diseases have also increased: eczema from 5% to 16% to 16.4%, and hay fever from 9% to 15% to 18.2% over the same period (11–13). Diagnostic transfer does not explain this, as a very similar, if not identical, ascertainment was employed each time in these studies. Furthermore, there has been a considerable increase in hospital admissions for childhood asthma over the last 10 years with no reduction in severity on admission, no increase in readmission ratio and no evidence of diagnostic transfer (14). A relatively small shift in population susceptibility due to changes in the environment could account for the increasing frequency of disease and especially of severe disease.

While a large number of infants with wheeze do not go on to develop asthma, the one consistent factor predicting ongoing disease is the presence of atopy (15,16). Non-atopic wheezers have a disease of very different pathogenesis and long-term implication and often remit in early childhood (17). Thus, a focus on the factors that influence the development of atopy will in turn indicate which factors are important in the genesis of the airway inflammation component of asthma. However, while asthma is strongly associated with atopy, it cannot be explained by this alone. Indeed, the population-attributable risk of asthma from atopy is less than 50% (18). Other etiological factors are as, if not more, important to the development of asthma. Therefore it is essential to consider factors predisposing not only to the development of atopy but also to the increased risk of developing asthma. The additional component of asthma is abnormal lung function and/or BHR which in turn probably reflects alterations in the structure of the airway (19). While these occur independently of atopy, they commonly co-exist with atopy, particularly in persistent and severe disease (5).

III. The Atopic Immune Response and Pregnancy

The immunological paradigm associated with atopic disease is the expression of T-cell immunity to common environmental allergens that is biased towards a Th-2 cytokine profile Interleukin-4 (IL-4), Interleukin-5 (IL-5), and Interleukin-13 (IL-13) as opposed to a Th-1 profile (IL-2, Interferon gamma (IFN-γ)). Th-2 cytokines favor the production of immunoglobulin E (IgE) and the activation of relevant pro-inflammatory cells (e.g., eosinophils by IL-5). It has been recognized that fetal development occurs in an environment biased towards the Th-2 pathway of immune response, with additional contributions from cytokines associated with regulatory T cells (IL-10 and Transforming growth factor beta (TGF-β)) (20,21). Evidence from murine and human pregnancies reveal that Th-1 type cytokines mediate pregnancy loss (22,23). At the normal materno-fetal interface, there is an upregulation of IL-4 and IL-10 production with a concurrent down-regulation of IL-2 and IFN-γ (24,25). Therefore, the developing fetal immune system is exposed to factors that should promote a Th-2 pattern of response (26) and responses to allergen are universally Th-2 skewed at birth (27). Rapid postnatal maturation of Th-1 responsiveness counterbalances this.

Observations of an altered immune response at birth in children at risk (family history) of developing atopy and in the subset who do go on to develop disease in infancy highlights the contribution of the early life environment to the development of atopy and atopic disease (28). These have shown that allergen- or mitogen-induced IFN-γ production by cord blood mononuclear cells (CBMC) from at-risk newborns or those that went on to develop disease (27,29,30) was reduced compared to their low-risk counterparts or those who did not develop atopic disease in infancy. Thus it was postulated that impaired Th-1 cytokine production at birth was associated with the development of IgE mediated disease, presumably due to failure to prevent IgE production upon early postnatal allergen exposure. However, my group has shown that IL-13 (Th-2 cytokine) production at birth is similarly reduced (31), and it is now thought that an altered intrauterine environment has a much more widespread effect on the development of the fetal immune response. IL-13 is an important neonatal immune system regulator (32) and reduced levels might have pervasive effects on other aspects of immunological function at birth and in infancy.

The Th-1/Th-2 paradigm has become less convincing as it has become clear that Th-1 associated diseases such as insulin dependent diabetes mellitus (IDDM) have the same demographic and environmental associations as allergy. Indeed allergic diseases occur more frequently than

The new paradigm of T-cell regulation.

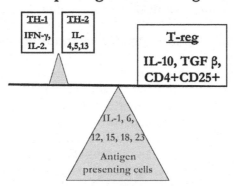

Figure 1   A concept of the new paradigm, which explains the current understanding of the balance of T-lymphocyte responses to antigen in relation to the peptide regulatory factors that they generate. Pivotal to the initiation of a T-cell response is antigen presentation by antigen presenting cells such as DC, macrophages and monocytes. The antigen is presenting as peptide fragments in association with the major histo-compatability complex molecules and is recognised by the T-cell receptor. Co-stimulatory signals in addition to the production of a range of cytokines by the antigen presenting cells then dictates the character of the T-cell response. These cytokines include IL-1, IL-6, IL-12, IL-15, IL-18, and IL-23. The old paradigm of a balance between T-helper 1 and T-helper 2 cells in which counter-regulation is initiated by IFN-γ and IL-4, respectively, must now be modified because a third group of T-cells is recognized which regulate both Th-1 and Th-2 activities. There are three varieties of regulatory cells, those generating IL-10, those generating TGF-β and those expressing CD-4 and CD-25 which regulate T-helper cell activity by cell–cell contact

by chance in association with IDDM (33). The current view is that both Th-1 and Th-2 activity is under the control of a third set of helper T-cells Th-3 and T-reg1, which generate TGF-β and IL-10, respectively. A defect in interactions between the three sets of T-helper lymphocytes may therefore be the common underlying malfunction (Fig. 1).

My groups have shown that the amniotic fluid of atopic mothers has higher levels of IL-10 than non-atopic mothers (34). Thus infants of atopic mothers who are at high risk of developing allergy themselves, will be subjected, in utero, to a greater regulatory influence, tending to suppress Th-1 and Th-2 cytokine production. This could explain the apparent immaturity of neonatal T-cell responses in infants destined to develop allergic disease.

IV. The Hygiene Hypothesis

Although both Th-1 and Th-2 responses are impaired at birth it appears that the failure to up-regulate IFN-γ production postnatally while consolidating Th-2 (IL-4, IL-5, and IL-13) activity is particularly associated with the development of atopic disease in infancy (35,36). One of the most compelling explanations for the increasing prevalence of atopic diseases in the developed world is the "hygiene hypothesis." Not only is there a credible immune mechanism to explain the hypothesis, namely up-regulation of Th-1 activity by microbes, but also diverse influences on hygiene have been associated with an altered prevalence of atopy (37). Most studies have focused on the inverse relationship between prevalence of infections and atopy. For example, the infectious diseases typhoid and tuberculosis occur rarely in countries with a high prevalence of allergic disease and it has been suggested that this explains the variation in disease prevalence around the world (38).

The composition of the gastrointestinal flora may be more important (39). Differences have been shown in the microflora from the feces of allergic compared with non-allergic infants (40,41), and alterations in gut microbial flora may explain both the inverse relationship between exposure to farm animals (42–45), and the positive association with antibiotic use in early life (46,47). There is even an effect of antibiotic usage during pregnancy increasing allergy in the offspring (48). This will have a potent influence on the type of organisms coming from the mother to colonize the newborn infant's gut. Normal priming to induce a change in the newborn infant's Th-2 biased response back to a more balanced Th-1/Th-2 type response by ensuring up-regulation of Th-1 reactivity during the first few years of life might well be initiated by particular gut flora (39). However, as impairment of immunological responsiveness at birth is common to children at risk of developing atopy (reduced IFN-γ and IL-13 production as already discussed), such children will also have a reduced ability to respond to the commensal flora, fail to up-regulate Th-1 responsiveness postnatally, and thereby consolidate the Th-2-mediated pattern of response. One microbial component considered to be of importance in initiating a Th-1 response is endotoxin or lipo polysaccharide (LPS), a product of gram-negative organisms. Many studies have highlighted an inverse relationship between early LPS exposure and both allergy and allergic disease. Indeed this might explain the paradoxical low prevalence of allergy and asthma in children born on farms (42–45). However, there may be additional effects from drinking unpasteurized milk (49). Similarly endotoxin exposure has been implicated in increasing infant wheeze associated with infections, but decreasing later allergic asthma in infants who attend day care from very early life or have older siblings (50). Indeed the original observations of higher sibship order being associated with less allergy led to the hygiene hypothesis being proposed (37).

V. Genetic Polymorphisms and Allergy

One component of the response to endotoxin is its binding to the cluster of differentiation marker-14 (CD-14) molecule either in a soluble form in biological secretions or on monocytes and macrophages (51). The gene for CD-14 gene is located in the 5q31–33 cytokine gene cluster, and polymorphisms at this location have been associated with high IgE levels in some but not all linkage studies (52–54). One of the studies also showed an inverse relationship between soluble CD-14 and IFN-γ levels (52). CD-14 is poorly expressed by monocytes in the fetus and neonate but is present as sCD-14 in amniotic fluid and at very high levels in human breast milk. Reduced supply from the mother in either the amniotic fluid or breast milk is associated with early-onset atopic eczema (55). Thus it is possible that the CD-14 polymorphism in the mother results in a failure of priming of the fetal and neonatal Th-1 immune response.

The ranges of genetic polymorphisms, which directly affect the mechanisms of IgE production, have been associated with raised IgE and sometimes atopic disease. The greatest focus has been on the cytokine gene cluster on 5q31–33, which not only contains CD-14, but also Th-2 cytokine IL-4, IL-9, and IL-13 genes (56). However, there are much stronger associations with atopy rather than asthma and some studies have used the presence of markers of allergy as a surrogate for disease.

It is not surprising that associations have been identified on most chromosomes with little uniformity between studies (57). The different results may be a consequence of genuine genetic variations between ethnic groups but are often due to differences in pheno-typing the populations. Other mechanistically credible associations have been with a common subunit of the IL-4 and IL-13 receptor on chromosome 16p12 (56), those for IFN-γ on 12q, the major histo-compatability complex molecules, TNF-α and -β on 6p21; IgE receptor on 11q12–13 (57), and IL-18 on 11q22 (58). The latter is particularly interesting because IL-18 has complex actions in initiating both Th-1 and Th-2 activity dependent on the antigenic stimulus. The impact of some of the polymorphisms may only be apparent at critical stages during development of the immune response, such that very minor perturbations particularly during pregnancy will alter outcomes. Until huge multi-national longitudinal pregnancy cohort studies are conducted it will not be possible to disentangle the relative importance of genetic and environmental factors.

VI. Ante-natal Origins of Allergic Sensitization

The Th-2 biased ante-natal environment will only be relevant to allergy if the fetus is also exposed to allergen and has sufficiently mature immune mechanisms for sensitization to occur. We have identified maternally derived allergen either free or complexed with IgG or IgE in amniotic fluid in the second trimester (59), and it is actively transported across the placenta directly into the fetal circulation mostly complexed with IgG in the third trimester (60). The IgE in amniotic fluid is of maternal origin and approximately 10% of circulating levels. Thus the fetus is exposed to higher concentrations if the mother has parasitosis or is atopic herself (61). The fetus is therefore, bathed in allergen, Th-2 and regulatory cytokines, and IgE. While the fetal circulating immune cells are very immature (62,63), those in the fetal small bowel are not only mature, but antigen-presenting cells show evidence of having picked up antigen and to have then sensitized T-cells, in regional lymphoid accumulations from as early as 14–16 weeks gestation (64). One very credible mechanism for sensitization to remarkably low doses of allergen is through IgE-facilitated antigen focusing, because there is ample CD-23 (low affinity IgE receptors) on antigen-presenting cells in the fetal small bowel (61). This promotes sensitization to 100–1000-fold lower concentrations of allergen than would be the case in the absence of IgE. It is, therefore, not surprising that the majority if not all neonates have a peripheral blood mononuclear cell response to common environmental allergens such as house dust mites (65).

While the Th-2 biased ante-natal environment has been assumed to be a mechanism which protects the pregnancy from maternal Th-1 immune responses it is possible that this process has evolved to protect the newborn infant against its mother's intestinal parasites (61). The newborn has an inevitable exposure to maternal gut organisms but virtually never is infected by its mother's parasites (66). Furthermore, the neonate of a parasitized mother has high parasite-specific IgE which can only have been generated by the infant, as IgE does not cross the placenta, and a Th-2 biased proliferative response to parasite antigens (67).

In summary, the newborn infant has already been exposed to many antigens and developed a primary Th-2 biased, but not committed, immune response to common environmental allergens. Normally postnatal maturation of immune responses, in part, as a consequence of exposure to microbial products leads to Th-1:2 balance. However, if the mother is atopic she will expose her fetus to higher IgE, Th-2, and regulatory cytokine levels which will lead to the genetically predisposed infant having a more committed, but immature, Th-2 response. She will also be less likely to be able to prime her infant with sCD-14 to enable a balanced response to LPS and other microbial products.

VII. Early Life Origins of Remodeling

Airway remodeling, which is now viewed as a pathognomonic feature of asthma, is postulated to result from damage to the airway epithelial layer with subsequent hypertrophy of airway smooth muscle (ASM) and deposition of collagen in the *lamina reticularis* below the true epithelial basement membrane. Features of asthma-associated tissue remodeling and inflammation in children are identical to those in the asthmatic adult with loss of epithelium, and cellular infiltration dominated by eosinophils and mast cells. Thickening and hyalinization of the sub-basement membrane in children aged 5 to 14 years old who had moderate asthma has been observed (68), but the thickness does not correlate with the duration of the disease or atopic status (69). We have found that there are more eosinophils in the bronchial mucosa and the thickness of the sub-epithelial *lamina reticularis* was greater in children with bronchial asthma. This had been diagnosed 22–80 months after the original bronchoscopy had been performed, at a time when the children had indeterminate respiratory symptoms not clearly diagnosed as asthma and were compared with those who presented with similar symptoms but did not progress to asthma (70). Thus, alterations in airway structure evolve in parallel with eosinophilic inflammation and are likely to occur before first symptoms are manifest. This would be in keeping with the association between BHR at four weeks of age and asthma at six years (8).

Diminished lung function in early infancy has been associated with later infant wheeze both in those with and without a high risk for atopy (71,72). However, many such infants do not progress to later asthma and constitute a group of children with transient, usually virus infection–associated, wheeze (73). As atopy remains the most important association with later asthma it is likely that there is a two-stage process in its development. Based on the above data linking very early BHR with later asthma, the first step is likely to be a change in airway morphology which will only persist at the second stage, in the presence of continuing inflammatory insults which are most commonly allergic in nature. The non-atopic infant wheezer with airway morphological changes alone will lose the susceptibility to respiratory symptoms as the airways grow through the first few years of life. Such individuals may be at risk of late adult-onset chronic obstructive pulmonary disease (COPD) as loss of elastic recoil exacerbates the subtle airway changes. Those infants with atopy alone either do not develop asthma or by virtue of persistant inflammation have a late onset of asthma, but this is of significantly less severity, associated with less BHR and is more likely to remit in adolescence (74) (Fig. 2).

If eosinophilic inflammation associated with allergy is not the primary stimulus for remodeling, alternative mechanisms require investigation. Elite cross-country skiers commonly develop asthma symptoms and bronchial biopsies have shown evidence of remodeling in the absence of eosinophils but the presence of neutrophils (75). Many asthmatics, particularly with more severe disease, both in infancy (76) and adulthood (77), have a predominance of neutrophils. Furthermore, the number of neutrophils correlates with levels of the major neutrophil chemokine, IL-8 (78), which is released by a host of lung cells, including macrophages and airway epithelium, when stressed. My groups have found raised levels of Matrix Metallo-Protease 9 (MMP-9) and TGF-β in broncho-alveolar lavage (BAL) of asthmatics and infant wheezers. Neutrophil MMP-9 exists in a high molecular weight form, which renders it relatively resistant to the effects of its inhibitor tissue

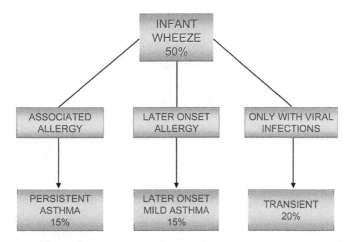

Figure 2 A diagrammatic representation of the outcome of infant wheeze. In some populations this effects of up to 50% of all infants. Where this is associated with allergy, asthma is likely to be the outcome and given its early age of onset is often persistent and provides the hard core of asthma requiring inhaled cortico-steroids and constitutes up to 15% of the total child population. There are other infant wheezers who only at a later stage show signs of allergy. Later onset allergy in association with asthma has a better prognosis and may well constitute the milder end of the asthma spectrum but still contributes up to 15% of the total child population. Finally there are a group of infant wheezers who only have problems with viral infections and have no evidence of underlying allergy. The vast majority of these infants lose their symptoms over the first few years of life. They may be classified as transient wheeze of infancy and constitute 20% of the infant population.

inhibitors of metal protinases (TIMP-1) (79). We have found that raised TIMP-1 predicts ongoing symptoms in infant wheezers, which is perhaps, generated in a frustrated attempt to counteract the effects of neutrophil MMP-9. TIMP-1 will inhibit matrix turnover leading to accumulation of collagens as seen in the remodeled airway of asthma. The TGF-β is a direct trigger of fibroblast activity and is released from the extra-cellular matrix (ECM) as it is degraded by MMPs, as well as being produced by regulatory T-cells. These associations suggest that the neutrophil may have a more important role in the pathogenesis of asthma than has hitherto been considered the case. In this respect, it is interesting to note that neutrophils appear in the airway at the onset of the late allergen-induced response, eosinophils are only evident when the late reaction is well established some 12 hr after allergen challenge (80). Thus many airway insults—allergic, infectious, or non-specific—could initiate the remodeling process (Fig. 3).

The unresolved issue is to establish how early the process begins. The association between BHR at four weeks and asthma at six years (8) suggests that the changes may have already occurred by birth. Our preliminary

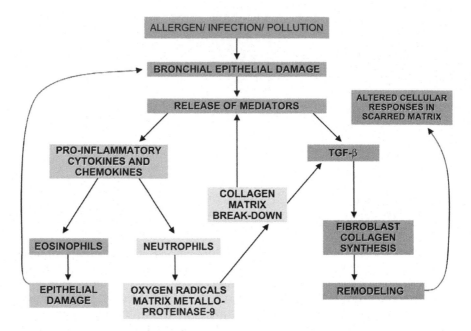

Figure 3 A diagrammatic representation of the sequence of events that constitute the current paradigm of histopathological changes in asthma. Exposure to allergens in allergic subjects, to various pollutants, and to infections in the airways leads to epithelial damage, which in turn results in the release of mediators. These include pro-inflammatory cytokines and chemokines. Eosinophils attracted to the site of damage themselves generate basic proteins which are intensely toxic to cells and induce more epithelial damage. Neutrophils are the main source of matrix metallo-proteinase-9 (MMP-9) and oxygen radicals, which will directly induce collagen matrix breakdown with the release of more mediators and a vicious cycle of inflammation. The TGF-β is present in the collagen matrix, as well as being released by a range of cells within the airway will induce fibroblast collagen synthesis, and thereby, a remodeling process. The altered matrix will then impact on inflammatory cells and change their responses thereby having an additional effect in potentiating the inflammatory process.

observations of second trimester fetal tissues suggests that a thick *lamina reticularis* may be a normal feature of the immature airway. Is remodeling, therefore, a misnomer, because it is a failure of remodeling of the immature airway that causes the initial changes of asthma? Postnatally, inflammatory stimuli induce cell influx into a subtly different matrix, which in turn leads to modified activity and a greater potential for persistent disease (Fig. 4). There is compelling evidence that inflammatory cells do behave differently in an altered matrix (81). If indeed, the pathological changes of asthma are initiated while the airways are developing, we need to understand the embryology of the lung.

A new paradigm – the un-
remodeled airway!

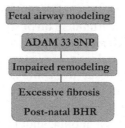

Figure 4 The paradigm of the histopathology within the airways of the asthmatics requires review and this figure suggests an alternative hypothesis. The processes, which result in the remodeled airway, are the same as the processes, which are involved with the modeling of the airway as it develops in the embryo in the first trimester of pregnancy. A number of genetic polymorphisms, of which the most noticeable is that related to ADAM-33 are directly implicated in affecting the airway wall structure. Such polymorphisms are likely to have significant effects on the way in which the airway is modeled in the first place. There is a continuous interaction between the epithelium and the mesenchyme with collagen being laid down and progressively remodeled to achieve a mature airway wall structure. Rather than implying that the polymorphism is associated with an excessive remodeling postnatally it is equally possible that there is impairment of remodeling during the airway-wall formation leading to abnormalities in matrix structure. This will lead to increases in bronchial hyper-responsiveness postnatally and the altered matrix will effect inflammatory cell activity and thereby set the scene for the development of the asthmatic processes.

VIII. Embryology of the Lung

Development of the lungs can be divided into four phases. During the embryonic phase, which begins at approximately day 26 of gestation, the lung bud is formed from the foregut. The pseudoglandular phase (weeks 5–17) is when the branching pattern of the airways develops. This well-coordinated event requires the interaction of both the epithelium and mesenchyme (the epithelial-mesenchymal trophic unit), with the release of factors that promote epithelial cell proliferation and branch growth [e.g. epidermal growth factor (EGF)], and those that promote electronic counter measures (ECM) formation (e.g. TGF-β). Vascularization also begins at this stage. The airways then enlarge, and an acinar framework is formed with development of saccules (canalicular phase: weeks 17–24). During the final saccular phase (week 24–term) the gas exchange surface area and lung volume increase, and although alveoli are recognizable from week 32, the development of alveoli is essentially a postnatal event. Thus, formation of the airways is complete by mid-gestation, but growth continues after birth with the diameter and length increasing into early adulthood (82–86). Each phase has susceptibility to altered developmental influences such as the balance of TGF-β isoforms, which, in turn, will have functional consequences postnatally.

Numerous epidemiological studies highlight the negative impact of a compromised intrauterine environment on postnatal pulmonary gas exchange and airway function. It is well recognized that maternal smoking during pregnancy restricts fetal growth and induces respiratory ill health in the offspring. Examination of respiratory tissue from infants (who died of sudden infant death syndrome (SIDS) of smoking mothers revealed increased inner airway wall thickness that would exaggerate airway narrowing compared with infants (who also died of SIDS) of non-smoking mothers (87). Thus the over-expression of growth factors and cytokines that enhance fibroblast proliferation and activity leading to increased deposition of fibrillar collagen species and other components of the ECM, might have a detrimental effect on intrauterine lung development and later respiratory function. Growth factors with these biological effects include TGF-β1, platelet derived growth factor beta (PDGF-β) and EGF (88–90). Many of these growth factors have been identified by immuno-histochemistry and/or reverse tramscriptase polymerase chain reaction (RT-PCR) of tissue RNA extracts in the fetal airways, leading to the postulate that they do indeed have roles in the growth and development of the human airways during fetal life.

Placental insufficiency may also compromise lung development, so factors that affect placental growth and development could impact indirectly on lung development and subsequent respiratory function. Altered vascular function has been observed in the placenta of asthmatic women but it remains unclear if these changes are associated with maternal asthma or the use of glucocorticoids during pregnancy or what the consequences are for the child (91). Vascular endothelial growth factor (VEGF) is central to placental vascular growth and remodeling. Interestingly, VEGF has been postulated to also directly affect fetal lung development with immuno reactivity for both VEGF and one of its receptors occurring in distal lung epithelial cells from human fetal lung at 16–20 weeks of gestation. Moreover, in an in vitro model, it was shown that VEGF induced the proliferation of human fetal lung epithelial cells (92). Thus VEGF may have a dual role in human lung development, mediating the formation and maintenance of both the capillary network and the thin layer of alveolar epithelial cells that are in close proximity.

TGF-β, which occurs as three isoforms in humans, is a key growth factor involved in the regulation of lung branching morphogenesis during the pseudoglandular phase. It can enhance ECM deposition and inhibit both EGF-induced proliferation and MMP synthesis (93). MMPs are a family of zinc metallo-endopeptidases secreted by cells and responsible for much of the turnover of matrix components. There is differential spatial expression of the different TGF-β isoforms during lung morphogenesis (94,95). TGF-β1 co-localizes at the branch clefts with collagens I and III, and fibronectin

(96), while TGF-β2 and β3 are expressed in epithelial cells at the tips of the growing lung buds (94,95). TGF-β1 stimulates the transcription of mRNA for collagen I and fibronectin (97) and primary human lung fibroblasts secrete more collagen and TIMP-1 (tissue inhibitors of metalloproteinases) in response to both TGF-β1 and β3 (98). TGF-β1 and β3 can also lead to a decrease in the secretion of MMP-1 and TIMP-2 by lung fibroblasts (98).

TGF-β regulates cellular processes via three high-affinity cell surface receptors designated types I, II, and III. TGF-β binds either directly to the type II receptor or to TGF-βRIII, which then presents TGF-β to the type II receptor. Once activated by TGF-β, type II receptors recruit, bind and trans-phosphorylate the type I receptor. This activates the intracellular serine–threonine protein kinase on the type I receptor leading to phosphorylation of either Smad 2 or 3 transcription factors. Phosphorylated Smad 2/3 then binds to Smad 4 and the complex translocates to the nucleus where it interacts in a cell-specific manner with other transcription factors to regulate the transcription of TGF-β responsive genes. The transcription of the inhibitory Smads 6 and 7 is also induced. Smad 6/7 lack the region that is phosphorylated by the type I protein kinase and they form a stable association with the TGF-β receptor complex, and thus block the phosphorylation of Smad 2/3 and subsequent signal transduction providing negative autocrine feedback (99).

Immuno-histochemical studies of embryonic mouse lung have shown that the expression of Smads 2 and 3 is localized to the basolateral region of epithelial cells in the distal airways, especially in areas undergoing branching (100,101). Intense staining of Smad 7 was similarly observed in the distal airways (101). Expression of Smad 7 was low in the proximal airway epithelial cells and no staining was evident in the mesenchyme (101). Similarly, phosphorylation of Smad 2 occurs in the bronchial epithelium and infiltrating inflammatory cells in an experimental model of ovalbumin-induced allergic airway inflammation (102). Thus, TGF-β activity (the balance of isoforms, binding proteins, receptors, and transcription factors) might have a role in lung branching morphogenesis and dictate the thickness of the sub-epithelial *lamina reticularis*. Whether the remodeled asthmatic airway is a consequence of inappropriate postnatal re-activation of pathways normally only operative during embryonic airway development, or is due to abnormal airway modeling in the first place, remains to be established. Depending on the phenotype of asthma and age of onset, it may well be a combination of both events.

IX. Genetic Polymorphisms and Airway Structure

Associations between genes and airway structure have become a recent focus of interest with the identification of a novel gene, a disintegrin and metalloprotease 33 (ADAM33) on the short arm of chromosome 20 (20p13), as a susceptibility factor for asthma (LOD 2.24). The strength of the association was increased using additional genetic markers (LOD 2.94). It was stronger still when BHR was included in the definition of asthma (LOD3.93) and weakest if raised total IgE (LOD 2.3) or specific IgE (LOD 1.87) were factored into the analysis (103). Confirmation of linkage on 20p13 has come from studies on other United Kingdom (UK), Dutch and United States (US) outbred populations (103,104). By physical mapping, direct cDNA selection, SSCP analysis and sequencing, polymorphisms in the ADAM33 gene have been identified which by haplotype and transmission disequilibrium test analysis have shown very strong associations with asthma.

The significance of this finding in relation to airway development and BHR is highlighted by a number of other observations. A syntenic region on mouse chromosome 2 with 70% homology with the human counterpart has been linked to BHR (105). ADAM33 is a member of a group of zinc-dependent matrix metalloproteases which is selectively expressed in mesenchymal cells such as ASM, myofibroblasts, and fibroblasts, but not epithelial T-cells or inflammatory leukocytes (106). ADAM33 is rapidly but transiently up-regulated during TGF-β induced myofibroblast differentiation (107). As the cells expressing ADAM33 share a common fibroblastic progenitor whose maturation is directed by growth factors such as TGF and both ADAMs 33 and 17 are expressed during murine tissue morphogenesis (108,109), this genetic factor may play a critical role in airway development. It appears that ADAM33 expression is increased in murine embryonic day 5 lungs undergoing branching morphogenesis in culture (110). These data suggest that ADAM33 polymorphisms may modulate airway growth and development in utero and lead to altered airway function postnatally with an increased risk of developing asthma. This is likely to be most important for the early-onset and most persistent form of the disease (74). It is also remarkable that common pathways appear to exist between airway growth and development and immune regulation through the mediation of TGF-β.

Another genetic polymorphism has recently been specifically associated with BHR in asthmatic children from two German cohorts-namely the Clara cell protein 16 (CC16) genes on 11q12–13 (111). Polymorphisms have been associated with lower serum levels of CC16 and asthma (112,113). This protein, also known as uteroglobulin or CC10, is expressed in bronchiolar epithelium and has several immuno-modulatory and anti-inflammatory functions (114). Lower levels have also been found in the BAL of patients with (COPD) (115). This again raises the issue of whether this gene has an impact on airway morphology.

Investigation of gene environment interactions have highlighted that asthma may be the consequence of environment tobacco smoke (ETS) exposure only when associated with a polymorphism in the glutathione S transferase M and T genes (GSTM1 and GSTT1), respectively (116,117). There is also an interaction between ozone exposure and the GSTM1 null genotype and greater reductions in lung function in asthmatic children. Futhermore, supplementation of the children's diet with anti-oxidants (vitamins C and E) may protect against this interaction (118). While the null genotypes may lead to reduced protection of the airway against postnatal oxidative stress, there is a suggestion that there may also be an impact on the developing lung, with an interaction between ante-natal ETS exposure and wheezing in childhood (117). It is likely that other such interactions will be identified in the future.

X. Fetal Programming

Although maternal smoking severely compromises fetal health, it remains unknown if a sub-optimal, rather than an extremely compromised, intra-uterine environment linked to other aspects of maternal and/or fetal health is associated with altered immunologic and lung function in childhood and beyond. However modest deficiencies in nutritional factors or minor perturbations in the delicate immunological balance postulated to ensure pregnancy success (each with possible downstream effects on placental function) could also be associated with long-term, impaired lung function. In a rat model, mild maternal vitamin A (retinol) deficiency was associated with reduced expression of fatty acid synthase and lung surfactant (lipids and proteins) (119). Thus vitamin A deficiency during pregnancy may not need to be severe to delay maturation of lung function via reducing the pre-natal accumulation of surfactant proteins. Low birth weight has clearly been shown to affect lung function both in infancy (120) and later adult life (121) with complex interactions with social disadvantage, ante-natal ETS exposure and maternal height. The latter influence may be genetic or a general reflection of maternal health. These effects on lung function have clear consequences for the risk of respiratory illnesses throughout life (122).

There is an association between large head circumference at birth and elevated IgE at birth (123), in childhood (124,125), or at 50 years of age (126). Thus it has been postulated that a pregnancy-associated environment that supports neuronal (brain) development to the detriment of immunological (thymic) development might be common to infants at high risk of developing IgE-mediated allergy (126). However, this hypothesis has been challenged (127). Alternatively, the cytokine imbalance that favors the development of allergy might also mediate disproportionate fetal growth. It is perhaps more likely that other organ systems, specifically the respiratory tract, might also suffer impaired growth as a consequence of a compromised intrauterine environment. Indeed the strongest relationship with birth head circumference was more frequent asthma requiring medical attention irrespective of atopy (124). Epidemiological studies highlight that a number of adult diseases originate in the womb as a consequence of fetal programming (128). Such observations underscore the impact of maternal health during pregnancy and immediately postpartum on the ongoing health of the child and raise the intriguing possibility that peculiarities of maternal health, such as atopic status and nutrition, impact on the asthmatic susceptibility of the child. In particular, nutritional factors might modify fetal airway development. Restricted maternal protein intake during pregnancy was associated with enhanced expression of glucocorticoid receptor in kidney, liver, lung, and brain during fetal/neonatal life and juvenile/adult life in a rat model and was postulated to contribute to raised systolic blood pressure throughout life in these offspring (129). The impact of altered nutritional status on immunological and pulmonary development has received little attention. However, high maternal intake of vitamin E in pregnancy has been associated with a decreased CBMC response to allergens (130).

Other studies have suggested an association between population changes in atopy prevalence and dietary intake of anti-oxidants such as selenium, vitamin C (131), and/or lipids (132). Supplementation of the maternal diet in pregnancy with fish oils reduced IL-13 in the infants, cord blood (133), and follow-up of the infants suggests that there may be an associated reduced risk of allergy (134). A large prospective birth cohort study has suggested an association between high milk fat intake at two years of age and a lower prevalence of asthma at three years (135). It is highly improbable that this is a direct causal relationship but it could reflect the dietary habits of the mother, which would have had its greatest impact during pregnancy.

There has been a recent interest in the association between obesity and asthma. There have been numerous reports of a striking relationship between body mass index and asthma risk in both children and adults (136). There is dispute on the reasons for the association, which is much more consistent in females compared with males. Obesity could have an impact on lung function (137), or on allergic immune responses (138). However, some form of confounding of the association is equally possible. In this respect early life influences could be important. We have found that smaller size at birth, even within the normal range of birth weights, was associated with lower lung function representing airway caliber at 6 to 13 weeks of age (by raised volume rapid thoracic compression technique—RVRTC). At all levels of birth weight, higher early infant weight gain was also associated with reduced lung function. The higher infant weight gain may reflect catch-up, as a consequence of late gestational faltering of fetal growth (139). Low birth weight and rapid postnatal weight gain may well translate into later obesity. Furthermore there is an association between rapid weight gain in the first six months of life and increased IgE in adolescence (140). No doubt many more studies will be required to disentangle the relevant factors.

XI. Early Infection and Asthma

The impact of respiratory tract infection in infancy on the subsequent development of asthma has been controversial. There now appears to be a differ-

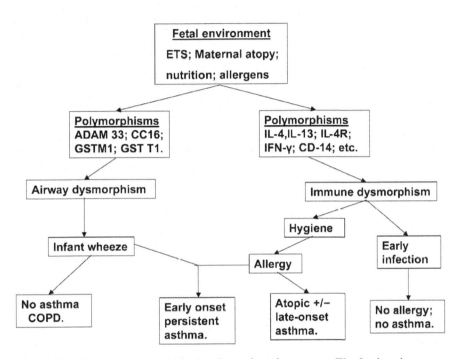

Figure 5 This figure summarizes the chapter's main message. The fetal environment is effected by such factors as maternal ETS exposure, maternal allergic status, nutrition and allergen exposure which will interact with a range of genetic polymorphisms. There are two groups of polymorphisms likely to be relevant to asthma. One group are associated with mechanisms involved with airway wall structure and remodeling such as ADAM-33, Clara cell protein-16 (CC-16), Glutathione S methyl-tranferase (M1 and T1). These polymorphisms confer susceptibility to abnormalities in the airway, which might be described as airway dysmorphism, which will be associated with the propensity to infant wheeze. In those without allergy this is a transient phenomenon in infancy but may be associated with later COPD. The second group of polymorphisms effect immune responsiveness such as those involved with the cytokine gene cluster, the generation of interferon-gamma and the CD-14 molecule. Abnormalities here could be described as causing immune dysmorphism. This will increase susceptibility to early infection but such early infections may switch off allergic immune responses and thereby not be associated with either allergy or asthma. However in the absence of relevant microbial stimuli allergy develops which if associated with airway dysmorphism will lead to early onset persistent asthma. In the absence of airway dysmorphism there will either be allergy without asthma or possibly a later onset milder form of asthma.

ential impact of infection on disease development such that repeated upper respiratory tract viral infections in early life might reduce the risk of developing asthma (141). However, it remains unknown if the associations between lower respiratory tract infection (e.g., respiratory syncytial virus (RSV)-associated bronchio litis) and increased risk of asthma is one of reverse causation, i.e., the child who will develop asthma is more prone to lower respiratory tract infection. Recent data shows that RSV protein F shares a receptor with LPS (CD14/TLR4) (142). It is possible that an impaired response via these receptors or a sustained reduction in the ability to produce IFN-γ and other anti-viral cytokines occurs in at-risk children? Thus, does the occurrence of lower respiratory tract infection in infancy identify those children with an immature host response unable to mount an efficient anti-viral response to clear the infection? Could ante-natal exposure to "switch factors" regulate postnatal responses?

In support of ante-natal exposure to potential switch factors we found significantly higher proliferative response rates to UV-inactivated RSV in those infants exposed in utero to the RSV epidemic after 22 weeks of gestation. UV-inactivated RSV stimulation induced significantly higher IFN-γ production from specimens with a positive proliferative response than those with a negative response. Intrauterine priming of the fetal immune system to RSV might result in reduced severity of subsequent RSV-mediated disease in these individuals and explain the clinical diversity of such disease (143). We have followed a cohort of 88 infants through their first RSV season. About 28 developed RSV infection, 19 upper respiratory tract infection (URTI) alone and nine with bronchiolitis. On day one of the illness before signs of lower respiratory tract infection (LRTI) had appeared, those who developed bronchiolitis had lower IFN-γ:IL-4 and IL-12:IL-10 ratios in nasal lavage fluid and lower IL-18 expression in stimulated PBMCs than those with URTI alone (144). As CD-14 and TLR-4 are key binding molecules which initiate the normal Th-1 pattern of immune response to RSV, it is possible that pre-existing polymorphisms for these molecules accounts for the differences, which would also explain associations between RSV bronchiolitis and asthma (Fig. 5).

XII. Conclusions

The apparently ever-increasing prevalence of asthma in the Western world calls for a novel approach to treatment and ultimately, prevention. Much evidence suggests that pregnancy and early postnatal life is the critical time for intervention (145). This requires elucidation of the gestation-associated gene and environment interactions that impact on the development of allergic immune responses and airway function leading eventually to asthma. By identifying the pathway(s) of altered immunological and pulmonary development in utero, as well as targets for manipulation (e.g. maternal diet, allergen exposure, and microbial load), therapeutic strategies will eventually be devised which will have considerable effects in reducing the burden of the disease, asthma.

References

1. Tattersfield AE, Knox AJ, Britton JR, Hall IP. Asthma. Lancet 2002; 360: 1313–1322.
2. Möller C, Dreborg S, Ferdousi HA, et al. Pollen immunotherapy reduces the development of asthma in children with seasonal rhinoconjunctivitis (the PAT-study). J Allergy Clin Immunol 2002; 109:251–256.
3. Martinez FD. Towards asthma prevention—Does all that really matters happen before we learn to read? New Eng J Med 2003; 349:1473–1475.
4. Roorda RJ, Gerritsen J, van Aalderen WM, et al. Follow-up of asthma from childhood to adulthood: influence of potential childhood risk factors on the outcome of pulmonary function and bronchial hyper responsiveness in adulthood. J Allergy Clin Immunol 1994; 93:575–584.
5. Sears MR, Greene JM, Willan AR, et al. A longitudinal, population-based, cohort study of childhood asthma followed to adulthood. New Eng J Med 2003; 349:1414–1422.
6. Holloway JW, Beghé B, Holgate ST. The genetic basis of atopic asthma. Clin Exp Allergy 1999; 29:1023–1032.
7. Lawrence S, Beasley R, Doull I, et al. Genetic analysis of atopy and asthma as quantitative traits and ordered ploychotomies. Ann Human Genet 1994; 58:359–368.
8. Palmer LJ, Rye PJ, Gibson NA, et al. Airway responsiveness in early infancy predicts asthma, lung function, and respiratory symptoms by school age. Am J Respir Crit Care Med 2001; 163:37–42.
9. Holgate ST. Asthma and allergy—disorders of civilization? Q J Med 1998; 91:171–184.
10. Persson CGA. Centenial notions of asthma as an eosinophilic desquamative exudative and steroid sensitive disease. Lancet 1997; 349:1021–1024.
11. Burr ML, Butland BK, King S, Vaughan Williams E. Changes in asthma prevalence: two surveys 15 years apart. Arch Dis Child 1989; 64:1452–1456.
12. Kaur B, Anderson HR, Austin J, Burr M, Harkins L, Strachan DP, Warner JO. Prevalence of asthma symptoms, diagnosis and treatment in 12–14-year-old children across Great Britain (International Study of Asthma and Allergies in Childhood, UK). Brit Med J 1998; 316:118–124.
13. Austin JB, Kaur B, Anderson RH, Burr M, Harkins LS, Strachan DP, Warner JO. Hay fever, eczema and wheeze—a nationwide UK survey (International Study of Asthma and Allergies in Childhood, ISAAC). Arch Dis Child 1999; 81:225–230.
14. Anderson HR. Increase in hospital admissions for childhood asthma: Trends in referral, severity and readmissions from 1970 to 1985 in a health region of the United Kingdom. Thorax 1989; 44:614–619.
15. Van Asperen PP, Mukhi A. Role of atopy in the natural history of wheeze and bronchial hyperresponsiveness in childhood. Pediatr Allergy Immunol 1994; 5:178–183.

16. Lombardi E, Morgan WJ, Wright AL, Stein RT, Holberg CJ, Martinez FD. Cold air challenge at age 6 and subsequent incidence of asthma: A longitudinal study. Am J Respir Crit Care Med 1997; 156:1863–1869.

17. Ross S, Godden DJ, Abdalla M, et al. Outcome of wheeze in childhood: the influence of atopy. Eur Respir J 1995; 8:2081–2087.

18. Pearce N, Pekkanen J, Beasley R. How much asthma is really attributable to atopy? Thorax 1999; 54:268–272.

19. Sont JK, van Krieken JH, Evertse CE, Hooijer R, Willems LNA, Sterk PJ. Relationship between the inflammatory infiltrate in bronchial biopsy specimens and clinical severity of asthma in patients treated with inhaled steroids. Thorax 1996; 51:496–451.

20. Power LL, Popplewell EJ, Holloway JA, et al. Immunoregulatory molecules during pregnancy and at birth. J Reprod Immunol 2002; 56:19–28.

21. Wegmann TG, Lin H, Guilbert L, Mosmann TR. Bi-directional cytokine interactions in the materno-fetal relationship: is successful pregnancy a Th-2 phenomenon. Immunol Today 1993; 14:353–356.

22. Raghupathy R. Th-1 type immunity is incompatible with successful pregnancy. Immunol Today 1997; 18:478–482.

23. Piccinni MP, Beloni L, Livi C, Maggi E, Scarselli G, Romagnani S. Defective production of both leukaemia inhibitory factor and type 2 T-helper cytokines by decidual T cells in unexplained recurrent abortions. Nat Medicine 1998; 4:1020–1024.

24. Jones CA, Williams KA, Finlay-Jones JF, Hart PH. Interleukin-4 production by human amnion epithelial cells and regulation of its activity by glycosaminoglycan binding. Biol Reprod 1995; 52:893–947.

25. Roth I, Corry DB, Locksley RM, Abrams JS, Litton MJ, Fisher SJ. Human placental cytotrophoblasts produce the immunosuppressive cytokine IL-10. J Exp Med 1996; 184:539–548.

26. Kalinski P, Hilkens CM, Wierenga EA, Kapsenberg ML. T-cell priming by type 1 and type 2 polarised dendritic cells: the concept of a thirds signal. Immunol Today 1999; 120:561–567.

27. Prescott SL, Macaubas C, Holt BJ, Smallacombe TJ, Loh R, Sly PD, Holt PG. Transplacental priming of the human immune system to environmental allergens: universal skewing of initial T-cell responses towards Th-2 cytokine profile. J Immunol 1998; 160:4730–4737.

28. Jones CA, Holloway JA, Warner JO. Does atopic disease start in fetal life? Allergy 2000; 55:2–10

29. Tang MLK, Kemp AS, Thorburn J, Hill DJ. Reduced IFN-γ secretion in neonates—subsequent atopy. Lancet 1992; 344:983–985.

30. Warner JA, Miles EA, Jones AC, Quint DJ, Colwell BM, Warner JO. Is deficiency of interferon gamma production by allergen triggered cord blood cells a predictor of atopic eczema? Clin Exp Allergy 1994; 24:423–430.

31. Williams TJ, Jones CA, Miles EA, Warner JA, Warner JO. Fetal and neonatal interleukin-13 production during pregnancy and at birth and subsequent development of atopic symptoms. J Allergy Clin Immunol 2000; 105:951–959.

32. Ribiero-do-Couto LM, Boeije LCM, Kroon JS, Hooibrink B, Breur-Criesendorp BS, Aarden LA, Boog CJP. High IL-13 production by human

neonatal T-cells: neonate immune system regulator? Eur J Immunol 2001; 31: 3394–3402

33. Simpson CR, Anderson WJA, Helms PJ, Taylor MW, Watson L, Prescott GJ, Godden DJ, Barker RN. Coincidence of immune-mediated diseases driven by Th-1 and Th-2 subsets suggests a common aetiology. A population-based study using computerized General Practice data. Clin Exp Allergy 2002; 32:37–42.

34. Warner JA, Jones CA, Jones AC, Miles EA, Francis T, Warner JO. Immune responses during pregnancy and the development of allergic disease. Pediatr Allergy Immunol 1997; 8(suppl 10):5–10.

35. Prescott SL, Macaubas C, Smallacombe T, Holt BJ, Sly PD, Holt PG. Development of allergen-specific T-cell memory in atopic and normal children. Lancet 1999; 353:196–200.

36. Van der Velden VHJ, Laan MP, Baert MRM, de Waal Malefyt R, Neijens HJ, Savelkoul HFJ. Selective development of a strong Th-2 cytokine profile in high-risk children who develop atopy: risk factors and regulatory role of IFN-γ, IL-4 and IL-10. Clin Exp Allergy 2001; 31:997–1006.

37. Strachan DP. Family size, infection and atopy: the first decade of the hygiene hypothesis. Thorax 2000; 55(suppl 1):S2–S10.

38. Jones PD, Gibson PG, Henry RL. The prevalence of asthma appears to be inversely related to the incidence of typhoid and tuberculosis: hypothesis to explain the variation in asthma prevalence around the world. Med Hypotheses 2000; 55:40–42.

39. Holt PG, Sly PD, Bjorksten B. Atopy versus infectious diseases in childhood; a question of balance. Pediatr Allergy Immunol 1997; 8:53–58.

40. Bottcher MF, Nordin EK, Sandin A, Midtvedt T, Bjorksten B. Microflora-associated characteristics in faeces from allergic and non-allergic infants. Clin Exp Allergy 2000; 30:1590–1596.

41. Bjorksten B, Naaber P, Sepp E, Mikelsaar M. The intestinal microflora in allergic Estonian and Swedish 2-year-old children. Clin Exp Allergy 1999; 29:342–346.

42. Von Ehrenstein OS, Von Mutius E, Illi S, Baumann L, Bohm O, Von Kries R. Reduced risk of hay fever and asthma among children of farmers. Clin Exp Allergy 2000; 30:187–193.

43. Riedler J, Eder W, Oberfeld G, Schreuer M. Austrian children living on a farm have less hay fever, asthma and allergic sensitization. Clin Exp Allergy 2000; 30:194–200.

44. Kilpelainen M, Terho EO, Helenius H, Koskenvuo M. Farm environment in childhood prevents the development of allergies. Clin Exp Allergy 2000; 30:201–208.

45. Downs SH, Marks GB, Mitakakis TZ, Leuppi JD, Car NG, Peat JK. Having lived on a farm and protection against allergic diseases in Australia. Clin Exp Allergy 2001:570–575.

46. Farooqi IS, Hopkin JM. Early childhood infection and atopic disorder. Thorax 1998; 53:927–932.

47. Wickens K, Pearce N, Crane J, Beasley R. Antibiotic use in early childhood and the development of asthma of cell stimulation. Clin Exp Allergy 1999; 29:766–771.

48. McKeever TM, Lewis SA, Smith C, Hubbard R. The importance of prenatal exposures on the development of allergic disease. Am J Respir Crit Care Med 2002; 166:827–832.

49. Riedler J, Braun-Fahrlander C, Eder W, et al. Exposure to farmong in early life and development of asthma and allergy: a cross-sectional survey. Lancet 2001; 358:1129–1133.

50. Ball TM, Castro-Rodriguez JA, Griffith KA, Holberg CJ, Martinez FD, Wright AL. Siblings, day-care and the risk of asthma and wheeze during childhood. N Engl J Med 2000; 343:538.

51. Ulevitch RJ, Tobias PS. Receptor-dependent mechanisms of cell stimulation by bacterial endotoxin. Annu Rev Immunol 1995; 13:437–457.

52. Baldini M, Lohman IC, Halonen M, Erickson RP, Holt PG, Martinez FD. A polymorphism in the flanking region of the CD-14 gene is associated with circulating soluble CD-14 levels and with total serum immunoglobulin E. Am J Respir Cell Mol Biol 1999; 20:967–983.

53. Koppelman GH, Reijmerink NE, Colin Stine O, et al. Association of a promoter polymorphism of the CD-14 gene and atopy. Am J Respir Crit Care Med 2001; 163:965–969.

54. Sengler C, Haider A, Sommerfeld C, Lau S, et al. Evaluation of the CD-14 C-159T polymorphism in the German Multicentre Allergy cohort. Clin Exp Allergy 2003; 33:166–169.

55. Jones CA, Holloway JA, Popplewell EJ, et al. Reduced soluble CD-14 levels in amniotic fluid and breast milk are associated with the subsequent development of atopy, eczema or both. J Allergy Clin Immunol 2002; 109:858–866.

56. Liu X, Beaty TH, Deindl P, et al. Associations between total IgE levels and six potentially functional variants within the genes IL-4, IL-13, and IL-4 RA in German children: The German Multicentre Atopy study. J Allergy Clin Immunol 2003; 112:382–388.

57. Wjst M, Fischer G, Immervoll T, et al. A genome-wide search for linkage to asthma. Genomics 1999; 58:1–8; J Allergy Clin Immunol 2003; 111:117–122.

58. Kruse S, Kuehr J, Moseler M, et al. Polymorphisms in the IL-18 gene are associated with specific sensitisation to common allergens and allergic rhinitis. J Allergy Clin Immunol 2003; 111:117–122.

59. Holloway JA, Warner JO, Vance GHS, et al. Detection of house dust mite allergen in amniotic fluid and umbilical cord blood Lancet 2000; 356:1900–1902.

60. Thornton CA, Vance GHS. The placenta: a portal of fetal allergen exposure. Clin Exp Allergy 2002; 32:1537–1539.

61. Thornton CA, Holloway JA, Popplewell EJ, et al. Fetal exposure to intact immunoglobulin E occurs via the gastrointestinal tract. Clin Exp Allergy 2003; 33:306–311.

62. Jones CA, Capristo CC, Power LL, et al. The effect of labour on neonatal T cell phenotype and function. Pediatr Res 2003; 54:1–5.

63. Thornton CA, Holloway JA, Warner JO. The expression of CD21 and CD23 during human fetal development. Pediatr Res 2002; 52:245–250.

64. Jones CA, Vance GHS, Power LL, et al. Co-stimulatory molecules in the developing human gastrointestinal tract: a pathway for fetal allergen priming. J Allergy Clin Immunol 2001; 108:235–241.

65. Prescott SL, Macaubas C, Smallacombe T, Holt BJ, Sly PD, Holt PG. Development of allergen-specific T-cell memory in atopic and normal children. Lancet 1999; 353:196–200.
66. D'Alauro F, Lee RV, Pao-in K, Khairallah M. Intestinal parasites and pregnancy. Ostet Gynecol 1985; 66:639–643.
67. King CL, Malhotra I, Mungai P, Wamachi A, Kioko J, Ouma JH, Kazura JW. B-cell sensitisation to helminthic infection develops in utero in humans. J Immunol 1998; 160:3578–3584.
68. Cokugras H, Akcakaya N, Seckin I, Camcioglu Y, Sarimurat N, Aksoy F. Ultrastructural examination of bronchial biopsy specimens from children with moderate asthma. Thorax 2001; 56:25–29.
69. Warner JO, Pohunek P, Marguet C, Clough JB, Roche WR. Progression from allergic sensitisation to asthma. Pediatr Allergy Immunol 2000; 11(suppl 13): 12–14.
70. Pohunek P, Warner JO, Turzikova J, Kudrmann J, Roche WR. Markers of eosinophilic inflammation and tissue re-modeling in children before clinically diagnosed bronchial asthma. Pediatr Allergy Immunol. 2005 Feb; 16(1):43–51.
71. Martinez FD, Morgan WJ, Holberg CJ, Taussig LM. Diminished lung function as a predisposing factor for wheezing respiratory illness in infants. N Engl J Med 1988; 319:1112–1117.
72. Murray CS, Pipis SD, McArdle EC, Lowe LA, Custovic A, Woodcock A. Lung function at one month of age as a risk factor for infant respiratory symptoms in a high-risk population. Thorax 2002; 57:388–392.
73. Martinez FD, Wright AL, Taussig LM, Holberg CJ, Halonen Mj, Morgan WJ. Asthma and wheezing in the first six years of life. The Group Health Medical Associates. New Engl J Med 1995; 332:133–138.
74. Peat JK, Salome CM, Woolcock AJ. Longitudinal changes in atopy during a 4-year period: relation to bronchial hyper-responsiveness and respiratory symptoms in a population sample of Australian school children. J Allergy Clin Immunol 1990; 85:65–74.
75. Karjalainen EM, Laitinen A, Sue-Chu M, Altraja A, Bjermer L, Laitinen LA. Evidence of airway inflammation and remodelling in ski athletes with and without bronchial hyperresponsiveness to methacholine. Am J Respir Crit Care Med 2000; 161:2086–2091.
76. Marguet C, Jouen-Boedes F, Dean TP, Warner JO. Broncho-alveolar cell profiles in children with asthma, infantile wheeze, chronic cough, or cystic fibrosis. Am J Respir Crit Care Med 1999; 159:1533–1540.
77. Jatakonen A, Uasuf C, Maziak W, Lim S, Chung KF, Barnes PJ. Neutrophilic inflammation in severe persistent asthma. Am J Respir Crit Care Med 1999; 160:1532–1539.
78. Marguet C, Dean TP, Basuyau JP, Warner JO. Eosinophil cationic protein and interleukin-8 levels in bronchial lavage fluid from children with asthma and infantile wheeze. Pediatr Allergy Immunol 2001; 12:27–33.
79. Cundall M, Sun Y, Miranda C, Trudeau JB, Barnes S, Wenzel SE. Neutrophil-derived matrix metalloproteinase-9 is increased in severe asthma and poorly inhibited by glucocorticoids. J Allergy Clin Immunol 2003; 112: 1064–1071.

80. Smith DL, Deshazo RD. Broncho-alveolar lavage in asthma: an update and perspective. Am Rev Respir Dis 1993; 148:523–532.

81. Adams JC, Watt FM. Regulation of development and differentiation by the extra-cellular matrix. Development 1993; 117:1183–1198.

82. Jeffery PK. The development of large and small airways. Am J Respir Crit Care Med 1998; 157:S174–S180.

83. Creagh T, Krausz. The respiratory system: normal structure and function. In: McGee JD, Isaacson PG, Wright NA, eds. Oxford textbook of pathology. Oxford University Press, Chapter 13.1, 1992:941–947.

84. Warburton D, Schwarz M, Tefft D, Flores-Delgado G, Anderson KD, Cardoso WV. The molecular basis of lung morphogenesis. Mech Dev 2000; 92:55–81.

85. Minoo P, King RJ. Epithelial–mesenchymal interactions in lung development. Annu Rev Physiol 1994; 56:13–45.

86. Stick S. The contribution of airway development to pediatric and adult lung disease. Thorax 2000; 55:587–594.

87. Elliot J, Vullermin P, Robinson P. Maternal cigarette smoking is associated with increased inner airway wall thickness in children who die from sudden infant death syndrome. Am J Respir Crit Care Med 1998; 158:802–806.

88. Khalil N, Bereznay O, Sporn M, Greenberg A. Macrophage production of transforming growth factor β and fibroblast collagen synthesis in chronic pulmonary inflammation. J Exp Med 1989; 170:727–737.

89. Martinet Y, Rom WN, Grotendorst GR, Martin GR, Crystal RG. Exaggerated spontaneous release of platelet-derived growth factor by alveolar macrophages from patients with idiopathic pulmonary fibrosis. N Engl J Med 1987; 317:202–209.

90. Ruocco S, Lallemand A, Tournier JM, Gaillard D. Expression and localization of epidermal growth factor, transforming growth factor-alpha, and localization of their common receptor in fetal human lung development. Pediatr Res 1996; 39:448–455.

91. Clifton VL, Giles WB, Smith R, Bisits AT, Hempenstall AJ, Kessell CG, Gibson PG. Alterations of placental vascular function in asthmatic pregnancies. Am J Respir Crit Care Med 2001; 164:546–553.

92. Brown KRS, England KM, Goss KL, Snyder JM, Acarregui MJ. VEGF induces airway epithelial cell proliferation in human fetal lung in vitro. Am J Physiol 2001; 281:L1001–L1010.

93. Ganser GL, Strciklin GP, Matrisian LM. EGF and TGF alpha influence in vitro lung development by the induction of matrix-degrading metalloproteinases. Int J Dev Biol 1991; 35:453–461.

94. Gatherer D, Ten Dijke P, Baird DT, Akhurst RJ. Expression of TGF-beta isoforms during the first trimester human enbryogenesis. Development 1990; 110:445–460.

95. Roberts AB, Sporn MB. Differential expression of the TGF-beta isoforms in embryogenesis suggests specific roles in developing and adult tissues. Mol Reprod Dev 1992; 32:91–98.

96. Heine UI, Munoz EF, Flanders KC, Roberts AB, Sporn MB. Colocalization of TGF-beta 1 and collagen I and III, fibronectin and glycosaminoglycans during lung branching morphogenesis. Development 1990; 109:29–36.

97. Ignotz RA, Endo T, Massague J. Regulation of fibronectin and type I collagen mRNA levels by transforming growth factor-β. J Biol Chem 1987; 262: 6443–6446.

98. Eickelberg O, Kohler E, Reichenberger F, Bertschin S, Woodtil T, Erne P, Perruchoud AP, Roth M. Extracellular matrix deposition by primary human lung fibroblasts in response to TGF-beta1 and TGF-beta3. Am J Physiol 1999; 276:L814–L824.

99. Blobe GC, Schiemann WP, Lodish HF. Role of transforming growth factor B in human disease. N Engl J Med 2000; 342:1350–1358.

100. Zhao J, Lee M, Smith S, Warburton D. Abrogation of Smad3 and Smad2 or of Smad4 gene expression positively regulates murine embryonic lung branching morphogenesis. Dev Biol 1998; 194:182–195.

101. Zhao J, Crowe DL, Castillo C, Wuenschell C, Chai Y, Warburton D. Smad7 is a TGF-β inducible attenuator of Smad2/3 mediated inhibition of embryonic lung morphogenesis. Mech Dev 2000; 93:71–81.

102. Rosendahl A, Checchin D, Fehniger TE, ten Dijke P, Heldin CH, Sideras P. Activation of the TGF-β/Activin-Smad 2 pathway during allergic airway inflammation. Am J Respir Cell Mol Biol 2001; 25:60–68.

103. Van Eerdewegh P, Little RD, Dupuis J, et al. Association of the ADAM33 gene with asthma and bronchial hyperresponsiveness. Nature 2002; 418:426–430.

104. Howard TD, Postma DS, Jongepier H, et al. Association of a disintegrin and metalloprotease 33 (ADAM33) with asthma in ethnically diverse populations. J Allergy Clin Immunol 2003; 112:717–722.

105. De Sanctis GT, Merchant M, Beier DR, et al. Quantitative locus analysis of airway hyper-responsiveness in A/J and C57BL/6J mice. Nat Genet 1995; 11:150–154.

106. Primakoff P, Myles DG. The ADAM gene family: surface proteins with adhesion and protease activity. Trends Genet 2000; 16:83–87.

107. Wicks J, Powell RM, Richter A. Transient up-regulation of ADAM33 by TGF-β precedes myofibroblast differentiation. Am J Respir Crit Care Med 2003; 167(7):A157.

108. Powell RM, Wicks J, Holloway JW, Davies DE, Holgate ST. Identification and quantification of novel splice variants of ADAM33 reveal distinct tissue expression profiles. Am J Respir Crit Care Med 2003; 167(7):A440.

109. Gunn TM, Azarani A, Kim PH, et al. Identification and preliminary characterisation of mouse Adam33. BMC Genet 2002; 3:2.

110. Haitchi HM, Powell RM, Wilson DI. ADAM33 expression in embryonic mouse. Am J Respir Crit Care Med 2003; 167:A377.

111. Stengler C, Heinzmann A, Jerkic M-P, et al. Clara cell protein 16 (CC16) gene polymorphism influences the degree of airway responsiveness in asthmatic children. J Allergy Clin Immunol 2003; 111:515–519.

112. Laing IA, Goldblatt J, Eber E, et al. A polymorphism of the CC16 gene is associated with an increased risk of asthma. J Med Genet 1998; 35: 463–467.

113. Laing IA, Hermans C, Bernard A, Burton PR, Goldblatt J, Le Souef PN. Association between plasma CC16 levels, the A38G polymorphism and asthma. Am J Respir Crit Care Med 2000; 161:124–127.

114. Singh G, Katyal SL. Clara cells and clara cell 10 kDa protein (CC10). Am J Respir Cell Mol Biol 1997; 17:141–143.

115. Bernard A, Marchndise FX, Delelchin S, Lauwerys R, Sibile Y. Claracell protein in serum and broncho-alveolar lavage. Eur Respir J 1992; 5: 1231–1238.

116. Kabesh M, Hoefler-Carr D, Leupold W, Weiland SK, von Mutius E. Glutathione S transferase deficiency and passive smoking increase childhood asthma. Thorax 2004; 59:569–573.

117. Gilliland FD, Li YF, Dubeau L, Berhane E, et al. Effects of glutathione S-transferase M1, maternal smoking during pregnancy and environmental tobacco smoke on asthma and wheezing in children. Am J Respir Crit Care Med 2002; 166:457–463.

118. Romieu I, Sienra-Monge JJ, Ramirez-Aguilar M, et al. Genetic polymorphism of GSTM1 and antioxidant supplementation influence lung function in relation to ozone exposure in asthmatic children in Mexico City. Thorax 2004; 59:8–10.

119. Chailley-Heu B, Chelly N, Lelievre-Pegorier M, Barlier-Mur A-M, Merlet-Benichou C, Bourbon JR. Mild Vitamin A deficiency delays fetal lung maturation in the rat. Am J Respir Cell Mol Biol 1999; 21:89–96.

120. Dezateux C, Lum S, Hoo A-F, Hawdon J, Costeloe K, Stocks J. Low birth weight for gestation and airway function in infancy: exploring the fetal origins hypothesis. Thorax 2004; 59:60–66.

121. Edwards CA, Osman LM, Godden DJ, Campbell DM, Douglas JG. Relationship between birth weight and adult lung function: controlling for maternal factors. Thorax 2003; 58:1061–1065.

122. Barker DJ, Godfrey C, Fall C, et al. Relation of birth weight and childhood respiratory infection to adult lung function and death from chronic obstructive airways disease. Brit Med J 1991; 303:671–675.

123. Oryszczyn MP, Annesi-Maesano I, Campagna D, Sahuquillo J, Huel G, Kauffmann F. Head circumference at birth and maternal factors related to cord blood total IgE. Clin Exp Allergy 1999; 29:334–341.

124. Gregory A, Doull I, Pearce N, Cheng S, Leadbitter P, Holgate S, Beasley R. The relationship between anthropometric measurements at birth: asthma and atopy in childhood. Clin Exp Allergy 1999; 29:330–333.

125. Leadbitter P, Pearce N, Cheng S, Sears MR, Holdaway MD, Flannery EM, Herbison GP, Beasley R. Relationship between fetal growth and the development of asthma and atopy in childhood. Thorax 1999; 54:905–910.

126. Godfrey KM, Barker DJP, Osmond C. Disproportionate fetal growth and raised IgE concentration in adult life. Clin Exp Allergy 1994; 24:641–648.

127. Katz KA, Pocock SJ, Strachan DP. Neonatal head circumference, neonatal weight, and risk of hay fever, asthma and eczema in a large cohort of adolescents from Sheffield, England. Clin Exp Allergy 2003; 33:737–745.

128. Barker DJP. Mothers, babies and health in later life. London: Churchill Livingstone, 1998.

129. Bertram C, Trowern AR, Copin N, Jackson AA, Whorwood CB. The maternal diet during pregnancy programs altered expression of the glucocorticoid receptor and type 2 11beta-hydroxysteroid dehydrogenase potential molecular

mechanisms underlying the programming of hypertension in utero. Endocrinology 2001; 142:2841–2853.

130. Devereux G, Barker RN, Seaton A. Antenatal determinants of neonatal immune responses to allergens. Clin Exp Allergy 2002; 32:43–50.

131. Fogarty A, Britton J. The role of diet in the aetiology of asthma. Clin Exp Allergy 2000; 30:615–627.

132. Calder PC. Polyunsaturated fatty acids and cytokine profiles: a clue to the changing prevalence of atopy. Clin Exp Allergy 2003; 33:412–415.

133. Dunstan JA, Mori TA, Barden A, et al. Maternal fish oil supplementation in pregnancy reduces interleukin-13 levels in cord blood of infants at high risk of atopy. Clin Exp Allergy 2003; 33:442–448.

134. Dunstan JA, Mori TA, Barden A, et al. Fish oil supplementation in pregnancy modifies neonatal allergen-specific immune responses and clinical outcomes in infants at high risk of atopy; a randomized controlled trial. J Allergy Clin Immunol 2003; 112:1178–1184.

135. Wijga AH, Smit HA, Kerkhof M, et al. Association of consumption of products containing milk fat with reduced asthma risk in pre-school children: the PIAMA birth cohort study. Thorax 2003; 58:567–572.

136. Chinn S. Asthma and obesity: where are we now? Thorax 2003; 58:1008–1010.

137. Tantisira KG, Litonjua AA, Weiss ST, Fuhlbrigge AL. CAMP management program research group. Association of body mass with pulmonary function in the Childhood Asthma Management Program (CAMP). Thorax 2003; 58:1036–1041.

138. Schachter LM, Peat JK, Salome CM. Asthma and atopy in overweight children. Thorax 2003; 58:1031–1035.

139. Lucas JS, Inskip HM, Godfrey KM, Foreman CT, Warner JO, Gregson RK, Clough JB. Small size at birth and greater postnatal weight gain: relationships to diminished infant lung function. Am J Crit Care Med 2004; 170:534–540.

140. McDade TW, Kuzawa CW, Adair LS, Beck MA. Prenatal and early postnatal environments are significant predictors of total immunoglobulin E concentration in Filipino adolescents. Clin Exp Allergy 2003; 34:44–50.

141. Illi S, von Mutius E, Lau S, Bergmann R, Niggermann B, Sommerfeld C, Wahn U, MAS Group. Early childhood infectious disease and the development of asthma up to school age: a birth cohort study. BMJ 2001; 322: 390–395.

142. Kurt-Jones EA, Popova L, Kwinn L, Haynes LM, Jones LP, Tripp RA, Walsh EE, Freeman MW, Golenbock DT, Anderson LJ, Finberg RW. Pattern recognition receptors TLR4 and CD14 mediate response to respiratory syncytial virus. Nat Immunol 2000; 1:398–401.

143. Legg JP, Jones CA, Warner JA, Johnston SL, Warner JO. A hypothesis: antenatal sensitization to respiratory syncytial virus in viral bronchiolitis. Arch Dis Child 2002; 86:431–433.

144. Legg JP, Hussain IR, Warner JA, et al. Type 1 and type 2 cytokine imbalance in acute respiratory syncytial virus bronchiolitis. Am J Respir Crit Care Med 2003; 168:633–639.

145. Martinez FD. Towards asthma prevention—Does all that really matters happen before we learn to read? New Engl J Med 2003; 349:1473–1475.

4

Developmental Features of Airway Remodeling

MERI K. TULIC, CÉLINE BERGERON, PATRICK DAIGNEAULT, and QUTAYBA HAMID

Meakins-Christie Laboratories, McGill University
Montréal, Québec, Canada

I. Introduction

Asthma was once regarded as a completely reversible disorder, and for many years the principal mechanisms thought to be responsible for this disease were airflow obstruction, airway edema, and mucous hypersecretion. For more than two decades now, asthma has been recognized as a chronic inflammatory disease involving inflammation of both the central and the peripheral airways. Despite aggressive treatment with anti-inflammatory drugs and bronchodilators, in some patients this obstruction cannot be completely reversed. Pathologic and morphometric studies have demonstrated structural changes in the airways of these patients when compared to healthy subjects (Fig. 1), and these changes are called airway remodeling. Structural changes identified as features of airway remodeling in asthma include airway smooth muscle (ASM) hyperplasia and hypertrophy, subepithelial fibrosis and thickening of basement membrane, mucous, and goblet cell hyperplasia, epithelial detachment and regeneration, and cartilage degradation, as well as increased size and number of microvessels in the submucosa. These structural changes in the airways collectively contribute

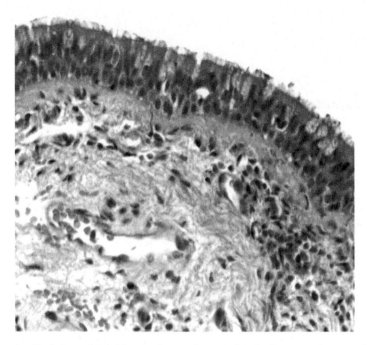

Figure 1 Endobronchial biopsy from the proximal airways of normal, non-asthmatic subject showing an intact epithelium containing a small number of goblet cells and inflammatory cells in the mucosa.

to thickening of the airway wall and are believed to be at least partially responsible for airflow obstruction, airway hyper-responsiveness (AHR) and mucous hypersecretion consistently observed among asthmatics (1–3). How inflammation leads to remodeling is currently unknown and has been a subject of intense investigation in the last few years.

In recent years, as a result of increased asthma prevalence, researchers have begun to study this disease more intensely in children. Pulmonary function testing, exhaled nitric oxide (NO), breath condensates, broncho-alveolar lavage (BAL) and bronchial biopsies are all used to better describe the asthmatic process in children, especially in terms of acute and chronic inflammation of the airways. However, very little has been detailed in terms of airway remodeling in young patients with asthma. Since it is considered unethical to obtain bronchial biopsies from healthy children, case-control studies are hence difficult to perform. Recently, however, it has been proposed that many of the characteristic features of airway remodeling may be observed at a very young age in susceptible children (4,5). Environmental and genetic factors could be implicated in this suspected susceptibility to airway remodeling. Bronchial biopsy-based case studies of young asthmatic patients in remission or with chronic symptoms have been published (6,7). These studies have shown that histological features of airway remodeling such as thickening of the basement membrane, peribronchial muscle hypertrophy, edema, goblet cell hyperplasia, epithelial shedding, and ciliary abnormalities are already present in children as young as three years of age. A recent case-control study has shown significant thickening of the basement membrane in young, difficult-to-treat asthmatics (5,8). Other studies in children who subsequently developed clinical asthma demonstrated early features of airway remodeling before the development of symptoms (9,10). A recent case study of six patients referred for difficult-to-control asthma who had bronchial biopsies showed that although five out of the six had normal forced expiratory volume in one second (FEV$_1$) all the patients had evidence of remodeling (4). Another recent study failed to show a difference in basement membrane thickness between symptomatic and non-symptomatic asthmatic children (11).

Studies based on pulmonary function testing show that lung growth is impaired during childhood in patients with severe and persistent symptoms of asthma (12). It is also well known that some young asthmatic patients have non-reversible airway obstruction. Other studies based on thoracic computerized tomodensitometry scans show early thickening of the airways in young asthmatics (13). In this chapter, we set out to describe the different components of airway remodeling and their contribution to asthma pathology and physiology in both adults and children. We will also discuss the potential mediators of airway remodeling, the proposed mechanisms which may be playing a role in the pathogenesis of these structural alterations, and the importance of airway remodeling in generating the asthma phenotype.

II. Epithelial Changes

Epithelial sloughing, fragility, and loss of surface epithelium are pathologic features of asthma, even in mild cases of the disease (Fig. 2). Fragile airway epithelium, severely damaged ciliated cells, and ciliogenesis have also been reported in young asthmatic children (14), and these structural changes are thought to begin in childhood or even at birth. Presence of epithelial cell clumps or Creola bodies in asthmatic sputum and increased number of epithelial cells in the BAL fluid of asthmatic patients (15) support these pathological findings. Epithelial desquamation has been described in postmortem specimens (16), endobronchial biopsies (17), and in expectorated sputum (15) from asthmatics. It has previously been shown that the extent of epithelial injury correlates with AHR (18). However, other studies have demonstrated epithelial shedding and desquamation to be present in not only biopsies from mild asthmatics (17) and non-asthmatic patients with allergic rhinitis (19), but also in healthy subjects (19).

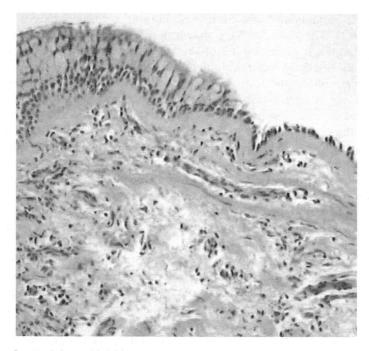

Figure 2 Endobronchial biopsy from proximal airways of an asthmatic patient showing epithelial detachment and goblet cell hyperplasia.

For these reasons, the presence or absence of epithelial desquamation as a phenotypic marker of asthma has been controversial. Whether the epithelial detachment results from weakened attachment of epithelial cells to the basement membrane as a result of extensive edema in the airways and release of free oxygen radicals from mast cell or eosinophil degranulation or whether it is simply an artifact of tissue sampling as a result of fiberoptic bronchoscopy procedures is widely debated.

One certain characteristic feature of the airway epithelium in asthma is goblet and mucous cell hyperplasia. Goblet cells secrete mucin glycoproteins, which are important for host defense. In asthmatic airways, mucous gland hyperplasia leads to excessive mucus secretion and plugging, leading to airway obstruction. These are well-documented features of chronic and fatal asthma in both adults and children ("mucus overproduction") and are almost always associated with airway occlusion from mucous plugs (16). Contributing to airway occlusion is the excess production and secretion of growth factors, cytokines, and chemokines by the epithelial cells. The airway epithelium is a major source of pro-inflammatory mediators, which perpetuate and accelerate the structural changes in the lungs.

Table 1 Cells Involved in Airway Remodeling in Asthma and their Respective Roles

Inflammatory cells	Role in remodeling
Eosinophils	Profibrotic cytokine production: TGF-β, IL-6, IL-11, and IL-17 Pro-inflammatory cytokine production: IL-4 and IL-5 Chemokine production: eotaxin, MCPs, MIP-1α. Production of MMP-9 Other mediators of inflammation such as leukotrienes and platelet-activating factor
Neutrophils	Production of TGF-β, MMP-9
Mast cells	Production of pro-inflammatory cytokines: IL-4, IL-5, and TNF-α Production of TGF-β Other mediators of inflammation such as leukotrienes, GM-CSF, histamine, and chemokines
Basophils	Production of pro-inflammatory cytokines: IL-4 and IL-13 Other mediators of inflammation such as leukotrienes and histamine
T-lymphocytes	Th-2 cytokine production: IL-4, IL-5, IL-9, and IL-13 Production of chemokines: eotaxin, RANTES, MCPs, and MIP-1α
Macrophages	Production of pro-fibrotic cytokines: IL-1β, TGF-β, and TNF-α
Epithelium	
Epithelial cells	Production of numerous pro-fibrotic and pro-inflammatory cytokines, chemokines, and growth factors Hyperplasia and hypertrophy, mucus overproduction
Goblet cells	Hyperplasia and hypertrophy, mucus overproduction
Submucosa	
Submucosal gland cells	Production of ECM proteins: collagens I–III–V, fibronectin, tenascin, lumican, and biglycan.
Fibroblasts	MMP-9/TIMP-1 imbalance

(Continued)

Table 1 Cells Involved in Airway Remodeling in Asthma and their Respective Roles (*Continued*)

Inflammatory cells	Role in remodeling
Smooth muscle	
ASM cells and activation	Smooth muscle hypertrophy, hyperplasia, migration
	Production of: Pro-inflammatory and pro-fibrotic cytokines: TNF-α, IL-1β, IL-5, IL-6, IL-11, and IFN-γ
	Chemokines: RANTES, eotaxin, IL-8, GM-CSF, and MCPs
	Lipid mediators: PGE2 and COX-2
	ECM proteins: laminin and fibronectin
Cartilage	
Chondrocytes	Cartilage degradation and remodeling
Blood vessels	
Endothelial vascular cells	Angiogenesis
	Production of pro-inflammatory cytokines, chemokines, leukotrienes, and prostaglandins

Abbreviations: TGF, transforming growth factor; IL, interleukin; ECM, extracellular matrix; MCP, macrophage chemattractant protein; MIP, macrophage infammatory protein; MMP, matrix metalloproteinase; TGF, tumor growth factor; IL, interleuin; RANTES, regulated on activation normal T cell expressed and secreted; TNF, tumor necrosis factor; IFN, interferon; TIMP, tissue inhibitor metallo proteinase; PGE, prostaglandin E; COX, cyclooxygenase; M-CSF, granulocyte macrophage-colony stimulating factor.

III. Subepithelial Fibrosis

In 1922, subepithelial fibrosis was first observed in autopsy samples of fatal asthma cases (reviewed in Ref. 20). Subepithelial fibrosis is now considered as a feature of asthma, not only in adult asthmatics but also in young children (4,5). Surprisingly, children with difficult-to-treat asthma have the same extent of subepithelial fibrosis as asthmatic adults (4,5). Airway remodeling and the fibrotic process are not restricted to large airways. The fibrosis process occurs in the *lamina reticularis* and involves increase in collagens I, III, V, fibronectin, tenascin, lumican, and biglycan (21–25) (Fig. 3).

Subepithelial fibrosis is believed to result from fibroblast activation. Airway fibroblasts are known to produce not only the extra-cellular matrix (ECM) proteins but also the ECM degradation enzymes. Subepithelial fibrosis is largely a result of the ongoing inflammatory process. ECM protein production is under control of many cytokines, the most relevant being transforming growth factor (TGF)-β, interleukin (IL)-17 and IL-11 (26–29).

Reduced collagen degradation is also an important cause of fibrosis. In asthma, it is believed that the protease/anti-protease balance favors the profibrogenic process. Interstitial cells, macrophages, and neutrophils are the major sources of proteases and anti-proteases. Activity of proteases is mainly regulated by anti-proteases. Matrix metalloproteinases (MMPs) are a family of proteases implicated in collagen degradation and were demonstrated to be expressed in asthmatic lung (30–33). Among these, MMP-9 has been strongly associated with asthma (32,34,35). MMP-9 level is significantly elevated in sputum of asthmatic patients when compared to healthy controls, however the level of MMP-9 inhibitor TIMP (tissue inhibitor metalloproteinase)-1 is similar between the two groups (32). This

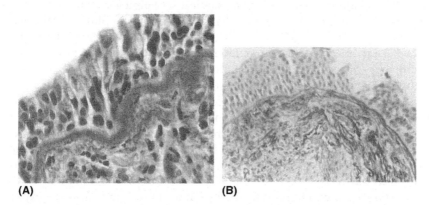

(A)   **(B)**

Figure 3 Endobronchial biopsies from asthmatic airways showing reticular membrane thickening, a milder form of subepithelial fibrosis in a mild asthmatic patient (**A**) and extensive subepithelial fibrosis in a severe asthmatic patient (**B**).

imbalance between MMP-9 and TIMP-1 leads to excessive deposition of collagen. Moreover, increased levels of MMP-9 have been demonstrated in asthmatics following exacerbation (30,36,37) or allergen challenge (38–40). This increase in macromolecules might not only lead to fibrosis but may also be a reservoir where adhesion molecules, cytokines, and other inflammatory mediators can be contained, perpetuating the inflammation process.

IV. Inflammation

In the 1980s, asthma was redefined as an inflammatory disease of the airways. The asthma phenotype is characterized by a Th-2 mediated inflammatory response and a complex interaction between a wide network of inflammatory and structural cells and the inflammatory mediators which they release. In both adult and young asthmatics, airway inflammation involves Th-2 cells, eosinophils, neutrophils, and mast cells (41–47). Mast cell hyperplasia is seen in mucosal epithelium and smooth muscle area in asthmatic airways (48). Mast cells are implicated in the immediate reaction of hypersensitivity by histamine and leukotrienes, leading to bronchoconstriction, vasodilatation, and tissue edema, and triggering leucocyte infiltration, collagen turnover, and resident cell growth through cytokines and proteinases released (44,48). Eosinophils release many potent proinflammatory mediators, which directly contribute to bronchoconstriction, mucus hypersecretion, and overall inflammation of the bronchial mucosa (42). Eosinophils have been increasingly recognized as important profibrotic cells due to their capacity to produce potent pro-fibrotic cytokines including TGF-β and IL-6 as well as proteases such as MMP-9 (28,49). MMP-9 promotes eosinophil inflammation by helping eosinophil trafficking (34). We have recently shown that asthmatic eosinophils constitutively express more TGF-β1, IL-11, and IL-17 than control eosinophils (unpublished data). Neutrophils are significantly increased in airways of severe asthmatics (50,51), in BAL of children with mild to moderate persistent asthma (41), and in induced sputum of children with acute asthma (46). This neutrophilic inflammation seems to be related to severity of the disease and may be a consequence of corticosteroid treatment. In vitro studies proposed that IL-17 may be responsible for neutrophil recruitment in severe asthmatics by its effect on IL-8 (52). Neutrophilic inflammation in asthma may reflect a role in injured tissue repair by MMP-9 and TGF-β production (53).

TGF-β is a potent pro-fibrotic cytokine. TGF-β increases the expression of ECM proteins including collagens I, III, and fibronectin (26,27), and decreases collagenase levels (54). Eosinophils are the main source of TGF-β in asthmatic airways (49). Expression of Smad 7, an intracellular antagonist of TGF-β signaling, is reduced in the bronchial epithelial cells of asthmatics compared to controls (55), suggesting that asthmatic epithelial cells are more susceptible to TGF-β stimulation than normal epithelial cells. Importantly, Smad 7 expression was inversely correlated with basement membrane thickness and ARH in these patients. IL-11 is another profibrotic cytokine. Using immunocytochemistry and in situ hybridization, we have demonstrated increased expression of IL-11 protein and IL-11 mRNA in the subepithelial and epithelial layer of bronchial biopsies from patients with severe asthma but not from mild asthmatics or healthy controls (29). Furthermore, IL-11 expression was inversely correlated with FEV_1 in severe asthmatics and the IL-11 mRNA-positive cells were localized to epithelial cells and myelin basic protein (MBP)-positive eosinophils (29). IL-17 is a newly described family of pro-fibrotic cytokines (IL-17A to IL-17E). We have recently shown increased IL-17 levels in the sputum and BAL fluid from asthmatic patients compared to healthy controls and this cytokine to be produced by T cells and eosinophils (28). Furthermore, IL-17 induces bronchial fibroblasts to increase their expression of IL-11 and IL-6 (28).

Along with inflammation, mechanical stimuli are believed to be important contributors to airway remodeling. Bronchoconstriction has been demonstrated to cause direct folding of airway wall leading to excess stress on the epithelial layer (56). Stress induces epithelial cells to produce an array of profibrotic cytokines, which then indirectly can stimulate fibroblasts and smooth muscle cells to perpetuate the inflammatory process. Fibroblasts are known to increase fibronectin, collagens III and V, and MMP-9 production following mechanical stress (57). Pressure stress on cultured rat tracheal epithelial cells can increase the expression of pro-fibrotic mediators such as TGF-β1 (58). Mechanical stress, along with inflammation, orchestrating synthesis, and degradation of matrix proteins, are the proposed mechanisms of airway remodeling.

V. Mucus Overproduction

Mucus overproduction is an important feature of asthma, as fatal cases are mostly the result of major mucus plugging of airways. Mucus plugging of the small and medium airways can contribute to airflow limitation and air trapping in severe asthma. Mucus plugging is also a feature of the disease in asthmatic children. Plugging can be found not only in children with severe asthma, but also in more stable patients (59).

In the human airway, mucus is produced by the goblet cells and the submucosal glands. The goblet cells' primary function is to secrete mucins onto the internal surface of the airways to form a liquid layer contributing to the host defense by protecting the epithelium. Goblet cells constitute up to 25% of the bronchial epithelial columnar cells, representing 30,000 to 50,000 cells per cubic millimeter of epithelial tissue (reviewed by Ref. 60). The relative contribution of goblet cells and submucosal glands to the mucin component of airway mucus in asthma is unknown. Prominence of the submucosal glands is usually not mentioned in bronchial biopsy studies of mild and moderate asthma, but increased submucosal gland volume is described in fatal cases of asthma. Airways of fatal and non-fatal asthmatic patients show goblet cell and submucosal gland hyperplasia, with strong predominance of these features in fatal asthmatic airways (16,61) (Fig. 4). Goblet cell hyperplasia can also be observed in patients with mild forms of the disease (62). Marked goblet cell hyperplasia is also found in the airways of children with severe asthma, in children with milder disease, and in those in remission (14,63). Goblet cell abundance can be heterogeneous, without clear hyperplasia of some smaller airways (64). Also present is submucosal gland hypertrophy (63) and development of intraepithelial glands in certain cases (14). Noticeably, submucosal glands were shown to be relatively more important in the airway wall of children without respiratory disease than in healthy adults (65,66). This relative gland hypertrophy in healthy children could contribute to mucus hypersecretion and airflow obstruction when airway disease is present.

Mucous cells are characterized by mucin production. Mucins are large, complex glycoproteins imparting rheological properties to the mucous, and secreted to trap foreign molecules in the airway lumen. The production of an optimal amount of mucus as well as an ideal viscoelasticity are important features ensuring efficient mucociliary clearance. Mucins are highly glycosylated peptide sequences, encoded by specific mucin (*MUC*) genes. Sixteen human *MUC* genes have been identified to date (60). Nine of these

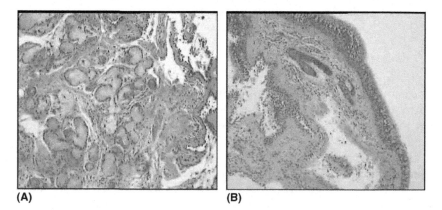

(A)   **(B)**

Figure 4   Endobronchial biopsies from asthmatic airways showing submucosal gland hyperplasia (**A**) and goblet cell hyperplasia (**B**).

genes are expressed in the respiratory tract (*MUC-1,-2,-4, -5AC,-5B,-7,-8,-11,* and *-13*) (67). The protein products of only four of these genes (*MUC2, MUC5AC, MUC5B,* and *MUC7*) have been identified in the respiratory tract (68). From these, *MUC5AC* (the major goblet cell mucin) and *MUC5B* (the major submucosal gland mucin) are considered the most clinically relevant in respiratory health and disease (69,70). *MUC5AC, MUC2,* and *MUC4* expression are increased in asthmatic patients, whereas decreased *MUC5B* expression was described in one study (64). Of course, much is still left to speculation as little data is available in this field. The epidermal growth factor receptor (EGFR) is implicated in increased expression of *MUC5AC* as well as in goblet cell hyperplasia (71). *MUC5AC* gene expression signals through the EGF cascade, involving EGFR up-regulation, and signaling via EGFR tyrosine kinase and mitogen activated protein (MAP) kinase.

Calcium-activated chloride channels (hCLCA1 in humans) are also implicated in mucus hypersecretion and their signaling is likely to occur via the EGFR-MAP pathway. Cytokines [mainly IL-4, IL-9, IL-13, tumor nerosis factor (TNF)-α, and platelet activating factor (PAF)], bacterial products (lipopolysaccharides and lipoteichoic acid), proteinases (elastase and cathepsin G), irritants (sulphur dioxide and cigarette smoke), and oxidants are known to promote goblet cell hyperplasia and mucin production, as well as EGFR overproduction (71,72). IL-13, a Th-2 cytokine, has been shown to induce mucus production in a murine model of allergic inflammation (73). We have shown that IL-9, another Th-2-type cytokine, plays an important role in mucus production in asthmatic airways (74,75). In addition, we have observed a strong correlation between IL-9 mRNA and protein expression, and a calcium-activated chloride channel (hCLCA1) in the asthmatic bronchial epithelium (76) suggesting that IL-9-induced up-regulation of hCLCA1 may be responsible for increased mucus overproduction in these patients. Furthermore, IL-4 has also been shown to increase *MUC5AC* gene expression, goblet cell metaplasia and mucus production in epithelial cell cultures as well as in a murine model of asthma (77).

Numerous therapeutic targets have been linked to the pathophysiology of airway mucus hypersecretion in experimental models of asthma or in asthmatic adults. Although inhaled corticosteroids (ICS) effectively reduce mucus production in asthmatic airways, the mechanism is yet to be elucidated (78). Importantly, we do not currently know if these agents have the same therapeutic effects in both adults and children and if the targets are similar in both populations. These targets range from the inflammatory cells themselves, to specific cellular elements such as EGFR tyrosine kinase, Bcl-2, p38 MAP kinase, proteinases, and CLCA channels (71). Some highly specific targets, such as hCLCA1, have recently been linked with airway mucus hypersecretion in adults. Clinical trials with specific blockers against hCLCA1, are awaited (60).

VI. Smooth Muscle Changes

ASM is the major effector cell responsible for airway tone. Asthmatic airways
are characterized by increased ASM size (hypertrophy) and increased ASM
number (hyperplasia) leading to a significant increase in ASM mass (Fig. 5).
The increase in ASM in asthma may contribute to airway wall thickening,
chronic airway obstruction, and bronchial hyper-responsiveness. These
changes are the major structural changes that are seen pathologically in asthmatic biopsies when compared to healthy individuals and are likely to be the
most important abnormality responsible for increased airway responsiveness
in asthmatics, as greater muscle thickness allows greater airway constriction
for a given amount of muscle stress. Increased ASM mass appears to be associated with more severe disease (79) and similar ASM changes have been
documented in young children who died from *status asthmaticus* (63) and children with difficult-to-treat asthma (4).

It has been repeatedly shown that the percentage of the bronchial wall
occupied by bronchial smooth muscle is increased in fatal asthma. Pare
et al. have demonstrated that in airways larger than 2 mm in diameter, there
is two- to four-fold increase over normal in the area of the wall occupied by

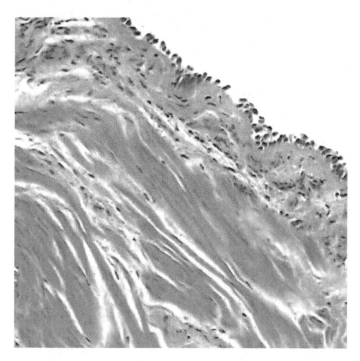

Figure 5   Endobronchial biopsy from asthmatic airways showing increased smooth
muscle mass and proximity of smooth muscle layer to the epithelium.

bronchial smooth muscle (80). Although some studies reported that the degree of ASM increase is greatest in those asthmatics with a long history of the disease (81) and increased ASM seems to be a more obvious pathologic feature of severe asthmatics compared to mild asthmatics, these results are inconsistent in the literature. Literature suggests that increased ASM mass in the larger airways is caused by hyperplasia, whereas increases in smaller airways are more likely to be caused by hypertrophy of the ASM cells (82). A more recent study has shown that the hyper-reactivity associated with asthma is not a consequence of increased ASM in large airways because no difference in the ASM mass was observed between asthmatic and non-asthmatic subjects (83). Their results suggest that the differences in mechanical responses of asthmatic airways cannot be explained solely by the amount of smooth muscle.

Traditionally, ASM has been viewed as a structural effector tissue, however, new evidence suggests that ASM is also capable of secreting pro-inflammatory cytokines [tumor necrosis factor (TNF)-α, IL-1β, IL-5, and IL-6, and granulocyte/monocyte-colony stimulating factor (GM-CSF)], chemokines (RANTES, eotaxin, and IL-8), lipid mediators (PGE2 and COX-2), and ECM proteins (laminin and fibronectin) and can migrate, proliferate and express cellular adhesion molecules (ICAM-1, VCAM-1, CD40, CD44, and integrins) as well as cytokine receptors (TNFR, IL-2R, IL-12R, IFN-γR, IL-4R, and IL-5R) (reviewed in Ref. 84). Together these changes contribute to sustained ASM activation and proliferation. Those results suggest that ASM itself may play an important role in immunomodulation of the immune response and may be an integral player in perpetuation of the chronic inflammatory process in asthma.

VII. Microvascular Changes

Dilatation and proliferation of bronchial blood vessels (angiogenesis), congestion, and wall edema are known features of fatal asthma and account for significant swelling and stiffness of the airway wall. Although these vascular changes comprise an important aspect of airway remodeling (Fig. 6) and may play an important role in AHR and in sustaining inflammation, the literature on angiogenesis and microvascular remodeling in man, particularly in children, has not been well studied.

Endothelial cells play a key role in asthma by regulating the selectivity and specificity of the cell infiltrate into the airways. Endothelial cells are often described as targets for numerous cytokines; however, these cells are also capable of producing numerous cytokines, chemokines, leukotrienes, and prostaglandins themselves. Using computerized image analysis to measure the vascularity of mucosa, Li and Wilson have demonstrated that the airways of patients with mild asthma were more vascularized, had

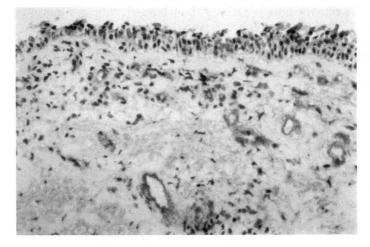

Figure 6   Endobronchial biopsy from asthmatic airways showing increased vascularity in the submucosal layer.

significantly greater numbers of blood vessels per mm^2 of submucosa and that these vessels were larger compared to airways of healthy non-asthmatic controls (85). These gross structural changes are likely to contribute to reduced lumen diameter and vascular obstruction of these vessels.

The mechanism responsible for microvascular remodeling in asthma and the consequences of these changes are just beginning to be elucidated. Vascular endothelial growth factor (VEGF) and angiopoietin-1 (Ang1) are two endothelial cell-specific growth factors that are likely to be important in the formation of new vessels and their remodeling. VEGF and Ang1 play complementary and coordinated roles in vascular growth and development, with VEGF acting early during vessel formation and Ang1 acting later during vessel remodeling, maturation, and stabilization. VEGF increases vascular permeability but Ang1 blocks plasma leakage. The literature on the effect of such growth factors on vascular changes in asthma is limited and conflicting. Increased levels of VEGF and Ang1 have been reported in sputum (86) and bronchial submucosa (87) of adult asthmatic patients. In the submucosa, VEGF immunostaining was associated with blood vessel area and the degree of vascularity was inversely correlated with airway caliber and airway responsiveness (87). In contrast to those results however, Demoly et al. have reported similar VEGF levels in the BAL fluid of asthmatics and controls and no correlation to exist between VEGF and BAL albumin and immunoglobulin A (IgA) (measures of vascular permeability) (88). Recent advances in the imaging of angiogenesis, which enables us to quantify the number of blood vessels, and measure blood flow and vascular permeability, as well as analyze abnormalities in blood vessel walls (89,90), is expected to significantly add to our understanding of these microvascular changes in both adults and children.

VIII. Cartilage Changes

Airway cartilage is an important structural contributor to the airway wall, making up to 60% of the total wall area in the large airways and up to 10% in smaller airways. The data concerning the structural modifications of airway cartilages in asthma is limited; however, there is some evidence that suggests that in asthmatic adults, the ECM is degraded and cartilage, volume is reduced (91,92). Cartilage proteoglycan (PG) degradation and cartilage remodeling has been described in cases of fatal asthma by Roberts (93). They have suggested that enzymes such as neutrophil elastase, mast cell tryptase, or cysteine proteinases have the ability to degrade collagen, elastin, and PGs and are therefore likely to play an important role in these structural changes. Alternative mechanisms for cartilage degradation include IL-1-driven resorption of airway cartilage by chondrocytes (94). The consequence of ECM degradation is increased airway wall stiffness, allowing for exaggerated smooth muscle shortening. As normal lung development is dependent on normal interstitium and collagen architecture, it has been proposed that excessive positive pressure ventilation can severely compress the interstitium and damage the collagen network in young children, resulting in abnormal lung development, and may in fact be the origin of chronic lung disease in this group of patients (95).

IX. Clinical Significance of Airway Remodeling

Irreversible airway obstruction and airway hyperresponsiveness in asthmatics have been attributed to airway remodeling (1,2,96). Furthermore, the duration of asthma has been associated with reduced lung function, increased hyper-responsiveness, more asthma symptomatology and greater use of medication in children (97). Airway remodeling attempts to explain these functional abnormalities. To date, many correlations have been shown to exist between the various pathological features of airway remodeling and the severity of asthma. We (29) and others (3,98) have demonstrated a direct correlation between subepithelial thickening and collagen types I and III deposition in the airways with the severity of the disease, but Chu et al. have suggested that in the large airways, collagen deposition and TGF-β immunostaining alone are not sufficient to differentiate severe asthmatics from milder forms of the disease (99). Furthermore, PG expression by bronchial fibroblasts correlates with airway responsiveness in asthmatics (25,100). Tenascin production per se has been directly associated with asthma disease activity (23), and increased smooth muscle mass in both large and small asthmatic airways has been linked to asthma severity. Functional consequences of increased ASM mass include airflow obstruction and increased airway responsiveness (79). There exists a second school of thought, however, which suggests that airway wall thickening may in fact prevent bronchoconstriction and smooth muscle shortening by creating stiffer airways (101,102). Despite the fact that decreased lung function appears to be associated with airway remodeling in asthmatic adults, no correlation has been found with age of patients, symptom duration, lung function, eosinophilic inflammation, or intensity of reticular basement membrane (RBM) thickness in these patients (4,5). Further studies are needed to look at the long-term effect of airway remodeling on lung function in asthmatic patients, particularly in children.

ICS are the recommended treatment for asthma and are currently the most effective in controlling inflammation (Fig. 7) but they are much less effective in reversing airway remodeling. Jeffery (103), Lundgren et al. (104), and Boulet et al. (105) reported no changes in basement membrane thickness following long (mean of 3,7, and 10 years) or short-term (eight weeks) use of ICS in asthmatics. In other studies, ICS courses of six weeks (106), four months (107), six months (108), one year (109), and two years' duration (110) resulted in modest decreases in basement membrane thickness in asthmatics. In a subsequent study, Sont et al. (110) described a

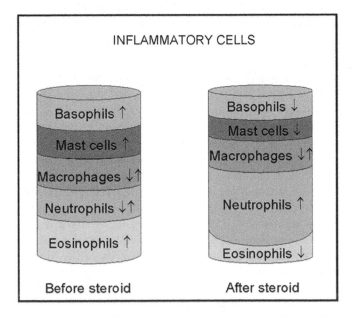

Figure 7   Inflammatory cells before and after treatment with corticosteroids in airway remodeling. There is a decrease in the number of eosinophils, mast cells and basophils and an increase in the number of neutrophils.

decrease in RBM thickness in a group of patients receiving a higher dose of ICS. This finding has led to the hypothesis that ICS might be effective in reducing RBM thickness when used for a long period of time and at higher dose. Tenascin, an ECM glycoprotein, appears to be more responsive to ICS treatment, as a short course of steroids (4–6 weeks) significantly decreasing tenascin immunoreactivity in the airways of chronic asthmatics (23). In a group of moderate to severe asthmatics, we failed to show any significant difference in types I and III collagen immunoreactivity after a two-week course of oral corticosteroids (111). In that study we further demonstrated steroids to be effective in reducing IL-17 and IL-11 expression in these patients, but interestingly, corticosteroids had no effect on TGF-β immunoreactivity (111). It is likely that the inability of ICS to inhibit TGF-β expression may be responsible for persistent fibrosis despite steroid treatment in this group of severe asthmatics.

The lack of effectiveness of ICS on airway remodeling has turned the attention to other agents, which may have a possible role in the improvement of airway morphology and function in asthmatic patients. In a study comparing salmeterol alone, fluticasone alone, and a placebo, a significant improvement in airway vascularity was observed only in the salmeterol-treated group (112). Therefore, long acting β2-agonists might have a beneficial effect on this feature of airway remodeling. Cysteinyl leukotrienes may also play an important role in the pathogenesis of airway remodeling. Henderson et al. have recently shown that a cysteinyl leukotriene 1 (CysLT1) receptor antagonist, montelukast, significantly inhibited ovalbumin (OVA)-induced ASM hyperplasia and subepithelial fibrosis in sensitized mice (113). In addition, a phosphodiesterase (PDE)-3 inhibitor, siguazodan, has been shown to reduce in vitro proliferation of human ASM (114) and, very recently, monoclonal antibodies to IL-5 were shown to be effective in reducing deposition of ECM proteins tenascin, lumican, and procollagen in the basement membrane of mild asthmatics (115). These data clearly suggest that some of the non-corticosteroid drugs have potent anti-remodeling effects. Their therapeutic effects in preventing or even reversing airway remodeling need to be investigated to correlate in vitro and animal anti-remodeling effectiveness.

X. Recent Advances

For many years it has been proposed that the production of excess NO by inducible NO synthase (iNOS) plays an important role in asthma. Both beneficial and detrimental actions of NO have been reported in the lung but whether excess NO in asthma is a result of the body's natural defense or NO is an active inflammatory mediator in the airways is the subject of an intense debate. Recent advances in the literature have identified arginase

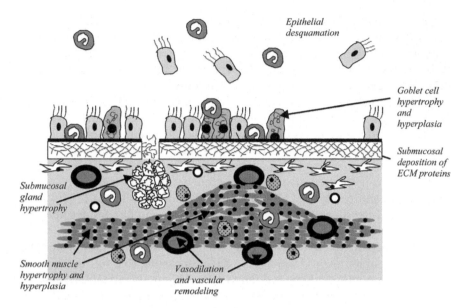

Figure 8   Features of airway remodeling in asthma.

as an important candidate gene and/or a marker of asthmatic phenotype (116). Arginase and NOS compete for the same substrate L-arginine and hence can interfere with each other's activity. Arginases I and II contribute to the development of bleomycin-induced lung fibrosis in mice (117) and increased airway responsiveness in a guinea-pig model of asthma (118). Increased arginase I mRNA and protein were detected in human asthmatic biopsies compared to controls and arginase expression is controlled by Th-2 cytokines via a STAT-6 dependent intracellular signaling pathway (116). Such increase in arginase expression in the lung would significantly affect arginine metabolism in the lung and indirectly have profound effects on the inhibition of NO production. Arginase converts arginine to ornithine, which gives proline and polyamines. Proline is used in collagen and mucus production, while polyamines increase cell proliferation. High activity of arginase might contribute to airway remodeling by increased collagen deposition and cell proliferation. Moreover, it is proposed that a substrate competition occurs between arginase and NOS. Enhanced arginase and activity leads to less substrate for NOS and thus less NO production. NO has beneficial bronchodilating effects on ASM (119). A decrease in NO production by constitutive NOS (cNOS) leads to increased AHR, a feature of asthma phenotype (118). Following these observations, arginase seems to be directly linked to asthma pathogenesis (120). The interaction between arginase and NOS as well as genetic studies looking at the arginase polymorphism in asthma is currently under investigation.

The second area of advances in asthma research involves the ADAMS (a disintegrin and metalloproteinase) family. A genome-wide screen used in an attempt to define the genetic origin of bronchial hyper-responsiveness lead to the identification of ADAM33 as a novel asthma susceptibility gene (121). ADAM33 is a member of the Zn^{2+}-dependent MMPs and it is expressed in ASM cells, myofibroblasts, and fibroblasts, but not epithelial cells or T-lymphocytes (122,123). Its selective expression in structural cells, but not in inflammatory cells, suggests this enzyme may play an important regulatory role in control of ASM responsiveness and/or fibroblast function and hence airway remodeling (121). ADAM33 catalytic activity is inhibited moderately by TIMP-3 and TIMP-4 and weakly by TIMP-2 (124). ADAM33 is a cell surface transmembrane protein with metalloproteinase-like activity and a disintegrin-like domain. This domain facilitates cell–cell and cell–matrix interactions (125). Polymorphisms have been identified in the ADAM33 gene (126) and linked with asthma in African American, U.S. Caucasian, U.S. Hispanic and Dutch populations (127), but not in Puerto Rican or Mexican populations (128). More detailed analysis of ADAM33 activity and its contribution to asthma severity is warranted. Identifying a major new candidate gene for asthma creates an imperative to determine its function and to understand how its disordered function translates into disease.

IL-25 is a newly identified cytokine mainly produced by Th-2 and mast cells with the capacity to increase IL-4, IL-5, and IL-13 gene expression (129,130). IL-25 (or IL-17E) is also an important remodeling-associated cytokine in experimental animal models of asthma whereby intranasal administration of IL-25 triggers epithelial cell hyperplasia and increased mucus secretion in these animals (130,131). Further studies are needed to understand the exact role of IL-25 in asthma.

Acknowledgments

Our laboratory is supported by grants from the Canadian Institutes of Health Research (CIHR). Dr. Meri K. Tulic is an NH&MRC Peter Doherty Postdoctoral Research Fellow, Dr. Céline Bergeron is a Merck-Frosst/CIHR/CAAIF Fellow and Dr. Patrick Daigneault a recipient of the Duncan L. Gordon Postdoctoral Fellowship of the Sick Children Foundation, Toronto, Canada. Dr. Q. Hamid is a recipient of the Senior Fonds de la Recherche en Santé du Québec (FRSQ) Chercheur-Boursier Award.

References

1. Elias JA, Zhu Z, Chupp G, Homer RJ. Airway remodeling in asthma. J Clin Invest 1999; 104(8):1001–1016.
2. Boulet LP, Laviolette M, Turcotte H, et al. Bronchial subepithelial fibrosis correlates with airway responsiveness to methacholine. Chest 1997; 112:45–52.

3. Chetta A, Foresi A, Del Donno M, Bertorelli G, Pesci A, Olivieri D. Airways remodeling is a distinctive feature of asthma and is related to severity of disease. Chest 1997; 111:852–857.

4. Jenkins HA, Cool C, Szefler SJ, et al. Histopathology of severe childhood asthma: a case series. Chest 2003; 124(1):32–41.

5. Payne DN, Rogers AV, Adelroth E, et al. Early thickening of the reticular basement membrane in children with difficult asthma. Am J Respir Crit Care Med 2003; 167:78–82.

6. Martinez FD, Wright AL, Taussig LM, Holberg CJ, Halonen M, Morgan WJ. Asthma and wheezing in the first six years of life. The Group Health Medical Associates. N Engl J Med 1995; 332(3):133–138.

7. Heino M, Juntunen-Backman K, Leijala M, Rapola J, Laitinen LA. Bronchial epithelial inflammation in children with chronic cough after early lower respiratory tract illness. Am Rev Respir Dis 1990; 141(2):428–432.

8. Barbato A, Turato G, Baraldo S, et al. Airway inflammation in childhood asthma. Am J Respir Crit Care Med 2003; 168(7):798–803.

9. Pohunek P RW, Turzikova J, Fudrmann J, Warner JO. Eosinophilic inflammation in the bronchial mucosa of children with bronchial asthma. Eur Respir J 1997; 11:1605.

10. Humbert M, Menz G, Ying S, et al. The immunopathology of extrinsic (atopic) and intrinsic (non-atopic) asthma: more similarities than differences. Immunol Today 1999; 20(11):528–533.

11. de Blic J, Tillie-Leblond I, Tonnel AB, Jaubert F, Scheinmann P, Gosset P. Difficult asthma in children: an analysis of airway inflammation. J Allergy Clin Immunol 2004; 113(1):94–100.

12. Peat JK, Woolcock AJ, Cullen K. Rate of decline of lung function in subjects with asthma. Eur J Respir Dis 1987; 70(3):171–179.

13. Marchac V, Emond S, Mamou-Mani T, et al. Thoracic CT in pediatric patients with difficult-to-treat asthma. AJR Am J Roentgenol 2002; 179(5): 1245–1252.

14. Konradova V, Copova C, Sukova B, Houstek J. Ultrastructure of the bronchial epithelium in three children with asthma. Pediatr Pulmonol 1985; 1(4):182–187.

15. Naylor B. The shedding of the mucosa of the bronchial tree in asthma. Thorax 1962; 17:69–72.

16. Carroll N, Elliot J, Morton A, James A. The structure of large and small airways in nonfatal and fatal asthma. Am Rev Respir Dis 1993; 147: 405–410.

17. Laitinen LA, Heino M, Laitinen A, Kava T, Haahtela T. Damage of the airway epithelium and bronchial reactivity in patients with asthma. Am Rev Respir Dis 1985; 131:599–606.

18. Jeffery PK, Wardlaw AJ, Nelson FC, Collins JV, Kay AB. Bronchial biopsies in asthma. An ultrastructural, quantitative study and correlation with hyper-reactivity. Am Rev Respir Dis 1989; 140(6):1745–1753.

19. Boulet LP, Turcotte H, Carrier G, Boutet M, Laviolette M. Increased maximal airway response to methacholine during seasonal allergic rhinitis in nonasthmatic subjects: relationships with airway wall thickness and inflammation. Eur Respir J 1995; 8:913–921.

20. Redington AE, Howarth PH. Airway wall remodelling in asthma. Thorax 1997; 52(4):310–312.
21. Roche WR, Beasley R, Williams JH, Holgate ST. Subepithelial fibrosis in the bronchi of asthmatics. Lancet 1989; 1:520–524.
22. Wilson JW, Li X. The measurement of reticular basement membrane and submucosal collagen in the asthmatic airway. Clin Exp Allergy 1997; 27(4): 363–371.
23. Laitinen A, Altraja A, Kampe M, Linden M, Virtanen I, Laitinen LA. Tenascin is increased in airway basement membrane of asthmatics and decreased by an inhaled steroid. Am J Respir Crit Care Med 1997; 156: 951–958.
24. Karjalainen EM, Lindqvist A, Laitinen LA, et al. Airway inflammation and basement membrane tenascin in newly diagnosed atopic and nonatopic asthma. Respir Med 2003; 97(9):1045–1051.
25. Huang J, Olivenstein R, Taha R, Hamid Q, Ludwig M. Enhanced proteogly-can deposition in the airway wall of atopic asthmatics. Am J Respir Crit Care Med 1999; 160:725–729.
26. Fine A, Goldstein RH. The effect of transforming growth factor-beta on cell proliferation and collagen formation by lung fibroblasts. J Biol Chem 1987; 262:3897–3902.
27. Ignotz RA, Massague J. Transforming growth factor-beta stimulates the expression of fibronectin and collagen and their incorporation into the extra-cellular matrix. J Biol Chem 1986; 261:4337–4345.
28. Molet S, Hamid Q, Davoine F, et al. IL-17 is increased in asthmatic airways and induces human bronchial fibroblasts to produce cytokines. J Allergy Clin Immunol 2001; 108:430–438.
29. Minshall E, Chakir J, Laviolette M, et al. IL-11 expression is increased in severe asthma: association with epithelial cells and eosinophils. J Allergy Clin Immunol 2000; 105:232–238.
30. Lemjabbar H, Gosset P, Lamblin C, et al. Contribution of 92 kDa gelatinase/ type IV collagenase in bronchial inflammation during status asthmaticus. Am J Respir Crit Care Med 1999; 159(4 Pt 1):1298–1307.
31. Prikk K, Maisi P, Pirila E, et al. Airway obstruction correlates with collage-nase-2 (MMP-8) expression and activation in bronchial asthma. Lab Invest 2002; 82(11):1535–1545.
32. Vignola AM, Riccobono L, Mirabella A, et al. Sputum metalloproteinase-9/ tissue inhibitor of metalloproteinase-1 ratio correlates with airflow obstruc-tion in asthma and chronic bronchitis. Am J Respir Crit Care Med 1998; 158:1945–1950.
33. Suzuki R, Kato T, Miyazaki Y, et al. Matrix metalloproteinases and tissue inhibitors of matrix metalloproteinases in sputum from patients with bron-chial asthma. J Asthma 2001; 38(6):477–484.
34. Wenzel SE, Balzar S, Cundall M, Chu HW. Subepithelial basement membrane immunoreactivity for matrix metalloproteinase 9: association with asthma severity, neutrophilic inflammation, and wound repair. J Allergy Clin Immunol 2003; 111(6):1345–1352.

35. Mautino G, Oliver N, Chanez P, Bousquet J, Capony F. Increased release of matrix metalloproteinase-9 in bronchoalveolar lavage fluid and by alveolar macrophages of asthmatics. Am J Respir Cell Mol Biol 1997; 17(5):583–591.

36. Lee YC, Lee HB, Rhee YK, Song CH. The involvement of matrix metalloproteinase-9 in airway inflammation of patients with acute asthma. Clin Exp Allergy 2001; 31(10):1623–1630.

37. Tanaka H, Miyazaki N, Oashi K, Tanaka S, Ohmichi M, Abe S. Sputum matrix metalloproteinase-9: tissue inhibitor of metalloproteinase-1 ratio in acute asthma. J Allergy Clin Immunol 2000; 105(5):900–905.

38. Warner JA, Julius P, Luttmann W, Kroegel C. Matrix metalloproteinases in bronchoalveolar lavage fluid following antigen challenge. Int Arch Allergy Immunol 1997; 113(1–3):318–320.

39. Kelly EA, Busse WW, Jarjour NN. Increased matrix metalloproteinase-9 in the airway after allergen challenge. Am J Respir Crit Care Med 2000; 162(3 Pt 1):1157–1161.

40. Cataldo DD, Bettiol J, Noel A, Bartsch P, Foidart JM, Louis R. Matrix metalloproteinase-9, but not tissue inhibitor of matrix metalloproteinase-1, increases in the sputum from allergic asthmatic patients after allergen challenge. Chest 2002; 122(5):1553–1559.

41. Barbato A, Panizzolo C, Gheno M, et al. Bronchoalveolar lavage in asthmatic children: evidence of neutrophil activation in mild-to-moderate persistent asthma. Pediatr Allergy Immunol 2001; 12(2):73–77.

42. Kroegel C, Virchow JC Jr, Luttmann W, Walker C, Warner JA. Pulmonary immune cells in health and disease: the eosinophil leucocyte (Part I). Eur Respir J 1994; 7(3):519–543.

43. Le Gros G, Ben-Sasson SZ, Seder R, Finkelman FD, Paul WE. Generation of interleukin 4 (IL-4)-producing cells in vivo and in vitro: IL-2 and IL-4 are required for in vitro generation of IL-4-producing cells. J Exp Med 1990; 172(3):921–929.

44. Metcalfe DD, Baram D, Mekori YA. Mast cells. Physiol Rev 1997; 77(4): 1033–1079.

45. Mosmann TR, Cherwinski H, Bond MW, Giedlin MA, Coffman RL. Two types of murine helper T cell clone. I. Definition according to profiles of lymphokine activities and secreted proteins. J Immunol 1986; 136(7): 2348–2357.

46. Twaddell SH, Gibson PG, Carty K, Woolley KL, Henry RL. Assessment of airway inflammation in children with acute asthma using induced sputum. Eur Respir J 1996; 9(10):2104–2108.

47. Swain SL, Weinberg AD, English M, Huston G. IL-4 directs the development of Th2-like helper effectors. J Immunol 1990; 145(11):3796–3806.

48. Boyce JA. The role of mast cells in asthma. Prostaglandins Leukot Essent Fatty Acids 2003; 69(2–3):195–205.

49. Minshall EM, Leung DY, Martin RJ, et al. Eosinophil-associated TGF-beta1 mRNA expression and airways fibrosis in bronchial asthma. Am J Respir Cell Mol Biol 1997; 17:326–333.

50. Wenzel SE, Szefler SJ, Leung DY, Sloan SI, Rex MD, Martin RJ. Bronchoscopic evaluation of severe asthma. Persistent inflammation associated with high dose glucocorticoids. Am J Respir Crit Care Med 1997; 156(3 Pt 1):737–743.

51. Boulet LP, Turcotte H, Turcot O, Chakir J. Airway inflammation in asthma with incomplete reversibility of airflow obstruction. Respir Med 2003; 97(6):739–744.

52. Linden A. Role of interleukin-17 and the neutrophil in asthma. Int Arch Allergy Immunol 2001; 126(3):179–184.

53. Chu HW, Trudeau JB, Balzar S, Wenzel SE. Peripheral blood and airway tissue expression of transforming growth factor beta by neutrophils in asthmatic subjects and normal control subjects. J Allergy Clin Immunol 2000; 106(6): 1115–1123.

54. Edwards DR, Murphy G, Reynolds JJ, et al. Transforming growth factor beta modulates the expression of collagenase and metalloproteinase inhibitor. Embo J 1987; 6:1899–1904.

55. Nakao A, Sagara H, Setoguchi Y, et al. Expression of Smad7 in bronchial epithelial cells is inversely correlated to basement membrane thickness and airway hyperresponsiveness in patients with asthma. J Allergy Clin Immunol 2002; 110:873–878.

56. Tschumperlin DJ, Drazen JM. Mechanical stimuli to airway remodeling. Am J Respir Crit Care Med 2001; 164(10 Pt 2):S90–S94.

57. Swartz MA, Tschumperlin DJ, Kamm RD, Drazen JM. Mechanical stress is communicated between different cell types to elicit matrix remodeling. Proc Natl Acad Sci USA 2001; 98(11):6180–6185.

58. Ressler B, Lee RT, Randell SH, Drazen JM, Kamm RD. Molecular responses of rat tracheal epithelial cells to transmembrane pressure. Am J Physiol Lung Cell Mol Physiol 2000; 278(6):L1264–L1272.

59. Maxwell GM. The problem of mucous plugging in children with asthma. J Asthma 1985; 22(3):131–137.

60. Rogers DF. Pulmonary mucous: Pediatric perspective. Pediatr Pulmonol 2003; 36(3):178–188.

61. Aikawa T, Shimura S, Sasaki H, Ebina M, Takishima T. Marked goblet cell hyperplasia with mucous accumulation in the airways of patients who died of severe acute asthma attack. Chest 1992; 101:916–921.

62. Fahy JV. Goblet cell and mucin gene abnormalities in asthma. Chest 2002;122(suppl 6):S320–S6.

63. Cutz E, Levison H, Cooper DM. Ultrastructure of airways in children with asthma. Histopathology 1978; 2(6):407–421.

64. Ordonez CL, Khashayar R, Wong HH, et al. Mild and moderate asthma is associated with airway goblet cell hyperplasia and abnormalities in mucin gene expression. Am J Respir Crit Care Med 2001; 163(2):517–523.

65. Field WE. Mucous gland hypertrophy in babies and children aged 15 years or less. Br J Dis Chest 1968; 62(1):11–18.

66. Matsuba K, Thurlbeck WM. A morphometric study of bronchial and bronchiolar walls in children. Am Rev Respir Dis 1972; 105(6):908–913.

67. Copin MC, Buisine MP, Devisme L, et al. Normal respiratory mucosa, precursor lesions and lung carcinomas: differential expression of human mucin genes. Front Biosci 2001; 6:D1264–D1275.

68. Davies JR, Herrmann A, Russell W, Svitacheva N, Wickstrom C, Carlstedt I. Respiratory tract mucins: structure and expression patterns. Novartis Found Symp 2002; 248:76–88; discussion: 93, 277–282.
69. Davies JR, Russell, W, Svitacheva N'Wickstrom C, Carlstedt I. Respiratory tract mucins: structure and expression patterns. In: Mucus hypersecretion in respiratory disease. Chichester: Wiley, 2002.
70. Hovenberg HW, Davies JR, Herrmann A, Linden CJ, Carlstedt I. *MUC5AC*, but not *MUC2*, is a prominent mucin in respiratory secretions. Glycoconj J 1996; 13(5):839–847.
71. Rogers DF. The airway goblet cell. Int J Biochem Cell Biol 2003; 35(1):1–6.
72. Levine SJ, Larivee P, Logun C, Angus CW, Ognibene FP, Shelhamer JH. Tumor necrosis factor-alpha induces mucin hypersecretion and *MUC-2* gene expression by human airway epithelial cells. Am J Respir Cell Mol Biol 1995; 12(2):196–204.
73. Zhu Z, Lee CG, Zheng T, et al. Airway inflammation and remodeling in asthma. Lessons from interleukin 11 and interleukin 13 transgenic mice. Am J Respir Crit Care Med 2001; 164:S67–S70.
74. Longphre M, Li D, Gallup M, et al. Allergen-induced IL-9 directly stimulates mucin transcription in respiratory epithelial cells. J Clin Invest 1999; 104(10): 1375–1382.
75. Louahed J, Toda M, Jen J, et al. Interleukin-9 upregulates mucous expression in the airways. Am J Respir Cell Mol Biol 2000; 22(6):649–656.
76. Toda M, Tulic MK, Levitt RC, Hamid Q. A calcium-activated chloride channel (HCLCA1) is strongly related to IL-9 expression and mucous production in bronchial epithelium of patients with asthma. J Allergy Clin Immunol 2002; 109:246–250.
77. Dabbagh K, Takeyama K, Lee HM, Ueki IF, Lausier JA, Nadel JA. IL-4 induces mucin gene expression and goblet cell metaplasia in vitro and in vivo. J Immunol 1999; 162(10):6233–6237.
78. Laitinen LA, Laitinen A. Inhaled corticosteroid treatment and extracellular matrix in the airways in asthma. Int Arch Allergy Immunol 1995; 107:215–216.
79. Benayoun L, Druilhe A, Dombret MC, Aubier M, Pretolani M. Airway structural alterations selectively associated with severe asthma. Am J Respir Crit Care Med 2003; 167(10):1360–1368.
80. Pare PD, Wiggs BR, James A, Hogg JC, Bosken C. The comparative mechanics and morphology of airways in asthma and in chronic obstructive pulmonary disease. Am Rev Respir Dis 1991; 143:1189–1193.
81. Bai TR. Abnormalities in airway smooth muscle in fatal asthma. Am Rev Respir Dis 1990; 141:552–557.
82. Ebina M, Takahashi T, Chiba T, Motomiya M. Cellular hypertrophy and hyperplasia of airway smooth muscles underlying bronchial asthma. A 3-D morphometric study. Am Rev Respir Dis 1993; 148:720–726.
83. Thomson RJ, Bramley AM, Schellenberg RR. Airway muscle stereology: implications for increased shortening in asthma. Am J Respir Crit Care Med 1996; 154:749–757.
84. Halayko AJ, Solway J. Molecular mechanisms of phenotypic plasticity in smooth muscle cells. J Appl Physiol 2001; 90:358–368.

85. Li X, Wilson JW. Increased vascularity of the bronchial mucosa in mild asthma. Am J Respir Crit Care Med 1997; 156:229–233.
86. Asai K, Kanazawa H, Kamoi H, Shiraishi S, Hirata K, Yoshikawa J. Increased levels of vascular endothelial growth factor in induced sputum in asthmatic patients. Clin Exp Allergy 2003; 33:595–599.
87. Hoshino M, Takahashi M, Aoike N. Expression of vascular endothelial growth factor, basic fibroblast growth factor, and angiogenin immunoreactivity in asthmatic airways and its relationship to angiogenesis. J Allergy Clin Immunol 2001; 107:295–301.
88. Demoly P, Maly FE, Mautino G, et al. VEGF levels in asthmatic airways do not correlate with plasma extravasation. Clin Exp Allergy 1999; 29:1390–1394.
89. McDonald DM, Choyke PL. Imaging of angiogenesis: from microscope to clinic. Nat Med 2003; 9(6):713–725.
90. McDonald DM. Angiogenesis and remodeling of airway vasculature in chronic inflammation. Am J Respir Crit Care Med 2001; 164(10 Pt 2):S39–S45.
91. Maisel JC, Silvers GW, Mitchell RS, Petty TL. Bronchial atrophy and dynamic expiratory collapse. Am Rev Respir Dis 1968; 98:988–997.
92. Haraguchi M, Shimura S, Shirato K. Morphometric analysis of bronchial cartilage in chronic obstructive pulmonary disease and bronchial asthma. Am J Respir Crit Care Med 1999; 159:1005–1013.
93. Roberts CR. Is asthma a fibrotic disease? Chest 1995; 107:111S–117S.
94. Saklatvala J, Sarsfield SJ. How do interleukin-1 and tumour necrosis factor induce degradation of proteoglycan in cartilage? In: Glauert AM, ed. The control of tissue damage. New York: Elsevier, 1998:97–108.
95. Thibeault DW, Mabry SM, Ekekezie, II, Zhang X, Truog WE. Collagen scaffolding during development and its deformation with chronic lung disease. Pediatrics 2003; 111(4 Pt 1):766–776.
96. Shiba K, Kasahara K, Nakajima H, Adachi M. Structural changes of the airway wall impair respiratory function, even in mild asthma. Chest 2002; 122(5):1622–1626.
97. Zeiger RS, Dawson C, Weiss S. Relationships between duration of asthma and asthma severity among children in the Childhood Asthma Management Program (CAMP). J Allergy Clin Immunol 1999; 103:376–387.
98. Hoshino M, Nakamura Y, Sim JJ. Expression of growth factors and remodelling of the airway wall in bronchial asthma. Thorax 1998; 53(1):21–7.
99. Chu HW, Halliday JL, Martin RJ, Leung DY, Szefler SJ, Wenzel SE. Collagen deposition in large airways may not differentiate severe asthma from milder forms of the disease. Am J Respir Crit Care Med 1998; 158:1936–1944.
100. Westergren-Thorsson G, Chakir J, Lafreniere-Allard MJ, Boulet LP, Tremblay GM. Correlation between airway responsiveness and proteoglycan production by bronchial fibroblasts from normal and asthmatic subjects. Int J Biochem Cell Biol 2002; 34(10):1256–1267.
101. Lambert RK, Codd SL, Alley MR, Pack RJ. Physical determinants of bronchial mucosal folding. J Appl Physiol 1994; 77(3):1206–1216.
102. Milanese M, Crimi E, Scordamaglia A, et al. On the functional consequences of bronchial basement membrane thickening. J Appl Physiol 2001; 91(3):1035–1040.

103. Jeffery PK. Pathology of asthma. Br Med Bull 1992; 48:23–39.
104. Lundgren R, Soderberg M, Horstedt P, Stenling R. Morphological studies of bronchial mucosal biopsies from asthmatics before and after ten years of treatment with inhaled steroids. Eur Respir J 1988; 1(10):883–889.
105. Boulet LP, Turcotte H, Laviolette M, et al. Airway hyperresponsiveness, inflammation, and subepithelial collagen deposition in recently diagnosed versus long-standing mild asthma. Influence of inhaled corticosteroids. Am J Respir Crit Care Med 2000; 162:1308–1313.
106. Olivieri D, Chetta A, Del Donno M, et al. Effect of short-term treatment with low-dose inhaled fluticasone propionate on airway inflammation and remodeling in mild asthma: a placebo-controlled study. Am J Respir Crit Care Med 1997; 155:1864–1871.
107. Trigg CJ, Manolitsas ND, Wang J, et al. Placebo-controlled immunopathologic study of four months of inhaled corticosteroids in asthma. Am J Respir Crit Care Med 1994; 150(1):17–22.
108. Hoshino M, Takahashi M, Takai Y, Sim J. Inhaled corticosteroids decrease subepithelial collagen deposition by modulation of the balance between matrix metalloproteinase-9 and tissue inhibitor of metalloproteinase-1 expression in asthma. J Allergy Clin Immunol 1999; 104:356–363.
109. Ward C, Pais M, Bish R, et al. Airway inflammation, basement membrane thickening and bronchial hyperresponsiveness in asthma. Thorax 2002; 57(4):309–316.
110. Sont JK, Willems LN, Bel EH, van Krieken JH, Vandenbroucke JP, Sterk PJ. Clinical control and histopathologic outcome of asthma when using airway hyperresponsiveness as an additional guide to long-term treatment. The AMPUL Study Group. Am J Respir Crit Care Med 1999; 159(4 Pt 1): 1043–1051.
111. Chakir J, Shannon J, Molet S, et al. Airway remodeling-associated mediators in moderate to severe asthma: effect of steroids on TGF-beta, IL-11, IL-17, and type I and type III collagen expression. J Allergy Clin Immunol 2003; 111:1293–1298.
112. Orsida BE, Ward C, Li X, et al. Effect of a long-acting beta2-agonist over three months on airway wall vascular remodeling in asthma. Am J Respir Crit Care Med 2001; 164(1):117–121.
113. Henderson WR Jr, Tang LO, Chu SJ, et al. A role for cysteinyl leukotrienes in airway remodeling in a mouse asthma model. Am J Respir Crit Care Med 2002; 165:108–116.
114. Billington CK, Joseph SK, Swan C, Scott MG, Jobson TM, Hall IP. Modulation of human airway smooth muscle proliferation by type 3 phosphodiesterase inhibition. Am J Physiol 1999; 276:L412–L419.
115. Flood-Page P, Menzies-Gow A, Phipps S, et al. Anti-IL-5 treatment reduces deposition of ECM proteins in the bronchial subepithelial basement membrane of mild atopic asthmatics. J Clin Invest 2003; 112:1029–1036.
116. Zimmermann N, King NE, Laporte J, et al. Dissection of experimental asthma with DNA microarray analysis identifies arginase in asthma pathogenesis. J Clin Invest 2003; 111:1863–1874.

117. Endo M, Oyadomari S, Terasaki Y, et al. Induction of arginase I and II in bleomycin-induced fibrosis of mouse lung. Am J Physiol Lung Cell Mol Physiol 2003; 285:L313–L321.

118. Meurs H, McKay S, Maarsingh H, et al. Increased arginase activity underlies allergen-induced deficiency of cNOS-derived nitric oxide and airway hyper-responsiveness. Br J Pharmacol 2002; 136:391–398.

119. Meurs H, Maarsingh H, Zaagsma J. Arginase and asthma: novel insights into nitric oxide homeostasis and airway hyperresponsiveness. Trends Pharmacol Sci 2003; 24(9):450–455.

120. Vercelli D. Arginase: marker, effector, or candidate gene for asthma? J Clin Invest 2003; 111(12):1815–1817.

121. Van Eerdewegh P, Little RD, Dupuis J, et al. Association of the ADAM33 gene with asthma and bronchial hyperresponsiveness. Nature 2002; 418: 426–430.

122. Garlisi CG, Zou J, Devito KE, et al. Human ADAM33: protein maturation and localization. Biochem Biophys Res Commun 2003; 301:35–43.

123. Umland SP, Garlisi CG, Shah H, et al. Human ADAM33 messenger RNA expression profile and post-transcriptional regulation. Am J Respir Cell Mol Biol 2003; 29(5):571–582.

124. Zou J, Zhu F, Liu J, et al. Catalytic activity of human ADAM33. (A disintegrin and metalloproteinase). J Biol Chem 2003; 279:9818–9830.

125. Primakoff P, Myles DG. The ADAM gene family: surface proteins with adhesion and protease activity. Trends Genet 2000; 16(2):83–87.

126. Chae SC, Yoon KH, Chung HT. Identification of novel polymorphisms in the Adam33 gene. J Hum Genet 2003; 48:278–281.

127. Howard TD, Postma DS, Jongepier H, et al. Association of a disintegrin and metalloprotease 33 (ADAM33) gene with asthma in ethnically diverse populations. J Allergy Clin Immunol 2003; 112:717–722.

128. Lind DL, Choudhry S, Ung N, et al. ADAM33 is Not Associated with Asthma in Puerto Rican or Mexican Populations. Am J Respir Crit Care Med 2003; 168:1312–1316.

129. Ikeda K, Nakajima H, Suzuki K, et al. Mast cells produce interleukin-25 upon Fc epsilon RI-mediated activation. Blood 2003; 101(9):3594–3596.

130. Fort MM, Cheung J, Yen D, et al. IL-25 induces IL-4, IL-5, and IL-13 and Th2-associated pathologies in vivo. Immunity 2001; 15(6):985–995.

131. Hurst SD, Muchamuel T, Gorman DM, et al. New IL-17 family members promote Th1 or Th2 responses in the lung: in vivo function of the novel cytokine IL-25. J Immunol 2002; 169:443–453.

5

Asthma in Children and Adults—Natural Course of the Disease

RONINA COVAR and JOSEPH D. SPAHN

Department of Pediatrics, Divisions of Clinical Pharmacology and
  Allergy-Clinical Immunology, Ira J. and Jacqueline Neimark Laboratory of Clinical
  Pharmacology in Pediatrics, National Jewish Medical and Research Center, and
  University of Colorado Health Sciences Center
Denver, Colorado, U.S.A.

I. Introduction

Asthma is the most common chronic disease in childhood. According to the latest report from the National Center for Health Statistics, in 2001, of 31.1 million people who had ever been diagnosed with asthma during their lifetime, 9.2 million were children less than 18 years old (1). The annual prevalence of an episode of asthma during the 12 months in children younger than 15 years of age is approximately 100/1000 populations. The rate of current asthma prevalence for children younger than 18 is 87/1000 compared to 69/1000 adults. These statistics would suggest that a considerable number of patients who develop asthma in childhood "outgrow" the disease.

Epidemiologic cohort studies provide us with critical information on the natural history of asthma. Although they give us a wealth of information on the pattern of asthma, they have inherent limitations. First, we do not have a standardized definition of asthma. Second, we do not have readily available, non-invasive measures of airway inflammation. Third, we cannot readily measure lung function in children less than five years of age, and as such cannot quantify disease severity in young children based on airflow obstruction.

Lastly, the existing cohort studies do not control for the impact asthma controller therapy has on the pathogenesis and natural history of asthma.

Table 1 summarizes the main findings of several of the important epidemiologic studies that we will discuss in this chapter. It describes the design, the cohort studied (i.e., birth versus school age), the purpose, and major findings, in addition to the strengths and weaknesses of the studies.

This review will focus on our current understanding of the natural history of asthma by addressing a number of important questions including: Do all infants and toddlers with recurrent wheezing proceed to develop persistent asthma? Can a child "outgrow" asthma? And if so, who is likely to outgrow asthma? Does asthma follow a uniform pattern over time? In other words, will the mild always be mild and the severe always be severe? Can the development and persistence of asthma be predicted? And lastly, are there phenotypic differences in patients with early-onset (in childhood) and late-onset (in adulthood) asthma?

II. Question #1: Will All Young Children with Recurrent Wheezing Proceed to Have Asthma?

To best understand the natural history of asthma, cohort studies that enroll children at birth are among the most helpful. Among the difficulties of determining the prevalence of asthma in the first years of life, is the difficulty in making the diagnosis of asthma in this age group due to a multitude of other conditions that mimic asthma presentation. What is clear from the large population-based studies is that recurrent wheezing in infants and young children is quite common and comprises a heterogeneous group of conditions with different risk factors and prognoses (Table 1). For example, a population-based study of preschool children (mean age of 3.0 years) from Leicestershire, England compared children with a history of a wheeze and a randomly selected group of asymptomatic children, over a two-to-four-year period (2). Almost 50% of those with a history of earlier wheeze were symptom-free, and 7% of the asymptomatic group now reported current wheeze.

Of interest, the children with "recent wheeze" were likely to be atopic, while the children with persistent wheezing had the greatest degree of bronchial reactivity and lowest lung function at follow-up.

Martinez et al. enrolled over 1200 newborns whose health care was served by a large health maintenance organization in Tucson, Arizona to evaluate the natural history of wheezing in the first six years of life (3). At six years of age, almost half of the children had reported at least one episode of wheezing. Several different wheezing phenotypes were observed (Table 2). Twenty percent were thought to have "transient wheezing." These children had at least one episode of wheezing during the first three years of life, but were no longer wheezing by six years. Children with

Table 1 Cohort Studies and the Natural Course of Asthma in Childhood

Cohort type/site/important publications	Start of study collection and duration of follow-up and number	Purpose/key findings	Strengths	Weaknesses
Birth Tucson, AZ, USA, HMO clinic population (3), Taussig et al., J Allergy Clin Immunol 2003; 111:661–675.	1980 (n = 1246) 6-year follow-up 22-year follow-up	Aim: To investigate the interrelationships between potential risk factors, acute LRT illnesses in first 3 years of life, and the development of chronic lung disorders, especially asthma. Description of distinct wheezing phenotypes during childhood & identification of risk factors for each phenotype	Large cohort, outpatient population Extensive data collection relating to a large number of risk factors Lung function measures Immunologic, allergic, microbiologic and serologic parameters Long follow-up period with excellent retention rate	Identified heterogeneous wheezing subtypes, which are arbitrarily based on age-defined criteria
Birth UK (14)	Birth cohort British National Child Development Study—all children born March 3–6, 1958 18,559, complete data on 5801. Interviews at 7, 11, 16, 23, and 33 years	Aim: Describe the incidence and prognosis of asthma from birth to 33 years. Cumulative incidence of wheezing 18% by 7, 24% by 16, 43% by 33 years 25% of children who wheezed by 7 years reported wheeze at 33 years. Relapse occurred in 13% before 33 years and 15% at 33 years.	Huge population studied Several evaluations over 33 years Information on incidence and prognosis of asthma from childhood to adulthood	Only 31% of original birth cohort with complete data No objective measures of lung function, atopy, or BHR
Birth New Zealand (24, 40)	Birth cohort born 1972, 1973 1037/1139 participated in first assessment at	Aim: To determine the outcome of childhood asthma. 25% unselected cohort had wheezing that persisted from childhood to	Frequency of and extent of evaluation with: spirometry at 9, 11, 13, 15, 18, 21, and 26 years	Population-based, majority of asthmatics mild, follow-up too soon

(Continued)

Table 1 Cohort Studies and the Natural Course of Asthma in Childhood (*Continued*)

Cohort type/site/ important publications	Start of study collection and duration of follow-up and number	Purpose/key findings	Strengths	Weaknesses
	age 3 years 613/1037 complete data at 26 years	adulthood or that relapsed after remission. Risk factors for persistence: female sex, BHR, sensitization to HDM. Risk factors relapse: BHR, earlier age of onset, sensitization to HDM	Methacholine challenges at 9, 11, 13, 15, 21, SPTs at 13 and 21 years, Serum IgE at 11 and 21 years	to determine frequency of relapse, and adult-onset disease Initial lung function measurement performed too late to detect loss of lung function in early childhood
School-age Melbourne (15)	1964–1999 1964 (n = 401; 106 never wheezed and 295 wheezing history) 35-year follow-up (age 42)	Original aim: To determine the prevalence and natural history of asthma and wheezy bronchitis in children By 42 years: one death from asthma, 60% of the original wheezy bronchitis group were free of wheeze, 5% of those with wheezy bronchitis had persistent asthma. 70% of original asthma group & 90% of the severe asthma group had ongoing symptoms. Subjects in the no-recent asthma and persistent asthma groups were likely to be in the same group at subsequent review.	Longest community-based longitudinal study, 87% retention after 35 years of follow-up Physiologic assessment included lung function tests, skin test, and provocation challenges in adulthood (exercise at 21, methacholine at 28, and histamine at age 35 and 42 years).	Classification of asthma changed multiple times during the study, at time of study onset, inhaled GCs unavailable–thus no insight into effect of anti-inflammatory medications on progression Initial classification relied on maternal recall, and was based on parental

Study	Design/Subjects	Aim/Findings	Methods	Comments
		Subjects with mild wheezy bronchitis as children or with no recent asthma/infrequent asthma had normal FEV$_1$, FEV$_1$/FVC. Subjects in the original asthma groups or those with frequent or persistent asthma at review had airflow obstruction. Loss of lung function in the severe asthma group evident by age 14. The difference between severe and mild asthma groups did not increase over time		report of audible wheezing, small control group in which development of asthma after 7 years of age could be evaluated
School-age Netherlands Grol et al., Am J Respir Crit Care Med 1999;160: 1830–1837	1966–1969 119 children with allergic asthma from outpatient pulmonary clinic 30-year follow-up	Aim: To determine the outcome of childhood asthma Low FEV$_1$ and BHR predict low lung function in adulthood. Emphasizes importance of early intervention with anti-inflammatory agents.	30 year follow-up of children with asthma Extensive evaluation including: spirometry, TEC, serum IgE ± SPTs Histamine challenges	Small number of subjects Only three evaluations over 30 years
School-age Belmont, Australia Xuan W, et al., Thorax 2002; 57:104–109.	1982: 718 8–10 years old enrolled (51% male) Of the cohort of 718 subjects, 498 participated in two or more surveys between 1996 and 1997	Aim: To examine the onset and remission of atopy/asthma and to identify risk factors that influence the onset and progression of atopy/asthma during adolescence and young adulthood The proportions of subjects with late-onset wheeze (12.4% vs. 5.6%) and atopy (13.7% vs. 3.2%) was greater than the remission rates, respectively.	Atopy, BHR, and wheeze in the last 12 months were measured at each survey	Arbitrary definition of never, intermittent, late-onset, remission and persistent wheeze, BHR, and atopy based on initial and follow-up surveys

(*Continued*)

Table 1 Cohort Studies and the Natural Course of Asthma in Childhood (*Continued*)

Cohort type/site/ important publications	Start of study collection and duration of follow-up and number	Purpose/key findings	Strengths	Weaknesses
		Children with mod-severe BHR at 8–10 were likely to have BHR and respiratory symptoms requiring asthma medications in adolescence.		
		Risk factors for recent wheeze: atopy at age 8–12 years (OR 2.8); parental asthma (OR 2.1)		
		Risk factors for persistent wheeze: BHR at 8–12 years (OR 4.3)		
		Risk factor for late onset BHR: female gender (OR 1.9) risk factor for late-onset atopy: male gender (OR 1.9) the onset of BHR after 12 years was rare, but more likely in those with atopy at an early age		
		Atopy at age 8–10 years predicts the subsequent onset of wheeze.		

Abbreviations: **BHR**, bronchial hyperresponsiveness; **OR**, odds ratio; **GC**, glucocorticoid.

Table 2 History of Wheezing in Children during the First 6 Years of Life

Group	Definition	Percentage of study population ($n = 1200$)
Transient wheezers	At least one episode <3 years of age, but not wheezing at 6 years	20%
Late-onset wheezers	No wheezing <3 years of age, but wheezing at 6 years	15%
Persistent wheezers	Wheezing before 3 years of age and at 6 years of age	14%
Total	Any history of wheezing	49%

Source: From Ref. 3.

late-onset wheeze comprised 15% of the cohort. These children did not wheeze during the first three years of life, but had wheezing by six years. Those with persistent wheezing accounted for 14% and had wheezing before three years, which persisted at six years. Thus, only a minority of children who wheezed with viral respiratory tract infections during the first three years of life went on to develop asthma. The transient wheezers had diminished airway function in infancy, were less likely to be atopic, and had a history of maternal smoking. In contrast, the persistent wheezers were more likely to have a positive maternal history of asthma, elevated serum IgE levels' and diminished lung function at six years. The late-onset wheezers had a similar percentage of atopic children compared to persistent wheezers and were also likely to have mothers with asthma.

The prevalence of persistent wheezing varies depending on the cohort studied, as illustrated by a study from Delacourt et al. (4), who enrolled 129 children from a large hospital-based pediatric pulmonary clinic with history of wheezing before age two. The investigators found that 38% of these children were still wheezing four years later. A family history of atopy was associated with a higher risk of persistent wheezing.

In addition, 50% of persistent wheezers were atopic compared with 24% of all other children and 13% of asymptomatic children. Persistent wheezers had the lowest lung function [Vmax funtional residual capacity (FRC)] measured at mean age of 17 months compared to the intermittent wheezers, coughers, and asymptomatic children. This is in contrast to the Martinez study that showed compromised lung function in the transient wheezers, demonstrating that lung function abnormalities may not reliably predict which children will go on to develop persistent asthma.

From the previous studies we can conclude that not all infants and small children with recurrent wheezing will go on to develop asthma. In fact, less than 50% of children with early-onset wheezing will go on to develop asthma. This is important in that only those children at risk for subsequent asthma are likely to benefit from asthma controller therapy. At present, atopy appears to be the only consistent risk factor for subsequent asthma. There appears to be a similar genetic predisposition for the asthma phenotype characterizing both persistent and late-onset wheezers. Although these reports suggest the coexistence of different "phenotypes," it remains to be determined whether the late-onset wheezers are a distinct group from the persistent wheezers.

III. Question #2: Do Children "Outgrow" Their Asthma?

While there are only a few birth cohort studies available, there are a number of retrospective and prospective cohort studies that sought to evaluate the natural history of asthma from school-age children to adulthood. Depending on the population under study, the percentage of asthmatic children who undergo clinical remission ranges from less than 10% to over 70% (Table 3). For instance, in a population followed at a specialty clinic and a population pre-identified to have risk factors such as atopy, the rate of "outgrowing" asthma is much lower since these likely represent either a more severe or less heterogeneous population.

From an original group of 85 asthmatic children aged 5 to 15 years referred to the Allergy Clinic at the National University Hospital in Copenhagen, 70 subjects were re-evaluated after 10–12 years to determine the outcome in children with intrinsic ($n = 24$) or extrinsic asthma ($n = 46$) (5). Persistent asthma was found in 94% and 57% of females and males, respectively, with intrinsic asthma and in 82% and 92% of female and male extrinsic

Table 3 Remission Rates of Asthma in Children

Group	In remission at follow-up (%)	Notes
Asthma clinic cohort (5)	14	6% to 43% remission in subgroups by gender and "allergic" [intrinsic]/ "non-allergic" [extrinsic] asthma; 10- to 12-year follow-up
Early studies (before the development of current asthma medications) (6–10)	22–55	Studies took place >25 years ago; 14- to 31-year follow-up
Hospital-based cohorts (11,12)	28–57	20-year follow-up
Community-based cohorts		
Melbourne (13–16)	40–70	25- to 35-year follow-up
Dunedin (24)	27.4	26-year follow-up: subsequent relapse noted in 12.4

asthmatics. Over 85% had symptoms within the past year and 90% were on daily controller therapy.

Studies of asthmatic children followed in private clinics and hospitals from more than 25 years ago and prior to the use of currently available medications (6–10), reported as many as 22–55% of patients undergoing asthma remission with no asthma symptoms in early adulthood. Similar rates were found from recent hospital-based cohorts, in that 28–57% of school-aged children re-examined 20 years later were symptom-free (11,12). In general, higher "remission" rates were found in community-based studies, which have extended follow-up until adulthood. From these studies, the percentage of patients who undergo asthma remission ranges from 40% to 70% (13–16).

IV. Question #3: Does Asthma Follow a Uniform Pattern Over Time?

In 1964, the longest community-based longitudinal study from a 1957 birth cohort began; the most recent update from this cohort at age of 42 years was published in 2002 (15). From 30,000 seven-year-old school children in Melbourne, Australia, children were randomly selected and stratified to the following groups: mild wheezy bronchitis ($n = 74$; fewer than five episodes of wheezing associated with respiratory tract infection), wheezy bronchitis ($n = 104$; five or more episodes of wheezing associated with respiratory tract infections), asthma ($n = 113$; wheezing unassociated with respiratory tract infections), and controls ($n = 113$).

In 1967, 83 children with severe asthma (onset of symptoms before age three, persistent symptoms at 10 years of age, barrel chest deformity, reduction of FEV_1/FVC to 50% or less) were added to the cohort having been randomly selected from the same age stratum. At age 14, children were classified in five groups: A—no more than five episodes of wheezing before 14 years; B—more than five episodes but none within 12 months before; C—continuing history of episodic asthma for years, wheezed within 12 months; D—frequent or unremitting asthma; and control (no history of wheezing). At age 21, 331 children who had started to wheeze in childhood and a control group of 77 children were included in the analysis (17). The new classification is as follows: W—no recent asthma and no wheezing in the last three years' X—infrequent asthma or wheezing in the last three years' Y—frequent asthma or wheezing in the past three months of less than once per week' Z—persistent asthma or wheezing in the past three months of more than once per week.

Important findings from this study included: 55% of subjects who reported wheezing prior to seven years of age had no wheezing in adolescence, and remained wheeze-free at 21 years. Over half the subjects with infrequent wheezing in childhood (groups A and B) had not wheezed between 14 and 21 years of age. Forty percent with frequent wheezing in childhood (groups C and D) had no or infrequent wheezing between 14 and 21 years of age. Forty-five percent of subjects who had apparently ceased to wheeze at 14 years (groups A and B) had minor recurrences of wheezing between 14 and 21 years of age. Of those subjects who presented at age 14 with history of wheezing in the previous year (groups C and D), 60% and 80%, respectively, had frequent or persistent asthma by age 21. In other words, fewer than 20% of those with persistent symptoms in childhood (group D) had become totally wheeze-free during adolescence. About 20% of those who did not wheeze at age 14 reported wheezing by age 21. Of importance, patients with persistent wheezing at age 21 had significant lung function abnormalities, and those who had persistent wheezing at 28 years showed a greater deterioration in their lung function since age seven years (18). As of the last update at age 42, 87% of the original cohort who were still alive participated (15). This study showed that the majority of children with wheezy bronchitis at age seven had a benign course, with 60% having no asthma by adult life. In contrast, only 30% of those children who carried the diagnosis of asthma at age seven were wheeze-free at age 42, and 50% continued significant wheezing into adult life. In addition, the more severe the asthma was in childhood, the more likely symptoms continued into adulthood, with 80% of the severe asthma group continuing to have significant wheezing at age 42. In addition, less than 10% of the original severe asthma groups were wheeze-free at 42 years.

V. Question #4: Can We Predict Which Infants and Young Children Are Likely to Develop Persistent Asthma?

There are few studies that have sought to quantitate the likelihood of developing asthma. One such study came from Southampton General Hospital where 109 infants (mean age 10.9 months) with a history of wheeze within 12 weeks and at least one parent having a history of asthma or eczema and current allergen skin prick test reactivity were evaluated over a 12-month period to determine which factors or combination of factors will predict persistent asthma (19). Infants with their first episode of wheeze secondary to a presumed or established respiratory syncytial virus (RSV) bronchiolitis were excluded. The diagnosis of persistent asthma was based on the need for controller asthma medication upon completion of the 12-month follow-up period. Fifty percent of the children required a controller asthma medication. Using univariate logistic regression analysis, atopy, older age, and a history of atopy in both parents were risk factors for need for controller treatment (Table 4).

Using multivariate logistic regression and modeling techniques, the only risk factors were an increased age at presentation and elevated serum

Table 4 Risk Factors for Asthma That Persists into Childhood

Author	Study design	Factors that may predict persistent asthma
Clough et al. (19)	109 infants, mean age 11 months, recent history of wheeze, followed for 1 year	Using univariate analysis Atopy Older age at presentation History of atopy in both parents Using multivariate analysis Older age at presentation IL-2R concentration in serum
Castro-Rodriquez et al. (20)	1246 newborns, followed through age 13 years	*Stringent index* Frequent wheeze age 0–3 One major or two minor risk factors[a] *Loose index* Any wheezing during 0–3 years One major or two minor risk factors[a]
Sears et al. (24)	613 of original 1037 children with complete respiratory data; followed from 9 to 26 years	Sensitization to house dust mite (OR 2.18) Bronchial Hyperresponsiveness (OR 3.0) Female sex (OR 1.71) at age 21 years Smoking (OR 1.84) at age 21 years

[a]Major risk factors: Eczema or parental history of asthma; minor risk factors: eosinophilia, wheezing without colds, and allergic rhinitis

soluble IL-2R levels accounting for a positive predictive value of 76% and a negative predictive value of 92%. This study has many limitations including a short duration of follow-up, a small sample size, and inadequate diagnostic criteria for persistent asthma—that being need for controller medication. Another limitation for the application of this study is the fact that soluble IL-2R assays are not commercially available at present.

A clinically more useful study comes from the Tucson Children's Respiratory Study. The investigators sought to determine an asthma predictive index using a combination of clinical and easily available laboratory data to help identify pre-school age children at risk for developing persistent asthma (20). Information on parental asthma diagnosis and maternal smoking status was obtained at enrollment, while the child's history of asthma, wheezing, and physician-diagnosed allergic rhinitis or eczema was included in the surveys done at years 2, 3, 6, 8, 11, and 13. Blood eosinophil counts were obtained in infancy at mean age 10.9 ± 0.6 months. Two indices were chosen to classify the children (Table 4). The stringent index required recurrent wheezing in the first three years, plus one major (parental history of asthma or physician-diagnosed eczema) or two of three minor (eosinophilia, wheezing without colds, and allergic rhinitis) risk factors, while the loose index required any episode of wheezing in the first three years, plus one major or two of three minor risk factors. Information on 986 children was available to determine the loose index. Of these, 23.6% had a positive index with males more likely to have a positive index than females. Of the 1002 children with information for the stringent index, 6.3% had a positive index with males again more likely to have a positive index than females.

Children with a positive loose index were 2.6 to 5.5 times more likely to have active asthma some time during the school years than those with a negative index for the prediction of asthma. In contrast, risk of asthma increased to 4.3 to 9.8 times when the stringent criteria were used. Of note, 59% of children with a positive loose index, and 76% of those with a positive stringent index had active asthma at least once during their school years, while less than 5% of children with a negative stringent index had active asthma at any time between the ages of six and 13. The negative predictive values and specificity were consistently at or above 80% using either the "loose" or "stringent" indices at any of the school age year surveys. In other words, at least 90% of young children with a negative "loose" or "stringent" index did not develop "active asthma" in school age. The authors concluded that the subsequent development of asthma could be predicted with a reasonable degree of accuracy by using a simple, clinically based index (20).

VI. Question #5: Are There Risk Factors for Persistent Asthma from Childhood to Adulthood?

Several studies have provided important information on risk factors associated with persistence of asthma from childhood to adulthood. Jenkins et al. (13), from the Tasmania cohort study, reported that any of the following—being female [odds ratio (OR) 1.57], having a history of eczema (OR 1.45), parental asthma (OR 1.74), and childhood asthma symptoms (OR 1.59), especially if severe and with onset after two years of age, were significant independent risk factors for persistence of asthma into adulthood (13). In addition, female sex is an independent risk factor for bronchial hyperresponsiveness (BHR) in adulthood (21). A personal or family history of atopy is also a risk factor for current, late-onset, and persistent asthma symptoms (22). Symptom severity in childhood is also related to outcome in adulthood. Childhood lung function is also strongly associated with adult lung function (13,16), while socioeconomic status is associated with late-onset wheeze (22).

In children, it is important to identify with some accuracy who is at risk for the development of persistent asthma. Peat et al. (23) calculated the predictive accuracy of symptoms, BHR, and atopy in early life on later BHR, asthma, or wheeze from several cohort studies. In general, only 30–50% of individuals with asthma in early adulthood had experienced symptoms during childhood. In contrast, the sensitivity of BHR or atopy in childhood was about 50–70%, meaning that of the adults with persistent asthma, 50–70% had evidence of atopy or BHR in childhood. These tests have a higher true positive rate as markers of persistent asthma than symptom measurements (23). For a diagnosis of persistent asthma in early adulthood, the calculated likelihood ratios are much higher for atopy and higher still for BHR than symptoms of wheeze or asthma in early life.

A recent study, from Sears et al. (24), sought to evaluate risk factors associated with persistence of asthma from childhood to adulthood using the Dunedin Multidisciplinary Health and Development cohort study from New Zealand. Of the original 1037 members, 613 had complete respiratory data from the age of 9 to 26 years. The investigators found that nearly three-quarters (72.6%) of the cohort had reported wheezing on at least one occasion, while over one-half (51.4%) reported wheezing more than once. In addition, 14.5% had persistent wheezing from childhood to age 26 years, while 27.4% had a remission, and 12.4% had a remission followed by a relapse at 26 years. Risk factors for persistence of asthma included BHR (odds ratio 3.00), sensitization to dust mites (odds ratio 2.41), and female sex (odds ratio 1.71) (Table 3). Risk factors for relapse included BHR (OR 3.03), sensitization to dust mites (OR 2.18), and earlier age at asthma onset (OR 0.89 per year of increase in age at onset). Patients with persistent wheezing and those with relapse had lower lung function than those who never reported wheezing. Of importance, the loss of lung function in those with asthma had already occurred by the first lung function measurement at nine years of age (Fig. 1).

This study provides several important observations with respect to the natural history of asthma. First, it demonstrates that wheezing is a common occurrence in childhood. Second, the wheezing episodes are often mild and transient. Third, patients with persistent wheezing are more likely to have BHR, be sensitized to dust mites, and to be female. Fourth, those likely to have an asthma relapse are more likely to have BHR, to be sensitized to dust mites, and to have an earlier onset of wheezing. Fifth, loss of lung function in those with persistent wheezing occurred early in life as the impairment was present by nine years of age! Lastly, there did not appear to be progressive loss of lung function in those with persistent wheeze. This implies that not all asthmatics will have a progressive decline in lung function over time. It should be noted that the cohort studied had mild disease as reflected by a mean FEV_1 of 96.6% at 26 years in those with persistent wheezing. Whether the same conclusions can be drawn from patients with moderate or severe asthma is unknown.

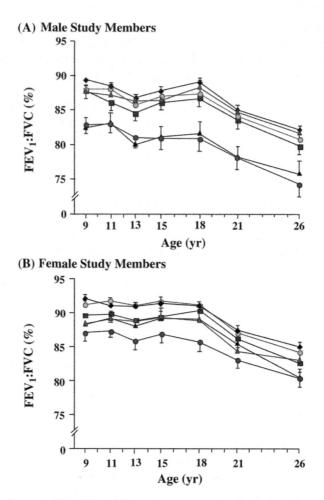

Figure 1 Mean (±SE) FEV$_1$:FVC ratios measured at 9, 11, 13, 15, 18, 21, and 26 years in males (panel A) and females (panel B) study members, according to pattern of wheezing. *Key*: ◆ No Wheezing Ever; ■ Intermittent Wheezing; ▲ Relapse; ○ Transient Wheezing; ▲ Remission; ● Persistent Wheezing. *Source*: Adapted from Ref. 24.

VII.   Question #6: Is Silent BHR a Risk Factor for Subsequent Asthma?

BHR is an essential feature of asthma, yet one can have BHR without respiratory symptoms. It is also known that asymptomatic or "silent" BHR is a risk factor for the subsequent development of asthma. Although several studies have shown associations between airway inflammation and BHR in patients with documented asthma, very little is known regarding the pathophysiology of silent BHR. In an intriguing study by Laprise et al. (25), 10 young adults with silent BHR, five of whom were atopic, were followed longitudinally over two years. Ten patients with mild asthma and ten non-asthmatics served as controls. All subjects underwent bronchoscopy with biopsy at baseline, while those with asymptomatic BHR had a repeat bronchoscopy after two years.

The subjects with asymptomatic BHR were similar to those with asthma in terms of their circulating eosinophil counts, serum IgE levels, baseline FEV_1, and degree of epithelial desquamation. Those with silent BHR differed from asthmatics in that their basement membranes showed areas of patchy fibrosis versus continuous thickening noted in the asthmatics. In addition, the asymptomatic BHR group had intermediate numbers of mucosal inflammatory cells (CD3, CD4, CD25, and EG2 cells) between those with asthma and the non-asthmatic controls.

Over the two-year study period, the FEV_1 tended to decline while BHR increased and serum IgE levels rose in those with asymptomatic BHR. In addition, four of the ten subjects with silent BHR went on to develop asthma. Those who developed asthma were atopic, had positive family histories of asthma, and were sensitized to and exposed to indoor allergens. In addition, their bronchial biopsies revealed increased basement membrane thickness and increased numbers of mucosal inflammatory cells, particularly CD25 and CD4 cells with a decrease in the number of CD8 cells.

This study suggests that airway inflammation is present in individuals with silent BHR at levels less than those associated with asthma. Second, progression of airway inflammation associated with airway remodeling occurred in subjects who went on to develop asthma. Third, the subjects who developed asthma were uniformly atopic, had positive family histories of asthma and were sensitized to and exposed to indoor allergens, suggesting that both genetic and environmental factors were required for the development of asthma. This study provides valuable insight into the natural history of asthma in that airway inflammation was evident in subjects with a "twitchy airway" but with no symptoms. It would appear as if a critical threshold in airway inflammation/remodeling must occur in subjects with silent BHR before the development of asthma. It also suggests that atopic individuals who are both sensitized to and exposed to perennial allergens are at greatest risk for crossing that threshold.

VIII. Question #7: Can We Predict Who Will Undergo an Asthma Remission?

The factors that determine whether a child with asthma will undergo remission have been investigated only to a limited degree. A random stratified cluster sample of children and adults from Arizona were followed up after nine years (26). Of the 2300 subjects, 136 had active asthma in the first survey with 22% of these individuals in remission at follow-up. The highest remission rate was found in adolescents with a remission rate of approximately 65% in subjects aged 10–19 years, while the lowest rate (6%) was seen in the 40–49-year-old group. The frequency and severity of wheeze and FEV_1 at initial survey were related to the remission rates. Although smoking appeared to have an effect on remission and relapse, this was found not to be statistically significant.

From a large cross-sectional study in Italy of over 18,000 subjects from 1998 to 2000, incidence and remission rates of asthma from birth to age 44 were determined (27). Subject was considered to be in remission if they did not require asthma treatment and had not experienced an asthma attack in the last 24 months. The overall remission rate was 45.8% (41.6% in women and 49.5% in men, $p < 0.001$). Of those who remitted, the last attack was on average 19 years before the interview. When adjusting for all the potential confounders, age at asthma onset was the main determinant of remission. Patients who underwent asthma remission had an earlier age at onset (7.4 vs. 15.9 years, $p < 0.001$) and a shorter duration of asthma (5.6 vs. 16.1 years, $p < 0.001$). The probability of remission was strongly ($p < 0.001$) and inversely related to the age at onset (62.8% and 15.0% in the <10 and ≥20 years age-at-onset groups, respectively). In addition, the likelihood of remission was quite high in the short term after onset (4–7 years), and decreased rapidly so that if the remission did not occur in the first years after the onset, the disease tended to persist. The minority of patients with early-onset asthma who do not remit represents more than 35% of patients with current asthma in the general young adult population.

IX. Question #8: Does the Lack of Symptoms Equate to Resolution of the Pathophysiologic Processes Associated with Asthma?

As previously discussed, many children with mild to moderate asthma will undergo a clinical remission of their asthma in their late adolescence and early adult lives. Previous studies have found individuals in a clinical remission to continue to have lung function abnormalities and heightened BHR. In addition, it is believed that a sizable number of these patients will have a relapse of their asthma later in their adult lives. What is not known is whether asthmatics in clinical remission have evidence for sub-clinical airway inflammation.

Van Den Toorn et al. (28,29) have published two provocative studies that suggest airway inflammation and remodeling persists in patients in asthma remission. In their first study (28), 20 young adults with asthma in clinical remission defined as having no symptoms for at least one year (median five years, range 1–12 years) were compared to 21 asthmatics and 18 non-asthmatic controls. Those in remission had significantly lower FEV_1 values compared to the controls (93% vs. 105% of predicted) while there was no difference in FEV_1 between those in remission and those with active asthma. In addition, patients in remission had elevated exhaled nitric oxide (eNo) levels compared to the controls, and had eNO levels similar to the asthmatics. Lastly, those in remission displayed an intermediate level of BHR compared to those with active asthma and the non-asthmatic controls. These data suggest that although these patients were in a clinical remission, they had evidence for airway inflammation as reflected by the lung function abnormalities, BHR, and elevated eNO levels.

In their second study, (29) the investigators attempted to more definitively address whether patients in remission had evidence for ongoing airway inflammation by performing endobronchial biopsies on 18 young adults in asthma remission, 19 young adults with asthma, and 17 non-asthmatic controls. Of little surprise based on their initial findings, the investigators found subjects whose asthma was in remission to have elevated numbers of T cells, eosinophils, mast cells, and elevated IL-5 levels compared to non-asthmatics. In addition, those in remission had thickening of the reticular basement membrane of similar magnitude as those with active asthma. These studies from Van Den Toorn clearly demonstrate physiologic (diminished lung function and presence of BHR) and histopathologic abnormalities (airway inflammatory infiltrate and thickening of the reticular basement membrane) in the absence of any active symptoms in patients with asthma in remission.

Several fundamental questions arise from the Van Den Toorn and Laprise studies. Why aren't these patients symptomatic? Patients studied by Van Den Toorn had asthma in clinical remission while the patients studied by Laprise had silent BHR. In both groups, the subjects had diminished lung function, BHR, and evidence for airway inflammation, yet they had no symptoms. Is there a critical threshold in airway inflammation that must be crossed for asthma symptoms to disappear or for that matter recur? Also, because they have evidence for sub-clinical inflammation, are these individuals at risk for subsequent relapse? And what can be gleaned from the Laprise study? Does a "threshold" of airway inflammation have to be crossed in subjects with silent BHR before they develop the disease we call asthma? These three studies clearly suggest that a certain amount of inflammation is required. In an asthmatic, if the inflammatory process diminishes past a certain level, that individual appears to undergo a clinical remission. On the other hand, in individuals with BHR but not asthma as inflammation passes that critical threshold, the individual becomes symptomatic and as such develops asthma.

X. Question #9: Are Children with Severe Asthma Different from Adults with Severe Asthma?

On the other end of the disease spectrum is severe asthma. Very little has been written regarding the clinical characteristics of severe childhood asthma, and even less is known whether severe asthma in childhood differs from that in adults. We sought to better understand these questions by evaluating 275 consecutive subjects referred to National Jewish Medical and Research Center for difficult-to-control asthma (30). The cohort consisted of 125 children and 150 adults. All of the subjects underwent a thorough evaluation including complete lung function studies, in addition to predniso-lone, pharmacokinetic study and lymphocyte stimulation assays in the presence and absence of glucocorticoids to evaluate for either diminished absorption or rapid metabolism of prednisolone or diminished glucocorticoid responsiveness in vitro. Children with severe asthma were as likely as their adult peers to have had a prior intubation, and to require high dose. inhaled glucocorticoid (GC) and chronically administered oral glucocorticoids but their daily requirement was smaller (19.2 vs. 32.9 mg/day), and they had required chronic oral GCs for a shorter period of time (2.3 vs. 5.3 years). Children were also more likely to be male (68% vs. 32%), and to have less lung function impairment as measured by FEV_1 (74% vs. 57.1% predicted), FEV_1/FVC ratio (72.5% vs. 66.9%), and Sgaw (44.2% vs. 64.4% predicted). In addition, prednisolone clearance was higher in children (220 vs. 189.4 ml/min/1.73 m^2) and they displayed significantly greater sensitivity to gluco-corticoids in vitro (log IC_{50} hydrocortisone 2.00 vs. 2.43 nM) than adults.

In summary, children with severe asthma had much less airflow obstruction and displayed greater responsiveness to glucocorticoids than their adult peers.

Of importance, even though the FEV_1 values were higher among the children than their adult peers, the slope of the decline in FEV_1 percent predicted per year of asthma duration was much steeper among the children than the adults (Fig. 2). This cross-sectional data in a cohort of severe asthmatics supports the findings of other studies that have noted that the decline in lung function in asthma may be greatest during childhood.

XI. Question #10: Are There Phenotypic Differences Between Adults with Early-Onset vs. Late-Onset Asthma?

In the past year, two studies have been published which sought to better understand the phenotypic differences between early-onset (childhood-onset) and late- or adult-onset asthma. Jenkins et al. (30) evaluated 150 adults who underwent an evaluation at National Jewish Medical and Research

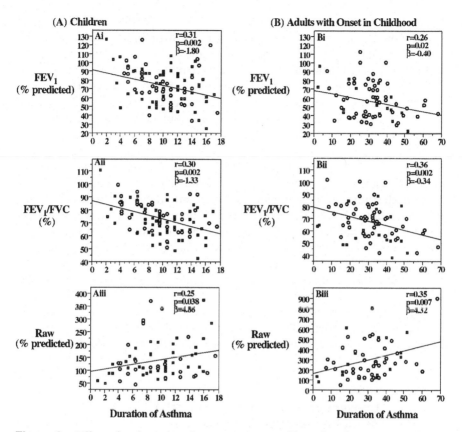

Figure 2 Effect of asthma duration on measures of lung function among children with severe asthma (A) and adults with onset of asthma in childhood (B). Figures Ai, Bi: The Y-axis is FEV_1 (% predicted), while the X-axis represents duration of asthma in years; figures Aii, Bii: The Y-axis represents the FEV_1/FVC ratio (%) while the X-axis represents duration of asthma in years; figures Aiii, Biii: The Y-axis represents Raw (% predicted) while the x-axis represents duration of asthma in years. Squares represent males, circles represent females. *Source*: From Jenkins et al. Chest 2003; 124: 1318–1324.

Center for poor asthma control over the past five years. Fifty-eight percent of the subjects had onset of asthma in childhood (early-onset), and they differed from adult-onset asthmatics in many ways. Childhood-onset asthmatics were younger (36.3 vs. 46.1 years old, $p = 0.0001$), had an earlier onset of asthma (5.2 vs. 35.4 years, $p = 0.0001$), and had a longer duration of asthma (31.0 vs. 11.0 years, $p = 0.0001$). Despite the much shorter duration of asthma, adult-onset asthmatics had similarly compromised lung function (FEV_1 58.2% vs. 56.3% predicted, $p = 0.59$; residual volume (RV) 204.3% vs. 191.2% predicted, $p = 0.47$; Sgaw 41.4% vs. 46.2% predicted, $p = 0.46$), were as likely to have had a prior intubation (31% vs. 25%, $p = 0.47$), displayed similar need for, and duration of, oral glucocorticoids (admission prednisolone dose 25.1 vs. 37.3 mg/day, $p = 0.24$; duration of prednisolone dependence 4.5 vs. 5.9 years, $p = 0.24$) as asthmatics with onset in childhood.

Miranda et al. (31), studied 80 adults—50 with early-onset and 30 with late-onset asthma—and found many of the same features. Their adults with early-onset asthma were younger and had an earlier onset of, and shorter duration of asthma compared to the adults with late-onset asthma.

Patients with early-onset asthma were more likely to be atopic, and had slightly less compromised FEV_1 values (56% vs 48% predicted, $p = 0.07$), and of some surprise, to have fewer airway eosinophils.

Both studies provide significant insight into the phenotypic differences between adults whose asthma began in childhood versus those whose asthma developed in adulthood. Both studies demonstrated that despite a much shorter duration of asthma among those with late-onset disease, lung function impairment was as great or worse than those with childhood asthma. This finding, and the greater amount of eosinophilic inflammation in those with late-onset disease, argue there may be two distinct forms of asthma. Differentiating asthma on the basis of disease onset has the potential to enhance our ability to isolate genetic differences, understand the pathophysiology, and ultimately improve our approach to treating patients with asthma.

XII. Question #11: Is Asthma Progression a Consequence of Airway Remodeling, Are All Asthmatics Affected, and Can Controller Medications Affect Disease Progression?

It may seem paradoxical that asthma on one hand is outgrown and on the other hand progressive. However, the concept of asthma as a progressive disease has been supported by recent findings of airway remodeling in endobronchial biopsy samples from both adult and pediatric asthmatics (32–34). In addition to pathologic evidence from the biopsy specimens, studies looking at lung function demonstrate asthma itself impacts attainment of peak lung growth in early adulthood and its subsequent decline (21,35,36). Roorda et al. have shown that FEV_1 in childhood impacts lung function in later years (21). A decline in lung function has already been shown to occur before age 18 in patients with asthma even prior to a steeper decline anticipated in adulthood. Results from the Coronary Artery Risk Development in Young Adults Study (CARDIA) study showed diagnosed and undiagnosed asthma prior to 18 years of age not only leads to lower peak FEV_1 values in early adulthood compared to a control healthy group, but also a more rapid rate of decline after 10 years (35).

In general and over time, asthmatics lose lung function at a greater rate than non-asthmatics. In children with asthma, the concern is that maximal lung or airway growth may not occur. As such, young adults with childhood-onset asthma may be starting out with diminished lung function, and thus at even greater risk of the development of significant airflow obstruction. Related to progressive loss of lung function is the concept of airway remodeling. The current paradigm states that chronic airway inflammation results in airway damage with an ongoing repair process that has been termed airway remodeling. The histologic features of a remodeled airway include basement membrane thickening, smooth muscle hyperplasia and hypertrophy, and goblet cell hyperplasia (Fig. 3). Many believe that these structural changes are associated with the progressive loss of lung function and the development of fixed airflow obstruction over time. Although a few studies have demonstrated associations between basement membrane thickness and lung function impairment (37), others have not (38). It is clear that airway remodeling occurs in asthmaitics (39) and can be present in children with severe asthma (30,32).

A recent study sought to evaluate risk factors associated with airway remodeling in a birth cohort studied longitudinally to 26 years (40). For this study, the investigators chose to use a low post-bronchodilator FEV_1/FVC ratio (-1.96 SD from the mean) as their measure of airway remodeling. Low ratios were seen in 7.4% and 6.4% of the subjects at 18 and 26 years while 4.6% had low ratios at both ages. Among asthmatics, 25% of males had persistently low ratios while 10% of females did. Risk factors for a low ratio included male sex, asthma, BHR, and low lung function in childhood. Subjects with a low ratio also had a more rapid decline in FEV_1 and FEV_1/FVC ratio from age 9 to 26 years, and they had become less responsive to β-agonists at 26 years. Inhaled glucocorticoid was used in a greater percentage among those with a diminished ratio (56% vs. 34%) compared to those with a normal ratio.

Of importance, the slope of decline in the FEV_1/FVC ratio was greatest in the first 18 years of life. Lastly, lung function appeared to track with age. Children with low lung function at 9 years were likely to have persistently low lung function.

This study suggests that clinically relevant airway remodeling does not occur in all patients with asthma. Approximately 25% of males and 10% of females with asthma developed airway remodeling. Thus, this process is not occurring in any functional way in the majority of asthmatics enrolled in a population-based study. Second, children with low lung function appeared to be at greatest risk of developing airway remodeling, and the steepest decline in the FEV_1/FVC ratio occurred in childhood. This reinforces the need for early intervention with the goal to prevent the development of airway remodeling. Third, airway remodeling and loss of β-agonist reversibility occurred despite inhaled glucocorticoid therapy. The investigators

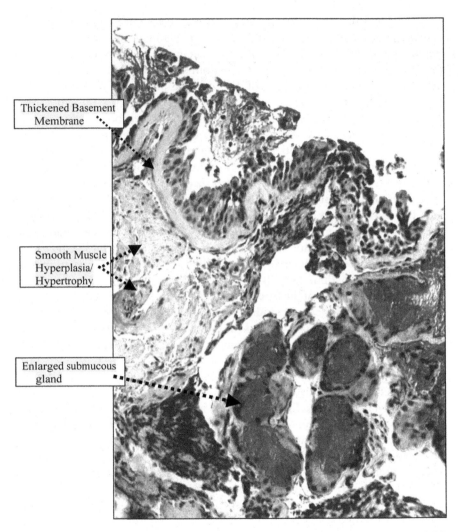

Figure 3 Endobronchial biopsy from a nine-year-old male with severe asthma. This Pentachrome stained slide (20x) demonstrates a greatly thickened basement membrane, massive smooth muscle hypertrophy, and goblet cell hyperplasia. In addition, a large submucous gland was noted as was mucus lining the epithelium. Minimal airway inflammation was noted with no eosinophils, neutrophils and only scanty patches of submucosal lymphocytes seen. *Source*: From Ref. 33.

also state that "at present, there is no direct evidence to demonstrate that early use of anti-inflammatory therapy will reduce the persistence of airway inflammation or prevent airway remodeling." This may be a result of the population of asthmatics studied—older children and adults. If we are to intervene, it must be early—as in the first couple years of disease onset!

Young children with recurrent wheezing and risk factors for persistent asthma such as a parent with asthma or the presence of eczema are obvious candidates for early intervention with long-term controller therapy. The National Heart, Lung, and Blood Institute (NHLBI) is currently funding an early intervention study in young children with recurrent wheezing. The results of this landmark study are likely to be available in 2005.

XIII. Summary

Wheezing occurs frequently in infancy and early childhood, but it is often mild and transient. Less than 50% of children who have recurrent wheezing in the first three years of life go on to develop persistent asthma later in childhood. Factors linked to persistence of asthma into childhood include atopy, eczema, older age at presentation, asthma in either or both parents, elevated serum IL-2R levels, eosinophilia, wheezing without colds, and allergic rhinitis. Factors linked to persistence of asthma from childhood into adult life include BHR, sensitization to house dust mites, atopy, female gender, parental asthma, and severe symptoms in childhood with onset after two years of age. Many children with asthma undergo a remission from their asthma in adolescence and early adulthood. Children likely to undergo remission are children diagnosed with asthma at a younger age, those with less frequent or less severe asthma, those with a normal FEV_1 at their initial visit, and males. Airway inflammation and subsequent airway remodeling are thought to contribute to disease progression over time, although there are few longitudinal studies that prove this paradigm. Whether any currently available asthma controller medication can prevent asthma progression or prevent or reverse airway remodeling remains an important but unresolved question.

References

1. National Center for Health Statistics Web Site. Health E-Stays—Asthma. Asthma prevalence, health care use and mortality, 2000–2001. Available at: http://www.cdc/nchs/products/pubs/pubd/hestats/asthma/asthma.htm.
2. Brooke AM, Lambert PC, Burton PR, Clarke C, Luyt DK, Simpson H. The natural history of respiratory symptoms in preschool children. Am J Respir Crit Care Med 1995; 152(6 Pt 1):1872–1878.
3. Martinez FD, Wright AL, Taussig LM, Holberg CJ, Halonen M, Morgan WJ. Asthma and wheezing in the first six years of life. The group health medical associates. N Engl J Med 1995; 332(3):133–138.
4. Delacourt C, Benoist MR, Waernessyckle S, Rufin P, Brouard JJ, de Blic J, Scheinmann P. Relationship between bronchial responsiveness and clinical evolution in infants who wheeze: a four-year prospective study. Am J Respir Crit Care Med 2001; 164(8 Pt 1):1382–1386.

5. Ulrik CS, Backer V, Dirksen A, Pedersen M, Koch C. Extrinsic and intrinsic asthma from childhood to adult age: a 10-yr follow-up. Respir Med 1995; 89:547–554.
6. Johnstone DE. A study of the natural history of bronchial asthma in children. Am J Dis Child 1968; 115(2):213–216.
7. Ryssing E, Flensborg EW. Prognosis after puberty for 442 asthmatic children examined and treated on specific allergologic principles. Acta Paediatr 1963; 52:97–105.
8. Buffum WP, Settipane GA. Prognosis of asthma in childhood. Am J Dis Child 1966; 112(3):214–217.
9. Blair H. Natural history of childhood asthma. 20-year follow-up. Arch Dis Child 1977; 52(8):613–619.
10. Rackemann FM, Edwards MC. Asthma in Childhood: a follow-up study of 688 patients after an interval of twenty years. N Engl J Med 1952; 246:815–863.
11. Gerritsen J, Koeter GH, Postma DS, Schouten JP, Knol K. Prognosis of asthma from childhood to adulthood. Am Rev Respir Dis 1989; 140: 1325–1330.
12. Kokkonen J, Linna O. The state of childhood asthma in young adulthood. Eur Resp J 1993; 6:657–661.
13. Jenkins MA, Hopper JL, Bowes G, Carlin JB, Flander LB, Giles GG. Factors in childhood as predictors of asthma in adult life. BMJ 1994; 309:90–93.
14. Strachan DP, Butland BK, Anderson HR. Incidence and prognosis of asthma and wheezing illness from early childhood to age 33 in a national British cohort. BMJ 1996; 312(7040):1195–1199.
15. Phelan PD, Robertson CF, Olinsky A. The Melbourne asthma study: 1964–1999. J All Clin Immunol 2002; 109(2):189–194.
16. Godden DJ, Ross S, Abdalla M, McMurray D, Douglas A, Oldman D, Friend JA, Legge JS, Douglas JG. Outcome of wheeze in childhood. Symptoms and pulmonary function 25 years later. Am J Respir Crit Care Med 1994; 149(1):106–112.
17. Martin AJ, McLennan LA, Landau LI, Phelan PD. The natural history of childhood asthma to adult life. Br Med J 1980; 280(6229):1397–1400.
18. Kelly WJ, Hudson I, Raven J, Phelan PD, Pain MC, Olinsky A. Childhood asthma and adult lung function. Am Rev Respir Dis 1988; 138(1):26–30.
19. Clough JB, Keeping KA, Edwards LC, Freeman WM, Warner JA, Warner JO. Can we predict which wheezy infants will continue to wheeze? Am J Respir Crit Care Med 1999; 160:1473–1480
20. Castro-Rodriguez JA, Holberg CJ, Wright AL, Martinez FD. A clinical index to define risk of asthma in young children with recurrent wheezing. Am J Respir Crit Care Med 2000; 162:1403–1406.
21. Roorda RJ, Gerritsen J, van Aalderen WMC, Schouten JP, Veltman JC, Weiss ST, Knol K. Follow-up of asthma from childhood to adulthood: influence of potential childhood risk factors on the outcome of pulmonary function and bronchial responsiveness in adulthood. J All Clin Immunol 1994; 93:575–584.
22. Withers NJ, Low L, Holgate ST, Clough JB. The natural history of respiratory symptoms in a cohort of adolescents. Am J Respir Crit Care Med 1998; 158:352–357.

23. Peat J, Toelle BG, Mellis CM. Problems and possibilities in understanding the natural history of asthma. J All Clin Immunol 2000; 106:S144–S152.
24. Sears MR, Greene JM, Willan AR, Wiecek EM, Taylor DR, Flannery EM, Cowan JO, Herbison GP, Silva PA, Poulton R. A longitudinal, population-based cohort of childhood asthma followed to adulthood. N Engl J Med 2003; 349:1414–1422.
25. Laprise C, Laviolette M, Boulet M, Boulet L-P. Asymptomatic airway hyper responsiveness: relationships with airway inflammation and remodeling. Eur Respir J 1999; 14:63–73.
26. Bronnimann S, Burrows B. A prospective study of the natural history of asthma: remission and relapse rates. Chest 1986; 90(4):480–484.
27. de Marco R, Locatelli F, Cerveri I, Bugiani M, Marinoni A, Giammanco G for the Italian Study on Asthma in Young Adults study group. Incidence and remission of asthma: a retrospective study on the natural history of asthma in Italy. J All Clin Immunol 2002; 110(2):228–235.
28. Van den Toorn LM, Prins J-B, Overbeek SE, Hoogsteden HC, De Jongste JC. Adolescents in clinical remission of atopic asthma have elevated exhaled nitric oxide levels and bronchial hyper responsiveness. Am J Respir Crit Care Med 2000; 162:953–957.
29. Van Den Toorn LM, Overbeek SE, DeJongste JC, Leman K, Hoogsteden HC, Prins J-B. Airway inflammation is present during clinical remission of atopic asthma. Am J Respir Crit Care Med 2001; 164:2107–2113.
30. Jenkins HA, Cherniack R, Szefler SJ, Covar R, Gelfand EW, Spahn JD. A comparison of the clinical characteristics of children and adults with severe asthma. Chest 2003; 124:1318–1324.
31. Miranda C, Busacker A, Balzar S, Trudeau J, Wenzel SE. Distinguishing severe asthma phenotypes: role of age at onset and eosinophilic inflammation. J All Clin Immunol 2004; 113:101–108.
32. Payne DNR, Rogers AV, Adelroth E, Bandi V, Guntupalli KK, Bush A, Jeffery PK. Early thickening of the reticular basement membrane in children with difficult asthma. Am J Respir Crit Care Med 2003; 167:78–82.
33. Jenkins HA, Cool C, Szefler SJ, Covar RA, Brugman S, Gelfand EW, Spahn JD. The histopathology of severe childhood asthma: a case series. Chest 2003; 124:32–41.
34. Ward C, Pais M, Bish R, Reid D, Feltis B, Johns D, Walters EH. Airway inflammation, basement membrane thickening, and bronchial hyper responsiveness in asthma. Thorax 2002; 57:309–316.
35. Apostol GG, Jacobs DR Jr, Tsai AW, Crow RS, Williams OD, Townsend MC, Beckett WS. Early life factors contribute to the decrease in lung function between ages 18 and 40: the coronary artery risk development in young adults study. Am J Respir Crit Care Med 2002; 166:166–172.
36. Lange P, Parner J, Vestbo J, Schnohr P, Jensen G. A 15-year follow-up study of ventilatory function in adults with asthma. N Engl J Med 1998; 339:1194–1200.
37. Chetta A, Foresi A, Del Donno M, et al. Bronchial responsiveness to distilled water and methacholine and its relationship to inflammation and remodeling of the airways in asthma. Am J Respir Crit Care Med 1996; 153:910–917.

38. Wenzel SE, Schwartz LB, Langmack EL, et al. Evidence that severe asthma can be divided pathologically into two inflammatory subtypes with distinct physiologic and clinical characteristics. Am J Respir Crit Care Med 1999; 160:1001–1008.
39. Chetta A, Foresi A, Del Donno M, et al. Airways remodeling is a distinctive feature of asthma and is related to severity of disease. Chest 1997; 111: 852–857.
40. Rasmussen F, Taylor DR, Flannery EM, JO Cowan, Greene JM, Herbison GP, Sears MR. Risk factors for airway remodeling in asthma manifested by a low post-bronchodilator FEV_1/vital capacity ratio: a longitudinal population study from childhood to adulthood. Am J Respir Crit Care Med 2002; 165: 1480–1488.

6

Growth and Development of the Child with Asthma

DAVID B. ALLEN

Professor of Pediatric Endocrinology and Residency Training,
    University of Wisconsin Children's Hospital
Madison, Wisconsin, U.S.A.

I. Introduction: Perspectives on Growth and Asthma

Normal childhood growth is a sensitive indicator of health, and there are few chronic diseases of childhood that do not adversely affect growth. Several mechanisms of growth suppression appear to be commonly involved in various diseases, although a clear understanding of which mechanisms are most important is still lacking. To evaluate the effects of any chronic disease on growth, three important aspects of the condition need to be considered: (1) how the natural history of the disease itself affects growth; (2) how medications required to treat the disease affect growth; (3) the clinical relevance of the growth effect—i.e., whether the growth impairment results in merely a delay in the normal tempo of growth with attainment of normal final height, or whether ultimate height is adversely affected.

The most common chronic disease of childhood is asthma, and various effects of asthma on growth have been described. However, the relative contributions to growth impairment of the disease process itself versus the medications required to treat the disease remain uncertain. Recently, attention has focused on the role of corticosteroids as both the most effective treatments for persistent asthma as well as likely growth suppressing agents.

This chapter will discuss normal physiology of growth during childhood, pathophysiology of growth suppression by the disease of asthma, abnormalities in growth and development observed in children with asthma, effects of oral and inhaled corticosteroids and other asthma medications on growth, and the clinical relevance of an effect of severe asthma and its treatment on final adult height.

II. Normal Growth

Although first examination of a childhood growth curve may suggest a simple and rather linear process, the regulation of normal growth is complex and the variations in normal growth substantial. A conceptual model that identifies three major periods of growth aids in understanding the various factors involved in the control of growth (Fig. 1): infancy, childhood, and puberty (1). The infancy period (first 2–3 years of life) is characterized by the distinctive combination of rapid yet rapidly decelerating growth rates. Control of growth during this period is primarily by nutrition-dependent factors (e.g., insulin and insulin-like growth factors) that are also critical for normal intrauterine growth. Consequently, caloric deprivation during infancy has a more significant growth-retarding effect than during later childhood. This slowing of the normal tempo of growth is reflected in delay

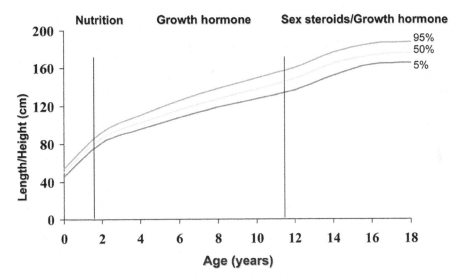

Figure 1 Phases of normal childhood growth (infancy-childhood-puberty) are depicted with the primary regulators of growth rate (nutrition-growth hormone-sex steroids plus growth hormone) during each phase.

in skeletal maturation. Conversely, overfeeding during this period can result in significant linear growth acceleration, which is accompanied by equal advancement in skeletal age.

During the early toddler years, a transition to dependency upon the endocrine system occurs, with the emergence of human growth hormone (GH) as the major growth-stimulating hormone. Accordingly, children who are severely GH-deficient typically experience failure of growth toward the end of the first year of life. The GH is secreted in pulsatile fashion from the anterior pituitary gland as a result of the interacting influences of hypothalamic growth hormone releasing hormone and somatostatin.

Two important observations regarding the childhood GH-dependent phase of growth are relevant to a discussion of influences of asthma on growth. First, the efficiency of the transition from the nutrition-dependent to GH-dependent phase of growth appears to vary among children, with some demonstrating excessive slowing of growth and downward crossing of percentiles on the growth curve usually between 15 and 30 months of age. Normal growth along this lower part of the growth curve usually resumes by three years of age, but the delay in body maturation which accompanies the growth delay results in late pubertal development (i.e., "late bloomers") and prolonged growth, with attainment of normal adult height. As discussed later, since chronic illness can slow the tempo of growth at any age, this pattern of growth delay is commonly observed in children with moderate to severe asthma. Second, the phase of childhood GH-dependent growth is marked by a gradual but consistent decline in growth rate, which reaches its nadir in the two to three years prior to puberty. In fact, provocative testing of GH secretion often reveals an apparent GH deficiency at this time. This waning resiliency of a child's growth axis may make the child unusually susceptible to growth-retarding effects of illness, medications, or psychological stress. Importantly, most studies of the effects of inhaled corticosteroids on growth in children with asthma have focused on children in the midst of this late childhood phase.

Sex steroids, particularly low serum concentrations of estrogen, stimulate the production and secretion of GH. Combined with growth promoting influences of rising levels of other hormones (insulin and androgens), these effects result in growth rate acceleration associated with puberty (2). Since growth plate maturation proceeds in the presence of sex steroids (particularly estrogen) even when growth rates are reduced by disease or medications, significant reductions in final height can occur if growth failure is not corrected promptly during adolescence.

III. Effects of Chronic Disease on Growth

Changes in endocrine function commonly occur during chronic illness. Although these changes represent an adaptation that benefits the individual in some way, the outcome in other systems (e.g., growth) is not always favorable. In general, endocrine adaptations to chronic illness reflect a reduction in either hypothalamic–pituitary output, peripheral conversion of hormones from inactive to more active forms, or development of some mechanism of peripheral hormone resistance that diminishes "nonessential" metabolic functions. As a result, growth, pubertal development, and peripheral thyroid hormone activity slow relatively early in the course of chronic illness, while adrenal function is maintained or even heightened (3).

Growth failure occurring during chronic illness can generally be attributed to factors related to both the primary illness and secondary disturbances in the endocrine growth axis (4). However, the mechanism through which asthma alone inhibits growth, and the relative importance of this effect, remains obscure. Physiologic stresses such as chronic hypoxia, infection, and poor nutritional status, thought to contribute to poor growth in children with cystic fibrosis, occur in only the most severe cases of intractable asthma. One attractive possibility is that a state of GH and insulin-like growth factor-1 (IGF-1) resistance develops during chronic illnesses such as severe asthma, which significantly reduces linear growth and other anabolic processes. Increased production of endogenous glucocorticoids observed during illness or stress has a direct inhibitory effect on protein synthesis in muscle and bone. In addition, protein degradation in chronic illnesses is enhanced by increased lysosomal activity and activity of the ubiquitin-proteasome pathway, mediated by the release of cytokines (5) and glucocorticoids (6), particularly in the midst of undernutrition (4).

Suppression of thyroid and gonadal function indirectly contributes to slowed growth during chronic illness by diminishing GH secretion and action. Illness-associated cytokines and glucocorticoids appear to exert suppressive effects on both central nervous system and peripheral control of these endocrine systems. For instance, preferential conversion of thyroxine (T4) to relatively inactive reverse triiodothyronine (rT3) rather than to the most active thyroid hormone, triiodothyronine (T3), occurs early and to varying degrees during chronic illnesses (7). Disruptions in the hypothalamic–pituitary-gonadal axis are commonly observed during illness, and are manifested by delayed or arrested pubertal development or, in females, menstrual abnormalities. While these compromises initially represent beneficial adaptations to stress, allowing diversion of limited metabolic resources to vital functions, long-term disruption of thyroid and sex steroid activity has important adverse consequences for linear growth, bone mineralization, and body composition.

Attention has recently turned to inflammatory cytokines as potential mediators of growth suppression during illness. In response to antigenic stimuli, a variety of cells secrete cytokines that are responsible for altering the host's metabolism. Three of these cytokines—tumor necrosis factor-α (TNF-α), interleukin-1 (IL-1), and interleukin-6 (IL-6)—have important neuroendocrine and metabolic effects (8). Each has been noted to stimulate muscle protein degradation and lipolysis, compromising anabolism and energy storage necessary for growth. Animal studies indicate that TNF-α, in particular, reduces food intake, increases cortisol secretion, and reduces growth hormone production when injected into the central nervous system (8). In children with cystic fibrosis, malnutrition and high levels of pro-inflammatory cytokines adversely affect IGF-1 production through interrelated mechanisms (9).

In vitro studies reveal that low concentrations of TNF-α create a state of IGF-1 resistance by impairing IGF-1-induced protein synthesis through reducing downstream activation signals of the IGF-1 receptor (10). Thus, there is substantial evidence that increased cytokine production due to immunological stress during childhood could inhibit growth directly (i.e., promoting catabolic responses) and indirectly (i.e., increasing cortisol and reducing growth hormone production).

IV. Effects of Severe Asthma on Growth

When compared with the general population, children with asthma have been reported to have mean heights and height velocities during childhood and adolescence that are less than children without asthma (11). Although it is well recognized that daily and alternate-day administration of glucocorticoids can impair growth, shorter stature for age has been observed in children with asthma who have not been treated with glucocorticoids (12–15). Mechanisms other than the effect of glucocorticoid treatment proposed to explain the impaired growth of children with asthma include chronic hypoxia, diminished lung function, chronic infection, undernutrition, sleep disturbance, and long-term stress (16–18). An assessment of the degree to which these factors may affect growth in the absence of glucocorticoid treatment depends upon early observations prior to the widespread use of glucocorticoid medications for asthma. One study revealed 77% of steroid-naïve children with severe asthma to be below the normal age-related mean for height, 30% were >1SD below the mean, and 8% were >2SD below the mean. By comparison, intermittent or continuous glucocorticoid treatment was associated with heights >2SD below the mean in 15% and 30% of children, respectively (11). Others have reported 74% of asthmatic children below the 50th percentile for height, 37% below the 25th, 27% below the 10th, and 7% below the third percentile (19).

Severity of growth retardation has been associated with early onset of asthma symptoms (i.e., before three years of age), disease severity sufficient to cause chronic hypoxemia, and poor nutrition (20). It is important to point out, however, that most children with mild to moderate persistent asthma do not experience growth retardation. This is verified by the normal heights and bone ages of children with asthma of this severity recruited into large prospective studies (21,22). Most convincingly, a cross-sectional study of 1041 children, 5 to 12 years old, with mild to moderate persistent asthma of four to seven-year duration, the mean ± SD height percentile was 56 + 28.5 percentile for the population (23). As expected, in more severely asthmatic children, a higher incidence of growth retardation is observed (24,25). One recent study, showed that only children with asthma in the lowest tertile for severity score showed a significant decrease in height SD score between ages 3 and 7.5 (26). Further, when children with asthma are separated according to disease severity, only the most severely affected group shows the development of a significant height deficit during adolescence (15).

Several explanations for the association between asthma and growth delay have been proposed, but none have been verified consistently. Reduced GH secretion has not been documented in slow-growing children with asthma (also receiving inhaled corticosteroids), even when markers of collagen synthesis were reduced (27). Alterations in thyroid hormone metabolism have been observed by some investigators (28) but not by others (17). Deficient nutrient intake was suggested by earlier reports (17,20), but not confirmed by more recent studies (29). Energy expenditure in asthmatic children was reportedly increased by 14% compared to healthy matched controls, but concomitant eczema or use of β-agonist medications may have been confounding factors (29).

The inability to identify mechanisms of asthma-related growth suppression most likely reflects failure to focus investigations on children with asthma of *sufficient severity to independently affect growth*. While such studies of severe asthma in the absence of glucocorticoid treatment are virtually impossible to ethically conduct today, information derived from children with cystic fibrosis are likely to be informative. That is, with disease of sufficient severity, cytokines and endogenous glucocorticoids released in response to chronic inflammation create an environment of GH resistance and reduced IGF-1 bioactivity, resulting in reduced protein synthesis and increased protein degradation (30).

Invariably, significant declines in height for age are accompanied by delayed skeletal maturation, indicating a slowing of the normal *tempo* of growth, but not necessarily a reduced long-term height prognosis. Relatively few data are available regarding the final height of individuals with asthma who did not receive glucocorticoid treatment. One study reported that final measured heights of 95 patients with asthma not treated with glucocorticoids differed negatively from mid-parental height by 4.8 ± 5.8 cm for females ($p = 0.18$) and 3.6 ± 6.0 cm for males ($p = 0.48$). However, in the unmatched analysis of this data set, mean height of patients with asthma, after adjusting for sex and mid-parental height, were not significantly different from a non-asthmatic comparison group (0.15 cm, $p = $ NS). Also, there was no difference in measured height between asthmatic subjects and matched non-asthmatic subjects (0.21 ± 9.42 cm, $p = 0.95$) (31). Reports of reduced final height of individuals with asthma tend to be confounded by prior long-term treatment with glucocorticoids (32). One exception is a recent study of adult height of women that grew up with asthma before inhaled corticosteroids became first-line therapy; compared with non-asthmatic women, girls with moderate to severe childhood asthma who grew up in this era attained 0.7–1.2 cm lower adult height (33).

In summary, while a delay in the growth process by severe asthma is well documented, it has not been shown that the disease of asthma itself, in the absence of glucocorticoid treatment, results in a clinically relevant reduced final height (31).

V. Effects of Asthma on Pubertal Development

Since the onset of puberty is more closely correlated with body maturation than with chronological age, delayed appearance of secondary sex characteristics is also observed more commonly in children with asthma (12). It is critical to account for this delayed growth pattern in assessing growth studies of children with asthma. As pointed out above, growth rates normally decline gradually throughout school-age years until pubertal growth acceleration occurs. Children experiencing a delayed growth pattern tend to show greater growth deceleration prior to puberty, and exaggerated disparities in growth rates compared with pubertal peers. Consequently, this pattern of delayed growth is often misinterpreted as disease- or medication-induced growth failure.

Because the prepubertal growth period in males is more prolonged compared to females, this period of growth slowing is often more pronounced in males and the susceptibility to further growth suppression by disease or medications enhanced. This difference between sexes in the normal tempo of growth and development is a likely explanation for observed variations in male and female sensitivity to growth suppression by asthma or medications. In most growth studies of peri-pubertal children with asthma, more pronounced growth deceleration is observed in males (34,35). On the other hand, one carefully designed study indicated that growth retardation observed in adolescent males with asthma was due to a delay in puberty but not to the prescription of 600 mcg of inhaled budesonide (BUD) daily (36). In most cases, although transient reductions in growth rate can result in detectable height differences between children with asthma and their peers, a more prolonged period of growth in the asthma group allows for "catch-up" and attainment of normal adult height appropriate for the subjects family (19,37).

VI. Effects of Glucocorticoids on Growth

Growth retardation is commonly experienced by children who receive long-term treatment with glucocorticoids (GC). While most disorders requiring such treatment are relatively rare, the expanding use of inhaled GC preparations for treatment of all degrees of persistent asthma has greatly increased the number of children chronically exposed to exogenous GC. Consequently, physicians today are likely to care for children treated with GC, and should be knowledgeable about potential growth effects of these medications.

The pathogenesis of growth suppression by GC is complex and multi-factorial, involving several steps in the cascade of events leading to linear growth (38) (Table 1). During childhood, the primary known mediator of epiphyseal growth and maturation is GH. Pulsatile, primarily nocturnal release of pituitary GH (39) occurs under the influence of interwoven hypothalamic stimulation (via growth-hormone-releasing hormone, GHRH) and inhibition (via somatostatin). In late childhood and adolescence, GH secretion is augmented by sex steroids produced by the adrenal glands and gonads. Growth-promoting effects of GH in epiphyseal cartilage occur both directly and indirectly through insulin-like-growth-factor-1 (IGF-1). Linear growth also requires synthesis of new type 1 collagen, which can be assessed through determination of blood levels of its precursor, type 1 procollagen.

Multiple catabolic effects of GC contribute to the profound impairment in linear growth associated with prolonged supra-physiologic GC therapy. Glucocorticoids interfere with nitrogen and mineral retention required for the growth process. Under the influence of GC excess, energy derived from protein catabolism is increased and the contribution from lipid oxidation is decreased (40).

This effect leads to characteristic changes in body habitus that are frequently associated with GC excess. Glucocorticoids inhibit bone formation directly (41), through inhibition of osteoblast function, and indirectly,

Table 1 Interference of Long-Term, High-Dose Glucocorticoid Treatment with the Integrity of the Somatrotropic Hormone Axis

Organ	Effect of Glucocorticoids
Hypothalamus	Somatostatin tone ↑
Hypophysis	GH secretion ↓
Liver	GH-induced IGF-1 mRNA ↓
Circulation	IGF-1 levels normal or ↑
	Induction of IGF-1 inhibitors
	IGFBP-2 ↑
Epiphyseal growth plate	Cell proliferation ↓
	Matrix production ↓
	Paracrine IGF-1 secretion ↓
	GH and type 1 IGF receptor ↓

by decreasing sex steroid secretion (in older children and adolescents). They also decrease intestinal calcium absorption (partially reversible with vitamin D therapy), increase urinary calcium excretion, and promote bone resorption due to secondary hyperparathyroidism. Osteopenia is particularly prominent in trabecular bone, such as the vertebrae (42). Skeletal maturation is delayed by long-term GC therapy. Particularly in GC-treated boys, suppression of bone age advancement may exceed that of height age advancement (13).

Glucocorticoids are capable of both inhibiting and stimulating endogenous GH secretion, an effect that arises from dichotomous action at the level of the pituitary and/or hypothalamus (Fig. 2). Cortisol facilitates pituitary GH synthesis by altering the affinity and density of pituitary GHRH receptors and interacting with a GC-responsive element on the GH gene (43). Thus, a minimum level of cortisol is essential for normal GH manufacture. Under conditions of eucortisolism, there is appropriate synthesis of GH as well as normal GHRH and somatostatin influence, resulting in the normal pulsatile release of GH. In the hypercortisolemic state, GH production is stimulated within the pituitary, but pulsatile release of GH is impaired, most likely through augmentation of hypothalamic somatostatin effect (44). Therefore, patterns of GH secretion in GC-treated

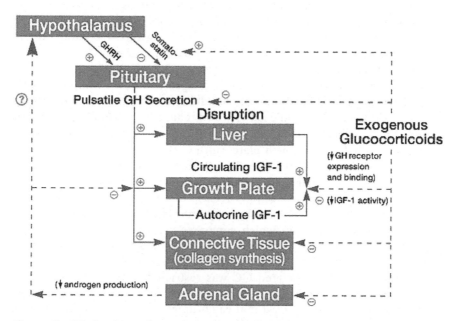

Figure 2 Mechanisms of growth suppression by glucocorticoids derived from both in vivo and in vitro studies. *Source*: From Ref. 38.

children can resemble "neurosecretory GH deficiency," where stimulated GH levels are normal, but spontaneous secretion of GH is subnormal (45). In the clinical setting, this attenuation of GH secretion associated with exposure to exogenous GC can be both rapid and profound (46).

In addition to altering GH output, GC reduce GH receptor expression and uncouple the receptors from their signal transduction mechanisms (47). Hepatic GH receptor binding and plasma levels of GH binding protein (GHBP) are markedly reduced in dose-dependent fashion by GC treatment, an effect accompanied by growth failure in treated animals (47). The GC also exert a depressive effect on rat liver GH receptor mRNA levels; this suppression can be partially reversed by co-treatment with estrogen or continuous exposure to GH. However, it is not clear that these effects on GH receptor synthesis and expression occur in non-liver tissues such as chondrocytes or muscle. However, circulating levels of GHBP, which are derived from the extra-cellular domain of the GH receptor, are reduced in GC-treated children compared with age-matched controls (48).

Levels of IGF-1 can be decreased, normal, or increased in GC-treated patients. Although GC do not consistently reduce circulating IGF-1 levels, they inhibit IGF bioactivity, possibly by increased production of IGF-1 inhibitors (49). IGF inhibitors, which have a molecular weight of 12–20 kDa and which clearly differ from IGF binding proteins, have been identified in in vitro investigations showing that cortisol increases IGF-1 inhibitor release by liver explants (50). Precise characterization of these "somatomedin inhibitors," however, remains elusive. Alterations in IGF binding proteins may also play a role; IGFBP-3, an IGF-1 binding protein thought to exert inhibitory effects on IGF-1 action, is increased in response to GC (51). Glucocorticoids also antagonize GH effects at target tissues by inhibiting chondrocyte mitosis and collagen synthesis. Studies of GC-treated rats show that inhibition of chondrocyte proliferation, diminishing of apoptosis, lower angiogenic activity, and reduced type II collagen mRNA expression contribute to the alterations in growth plate architecture and the significant reduction in growth plate width (52).

The GC also interferes directly with post-translational modifications of the precursor procollagen chains and increases collagen degradation (53).

Resumption of growth follows release of GC-induced growth inhibition. This "catch-up" growth has been hypothesized to result from a central nervous system mechanism which compares actual body size to an age-appropriated set point and adjusts growth rate accordingly (54). Recently, however, it was demonstrated that catch-up growth of a single growth plate exposed to locally administered GC was restricted to the affected growth plate, suggesting a mechanism intrinsic to the growth plate (55). While anecdotal reports often suggest that catch-up growth is complete, resulting in normal adult height, controlled studies of animals and humans indicate that growth deficits are often not fully compensated (56).

VII. Growth of Asthmatic Children Treated with Oral Glucocorticoids

The adverse effects of systemically administered GC on the growth of children with asthma have been well documented over the past 40 years (57). Dose, type of GC preparation, and timing of GC exposure each influence the degree of growth suppression observed. Large amounts of exogenous GC are not required for this adverse effect; relatively modest doses of prednisolone (3–5 mg/m^2/day) or hydrocortisone (12–15 mg/m^2/day) can impair growth, particularly in prepubertal children (57,58). Alternate day GC therapy reduces, but does not eliminate, the chances for growth failure. Children with asthma have reportedly received over 30 mg of prednisolone (mean 41.8 ± 3.9 mg/day) every other day for 6 to 50 months without experiencing growth suppression (59). However, in other more closely monitored studies, alternate-day doses of prednisolone above 15 mg cause slowed growth velocity in many patients and resumption of normal growth was not observed when children with existing growth failure were switched from daily to alternate-day prednisolone treatment (60).

Growth-retarding effects of prednisolone are greater than that of (equivalent doses of) hydrocortisone, most likely due to a comparatively longer half-life and sustained plasma concentration of prednisolone.

The effects of oral GC therapy on final adult height have been variable, most likely reflecting variations in dose, compliance, length of continuous exposure, and other individual factors. Most children treated with oral GC have severe underlying illness, making it difficult to distinguish growth effects of GC from those of the illness itself. However, in one study examining asthmatic children already growth suppressed prior to GC therapy, more growth delay was observed with GC therapy, with the severity of increased retardation correlated to the dose and duration of GC exposure (61). Children exposed to GC excess just prior to puberty may be particularly susceptible to growth suppression; childhood growth velocity is at its slowest and endogenous GH secretion is often transiently reduced during this period. Suppression of adrenal sex steroid secretion (adrenarche) by exogenous GC at this time may itself delay the activation of the hypothalamic–pituitary–gonadal axis and attenuate both the augmentation of GH release and direct growth stimulation by sex steroids normally observed in early puberty. Detrimental effects on final height, however, are more likely with GC treatment during puberty, since sex-hormone mediated growth plate maturation can occur in the midst of suppressed linear growth (62). While some studies demonstrate that short term (63) or intermittent (64) exposure to oral GC at supra-physiologic doses does not adversely affect final height, a meta-analysis of previous investigations found that long-term treatment of asthma with prednisolone was significantly correlated with adult height reduction (65).

VIII. Growth of Asthmatic Children Treated with Inhaled Corticosteroids (ICS)

Inhaled corticosteroids (ICS) offer several advantages over oral GC in the treatment of asthma: delivery of high potency GC directly to the target site in high concentrations, reduced total dosage, and the opportunity for frequent dosing. Although physical properties shared by ICS (e.g., rapid inactivation of absorbed drug) increase the ratio of topical anti-inflammatory to systemic activity, questions remain about whether some pulmonary effects of inhaled steroids may result from systemic actions.

Adverse effects from ICS should be anticipated if daily systemic exposure exceeds normal endogenous cortisol production ($\sim$12 mg hydrocortisone equivalent/m^2/day) or if the pattern of drug bioavailability significantly disrupts normal diurnal hormonal rhythms. Systemic GC effect is determined not only by the amount of ICS delivered to the airway and absorbed into circulation, but also the binding affinity and plasma half-life of the corticosteroid, the drug's volume of distribution, the potency and half-lives of its metabolites, the patient's sensitivity to and metabolism of the medication, and newly described factors such as protein binding of the drug, the duration of GC contact with the cell, or the rate of rise in steroid concentration. Consequently, individual risk for adverse effects from ICS varies widely and is difficult to predict.

Systemic bioavailability of ICS results from a combination of oral (swallowed fraction) and lung components. Significant amounts of IC are absorbed unaltered into the circulation following inhalation, [e.g., $\sim$30% for budesonide (BUD) (66), $\sim$30% for flunisolide (FLU) (67)], and the amount of drug available for absorption into the pulmonary vasculature is influenced by delivery vehicle (e.g., deposition following dry powder inhalation exceeds pressurized metered-dose inhalation for BUD but is less for FP) and technique. The bioavailability of swallowed drug varies significantly: beclomethasone dipropionate (BDP) 40–60%, triamcinolone acetonide (TA) 20–22%, BUD 10–15% (68), and fluticasone propionate (FP) 1% (69). These differences in inactivation of swallowed drug (which exerts little or no therapeutic effect) appear to be critical in determining a drug's therapeutic effect versus systemic effect profile. Plasma half-lives of most ICS are brief (e.g., 1.5–2 hr) due primarily to extensive first pass hepatic metabolism. For some ICS (e.g., BUD), higher clearance rates and shorter plasma half-lives have been shown in children when compared with adults, suggesting an increase in the ratio between local and systemic side effects (70). Intrapulmonary metabolism of ICS is also variable: BDP differs from other ICS because it is metabolized to potent active metabolites in the lung, which prolong the half-life of "BDP-effect" ($\sim$15 hr) and account for most of the systemic GC effect of inhaled BDP (71). Ciclesonide, a newer ICS, is also a prodrug that requires activation in the lung before interacting with the receptor.

Properties that make ICS extremely potent might increase risk for adverse effects as well. Two such factors are relative binding affinity for the glucocorticoid receptor compared with dexamethasone (e.g., 8:1 for racemic BUD and 20:1 for FP) and increased lipophilicity, which allows increased deposition in the lung lipid compartment, prolonged occupancy of the glucocorticoid receptor, and extended terminal elimination half-life with greater steady state drug accumulation. The ranked order of lipophilicity among currently used ICS is FP > BDP > BUD > TA > FLU, with FP being threefold and 300-fold more lipophilic than BDP and BUD, respectively (72). That receptor pharmacokinetics and lipophilicity are predictive of drug pharmacodynamics and potency is supported by the observed approximate 2–3:1 ratio in corticosteroid potency between FP and BDP when compared mcg for mcg. However, precise comparison of different ICS remains confounded by complexities of determining the *clinical therapeutic equivalence* of each compound and its delivery system. For instance, BUD delivered by metered-dose inhaler approximates BDP in potency, while delivery of BUD by dry powder inhaler may compare mcg-for-mcg in GC effect with FP, presumably due to greater lung deposition of the drug (73).

Consequently, well-designed studies are needed to more accurately assess the GC therapeutic equivalence of various ICS as well as dosing strategies designed to minimize adverse effects. Because efficacy dose-response curves of ICS flatten out at moderate to high doses after initial steepness at relatively low doses, comparisons of IC-plus-delivery-system therapeutic potency require determination of "minimal effective dosage" by step-down dosing within the steep part of the dose–response curve (73). While manipulations such as these may further reduce the relatively low risk of growth failure by ICS (compared to oral GC therapy), individual variations in absorption, responsiveness, and metabolism of ICS will continue to place some patients at risk of toxicity, requiring ongoing vigilance by prescribing physicians.

Do inhaled corticosteroids impair growth? A critical analysis of this question is complicated by two central factors. First, children with chronic asthma frequently exhibit growth retardation, manifested primarily by delays in skeletal maturation and pubertal growth acceleration, in proportion to either treatment with GC or severity of pulmonary disease (25). Second, substantial pharmacodynamic differences exist between specific ICS, and results obtained by studying one should not be extrapolated to another. In addition, non-steroid asthma treatments (e.g., β2-receptor activation) may also inhibit the GH axis (74).

Although administering corticosteroids via inhalation is associated with fewer systemic effects compared to oral administration, the *potential* of ICS to retard growth is clearly documented (75). This observation, however, is derived primarily from studies of BDP, whereas emerging data regarding BUD and FP suggest that ICS effects on growth might be reduced by the enhanced hepatic inactivation of swallowed drug exhibited by these preparations.

Until recently, most studies of growth in asthmatic children treated with ICS have suffered from flaws in study design. These include lack of evaluation of pubertal status, inappropriate stratification of pubertal status by age alone, lack of an adequate untreated control group, lack of baseline growth rate data, and baseline differences in age and height between treatment groups. However, during the past several years, prospective and, in some cases, well-controlled studies have overcome these confounding factors. In each case, growth inhibition by BDP was demonstrated.

Several recent studies have utilized knemometry, a sensitive technique of measuring growth of the lower leg, to assess short-term effects of higher dose IC therapy on growth. Studies using this technique have revealed dose-dependent inhibition of short-term lower leg growth (76) and reduced levels of type 1 procollagen (but not IGF-1, IGFBP-3, or osteocalcin) during IC therapy >400 mcg/day, suggesting a primary role for effects on collagen turnover in IC-induced growth retardation (77). However, while accurate and reproducible, the predictive value of lower leg growth velocity determinations for either overall height velocity (78) or long-term future growth is poor (79). Consequently, proposed advantages of knemometry (e.g., shortened observation periods allowing for controlled and double-blinded studies) are essentially nullified by these constraints (80,81). Biochemical markers of growth also correlate poorly with total body linear growth over time. The predictive value of studies for assessing clinically relevant effects of ICS on growth becomes more substantial with increasing duration of study (82). Consequently, prospective intermediate to long-term assessment of total body growth has yielded the most credible information regarding effects of ICS on growth, and only these studies are discussed here.

Longer-term prospective analysis of the effect of ICS on growth is available predominantly for BDP and BUD, and to a lesser extent, FP. A randomized clinical trial comparing BDP with oral theophylline in children, ages 6 to 17 years, with mild to moderately severe asthma demonstrated reduced growth in the BDP-treated children (34). A subsequent prospective parallel-group study compared growth effects of BDP (400 μg daily via dry powder device) to placebo in 94 prepubertal children (aged 7–9 years) with mild asthma. Over the seven-month study period, mean growth rate was significantly lower in the BDP group (0.79 mm/week, $p > 0.001$) and catch-up growth did not occur during the four-month wash-out period (83). In another well-designed prospective and randomized study, growth was significantly slower in BDP-treated children compared to those treated with salmeterol, although asthma exacerbations were less frequent during ICS therapy (84). These findings were recently confirmed by a similar comparison of long-term controller medications, in which mean linear growth was 3.96 cm/year in children receiving BDP compared with 5.40 cm/year in the salmeterol-treated group (85). Discontinuation of BDP in one trial restored a normal, but not accelerated, growth rate (83), highlighting the inconsistent occurrence of catch-up growth after cessation of GC therapy and a possible dampening of a supra-normal growth recovery phase by persistent mild asthma. Taken together, these four prospective, controlled studies reveal a remarkably similar effect of uninterrupted administration of 400 µg/day of BDP on growth: a reduction of ~1.5 cm gain in height per year. In other words, it has been clearly shown that conventional dose treatment with inhaled BDP, administered without interruption, is *capable* of suppressing linear growth.

Variations in the metabolism and pharmacokinetics of ICS predict different degrees of pulmonary versus systemic effects, i.e., ICS that have greater first-pass inactivation by the liver (e.g., BUD and FP) would theoretically be expected to have a reduced effect on the growth axis for a given degree of airway anti-inflammatory effect. Several studies examining BUD in children with asthma have shown no adverse effects on growth.

In a large, controlled, prospective study, 216 children followed for one to two years while not receiving inhaled BUD and then for three to six years while receiving inhaled BUD (mean daily dosage decreased from 710–430 µg over the course of the study) showed no significant changes in growth velocity (86). While this and other studies (87) provide reassurance regarding the "real world" experience with BUD, their conclusions are weakened by lack of control subjects, variations in dosage and delivery device, and poor documentation of consistency of drug administration.

One randomized, double-blind study examined 40 asthmatic adolescents (mean age 12.8 years) receiving salbutamol 600 µg daily and inhaled BUD 600 µg daily or placebo for a median period of 22 months. Growth rates were matched with those of 80 controls. Budesonide treatment was not associated with a significant effect on growth velocity compared to placebo. Interestingly, males treated with either BUD or placebo showed similar slowing of growth rates compared with controls, pointing again to a likely confounding effect of delayed puberty in the analysis of growth of children with asthma (36). With regard to FP, a double-blind, randomized, parallel-group multicenter study prospectively examined growth in 325 prepubescent children with persistent asthma treated with placebo or FP powder 50 µg or 100 µg administered twice daily. Over a period of one year, there was no significant difference in mean height increase (6.15 cm in the placebo group, 5.94 cm in the FP 50 µg (bid) group, and 5.73 cm in the FP 100 µg BID group). While the trend toward slower growth in FP-treated children could have reflected drop-out of ill, poorly-growing children from the placebo group, a small drug effect on growth could not be excluded. Compared with similarly designed studies administering clinically equivalent dosages of ICS, any potential growth effect of FP appeared to be 25–30% that associated with BDP (21). Further, a recent 24-month study comparing children treated with 200 μg/day FP or nedocrimil sodium (NS) showed no significant difference in growth between the two groups: adjusted mean growth rates were 6.1 cm/year with FP and 5.8 cm/year with NS (103). It is important to point out that available information regarding effects of ICS on growth derives from studies using low to medium doses of ICS. With the exception of anecdotal reports, there is a lack of information regarding the effect of high-dose ICS, as recommended for the treatment of severe asthma, on growth rates and final stature.

In addition to drug properties that influence the degree of systemic effects observed at a given dosage, patient characteristics also affect suscept-ibility to growth suppression. These include age and growth pattern of the child, underlying disease severity, and timing of drug administration. In some children, susceptibility to growth suppression by a variety of influences is increased during transitions from one growth phase (i.e., infancy-to-child-hood, or childhood-to-adolescent growth) to another. This is particularly true in the two to three years prior to puberty, when growth rates are low and the resiliency of the growth hormone axis is transiently, physiologically low. Significantly, most studies of growth effects of ICS have focused on chil-dren of this age, and results cannot confidently be extrapolated to infants or adolescents. As mentioned above, contributions of asthma disease itself can be over- and underestimated. Baseline characteristics of children with mild to moderate persistent asthma recruited into recent prospective trials shows them to have normal mean heights and skeletal ages for chronological age. Consequently, it appears that at least moderate to severe asthma is required to significantly slow the tempo of childhood growth and delay the onset of pubertal growth acceleration (15). With regard to dosing strategies, reducing the frequency of ICS administration to one inhalation per day might allow restoration of normal growth axis function between doses; although long-term growth studies have not examined this possibility, knemometry studies suggest that suppressed growth observed during bid. intranasal steroid treat-ment was not observed when similar doses were administered once a day (89). Selectively eliminating nighttime administration of ICS might also avoid GC-mediated blunting of nocturnal pituitary GH secretion and/or ACTH-induced adrenal androgen production (90).

Debate continues regarding the use of ICS in children <3 years of age. Potential benefit of early intervention with ICS is supported by one long-term study that showed that improvement in lung function was significantly greater in children who started BUD treatment within two years of diagnosis of asthma compared with those who started later (91). Other studies have not shown evidence of deterioration in lung function in the absence of anti-inflammatory treatment. More information is gradu-ally emerging regarding the influence of ICS on growth during infancy and early childhood. Six-month treatment with BDP 200 μg daily, administered via a metered dose inhaler (MDI) and spacer plus mask (Aerochamber®), had no effect on length/height in 12 very young children (mean age 1.22 years) (92). A subsequent study of children less than three years of age treated with nebulized BUD (1–4 mg/day) for 6 to 18 months showed no reduction in mean linear growth rates (93). A large study of children with ages six months to eight years treated with BUD inhalation suspension (0.5 mg once or twice daily) revealed a small, statistically significant decrease in growth velocity compared with children whose asthma was treated without the use of corticosteroids (94). Similarly, a short-term knemometry study showed that FP and BUD both resulted in reduced lower leg growth in children one to three years old when administered for four weeks from their dedicated spacer devices in daily doses of 400 µg with no difference between the two steroid regimens. On the other hand, a recent prospective one-year stadiometry study of one to three-year-old children with asthma showed equal gains in length/height during treatment with either FP (200 mcg/day) or cromolyn (95). These findings call for additional comparison studies of clinical side effects from various ICS/delivery device treatments of preschool children.

Traditionally, the *clinical relevance* of growth suppression by ICS has been judged more on ultimate effect on final height than short-term reductions in growth rate. A 1986 study followed 66 asthmatic children (mean age 7.5 years at entry) for a mean of 13.1 years, 26 of whom were receiving inhaled BDP up to 600 µg/day. Eleven children whose dosage of BDP exceeded 400 µg/day showed decelerating growth velocity during a period of delayed onset of puberty, but later demonstrated catch-up growth and achieved their predicted adult height. There was no significant difference between the final heights of children receiving BDP and those not receiving inhaled corticosteroids (12). Similar results have been recently reported for relatively small numbers of patients followed to final height following ICS treatment *alone* (31). In two retrospective studies, final adult height was not significantly different in young adults treated with ICS during childhood compared to those who were not treated with ICS during childhood (actual mean numeric differences were 1.22 cm (31) and 1.4 cm (96), $p = $ NS for both). However, there was also a small difference between the two groups for adult height minus target height (statistically significant in one study), suggesting mild permanent effects of growth retardation in ICS-treated patients. The authors could not exclude the possibility that differences in asthma severity accounted for this effect. In contrast, a follow-up study of 142 patients treated with BUD for a mean duration of 9.2 years during childhood revealed no significant differences between measured and target adult heights (+0.3 cm; 95% confidence interval, −0.6 to +1.2) (Fig. 3). The adult height depended significantly on the child's height before BUD treatment (97).

Another recent follow-up study of 356 asthmatic patients revealed no trend (compared with 384 healthy controls) toward a decrease in final height in relation to final height when inhaled budesonide treatment was initiated

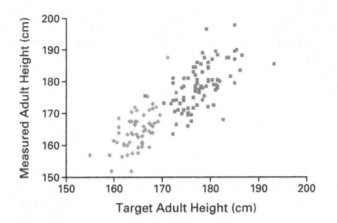

Figure 3 Measured adult height in relation to target adult height in 142 children treated with inhaled budesonide for 3–13 years. Diamonds represent girls, and squares, boys. *Source*: From Ref. (97).

prior to adolescence (98). A meta-analysis (of 21 studies in 810 asthma patients) of the effect of oral corticosteroid or inhaled BDP on growth showed a small but significant correlation between corticosteroid treatment in general and reduced final height. Growth impairment was linked to oral corticosteroid treatment, whereas inhaled BDP treatment was associated with reaching normal height. The statistical evidence did not suggest a link between growth impairment and BDP at higher doses, for more prolonged treatment durations, or among patients with more severe asthma (65).

These encouraging long-term final height data provide reassurance that long-term treatment of children with asthma with moderate-dose ICS does not significantly affect growth.

How can recent prospective studies showing growth suppression by inhaled BDP be reconciled with retrospective studies showing minimal or no effect on growth rate or height? One likely explanation stresses the differences between therapeutic efforts to achieve constant *disease control* versus *symptom control* (99). Closely monitored clinical trials designed to achieve disease control with consistent dosing indicate that BDP inhaled at a dosage of 400 mcg *every* day is capable of suppressing prepubertal growth. Most patients, on the other hand, reduce drug exposure by titrating medication to achieve symptom control rather than disease control (100), a fact that could account for the apparent absence of effect of "real life" prescriptions of BDP 400 mcg/day retrospective growth rates or final adult stature. Declining compliance over time is an inevitable confounding factor in accurately interpreting long-term studies of ICS and growth (101).

Nevertheless, studies cited above strongly suggest that long-term treatment with moderate-dose ICS (particularly those with lower systemic bioavailability than BDP) with sufficient consistency to achieve good disease control results in attainment of normal adult height.

Thus, following conclusions regarding the effects of ICS given in moderate therapeutic doses on childhood growth appear well substantiated: (1) detectable slowing of one-year growth in prepubertal children can occur with continuous, twice-daily treatment with BDP (400 mcg/day); (2) effects of fixed moderate-dose ICS on growth for two to four years is minimal or non-detectable for the vast majority of patients; (3) effects of moderate-dose ICS treatment during childhood on adult height is minimal in retrospective and prospective analyses; (4) in contrast, oral corticosteroid treatment is associated with reduced adult stature; (5) administration of ICS with more efficient first-pass hepatic inactivation of swallowed drug reduces risk of growth suppression; (6) because total systemic corticosteroid burden reflects absorption of exogenous corticosteroids administered by any route, the risk for growth-suppression is increased when ICS therapy is combined with intranasal or dermal steroid therapy; (7) titration to the lowest effective dose will minimize an already low risk of growth suppression by ICS; and (8) certain children (particularly those already short in stature, following a pattern of delayed growth and puberty, or on other growth-suppressing medications) demonstrate heightened sensitivity to growth suppressing effects of ICS.

Important questions remain about the potential long-term effects of ICS on bone growth. It is possible, as suggested by one recent report, that growth suppression is more prominent during early ICS treatment, and that recovery of normal growth occurs with longer-term treatment (102).

It is also possible that ICS effects on growth observed during the prepubertal years will not persist into puberty, during which the combined effects of sex steroids and increased growth hormone secretion normally increase growth rate. Predictions that time of day and/or frequency of dosing significantly affect risk of growth suppression by ICS require further confirmation. Finally, while studies examining bone metabolism in prepubertal children treated with moderate doses of ICS have not found a detrimental effect (103–105), treatment with higher dosages (mean 0.67 mg/ m^2/day) was associated with reduced acquisition of bone mineral (106). Long-term study of pubertal (a critical period of bone mineral accretion and linear growth) patients treated consistently with ICS is required to answer these questions.

IX. Effects of Other Asthma Medications on Growth

In contrast to the profound concern regarding potential effects of exogenous glucocorticoids on growth, other medications used to treat asthma have been assumed to have little or no effect on growth. However, few prospective studies directly examining growth effects of β-agonists, sodium cromoglycate, nedocrimil, and leukotriene receptor antagonists have actually been done. β-adrenergic receptors mediate the inhibitory influence of cathecolamines on GH secretion, probably via the stimulation of hypothalamic somatostatin release. Accordingly, β-adrenergic agonists and antagonists inhibit and increase, respectively, the GH response to many stimuli, including GHRH, in man. In healthy exercising volunteers (88), and in normal-weight and anorexic adult women (108), plasma growth hormone levels are significantly decreased after administration of salbutamol. In children with mild asthma, overnight integrated concentrations of GH and peak GH levels following GHRH diminished significantly after 24 hours of salbutamol therapy.

However, spontaneous and stimulated GH levels after three months of salbutamol were not different from baseline levels. These data suggest an inhibition of both spontaneous and stimulated GH secretion following short-term oral salbutamol ingestion, but this suppressive effect is not maintained with its long-term use. Growth studies of prepubertal children treated with salbutamol alone confirm the lack of any detectable effect during 12 months, administration (84). Further, in children treated with inhaled glucocorticoids, halving the dose and adding formoterol is associated with faster short-term growth and an increase in markers of collagen turnover, with no loss of asthma control (109). Thus, in spite of experimental evidence that acute β-adrenergic stimulation suppresses GH secretion, no evidence exists presently to support a clinical effect on linear growth.

Studies of other asthma medications have been similarly reassuring. Treatment of children with asthma with sodium cromoglycate for 12 months was associated with normal growth velocity adjusted for age and gender (110). Growth of children with asthma ages 5 to 12 treated with nedocrimil for four years was equal to that of children treated with placebo (mean 23.7 vs. 23.8 cm), with both groups demonstrating normal annual growth rates for age. In addition, markers of bone metabolism (serum carboxy-terminal telopeptide of type I collagen and urinary pyridinium cross links) returned to normal during six months of nedocrimil treatment, after showing decreases during the prior six months of budesonide therapy (111). With regard to commonly prescribed leukotriene antagonists, a MedLine search failed to reveal any citations cross-referenced with "growth."

X. Summary

Severe asthma, like all severe chronic diseases of childhood, can adversely affect growth. Mechanisms underlying this effect remain obscure, but growth-suppressing influences of endogenous cytokines and glucocorticoids produced in response to illness and inflammation appear likely.

Significant disease-related growth suppression occurs only when asthma is persistent and of at least moderate severity. This delay in the tempo of the growth process is commonly associated with delays in the timing of pubertal development, which can further exacerbate growth deceleration late in childhood.

Glucocorticoids are the most effective anti-inflammatory medications for asthma, but also interfere with the normal process of linear growth at multiple sites within the growth axis: secretion of GH, expression of GH receptors, IGF-1 bioactivity, chondrocyte proliferation, collagen synthesis, accretion of bone mineral, maintenance of positive nitrogen balance. Long-term treatment with oral glucocorticoids is associated with reduced growth rates and diminished adult stature. Inhaled corticosteroids have a high ratio of local to systemic activity, but, *in sufficient doses*, are capable of suppressing growth, particularly during prepubertal years. However, this effect on growth is markedly reduced when compared with clinically equivalent doses of oral glucocorticoids, and available retrospective final height analysis of ICS-treated individuals suggests a negligible effect on ultimate height. Persistent addition of other topical steroid therapy (e.g., intranasal or dermal) could magnify growth suppression in individual cases.

To date, other medications used for asthma therapy have not been shown to adversely affect growth. Whatever the *measurable* growth-suppressing effects of ICS might be for an individual child with asthma must be weighed against the possibility of growth suppression due to the disorder itself and the paramount objective of optimizing disease control and quality of life. Only then can the clinical relevance of potential systemic effects of ICS be placed in proper perspective.

References

1. Karlberg J, Engstrom I, Karlberg P, Fryer JG. Analysis of linear growth using a mathematical model. Acta Paediatr Scand 1987; 76:478–488.
2. Frank GR. Growth and estrogen. Growth Genet Hormones 2000; 16(1):1–5.
3. VandenBerghe G, de Zegher F, Bouillon R. Acute and prolonged critical illness as different neuroendocrine paradigms. J Clin Endocrinol Metab 1998; 83:1827–1834.
4. Zeitler PS, Travers S, Kappy MS. Endocrine complications of children with chronic illness. Adv Pediatr 1999; 46:101–149.
5. Vassilopoulou-Sellin R. Endocrine effects of cytokines. Oncology 1994; 8:43–49.
6. Umpleby AM, Russell-Jones DL. The hormonal control of protein metabolism. Baillieres Clin Endocrinol Metab 1996; 10:551–570.

7. Chopra IJ. Euthyroid sick syndrome: is it a misnomer? J Clin Endocrinol Metab 1997; 82:329–334.

8. Johnson RW. Inhibition of growth by pro-inflammatory cytokines: an integrated view. (Review) (22 refs). J Anim Sci 1997; 75(5):1244–1255.

9. Hankard R, Munck A, Navarro J. Nutrition and growth in cystic fibrosis. (Review) (28 refs). Hormone Res 2002; 58(suppl):20.

10. Broussard SR, McCusker RH, Novakofski JE, Strle K, Shen WH, Johnson RW, Freund GG, Dantzer R, Kelley KW. Cytokine–hormone interactions: tumor necrosis factor alpha impairs biologic activity and downstream activation signals of the insulin-like growth factor I receptor in myoblasts. Endocrinology 2003; 144(7):2988–2996.

11. Falliers CJ, Tan LS, Szentivanyi J, Jorgensen JR, Bukantz SC. Childhood asthma and steroid therapy as influences on growth. Am J Dis Child 1963; 105:127–137.

12. BalfourLynn L. Growth and childhood asthma. Arch Dis Child 1986; 61:1049–1055.

13. Morris HG. Growth and skeletal maturation in asthmatic children: effect of corticosteroid treatment. Pediatr Res 1975; 9:579–583.

14. Hauspie R, Susanne C, Alexander F. Maturational delay and temporal growth retardation in asthmatic boys. J All Clin Immunol 1977; 59:200–206.

15. Martin AJ, Landau LI, Phelan PD. The effect on growth of childhood asthma. Acta Paediatr Scand 1981; 70:683–688.

16. Cogswell JJ, El-Bishti MM. Growth retardation in asthma: role of calorie deficiency. Arch Dis Child 1982; 57:473–475.

17. Sole D, Castro AM, Naspitz CK. Growth in allergic children. J Asthma 1989; 26:217–221.

18. Morris HG. Growth of asthmatic children. J Asthma 1989; 26:215–216.

19. Hauspie R, Susanne C, Alexander F. A mixed longitudinal study of the growth in height and weight in asthmatic children. Hum Biol 1976; 48:271–283.

20. Murray AB, Fraser BM, Hardwick DF, Pirie GE. Chronic asthma and growth failure in children. Lancet 1976; 2(7989):801–802.

21. Allen DB, Bronsky EA, LaForce CF, Nathan RA, Tinkelman DG, Vandewalker ML, Konig P. Growth in asthmatic children treated with fluticasone propionate. J Pediatr 1998; 132:472–477.

22. The Childhood Asthma Management Program Research Group. Long-term effects of budesonide or nedocromil in children with asthma. N Engl J Med 2000; 343(15):1054–1063.

23. Kelly HW, Strunk RC, Donithan M, Bloomberg GR, McWilliams BC, Szefler S, et al. Growth and bone density in children with mild-moderate asthma: a cross-sectional study in children entering the Childhood Asthma Management Program (CAMP). J Pediatr 2003; 142(3):286–291.

24. Chang KC, Miklich D, Barwise G, Chai H. Growth of chronic asthmatic children. J All Clin Immunol 1978; 61:159.

25. Ninan T, Russell G. Asthma, inhaled corticosteroid treatment, and growth. Arch Dis Child 1992; 67:703–705.

26. Rotteveel J, Potkamp J, Holl H, Delemarre-Van de Waal HA. Growth during early childhood in asthmatic children: relation to inhalation steroid dose and clinical severity score. Hormone Res 2003; 59(5):234–238.

27. Crowley S, Hindmarsh PC, Matthews DR, Brook CGD. Growth and the growth hormone axis in prepubertal children with asthma. J Pediatr 1995; 126:297–303.
28. Ferguson AC, Murray AB, Tze W-J. Short stature and delayed skeletal maturation in children with allergic disease. J All Clin Immunol 1982; 69:217–221.
29. Zeitlen SR, Bond S, Wootton S, Gregson RK, Radford M. Increased resting energy expenditure in childhood asthma: does this contribute toward growth failure? Arch Dis Child 1992; 67:1366–1369
30. Taylor AM, Bush A, Thomson A. Relation between insulin-like growth factor-1, body mass index, and clinical status in cystic fibrosis. Arch Dis Child 1997; 76:304–309.
31. Silverstein MD, Yunginger JW, Reed CE, Petterson T, Zimmerman D, Li JT, O'Fallon WM. Attained adult height after childhood asthma: effect of glucocorticoid therapy. J All Clin Immunol 1997; 99:466–474.
32. Oberger E, Engstrom I, Karlberg J. Long-term treatment with glucocorticoids/ACTH in asthmatic children III. Effects on growth and adult height. Acta Paediatr Scand 1990; 79:77–83.
33. Norjavaara E, Gerhardsson d, V, Lindmark B. Adult height in women with childhood asthma—a population-based study. Pharmacoepidemiol Drug Safety 2001; 10(2):121–125.
34. Tinkelman DG, Reed CE, Nelson HS, Offord KP. Aerosol beclomethasone dipropionate compared with theophylline as primary treatment of chronic mild to moderately severe asthma in children. Pediatrics 1993; 92:64–77.
35. Heuck C, Wolthers OD, Kollerup G, Hansen M, Teisner B. Adverse effects of inhaled budesonide (800 micrograms) on growth and collagen turnover in children with asthma: a double-blind comparison of once-daily versus twice-daily administration. (See comments.) J Pediatr 1998; 133(5):608–612
36. Merkus PJFM, VanEssenZandvliet EEM, Duiverman EJ, VanHouwelingen HC, Kerrebijn KF. Long term effect of inhaled corticosteroids on growth rate in adolescents with asthma. Pediatrics 1993; 91:1121–1126.
37. Sohat M, Sohat T, Kedem R, Mimouni M, Danon YL. Childhood asthma and growth outcome. Arch Dis Child 1987; 62:63–65.
38. Allen DB, Julius JR, Breen TJ, Attie KM. Treatment of glucocorticoid-induced growth suppression with growth hormone. J Clin Endocrinol Metab 1998; 83:2824–2829.
39. Allen DB. Inhaled corticosteroids in children. In: Middleton E, Reed CE, Ellis EF, Adkinson NF, Yunginger JW, Busse WW, eds. Allergy: Principles and Practice. Vol 15. 4th ed. St. Louis: Mosby Yearbook, 1993:6–16.
40. Beaufrer B, Horber FF, Schwenk WF. Glucocorticoids increase leucine oxidation and impair leucine balance in humans. Am J Physiol 1995; 257:712–721.
41. Locascio V, Bonucci E, Imbimbo B. Bone loss in response to long term glucocorticoid therapy. Bone Miner 1990; 8:39–51.
42. Saville PD, Kharmosh O. Osteoporosis of rheumatoid arthritis: influence of age, sex, and corticosteroids. Arthritis Rheum 1967; 10:423–430.
43. Moore DD, Marks AR, Buckley DI, Kapler G, Payvar F, Goodman HM. The first intron of the human growth hormone gene contains a binding site for glucocorticoid receptor. Proc Natl Acad Sci USA 1985; 82:699–702.

44. Guistina A, Wehrenberg WB. The role of glucocorticoids in the regulation of growth hormone secretion—mechanisms and clinical significance. Trends Endocrinol Metab 1992; 3:306–311.
45. Spiliotis BE, August GP, Hung W. Growth hormone neurosecretory dysfunction. JAMA 1984; 257:2223–2226.
46. Kaufmann S, Jones KL, Wehrenberg WB, Culler FL. Inhibition by prednisone of growth hormone (GH) response to GH-releasing hormone in normal men. J Clin Endocrinol Metab 1988; 67:1258–1261.
47. Gabrielsson BG, Carmignac DF, Flavell DM, Robinson ICAF. Steroid regulation of growth hormone (GH) receptor and GH-binding protein messenger ribonucleic acids in the rat. Endocrinology 1995; 136:209–217.
48. Tonshoff B, Mehls O. In: Tejani AH, Fine RN, eds. Pediatric Renal Transplantation. New York, NY: John Wiley & Sons, 1994:441–459.
49. Unterman TG, Phillips LS. Glucocorticoid effects on somatomedins and somatomedin inhibitors. J Clin Endocrinol Metab 1985; 61:618–626.
50. Binoux M, Lassarre C, Seurin D. Somatomedin production by rat liver in organ culture. II. Studies of cartilage sulphation inhibitors released by the liver and their separation from somatomedins. Acta Endocrinol 1980; 93:83–90.
51. Hokken-Koelega ACS, Stijnen T, deMuinckKeizer-Schrama SMPF, Blum WF, Drop SLS. Levels of growth hormone, insulin-like growth factor I (IGF-1) and -II, IGF binding protein-1 and -3, and cortisol in prednisolone-treated children with growth retardation after renal transplantation. J Clin Endocrinol Metab 1993; 77:932–938.
52. Sanchez CP, He YZ. Alterations in the growth plate cartilage of rats with renal failure receiving corticosteroid therapy. Bone 2002; 30(5):692–698.
53. Ristelli J. Effect of prednisolone on the activities of intracellular enzymes of collagen biosynthesis in rat liver and skin. Biochem Pharmacol 1977; 26:1295–1298.
54. Mosier HD. The determinants of catch-up growth. Acta Paediatr Scand 1990; 367:126–129.
55. Baron J, Klein KO, Colli MJ, Yanovski JA, Novosad JA, Bacher JD, Cutler GB, Jr. Catch-up growth after glucocorticoid excess: a mechanism intrinsic to the growth plate. Endocrinology 1994; 135:1367–1371.
56. Tanner JM. Growth as a target-seeking function. In: Falkner F, Tanner JM, eds. Human Growth—A Comprehensive Treatise. Vol 1. New York, Plenum Press, 1990:167–179.
57. Van Metre TE, Pinkerton HL. Growth suppression in asthmatic children receiving prolonged therapy with prednisolone and methylprednisolone. J All 1959; 30:103–113.
58. Kerribijn KF, DeKroon JPM. Effect on height of corticosteroid therapy in asthmatic children. Arch Dis Child 1968; 43:556–561.
59. Sadeghi-Nelad A, Semor B. Adrenal function, growth, and insulin in patients treated with corticoids on alternate days. Pediatrics 1969; 43:277–283.
60. Reimer LG, Morris HG, Ellis EE. Growth of asthmatic children during treatment with alternate-day steroids. J All Clin Immunol 1975; 55:224–231.
61. Chang KC, Miklich D, Barwise G, Chai H, Miles EA, Lawrence R. Linear growth of chronic asthmatic children: the effects of disease and various forms of steroid therapy. Clin All 1982; 12:369–378.

62. Allen DB. Growth suppression by glucocorticoid therapy. In: Rosenfield RL, ed. Growth and Growth Disorders. Philadelphia: W.B. Saunders Company, 1996; 25(3):699–717.
63. Lam CN, Arneil GC. Long-term dwarfing effects of corticosteroid treatment for childhood nephrosis. Arch Dis Child 1968; 43:589–594.
64. Foote KD, Brocklebank JT, Meadow SR. Height attainment in children with steroid responsive nephrotic syndrome. Lancet 1985; 2:917–976.
65. Allen DB, Mullen M, Mullen B. A meta-analysis of the effects of oral and inhaled glucocorticoids on growth. J All Clin Immunol 1994; 93:967–976.
66. Agertoft L, Pedersen S. Lung deposition and systemic availability of fluticasone diskus and budesonide turbuhaler in children. Am J Resp Crit Care Med 2003; 168:779–782.
67. Chaplin MD, Cooper WC, Segre EJ. Correllation of flunisolide plasma levels to eosinopenic response in humans. J All Clin Immunol 1980; 65:445.
68. Ryrfeldt A, Edsbacker S, Pouwles R. Kinetics of epimeric glucocorticoid budesonide. Clin Pharmacol Therapeut 1984; 35:525–530.
69. Harding SM. The human pharmacology of fluticasone propionate. Respir Med 1990; 84(suppl A):25–29.
70. Pedersen S, Steffensen G, Ekman I, Tonnesson M, Borga O. Pharmacokinetics of budesonide in children with asthma. Eur J Clin Pharmacol 1987; 31:579–582.
71. Johansson SA, Andersson KE, Brattsand R. Topical and systemic glucocorticoid potencies of budesonide and beclomethasone dipropionate in man. Eur J Clin Pharmacol 1982; 22:523.
72. Johnson M. Pharmacokinetics and pharmacodynamics of inhaled glucocorticoids. J Clin All Immunol 1996; 98:169–176.
73. Agertoft L, Pedersen S. A randomized, double-blind dose reduction study to compare the minimal effective dose of budesonide Turbuhaler and fluticasone propionate Diskhaler. J All Clin Immunol 1997; 99(6):773–780.
74. Ghigo E, Valetto MR, Gaggero L, Visca A, Valente F, Bellone J, Castello D, Camanni F. Therapeutic doses of salbutamol inhibit the somatotropic responsiveness to growth hormone-releasing hormone in asthmatic children. J Endocrinol Invest 1993; 16:271–276.
75. Hollman GA, Allen DB. Overt glucocorticoid excess due to inhaled corticosteroid therapy. Pediatrics 1988; 81:452–455.
76. Wolthers OD, Pederson S. Controlled study of linear growth in asthmatic children during treatment with inhaled glucocorticoids. Pediatrics 1992; 89: 839–842.
77. Wolthers OD, Hansen M, Juul A, Nielsen HK, Pederson S. Knemometry, urine cortisol excretion, and measures of insulin-like growth factor axis and collagen turnover in children treated with inhaled glucocorticoids. Pediatr Res 1997; 41(1):44–50.
78. Wales JKH, Milner RDG. Knemometry in assessment of linear growth. Arch Dis Child 1987; 62:166–171.
79. Agertoft L, Pedersen S. Relationship between short-term lower leg growth and long-term statural growth in asthmatic children treated with budesonide [abstr]. Eur Respir J 1996; 9(suppl 23):294s.

80. Hermanussen M, Burmeister J. Standards for the predictive accuracy of short-term body height and lower leg length measurements on half annual growth rates. Arch Dis Child 1989; 64:259–263.
81. Karlberg J, Gelander L, Albertsson-Wikland K. Distinctions between short- and long-term human growth studies. Acta Paediatr 1993; 82:631–634.
82. Allen DB. Limitations of short-term studies in predicting long-term effects of inhaled corticosteroids. Allergy 1999; 54(suppl 49):29–34.
83. Doull IJM, Freezer NJ, Holgate ST. Growth of prepubertal children with mild asthma treated with inhaled beclomethasone dipropionate. Am J Respir Crit Care Med 1995; 151:1715–1719.
84. Verberne AAPH, Frost C, DipStat MA, Roorda RJ, van der Laag H, Kerribijn KF. One-year treatment with salmeterol compared to beclomethasone in children with asthma. Am J Resp Crit Care Med 1997; 156:688–695.
85. Simons FER. A comparison of beclomethasone, salmeterol, and placebo in children with asthma. N Engl J Med 1997; 337:1659–1665.
86. Agertoft L, Pederson S. Effects of long-term treatment with an inhaled cortico-steroid on growth and pulmonary function in asthmatic children. Respir Med 1994; 88:373–381.
87. Volovitz B, Amir J, Malik H, Kauschansky A, Varsano I. Growth and pituitary adrenal function in children with severe asthma treated with inhaled budesonide. N Engl J Med 1993; 329:1703–1708.
88. Collomp K, Candau R, Millet G, Mucci P, Borrani F, Prefaut C, De Ceaurriz J. Effects of salbutamol and caffeine ingestion on exercise metabolism and performance. Int J Sports Med 2002; 23(8):549–554.
89. Agertoft L, Pederson S. The importance of delivery system for the effect of Budesonide. Arch Dis Child 1993; 69:130–133.
90. Allen DB. Systemic effects of intranasal steroids: an endocrinologist's per-spective. J Allergy Clin Immunol 2000; 106(4 Suppl):S179–S190.
91. Pedersen S, Warner JO, Price JF. Early use of inhaled steroids in children with asthma. Clin Exp All 1997; 27:995–1006.
92. Teper AM, Kofman CD, Maffey AF, Vidaurreta S, Bergadi I, Heinrich J. Effect of inhaled beclomethasone dipropionate on pulmonary function, bron-chial reactivity and longitudinal growth in infants with bronchial asthma. Asthma 1995; 95(Theory to treatment.):13.
93. Reid A, Murphy C, Steen HJ, McGovern V, Shields MD. Linear growth of very young asthmatic children treated with high-dose nebulized budesonide. Acta Paediatr 1996; 85:421–424.
94. Skoner DP, Szefler SJ, Welch M, Walton-Bowen K, Cruz-Rivera M, Smith JA. Longitudinal growth in infants and young children treated with budesonide inhalation suspension for persistent asthma. J All Clin Immunol 2000; 105:259–268.
95. Bisgaard H, Allen D, Milanowski J, Kalev I, Willits L, Davies P. Twelve-month safety and efficacy of inhaled fluticasone propionate in children aged 1 to 3 years with recurrent wheezing. Pediatrics 2004;113(2):e87–94.
96. Van Bever HP, Desager KN, Lijssens N, Weyler JJ, Du Caju MVL. Does treatment of asthmatic children with inhaled corticosteroids affect their adult height? Pediatr Pulmonol 1999; 27:369–375.

97. Agertoft L, Pedersen S. Effect of long-term treatment with inhaled bude-sonide on adult height in children with asthma. [See comment.]. N Engl J Med 2000; 343(15):1064–1069.
98. Larsson L, Gerhardsson d, V, Lindmark B, Norjavaara E. Budesonide-treated asthmatic adolescents attain target height: a population-based follow-up study from Sweden. Pharmacoepidemiol Drug Safety 2002; 11(8):715–720.
99. Lemanske RF, Allen DB. Choosing a long-term controller medication in childhood asthma: the proverbial two-edged sword. Am J Respir Crit Care Med 1997; 156:685–687.
100. Milgrom H, Bender B, Ackerson L, Bowry P, Smith B, Rand C. Noncompli-ance and treatment failure in children with asthma. J All Clin Immunol 1996; 98:1051–1057.
101. Wolthers OD, Allen DB. Inhaled corticosteroids, growth, and compliance. N Engl J Med 2002; 347(15):1210–1211.
102. Doull IJM, Campbell MJ, Holgate ST. Duration of growth suppressive effects of regular inhaled corticosteroids. Arch Dis Child 1998; 78:172–173.
103. Roux C, Kolta S, Desfougeres JL, Minini P, Bidat E. Long-term safety of fluticasone propionate and nedocromil sodium on bone in children with asthma. Pediatrics 2003; 111(6:Pt 1):t-13.
104. Konig P, Hillman L, Cervantes C, Levine C, Maloney C, Douglass B, Johnson L, Allen S. Bone metabolism in children with asthma treated with inhaled beclo-methasone dipropionate. J Pediatr 1993; 122:219–226.
105. Agertoft L, Pedersen S. Bone mineral density in children with asthma receiv-ing long-term treatment with inhaled corticosteroids. Am J Respir Crit Care Med 1998; 157:178–183.
106. Allen HDW, Thong IG, Clifton-Bligh P, Holmes S, Nery L, Wilson KB. Effects of high-dose inhaled corticosteroids on bone metabolism in prepuber-tal children with asthma. Pediatr Pulmonol 2000; 29:188–193.
107. Giustina A, Malerba M, Bresciani E, Desenzani P, Licini M, Zaltieri G, Grassi V. Effect of two β2-agonist drugs, salbutamol and broxaterol, on the growth hormone response to exercise in adult patients with asthmatic bron-chitis. J Endocrinol Investig 1995; 18(11):847–852.
108. Gianotti L, Arvat E, Valetto MR, Ramunni J, Di Vito L, Maccagno B, Camanni F, Ghigo E. Effects of β-adrenergic agonists and antagonists on the growth hormone response to growth hormone-releasing hormone in anor-exia nervosa. Biol Psychiatry 1998; 43(3):181–187.
109. Heuck C, Heickendorff L, Wolthers OD. A randomised controlled trial of short-term growth and collagen turnover in asthmatics treated with inhaled formoterol and budesonide. Archiv Dis Childhood 2000; 83(4):334–339.
110. Price JF, Russell G, Hindmarsh PC, Weller P, Heaf DP, Williams J. Growth during one year of treatment with fluticasone propionate or sodium cromo-glycate in children with asthma. Pediatr Pulmonol 1997; 24(3):178–186.
111. Sorva R, Tahtela R, Turpeinen M, Juntunen-Backman K, Haahtela T, Risteli L, Risteli J, Sorva A. Changes in bone markers in children with asthma during inhaled budesonide and nedocromil treatments. Acta Paediatr 1996; 85(10): 1176–1180.

7

Viral Respiratory Infections and Asthma

JAMES E. GERN and ROBERT F. LEMANSKE

Division of Pediatric Allergy, Departments of Pediatrics and Medicine,
Immunology, and Rheumatology, University of Wisconsin Medical School
Madison, Wisconsin, U.S.A.

I. Introduction

Infections with respiratory viruses can cause wheezing in children of all ages (Fig. 1). The nature of this relationship, however, evolves with the age of the child. In infancy, viruses are overwhelmingly the most common cause of wheezing illnesses, and in fact, age itself is an important risk factor for wheezing with respiratory syncytial virus (RSV) infection in the first year of life. Conversely, repeated exposure to infectious viruses in day care centers increases the number of respiratory infections, but in doing so, may paradoxically reduce the long-term risk of allergies and asthma. For most children, virus-induced wheezing is largely confined to infancy; however, there are subsets of children who continue to have virus-induced episodes of wheezing during the first decade of life. Finally, for children who go on to develop asthma requiring daily controller medications, common cold infections are one of the most common causes of acute exacerbations.

Although these associations have been recognized for a number of years, there are lingering questions regarding the nature of the relationship between viral infections and the onset and activity of asthma. Do early

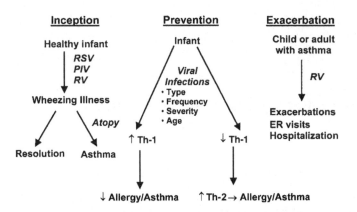

Figure 1 Relationship of viral respiratory infections to allergy and wheezing in children. *Abbreviations*: RSV, respiratory syncytial virus; RV, rhinoviruses; PIV, parainfluenza viruses; ER, emergency department; Th-1, T helper-1; Th-2, T helper-2.

infections with viruses such as RSV cause asthma? Can infections with some viruses actually reduce the likelihood of developing allergic diseases and asthma? What role do common cold viruses play in exacerbations of asthma? How do viral infections cause bronchospasm and mucus plugging, leading to airway obstruction and wheezing? And finally, what are the genetic, environmental, and immunological risk factors for the development of more severe lower respiratory tract infections in childhood? In this review, current concepts related to these questions will be explored, and implications for the treatment of virus-induced wheezing will be discussed.

II. Do Early Infections with Viruses Such as RSV Cause Asthma?

In infants, infection with RSV has received much attention because of its predilection to produce a pattern of symptoms termed "bronchiolitis," which parallels many of the features of childhood and adult asthma (1). From 1980 to 1996, rates of hospitalization of infants with acute virus-induced wheezing and respiratory distress (bronchiolitis) increased substantially, as did the proportion of total and lower respiratory tract hospitalizations associated with bronchiolitis; RSV causes about 70% of these episodes. However, RSV bronchiolitis represents only the most severe fraction of cases in that by age one, 50–65% of children will have been infected with this virus and, by age two, nearly 100% (2). Children aged three to six months are most prone to develop lower respiratory tract symptoms, suggesting that a developmental component (e.g., lung and/or immunological maturation) may be involved as well (3). Although controversy exists regarding the relevance of antecedent infections and the development of recurrent wheezing (4), a recent long-term prospective study of large numbers of children has demonstrated that RSV bronchiolitis is a significant independent risk factor for subsequent frequent wheezing at least within the first decade of life (5). It remains to be established, however, how RSV infections produce these outcomes due to the fact that virtually all children have been infected with this virus before their second birthday. Some of the factors, that have been evaluated include the immune response (both innate and adaptive) to the virus and host-related differences,—gender, lung size, and passive smoke exposure (6–8)—which may predispose an infant or child to lower airway physiologic alterations as a consequence of the infection.

Recently, additional insight into these areas has been provided by the results of an 11-year prospective study involving 880 children who were enrolled at birth, followed for the development of lower respiratory tract illnesses (LRIs) in the first three years of life, and then evaluated for the presence or absence of physician-diagnosed asthma and/or a history of current wheezing at ages 6 and 11 years (7,9). Most importantly, lung function was evaluated in the first few months of life in a subset of these children prior to the development of a documented LRI. During the first three years of life, 7.4% had pneumonia documented radiographically and 44.7% had a significant LRI without pneumonia. The RSV and parainfluenza virus were identified in 36.4% and 7.3%, respectively, in the subjects with pneumonia, and in 35.6% and 15.2%, respectively, of the subjects with an LRI. At age six, physician-diagnosed asthma was present in 13.6% [Odds Ratio (OR) = 3.3], 10.2% (OR = 2.4), and 4.6% of the subjects with pneumonia, LRI, and no LRI, respectively. By age 11, these values increased to 25.9% (OR = 2.8), 16.1% (OR = 1.6), and 11%, respectively. Mean values of V_{max} functional residual capacity (FRC) before any LRI were lower in children with pneumonia and with LRIs than in children with no LRIs. These latter results favor the hypothesis that inherent abnormalities in pulmonary function predispose infants to more severe lower respiratory tract symptoms, i.e., association versus causation (10). When pulmonary function measurements were evaluated at ages 6 and 11, similar group relationships persisted. Interestingly, despite the persistence of lowered baseline lung function in both the pneumonia and LRI groups, many of these deficits were markedly (but not completely) reduced following administration of albuterol.

In a second report, further follow-up of this large cohort of children demonstrated that the risk for both frequent (>3 episodes of wheezing per year) and infrequent (three episodes of wheezing per year) wheezing in relation to RSV lower respiratory illnesses decreased markedly with age and became non-significant by age 13 (5).

A decrease in the frequency of wheezing with increasing age following documented RSV infections has been observed by other investigators as well (1,10,11). These data suggest that, although RSV infections contribute substantially to the expression of the asthmatic phenotype, other cofactors (e.g., genetic, environmental, and developmental) also appear to contribute either in terms of its initial expression, or the modification of the phenotype over time.

From a number of epidemiological observations, it appears that other viral infections during infancy and early childhood that have a predisposition for lower airway involvement (e.g., parainfluenza, influenza A, and metapneumovirus) can also be associated with chronic lower respiratory tract symptoms including asthma (1,9,12–15). The recent discovery of a previously unrecognized pathogen, metapneumovirus, indicates that it has contributed significantly to lower respiratory tract illnesses in early childhood (15). The precise contribution of these infections to the development of asthma remains to be determined.

As previously stated, premorbid measurements of lung function indicate that children with reduced levels of lung function in infancy appear to be at increased risk of chronic lower respiratory tract sequelae following viral infections (9). It is doubtful that this defect is solely responsible for the development of chronic lung disease, and other host factors are now being evaluated. Further, the ability of one virus (i.e., RSV) to be more likely responsible for these outcomes (due to either virus- or host-specific factors) has also not been well defined. Indeed, recent data would indicate that rhinovirus-induced bronchiolitis may be associated with a particularly high risk of recurrent wheezing and asthma during infancy and early childhood (16,17).

III. What Is the Role of Common Cold Infections in Causing Acute Exacerbations of Asthma?

The relationship between viral infections and wheezing illnesses in older children and adults has been clarified by the advent of sensitive diagnostic tests, based on the polymerase chain reaction (PCR), for picornaviruses such as rhinovirus (RV). With the advent of these more sensitive diagnostic tools, information linking common cold infections with exacerbations of asthma has come from a number of sources. Prospective studies of subjects with asthma have demonstrated that up to 85% of exacerbations of asthma in children, and close to half of such episodes in adults, are caused by viral infections (18). Although many respiratory viruses can provoke acute asthma symptoms, RV are most often detected, especially during the spring and fall RV seasons. In fact, the spring and fall peaks in hospitalizations due to asthma closely coincide with patterns of RV isolation within the community (19). Influenza and RSV are somewhat more likely to trigger acute asthma symptoms in the wintertime, but appear to account for a smaller fraction of asthma flares. RV infections are also frequently detected in children over the age of two years who present to emergency departments with acute wheezing (20,21), and in adults, account for approximately half of asthma-related acute care visits (22). Together, these studies provide evidence of a strong relationship between viral infections, particularly those due to RV, and acute exacerbations of asthma.

Individuals with asthma do not necessarily have more colds, and neither the severity nor duration of virus-induced upper respiratory symptoms is enhanced by respiratory allergies or asthma (23,24). In contrast to findings in the upper airway, a prospective study of colds in couples consisting of one asthmatic and one normal individual demonstrated that colds cause greater duration and severity of lower respiratory symptoms in subjects with asthma (24). These findings suggest that there are fundamental differences in the lower airway effects of respiratory viral infections related to asthma.

Although viral infections alone can promote lower airway symptoms, there is evidence that viral infections may exert synergistic effects together with other known triggers for asthma. For example, there is evidence that the effects of colds on asthma may be amplified by exposure to allergens (25), and possibly by exposure to greater levels of air pollutants (26).

In addition to provoking asthma, RV infections can also increase lower airway obstruction in individuals with other chronic airway diseases (e.g., chronic obstructive lung disease and cystic fibrosis) (27,28), and in infants (29) and the elderly (30). Thus, common cold viruses that produce relatively mild illnesses in most people can cause severe pulmonary problems in selected individuals.

IV. How Do Viral Infections Cause Bronchospasm and Plugging, Leading to Airway Obstruction and Wheezing?

A. Extension of Viral Infections into the Lower Airway

There is little doubt that pathogens such as RSV and influenza virus infect lower airway tissue, and are capable of causing a local inflammatory response that leads to airway obstruction and in some individuals, bronchospasm. In contrast, efforts to explain the relationship between common cold infections and acute exacerbations of lower airway symptoms have been difficult due to the assumption that common cold infections are restricted to the upper airway.

For example, RV has traditionally been considered to be an upper airway pathogen due to its association with common cold symptoms, and the observation that RV replicates best at 33–35°C, which approximates temperatures in the upper airway. There is evidence to indicate, however, that temperature may not be a barrier to RV replicating in lower airway tissues. In fact, lower airway temperatures have been directly mapped using a broncho-scope equipped with a thermister (31). During quiet breathing of air at room temperature, airway temperatures are conducive to RV replication down to fourth-generation bronchi and only exceed 35°C in the periphery of the lung. Moreover, RV appears to replicate equally well in cultured epithelial cells derived from either upper or lower airway epithelium (32). Although RV has been difficult to culture from the lower airway it has been detected in lower airway cells and secretions by RT-PCR (33) and in mucosal biopsies by in situ hybridization and immunohistochemistry (34,34a). Finally, experi-mentally-induced RV infections can produce lower airway inflammation, including increased neutrophils in bronchial lavage fluid (35), influx of T cells and eosinophils into lower airway epithelium (36), and enhanced epithelial expression of ICAM-1 (37). These findings provide strong evidence that RV can replicate in the large lower airways.

Remaining challenges include determining whether viral replication in the lower airway is a sufficient stimulus to provoke exacerbations of asthma. RV replication in large lower airways appears to be substantial (34a,38), suggesting that the virus-induced cellular inflammation, mucus, and tissue edema could directly induce airway obstruction and closure. Other mechan-isms that may also contribute to virus-induced exacerbations include sys-temic immune activation, the existence of reflex bronchospasm triggered by upper airway inflammation, and the aspiration of inflammatory cells and mediators that are generated in the upper airway (39).

B. Virus-Induced Cellular Inflammation

The epithelial cell is of primary importance during viral respiratory infec-tions because it serves as the host cell for viral replication, and also initiates innate immune responses. It has been hypothesized that other cells may become infected during viral infections. For example, airway smooth mus-cle cells can be infected by virus in tissue culture, suggesting a potential mechanism for viral infections to cause bronchospasm and airway hyperre-sponsiveness (40,41), although this has not yet been verified in vivo.

Damage to the epithelial cells can disturb airway physiology through a number of different pathways. For example, epithelial edema and shedding together with mucus production can cause airway obstruction and wheezing. The immune response to the virus can also contribute to the pathogenesis of respiratory symptoms. For viruses such as RV, which infect relatively few cells in the airway, this may be the primary mechanism for airway symptoms and lower airway dysfunction (42). Virus-induced epithelial damage can also increase the permeability of the mucosal layer (43,44), per-haps facilitating allergen contact with immune cells, and exposing neural elements to promote neurogenic inflammation. Finally, experiments with cultured cells indicate that well-differentiated epithelial cells are relatively resistant to infection with RV, and suggest that cells that are damaged by inflammation or environmental irritants are more susceptible to viral infection (45).

The processes associated with viral replication trigger both innate and adaptive immune responses within the epithelial cell. Virus attachment to cell surface receptors may initiate some immune responses. For example, RSV infection activates signaling pathways in airway epithelial cells through the surface molecule toll-like receptor 4 (TLR-4) (46). There is also evidence of receptor-independent pathways for virus activation of epithelial cells, such as the generation of oxidative stress (47).

Replication of viral RNA can also stimulate anti-viral responses in epithelial cells. Double-stranded RNA (dsRNA) that is synthesized in virus-infected cells can bind to TLR-3 receptors on the cell surface and within the cell (48).

Activation of TLR receptors or other RNA-binding enzymes, such as the dsRNA dependent protein kinase (PKR) and 2,5 oligoadenylate synthase, lead to a cascade of events that lead to the activation of innate anti-viral activity such as the generation of nitric oxide, activation of ribonuclease (RNase) L, and inhibition of protein synthesis within infected cells (49). Furthermore, dsRNA generated during viral infections also promotes the activation of chemokine genes such as interleukin-8 (IL-8) and regulated on activation normal T cell expressed and secreted (RANTES), which recruit inflammatory cells into the airway (32). Thus, host cell recognition of dsRNA initiates both anti-viral and pro-inflammatory pathways within the cell.

Viral respiratory infections are generally spread by a small number of viruses via either aerosols or contact with infected material. After several days of replication, however, viral titers in respiratory secretions can markedly increase (50), leading to the activation of mononuclear cells in the area or in regional lymph nodes. Monocytes, macrophages, and presumably dendritic cells are drawn into the area of infection by chemokines and local inflammation, and are in turn activated by viruses to secrete pro-inflammatory cytokines such as IL-1, IL-8, TNF-α, IL-10, and IFN-α and IFN-γ (51–53). These responses amplify the inflammatory response, and are also important anti-viral effectors. In addition to mononuclear cells, neutrophils are recruited early in the course of infection, and these are the predominant cells in airway secretions (35,54). Of particular interest is evidence that activated neutrophils, through the release of the potent secretagogue elastase, can up-regulate goblet cell secretion of mucus (55). In addition, changes in IL-8 levels in nasal secretions have been related to respiratory symptoms and virus-induced increases in airway hyperresponsiveness (56,57). These findings suggest that neutrophils and neutrophil activation products contribute to airway obstruction and symptoms during viral infections and exacerbations of asthma.

C. Neural Inflammation and Effects on Airway Responsiveness

Information derived from animal models, as well as clinical studies of natural or experimentally-induced viral infections, indicate that viruses can enhance airway hyperresponsiveness, which is one of the key features of asthma. The clinical studies have generally shown that viral infections cause mild increases in airway responsiveness during the time of peak cold symptoms, and that these changes can sometimes last for several weeks. A heightened sensitivity to inhaled irritants, as well as greater maximum bronchoconstriction in response to these stimuli have both been observed. The mechanism of virus-induced airway responsiveness is likely to be multifactorial, and contributing factors are likely to include impairment in the inactivation of tachykinins, virus effects on nitric oxide production, and virus-induced changes in neural control of the airways (58).

Tachykinins, which are synthesized by sensory nerves, are potent bronchoconstrictors and vasodilators, and through these effects have the potential to cause severe airway obstruction. Since airway epithelial cells help to regulate tachykinin levels through the production of the enzyme neutral endopeptidase, loss of this enzyme activity in epithelium that has been damaged by viral infection could lead to airway obstruction (59). Nitric oxide (NO) can regulate both vascular and bronchial tone, and can interfere with the replication of some viruses (60). Nitric oxide synthesis is enhanced by viral infections (61), but because of the many potential effects of NO on the lower airways, it is uncertain as to whether this is beneficial to lower airway function in asthma.

Viruses can also affect airway tone and responsiveness by enhancing vagally mediated reflex bronchoconstriction, and this has been demonstrated in humans and in animal models. One potential mechanism for this effect is virus interference in the function of the M2 muscarinic receptor (62).

Experiments in guinea pigs infected with a parainfluenza virus indicate that the M2 receptor is part of an important negative feedback loop that limits the release of acetylcholine from vagal nerve endings. When the M2 receptor is damaged by viral infection or virus-induced interferon (63,64), bronchoconstriction is enhanced, leading to increased airway obstruction. This effect is likely to involve neurokinin-1 (NK-1) receptors, and is amenable to treatment with dexamethasone (64,65). Further delineation of this pathway may lead to novel treatments for virus-induced asthma symptoms that are refractory to standard therapy.

D. Viral Infections and Airway Remodeling

Asthma is associated with distinctive changes in the structure of the airways, and these morphologic alterations contribute to airflow limitation and bronchospasm. These changes include thickening of the basement membrane and the airway wall, hypertrophy of smooth muscle, and fibrosis (66).

Although it is clear that remodeling can be a progressive process, some of these changes have been documented in biopsy specimens of young children (67). This raises the possibility that some of the abnormalities are either congenital, or are caused by an environmental insult at a very early age.

Along this line of reasoning, viral lower respiratory infections in infancy occur during a period of ongoing lung development. It is certainly possible that damage to small airways during this vulnerable period of lung development could lead to long-term changes in lung structure. Alternately, the release of high levels of pro-inflammatory cytokines could affect development processes such as airway budding and branching that continue to occur during the first months of life. In animal models of viral infection, infection of young mice with a paramyxovirus induces goblet cell hyperplasia and airway hyperresponsiveness that persist for many months after clearance of the virus (68).

Indicators of lung function such as FEV_1 and airway responsiveness can be abnormal for as long as 10 years after a severe viral infection such as RSV bronchiolitis. This information is difficult to interpret, however, given that low lung function in infancy is actually a risk factor for the development of lower respiratory symptoms and infection with viruses such as RSV (69). In the Tucson Children's Respiratory Study, children who had RSV bronchiolitis in infancy continued to have low lung function and responsiveness to bronchodilators for up to age 11 years (5). Notably, postbronchodilator FEV_1 was not different in children who had suffered RSV bronchiolitis, suggesting that there was no fixed airway narrowing.

Several animal models have evaluated the types of changes that occur in the airways as a result of infections with respiratory viruses. The RSV infections have been most extensively studied in mice, which result in airway inflammatory and physiologic changes reminiscent of human asthma. The results of these evaluations indicate that RSV has the potential of inducing polarized cytokine response patterns based on differential responses to two of its structural constituents (F and G proteins) (70), and this may be particularly likely if the animals are infected at a young age (71). (IL-13) seems to be important in inducing a state of airway hyperresponsiveness following infection (72), while prior airway exposure to allergen increases viral-induced airway hyperresponsiveness (73). Parainfluenza 1 (another member of the paramyxovirus family) infections in weanling rats can induce the development of a chronic asthma phenotype (74,75). To induce this response, the infection must occur in a genetically susceptible strain (Th-2 skewed) at a critical time point in the development of the animal (76). Interestingly, the selective administration of (IFN-γ) to these animals following infection inhibits the development of the chronic airway dysfunction (77).

Cytokine dysregulation in these rats is related to aberrancies in natural killer cell numbers and function as part of the innate immune response to viral infection (78). These findings strongly support the concept that viral infections may have to occur in a genetically susceptible host at a critical time period in either the development of the immune system or the lung for asthma inception to occur in early childhood.

V. What Are the Genetic, Environmental, and Immunological Risk Factors for More Severe Respiratory Infections in Childhood?

As mentioned previously, both young age and small lung size were some of the first factors to be identified for the development of wheezing illnesses such as bronchiolitis in infancy. Since these initial observations, a number of other risk factors have been identified that affect the likelihood of developing a lower respiratory infection or wheezing with viral infections (Fig. 2). Many of the recently identified factors relate to immune responses that regulate inflammatory or anti-viral responses.

A. Allergy and Atopy

In addition to premorbid lung function, the influence of atopy on the development of the asthmatic phenotype in relationship to viral infections has also been evaluated. Interactions between these two factors appear to

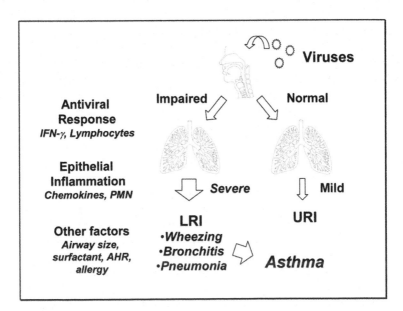

Figure 2   Pathogenesis of virus-induced wheezing and asthma (see text).

be bidirectional and dynamic in that the atopic state can influence the lower airway response to viral infections (69,79), viral infections can influence the development of allergen sensitization (80–82), and interactions can occur when individuals are exposed simultaneously to both allergens and viruses (83–85).

Atopy can be defined as the genetic predisposition to the preferential development of an IgE antibody response to a variety of environmental allergens. As stated previously, atopy has been considered to be a risk factor for the development of childhood asthma and its influence on the pattern of responses following viral infections has been of interest to many investigative groups.

It has also been suggested that atopy could be a significant predisposing factor for the development of acute bronchiolitis during RSV epidemics (86). While some have found that those children most likely to have persistent wheezing were children born to atopic parents (86–88), others have not (89,90). Although some have found that personal atopy is not more prevalent in symptomatic children *after* bronchiolitis (5,90), others have found that documented RSV bronchiolitis significantly increases a child's chances (32% vs. 9% in controls) of subsequently developing IgE antibody (80) or lymphocyte proliferative responses (91) to both food and aeroallergens.

Respiratory syncytial virus infections may interact with immuno-inflammatory mechanisms involved in immediate hypersensitivity responses in a number of ways (92). First, it has been suggested that viruses capable of infecting lower airway epithelium may lead to enhanced absorption of aeroallergens across the airway wall predisposing to subsequent sensitization (93,94). Second, RSV-specific IgE antibody formation may lead to mast cell mediator release within the airway, resulting in the development of bronchospasm and the ingress of eosinophils (95–100). Third, airway resident and inflammatory cell generation of various cytokines (TNF-α, IFN-γ, IFN-α, IL-1β, IL-6, and IL-9) (101–106), chemokines [macrophage inflammatory protein (MIP)-1α, RANTES, macrophage chemoattractant protein (MCP)-1, and IL-8] (107–109), leukotrienes (110), and adhesion molecules (ICAM-1) (101) may further upregulate the ongoing inflammatory response. Finally, similar to various allergenic proteins (111), the processing of RSV antigens and their subsequent presentation to lymphocyte subpopulations may provide a unique mechanism of interaction to promote a Th-2-like response in a predisposed host.

Studies have been performed using the techniques of bronchoscopy and experimental viral inoculation to try to understand RV-induced inflammation in the lower airway and interactions with allergen-induced inflammation. These studies have demonstrated that RV infections can enhance lower airway histamine responses and eosinophil recruitment in response to allergen challenge (85,112). In addition, during an RV infection, study subjects had enhanced immediate responses to allergen and were more likely to have a late asthmatic response after allergen challenge (83). These findings suggest that RV can enhance both the immediate and the late-phase response to allergen.

Other interactions between allergy and RV infections have been observed in clinical studies involving natural infections. For example, experimental inoculation with RV is more likely to increase airway responsiveness in allergic individuals rather than non-allergic individuals (113). In a study of children who presented to an emergency department (21,114), individual risk factors for developing wheezing included detection of a respiratory virus, most commonly RV, allergen-specific IgE, and evidence of eosinophilic inflammation in nasal secretions. Notably, there was also evidence of a synergism between viral infections and allergic inflammation [eosinophilia or positive, radioallergosorbent (RAST) tests] in determining the risk of wheezing (21). Accordingly, the risk of hospitalization among virus-infected individuals is increased in patients who are both sensitized and exposed to respiratory allergens (25). When considered together, these findings provide strong evidence that individuals either with respiratory allergies or eosinophilic airway inflammation have an increased risk for wheezing with viral infections. These concepts have proven difficult to model in the laboratory, however, as inflammation secondary to allergen challenge had no effect on experimental RV infection in two carefully conducted studies (115,116). Although additional studies are required to solve this puzzle, these findings suggest that there may be additional cofactors, related to either the host or the environment, that help to drive the synergy between colds and allergic responses.

B. Cellular Immune and Cytokine Responses

Lymphocytes are recruited into the upper and lower airway during the early stages of a viral respiratory infection, and it is presumed that innate and adaptive immune responses serve to limit the extent of infection, and to clear virus-infected epithelial cells. This is consistent with reports of severe viral lower respiratory infections in immunocompromised patients (117).

For RSV, the G (attachment) and F (fusion) proteins are the major surface glycoproteins against which neutralizing antibody is directed. Interestingly, in both murine (118) and human (119) in vitro experiments, it has been noted that the G protein elicits a predominant Th-2 immune response, whereas the F protein and infectious RSV produce a predominant Th-1 response. This property of the G protein has led to speculation that this may be a mechanism by which RSV promotes allergen sensitization. In murine models, RSV infections are associated with the development of airway hyperresponsiveness (120) and an augmented allergic airway response (121). Some (72), but not all (122), investigators have demonstrated that these alterations are related to increased production of the Th-2-like cytokine IL-13 in the airway.

These and other animal models of respiratory viral infection suggest that cellular immune responses and patterns of cytokine production may be related to the outcome of respiratory infections. This same concept has been tested in a limited number of studies involving humans. Concentrations of IFN-γ in upper airway secretions are increased during episodes of viral-induced wheezing compared to Upper Respiratory infection Illness (URI) (110), indicating that more severe infections induce a greater antiviral immune response. In contrast, the capacity of peripheral blood mononuclear cells (PBMC) stimulated ex vivo to secrete IFN-γ is inversely related to the severity of respiratory illness in clinical studies. For example, PBMC production of IFN-γ both during and months following RSV has been observed in only those children who develop subsequent asthma (123).

In addition, in a birth cohort study of viral infections and immune development, the frequency of moderate to severe viral respiratory infections in the first year of life was inversely related to mitogen-induced IFN-γ from cord blood cells (124). This relationship was stronger in the subgroup of children with the greatest exposure to other children at home and day care, suggesting the presence of a gene-by-environment interaction.

Additional information has been obtained by evaluating immune responses in volunteers inoculated with a strain of RV. Peripheral blood mononuclear cell responses to RV-16 in vitro were assessed in a group of volunteers who were then inoculated with the same virus. Individuals who had strong IFN-γ responses to virus in peripheral blood cells shed less-virus during the peak of the cold (125). In addition, cytokine patterns in sputum have been compared to the outcome of experimentally induced RV infection. A stronger Th-1-like response in sputum cells (higher IFN-γ/IL-5 mRNA ratio) during the acute cold was associated with milder cold symptoms, and also more rapid clearance of the virus (50). In asthmatics, stronger Th-1-like responses to virus ex vivo correlated with better lung function and less airway responsiveness to methacholine (126). Together, these experimental findings suggest that the cellular immune response to respiratory viruses, and IFN-γ production in particular, can influence the clinical and virologic outcomes of infection. This is of special interest in light of experimental findings indicating that Th-1 responses to viruses could be impaired in asthma (127).

Finally, PBMC secretion of the anti-inflammatory cytokine IL-10 has also been evaluated in relationship to RSV-induced bronchiolitis resulting in hospitalization (128). During the convalescent phase three to four weeks after illness onset, IL-10 responses were significantly increased in patients as compared with those in healthy control subjects. At follow-up, 58% of the children had recurrent episodes of wheezing. IL-10 levels, measured during the convalescent phase, were significantly higher in patients who developed recurrent wheezing during the year after RSV bronchiolitis than in patients without recurrent episodes of wheezing. Moreover, IL-10 responses during the convalescent phase correlated significantly with the number of wheezing episodes. Interestingly, no association was found between IFN-γ responses, IL-4 responses, or IFN-γ/IL-4 ratios and recurrent wheezing. Unfortunately, in all of the studies reported thus far, the pattern of cytokine response these infants had prior to infection was not evaluated, begging the question as to which of the observed results may be cause and which effect.

Finally, risk factors for RSV infection have been evaluated in a limited number of genetic studies. This provides an attractive model for study: although practically all children contract RSV infection by the age of three years, only a subset of these children develop wheezing, and hospitalization is generally limited to 1–2% of the general population. Several different genes have been related to adverse outcomes with RSV infection (Table 1) (129–135), and this has spurred intensive efforts to determine the mechanisms underlying these relationships.

VI. Treatment of Virus-Induced Wheezing and Asthma

A. Virus-Induced Wheezing in Infancy

Standard therapy for virus-induced wheezing in young children generally includes a stepwise addition of medications, typically commencing with a bronchodilator. If lower respiratory tract symptoms become increasingly severe or respiratory distress develops, oral corticosteroids are often added. Recent clinical trials in the management of these wheezing episodes also have included the use of high dose inhaled corticosteroids (both prophylactically and/or as an acute intervention) and leukotriene receptor antagonists.

The efficacy of various therapeutic interventions for the acute symptoms of wheezing, tachypnea, retractions, and hypoxemia that occur as a result of bronchiolitis has been controversial due to variations in study design, the inability to rapidly and conveniently measure pulmonary physiologic variables, the confounding of results by the inclusion of children with a history of multiple wheezing episodes (i.e., asthmatic phenotypes), and the choice of outcome measures that have been evaluated. In a recent Cochrane meta-analysis of this subject (136), bronchodilators were found to produce modest short-term improvements in clinical features of mild or moderately severe bronchiolitis; no differences in the rate or duration of hospitalization were noted. However, given the high costs and uncertain benefit of this therapy, the authors concluded that bronchodilators could not be recommended for routine management of first-time wheezers. They further recommended that prior to conducting future treatment trials, an outcome measure that reflects pulmonary status independent of the level of alertness needs to be validated.

The efficacy of therapy with either oral or parenteral corticosteroids has recently been reviewed by a number of authors (137,138). In one

Table 1 Genetic Associations with More Severe RSV Infections

Gene	Function	Associated Outcome	Study Design	References
CCR5	Receptor for chemokines (RANTES)	More severe hospitalized patients	Case control and transmission disequilibrium	132
IL-4	Th-2 differentiation, promotes IgE synthesis	Hospitalization	Case control	131, 133
IL-4RA	Receptor subunit for IL-4 and IL-13	Hospitalization	Case control and transmission disequilibrium	133
IL-8	Neutrophil chemoattractant		Transmission disequilibrium	129
IL-10	Anti-inflammatory cytokine	Hospitalization	Case control and transmission disequilibrium	130
Surfactant protein D	Airway surfactant	Hospitalization		134
TGFB1	Fibrosis, anti-inflammatory effects	Wheezing	Birth cohort	135

Abbreviations: RANTES, regulated on activation normal T cell expressed and secreted.

meta-analysis (137) of twelve relevant publications, six met the selection criteria and had relevant data available. Corticosteroid therapy (prednisone, prednisolone, methylprednisone, hydrocortisone, dexamethasone; with routes of administration being oral, intramuscular, or intravenous; dose ranges = 0.6–6.3 mg/kg/day of prednisolone equivalents) was associated with a statistically significant reduction in clinical symptom scores and length of hospital stay. The effects of corticosteroids on improving clinical symptom scores were apparent within 24 hours of treatment initiation. The authors also indicated that their analyses suggested that corticosteroid treatment might have its greatest effects in more severe cases.

B. Effect of Corticosteroids for the Prophylactic Treatment of Chronic Respiratory Tract Symptoms Associated with RSV-Induced Bronchiolitis

Several placebo-controlled trials (4,139–147) that address the question as to whether corticosteroid treatment can influence the degree of respiratory sequelae after RSV bronchiolitis have recently been reviewed (1). The majority (7 out of 10) of these trials did not show any long-term effects (follow-up time from 6 months to 5 years) on postbronchiolitic wheezing, the development of various wheezing phenotypes (transient, persistent, or late-onset), or a subsequent diagnosis of asthma. In the three trials that did show some benefit, the positive effects observed were mainly over shorter time intervals following infection. One study (147) concluded that the greatest benefit was more likely to be seen in atopic children.

C. Role of Oral Corticosteroids in Acute Exacerbations of Asthma in Young Children

Numerous studies have been undertaken to assess the role of corticosteroid therapy in acute episodes of asthma in children and adults. A meta-analysis of these studies supports the early use of systemic corticosteroids in acute exacerbations based upon a reduction in the admission rate for asthma and prevention of relapse in the outpatient treatment of exacerbations (148). As a reflection of such information, the most recent National Heart, Lung, and Blood Institute (NHLBI) Guidelines for the Diagnosis and Management of Asthma recommend the addition of corticosteroids for asthma exacerbations unresponsive to bronchodilators. These guidelines recommend the addition of oral corticosteroids for the management of moderate and severe exacerbations (149). Alternately, it was suggested that the dose of maintenance inhaled corticosteroids (ICS) could be doubled for mild episodes unresponsive to bronchodilators, although more recent information suggests that this approach does not reduce the risk of exacerbation

(150). Unfortunately, the applicability of these recommendations to young children and infants whose acute wheezing episode is primarily related to viral respiratory tract infections has not been as thoroughly evaluated.

However, results from a few clinical trials are noteworthy. Brunette et al. (151) explored the role of early intervention with oral corticosteroid therapy in 32 children under the age of six years (mean age 38.4 months) with asthma typically provoked by viral URIs. During the first year of this two-year study, acute exacerbations were treated with oral bronchodilators initially with the addition of prednisolone for more severe attacks. In the second year, oral prednisolone was initiated at the first sign of an upper respiratory infection to a group of patients whose parents and caretakers were unblinded to the treatment intervention. The group receiving prednisolone during the second year experienced fewer attacks, a 65% reduction in the number of wheezing days, a 61% decrease in emergency department (ED) visits, and a 90% decrease in hospitalizations. The administration of prednisolone at the first sign of URI was not associated with greater overall prednisolone usage. Although this study suggests that early intervention with oral corticosteroids has the potential to significantly impact the morbidity associated with acute viral-induced asthma episodes, the unblinded study design makes these results less convincing.

Tal et al. conducted an emergency department-based, double-blind, placebo-controlled trial of administration of a single dose of methylprednisolone intramuscularly and demonstrated a statistically significant decrease in hospitalization rate (20% in methylprednisolone group versus 43% in control group, $p < 0.05$ this effect was most pronounced in the group less than 24 months of age, 18% in methylprednisolone group versus 50% in control group, $p < 0.050$) (152). Taken together, the results of these two studies suggest that early corticosteroid therapy, ideally started at home, should impact on the progression of asthma episodes and decrease the rate of hospitalization for asthma.

D. Role of ICS in the Treatment of Acute Asthma Exacerbations

Young children who experience frequent exacerbations of asthma may receive several short courses of systemic corticosteroids during each viral season. Individual courses of oral corticosteroids may be associated with behavioral side effects. In addition, Dolan et al. reported that 20% of children who received four or more short courses of oral corticosteroids in the past year had impaired response to insulin-induced hypoglycemia (153). The potential toxicity of repeated courses of oral corticosteroids is a significant clinical concern and likely influences the behaviors of pediatricians faced with young children who wheeze following URI symptoms. The use of topical ICS in the treatment of acute exacerbations is likely to be accompanied by a greater safety profile and parental acceptance.

The efficacy of ICS intervention has been evaluated by at least six different research groups. First, Wilson and Silverman (154) examined the use of beclomethasone dipropionate [750 μg three times daily for five days administered via metered dose inhaler (MDI)] at the first sign of an asthma episode in children one to five years of age. Although failing to alter the need for additional therapy, ICS therapy was associated with improvement in asthma symptoms during the first week of the episode. Second, Daugbjerg et al. (155) conducted a double-blind placebo-controlled trial comparing the effects of inhaled bronchodilator alone or in combination with either high dose ICS (budesonide nebulization, 0.5 mg every four hours until discharge) or systemic corticosteroid (prednisolone) in children below 18 months of age admitted to a hospital with acute wheezing. Their results demonstrated earlier discharge from hospital in both the inhaled and systemic corticosteroid-treated groups, as well as a significantly accelerated rate of clinical improvement in the budesonide-treated group compared to the oral corticosteroid and non-corticosteroid treated groups.

Third, Connett and Lenney (156) compared the efficacy of two doses of budesonide (800 or 1600 μg twice daily) via MDI and a spacer device initiated at the onset of upper respiratory tract symptoms in preschool aged children with recurrent wheezing with URIs. Therapy was continued for up to seven days or until patients were asymptomatic for 24 hours. Budesonide therapy was associated with decreased symptom scores during the first week of infection. Fourth, a double-blind, placebo-controlled crossover study by Svedmyr et al. (157) involved administration of budesonide (200 μg qid for three days, tid for three days and bid for three days) via MDI and spacer or placebo to children 3 to 10 years of age with a history of URI-associated deterioration of asthma. While having no significant impact on symptom scores, budesonide therapy was associated with significantly higher peak expiratory flow (PEF) rates. Fifth, in a recent ED-based study, Volovitz et al. compared the effect of inhaled budesonide and oral prednisolone in children aged 6 to 16 years with acute asthma exacerbations (158). Patients received either budesonide 1600 μg by turbuhaler or 2 mg/kg of oral prednisolone in the ED followed by a tapering dose of medication over the next six days. Both treatment groups had similar rates of improvement in the ED in terms of symptom scores and PEF. However, over the next week, the budesonide treated group had a more rapid improvement in asthma symptoms. Serum cortisol levels and response to adreno corticotropic hormone (ACTH) were significantly decreased in the prednisolone group at the end of the week of therapy compared to the budesonide group but returned to the normal range two weeks later. This study suggests that high dose therapy with a potent ICS may be as effective as oral prednisolone and avoids hypothalamic pituitary adrenal axis (HPA) axis suppression. Sixth, a recent study comparing the effects of high dose ICS and oral corticosteroids in children seen in an ED for acute severe asthma (mean

$FEV_1 < 40\%$ predicted upon presentation) found oral corticosteroids superior in terms of improvement in lung function and hospitalization rate (159).

However, these patients were clearly in the midst of severe exacerbations, and ICS were not utilized early in the course of the illness.

In summary, ICS appear to improve asthma symptoms when given for acute exacerbations of asthma. While providing useful information, all of these studies are limited by small numbers of patients and do not delineate features predictive of patients who would be expected to respond to a given therapy. In addition, the ideal drug, dosage, delivery system, and duration of therapy remain unclear. Improved delivery of a potent drug to the lower airways may be associated with a more favorable clinical response.

E. Role of Leukotrienes in Viral-Induced Wheezing

The cysteinyl leukotrienes have been identified as important mediators in the complex pathophysiology of asthma. Leukotrienes are detectable in the blood, urine, nasal secretions, sputum, and bronchoalveolar lavage fluid of patients with chronic asthma. In addition, leukotrienes are released during acute asthma episodes. Volovitz and colleagues demonstrated elevated levels of leukotriene C4 (LTC4) in nasopharyngeal secretions from infants with acute bronchiolitis due to RSV compared with children with upper respiratory illnesses alone (98). A recent study by van Schaik et al. (110) also examined leukotriene levels in nasopharyngeal samples from infants and young children with either upper respiratory infections without wheezing, bronchiolitis (first-time wheezers), or acute episodes of wheezing in children with a prior wheezing episode(s). These investigators found elevated levels of leukotrienes in nasopharyngeal samples from both first-time and recurrent viral wheezers compared with children with non-wheezing URIs. Finally, bronchoalveolar lavage samples obtained from recurrently wheezing young children (median age = 14.9 months) have been found to contain not only an increase in numbers of epithelial and inflammatory cells, but increased levels of cyclooxygenase and lipoxygenase pathway mediators as well (160).

Interestingly, levels of these cells and mediators were unaffected by concurrent treatment with ICS. These studies, when combined with in vitro data demonstrating increased 5-lipoxygenase activity with RSV infection of bronchial epithelial cell lines (161), or reductions in RSV-induced airway edema in rats following treatment with a leukotriene receptor antagonist (162), suggest a potential role of leukotrienes in acute episodic viral-induced wheezing.

A recent prospective clinical trial indicates that leukotrienes may contribute to more chronic sequelae as well (163). The authors enrolled infants, 3 to 36 months old (median age = 9 months), who were hospitalized with acute RSV bronchiolitis. They were randomized into a double-blind, parallel comparison of 5 mg montelukast or matching placebo given for 28 days starting within seven days of the onset of symptoms. Infants with a suspected history of asthma were excluded. Infants on montelukast had significantly more days free of day and nighttime symptoms compared to those on placebo (22% vs. 4%). Exacerbations were significantly delayed following montelukast treatment compared with placebo as well. These findings indicate that LTRA treatment reduces lung symptoms subsequent to RSV bronchiolitis. Whether more prolonged treatment could influence asthma inception in infants at risk remains to be determined.

VII. Future Directions

Viral infections are important causes of wheezing illnesses throughout childhood. There has been progress in understanding how viral infections produce wheezing, and in identifying risk factors for severe respiratory symptoms, and in particular, wheezing. The precise role of viral infections in causing asthma, however, is still incompletely understood. This is largely a result of the difficulty in ascertaining risk factors, including lung function, during early infancy before the onset of virus-induced wheezing, and in differentiating risk factors for wheezing from those associated with asthma.

A more thorough understanding of risk factors and associated mechanisms could lead to new and more effective strategies for the prevention of virus-induced wheezing, and perhaps the ability to intervene in the early stages of this process to block the transition from virus-induced wheezing to asthma.

Given the close relationship between viral infections and wheezing illnesses in children, it would be attractive to apply anti-viral strategies to the prevention and treatment of asthma, and both RV and RSV are obvious targets. Unfortunately, attempts at developing an RSV vaccine have so far been unsuccessful, and vaccination to prevent RV infection does not seem to be feasible due to the large number of serotypes. As an alternative, several types of anti-viral agents are in development, and several compounds with activity against RV have been tested in clinical trials. These include molecules such as soluble ICAM and capsid-binding agents, which either hinder RV binding to cellular receptors or inhibit uncoating of the virus to release RNA inside the cell (164–167), and inhibitors of RV 3C protease (168). One problem with the use of antiviral medications is that once the clinical signs and symptoms appear, viral replication is well underway. As a result, reductions in respiratory symptoms or the duration of illness are modest (167).

The other potential therapeutic approach for respiratory viral infections would be to selectively inhibit pro-inflammatory immune responses induced by the virus. The beneficial effects of systemic glucocorticoids indicate that this approach is valid; the challenge will be to develop treatments with greater efficacy and a reduced potential for adverse effects. It remains to be demonstrated whether more focused inhibition of specific components of virus-induced inflammation, such as pro-inflammatory cytokines (e.g., IL-8) or mediators (leukotrienes and bradykinin), will successfully reduce the severity of viral respiratory infections or exacerbations of asthma.

Acknowledgments

Supported by NIH Grants AI34891, HL56396, 1RO1HL61879, and P01HL070831.

References

1. Wennergren G, Kristjansson S. Relationship between respiratory syncytial virus bronchiolitis and future obstructive airway diseases. Eur Respir J 2001; 18(6):1044–1058.
2. Openshaw PJM. Immunological mechanisms in respiratory syncytial virus disease. Springer Semin Immunopathol 1995; 17:187–201.
3. Welliver RC. Respiratory syncytial virus and other respiratory viruses. Pediatr Infect Dis J 2003; 22(2 suppl):S6–S10.
4. Reijonen TM, Kotaniemi-Syrjänen A, Korhonen K, Korppi M. Predictors of asthma three years after hospital admission for wheezing in infancy. Pediatrics 2000; 106:1406–1412.
5. Stein RT, Sherrill D, Morgan WJ, Holberg CJ, Halonen M, Taussig LM, Wright AL, Martinez FD. Respiratory syncytial virus in early life and risk of wheeze and allergy by age 13 years. Lancet 1999; 354:541–545.
6. Openshaw PJ, Dean GS, Culley FJ. Links between respiratory syncytial virus bronchiolitis and childhood asthma: clinical and research approaches. Pediatr Infect Dis J 2003; 22(2 Suppl):S58–S64.
7. Taussig LM, Wright AL, Holberg CJ, Halonen M, Morgan WJ, Martinez FD. Tucson children's respiratory study: 1980 to present. J All Clin Immunol 2003; 111(4):661–675.
8. Martinez FD. Respiratory syncytial virus bronchiolitis and the pathogenesis of childhood asthma. Pediatr Infect Dis J 2003; 22(2 suppl):S76–S82.
9. Castro-Rodríguez JA, Holberg CJ, Wright AL, Halonen M, Taussig LM, Morgan WJ, Martinez FD. Association of radiologically ascertained pneumonia before age 3 yr with asthmalike symptoms and pulmonary function during childhood: a prospective study. Am J Respir Crit Care Med 1999; 159(6):1891–1897.
10. McBride JT. Pulmonary function changes in children after respiratory syncytial virus infection in infancy. J Pediatr 1999; 135(2 Pt 2):28–32.

11. Kneyber MCJ, Steyerberg EW, De Groot R, Moll HA. Long-term effects of respiratory syncytial virus (RSV) bronchiolitis in infants and young children: a quantitative review. Acta Paediatr 2000; 89(6):654–660.

12. Korppi M, Reijonen T, Poysa L, Juntunen-Backman K. A 2- to 3-year outcome after bronchiolitis. Am J Dis Child 1993; 147(6):628–631.

13. Wennergren G, Amark M, Amark K, Oskarsdottir S, Sten G, Redfors S. Wheezing bronchitis reinvestigated at the age of 10 years. Acta Paediatr 1997; 86(4): 351–355.

14. Eriksson M, Bennet R, Nilsson A. Wheezing following lower respiratory tract infections with respiratory syncytial virus and influenza A in infancy. Pediatr All Immunol 2000; 11(3):193–197.

15. Williams JV, Harris PA, Tollefson SJ, Halburnt-Rush LL, Pingsterhaus JM, Edwards KM, Wright PF, Crowe JE, Jr. Human metapneumovirus and lower respiratory tract disease in otherwise healthy infants and children. N Engl J Med 2004; 350(5):443–450.

16. Kotaniemi-Syrjanen A, Vainionpaa R, Reijonen TM, Waris M, Korhonen K, Korppi M. Rhinovirus-induced wheezing in infancy—the first sign of childhood asthma?. J All Clin Immunol 2003; 111(1):66–71.

17. Lemanske RF, Jr., Jackson DJ, Gangnon RE, Evans ME, Li Z, Shult P, Kirk CJ, Reisdorf E, Roberg KA, Anderson EL, Carlson-Dakes KT, Adler KJ, Gilbertson-White S, Pappas TE, DeSilva DF, Tisler CJ, Gern JE. Rhinovirus illnesses during infancy predict subsequent childhood wheexzing. J Allergy Clin Immunol. In press.

18. Johnston SL, Pattemore PK, Sanderson G, Smith S, Lampe F, Josephs L, Symington P, O'Toole S, Myint SH, Tyrrell DA, Holgate ST. Community study of role of viral infections in exacerbations of asthma in 9–11 year old children. BMJ 1995; 310(6989):1225–1229.

19. Johnston SL, Pattemore PK, Sanderson G, Smith S, Campbell MJ, Josephs LK, Cunningham A, Robinson BS, Myint SH, Ward ME, Tyrrell DAJ, Holgate ST. The relationship between upper respiratory infections and hospital admissions for asthma: a time-trend analysis. Am J Respir Crit Care Med 1996; 154(3 Pt 1):654–660.

20. Ingram JM, Rakes GP, Hoover GE, Platts-Mills TA, Heymann PW. Eosinophil cationic protein in serum and nasal washes from wheezing infants and children. J Pediatr 1995; 127(4):558–564.

21. Rakes GP, Arruda E, Ingram JM, Hoover GE, Zambrano JC, Hayden FG, Platts-Mills TA, Heymann PW. Rhinovirus and respiratory syncytial virus in wheezing children requiring emergency care. IgE and eosinophil analyses. Am J Respir Crit Care Med 1999; 159(3):785–790.

22. Atmar RL, Guy E, Guntupalli KK, Zimmerman JL, Bandi VD, Baxter BD, Greenberg SB. Respiratory tract viral infections in inner city asthmatic adults. Arch Intern Med 1998; 158(2453):2459.

23. Skoner DP, Doyle WJ, Seroky J, Vandeusen MA, Fireman P. Lower airway responses to rhinovirus 39 in healthy allergic and nonallergic subjects. Eur Respir J 1996; 9(7):1402–1406.

24. Corne JM, Marshall C, Smith S, Schreiber J, Sanderson G, Holgate ST, Johnston SL. Frequency, severity, and duration of rhinovirus infections in asth-

matic and non-asthmatic individuals: a longitudinal cohort study. Lancet 2002; 359(9309):831–834.

25. Green RM, Custovic A, Sanderson G, Hunter J, Johnston SL, Woodcock A. Synergism between allergens and viruses and risk of hospital admission with asthma: case-control study. BMJ 2002; 324(7340):763.

26. Tarlo SM, Broder I, Corey P, Chan-Yeung M, Ferguson A, Becker A, Rogers C, Okada M, Manfreda J. The role of symptomatic colds in asthma exacerbations: Influence of outdoor allergens and air pollutants. J Allergy Clin Immunol 2001; 108(1):52–58.

27. Smyth AR, Smyth RL, Tong CYW, Hart CA, Heaf DP. Effect of respiratory virus infections including rhinovirus on clinical status in cystic fibrosis. Arch Dis Child 1995; 73:117–120.

28. Seemungal T, Harper-Owen R, Bhowmik A, Moric I, Sanderson G, Message S, et al. Respiratory viruses, symptoms, and inflammatory markers in acute exacerbations and stable chronic obstructive pulmonary disease. Am J Respir Crit Care Med 2001; 164(9):1618–1623.

29. Hegele RG, Ahmad HY, Becker AB, Dimich-Ward H, Ferguson AC, Manfreda J, Watson WT, Chan-Yeung M. The association between respiratory viruses and symptoms in 2-week-old infants at high risk for asthma and allergy. J Pediatr 2001; 138(6):831–837.

30. Nicholson KG, Kent J, Hammersley V, Cancio E. Risk factors for lower respiratory complications of rhinovirus infections in elderly people living in the community: prospective cohort study. BMJ 1996; 313:1119–1123.

31. McFadden ER, Jr. Improper patient techniques with metered dose inhalers: clinical consequences and solutions to misuse. J All Clin Immunol 1995; 96:278–283.

32. Konno S, Grindle KA, Lee WM, Schroth MK, Mosser AG, Brockman-Schneider RA, Busse WW, Gern JE. Interferon-gamma enhances rhinovirus-induced RANTES secretion by airway epithelial cells. Am J Respir Cell Mol Biol 2002; 26(5):594–601.

33. Gern JE, Galagan DM, Jarjour NN, Dick EC, Busse WW. Detection of rhinovirus RNA in lower airway cells during experimentally induced infection. Am J Respir Crit Care Med 1997; 155:1159–1161.

34. Papadopoulos NG, Bates PJ, Bardin PG, Papi A, Leir SH, Fraenkel DJ, Meyer J, Lackie PM, Sanderson G, Holgate ST, Johnston SL. Rhinoviruses infect the lower airways. J Infect Dis 2000; 181(6):1875–1884.

34a. Mosser AG, Urtis R, Ruchell L, Lee WM, Dick CR, Weissman E, Bock D, Swenson CA, Cornwell RD, Meyer KC, Jarjour NN, Busse WW, Gern JE. Quantitative and qualitative analysis of rhinovirus infection in bronchial tissues. Am J Respir Crit Care 2005; 171:645–651.

35. Jarjour NN, Gern JE, Kelly EAB, Swenson CA, Dick CR, Busse WW. The effect of an experimental rhinovirus 16 infection on bronchial lavage neutrophils. J All Clin Immunol 2000; 105:1169–1177.

36. Fraenkel DJ, Bardin PG, Sanderson G, Lampe F, Johnston SL, Holgate ST. Lower airway inflammation during rhinovirus colds in normal and in asthmatic subjects. Am J Respir Crit Care Med 1995; 151:879–886.

37. Grünberg K, Sharon RF, Hiltermann TJN, Brahim JJ, Dick EC, Sterk PJ, Van Krieken JHJM. Experimental rhinovirus 16 infection increases intercellular adhesion molecule-1 expression in bronchial epithelium of asthmatics regardless of inhaled steroid treatment. Clin Exp Allergy 2000; 30(7):1015–1023.

38. Horn MEC, Reed SE, Taylor P. Role of viruses and bacteria in acute wheezy bronchitis in childhood: a study of sputum. Arch Dis Child 1979; 54:587–592.

39. Bardin PG, Johnston SL, Pattemore PK. Viruses as precipitants of asthma symptoms. II. Physiology and mechanisms. Clin Experiment All 1992; 22:809–822.

40. Hakonarson H, Carter C, Maskeri N, Hodinka R, Grunstein MM. Rhinovirus-mediated changes in airway smooth muscle responsiveness: induced autocrine role of interleukin-1b. Am J Physiol Lung Cell Mol Physiol 1999; 277(1):L13–L21.

41. Grunstein MM, Hakonarson H, Whelan R, Yu Z, Grunstein JS, Chuang S. Rhinovirus elicits proasthmatic changes in airway responsiveness independently of viral infection. J All Clin Immunol 2001; 108(6):997–1004.

42. Hendley JO. The host response, not the virus, causes the symptoms of the common cold. Clin Infect Dis 1998; 26(4):847–848.

43. Igarashi Y, Skoner DP, Doyle WJ, White MV, Fireman P, Kaliner MA. Analysis of nasal secretions during experimental rhinovirus upper respiratory infections. J All Clin Immunol 1993; 92:722–731.

44. Ohrui T, Yamaya M, Sekizawa K, Yamada N, Suzuki T, Terajima M, Okinaga S, Sasaki H. Effects of rhinovirus infection on hydrogen peroxide-induced alterations of barrier function in the cultured human tracheal epithelium. Am J Respir Crit Care Med 1998; 158(1):241–248.

45. Lopez-Souza N, Dolganov G, Dubin R, Sachs LA, Sassina L, Sporer H, Yagi S, Schnurr D, Boushey HA, Widdicombe JH. Resistance of differentiated human airway epithelium to infection by rhinovirus. American Journal of Physiology - Lung Cellular & Molecular Physiology 2004; 286(2):L373–L381.

46. Kurt-Jones EA, Popova L, Kwinn L, Haynes LM, Jones LP, Tripp RA, Walsh EE, Freeman MW, Golenbock DT, Anderson LJ, Finberg RW. Pattern recognition receptors TLR4 and CD14 mediate response to respiratory syncytial virus. Nature Immunology 2000; 1(5):398–401.

47. Kaul P, Biagioli MC, Singh I, Turner RB. Rhinovirus-induced oxidative stress and interleukin-8 elaboration involves p47-*phox* but is independent of attachment to intercellular adhesion molecule-1 and viral replication. J Infect Dis 2000; 181:1885–1890.

48. Alexopoulou L, Holt AC, Medzhitov R, Flavell RA. Recognition of double-stranded RNA and activation of NF-kappaB by Toll- like receptor 3. Nature 2001; 413(6857):732–738.

49. Williams BRG. PKR: a sentinel kinase for cellular stress. Oncogene 1999; 18:6112–6120.

50. Gern JE, Vrtis R, Grindle KA, Swenson C, Busse WW. Relationship of upper and lower airway cytokines to outcome of experimental rhinovirus infection. Am J Respir Crit Care Med 2000; 162:2226–2231.

51. Gern JE, Vrtis R, Kelly EAB, Dick EC, Busse WW. Rhinovirus produces nonspecific activation of lymphocytes through a monocyte-dependent mechanism. J Immunol 1996; 157:1605–1612.

52. Panuska JR, Merolla R, Rebert NA, Hoffmann SP, Tsivitse P, Cirino NM, et al. Respiratory syncytial virus induces interleukin-10 by human alveolar macrophages. Suppression of early cytokine production and implications for incomplete immunity. J Clin Invest 1995; 96(5):2445–2453.

53. Johnston SL, Papi A, Monick MM, Hunninghake GW. Rhinoviruses induce interleukin-8 mRNA and protein production in human monocytes. J Infect Dis 1997; 175(2):323–329.

54. McNamara PS, Smyth RL. The pathogenesis of respiratory syncytial virus disease in childhood. Br Med Bull 2002; 61:13–28.

55. Cardell LO, Agusti C, Takeyama K, Stjarne P, Nadel JA. LTB(4)-induced nasal gland serous cell secretion mediated by neutrophil elastase. Am J Respir Crit Care Med 1999; 160(2):411–414.

56. Grünberg K, Timmers MC, Smits HH, De Klerk EPA, Dick EC, Spaan WJM, Hiemstra PS, Sterk PJ. Effect of experimental rhinovirus 16 colds on airway hyperresponsiveness to histamine and interleukin-8 in nasal lavage in asthmatic subjects *in vivo*. Clin Exp Allergy 1997; 27:36–45.

57. Gern JE, Martin MS, Anklam KA, Shen K, Roberg KA, Carlson-Dakes KT, Adler K, Gilbertson-White S, Hamilton R, Shult PA, Kirk CJ, Da Silva DF, Sund SA, Kosorok MR, Lemanske RF, Jr. Relationships among specific viral pathogens, virus-induced interleukin-8, and respiratory symptoms in infancy. Pediatric Allergy & Immunology. 2002;13:386–393.

58. Jacoby DB. Virus-induced asthma attacks. J Am Med Assoc 2002; 287(6): 755–761.

59. Jacoby DB, Tamaoki J, Borson DB, Nadel JA. Influenza infection causes airway hyperresponsiveness by decreasing enkephalinase. J Appl Physiol 1988; 64:2653–2658.

60. Sanders SP. Asthma, viruses, and nitric oxide. Review (162 refs). Proc Soc Exp Biol Med 1999; 220(3):123–132.

61. Sanders SP, Siekierski ES, Richards SM, Porter JD, Imani F, Proud D. Rhinovirus infection induces expression of type 2 nitric oxide synthase in human respiratory epithelial cells in vitro and in vivo. J All Clin Immunol 2001; 107(2):235–243.

62. Fryer AD, Jacoby DB. Parainfluenza virus infection damages inhibitory M2 muscarinic receptors on pulmonary parasympathetic nerves in the guinea pig. Br J Pharmacol 1991; 102:267–271.

63. Bowerfind WML, Fryer AD, Jacoby DB. Double-stranded RNA causes airway hyperreactivity and neuronal M_2 muscarinic receptor dysfunction. J Appl Physiol 2002; 92(4):1417–1422.

64. Jacoby DB, Yost BL, Elwood T, Fryer AD. Effects of neurokinin receptor antagonists in virus-infected airways. Am J Physiol Lung Cell Mol Physiol 2000; 279(1):L59–L65.

65. Moreno L, Jacoby DB, Fryer AD. Dexamethasone prevents virus-induced hyperresponsiveness via multiple mechanisms. Am J Physiol Lung Cell Mol Physiol 2003; 285(2):L451–L455.

66. Davies DE, Wicks J, Powell RM, Puddicombe SM, Holgate ST. Airway remodeling in asthma: new insights. J All Clin Immunol 2003; 111(2):215–225.
67. Çokugras H, Akçakaya N, Seçkin I, Camcioglu Y, Sarimurat N, Aksoy F. Ultrastructural examination of bronchial biopsy specimens from children with moderate asthma. Thorax 2001; 56(1):25–29.
68. Walter MJ, Morton JD, Kajiwara N, Agapov E, Holtzman MJ. Viral induction of a chronic asthma phenotype and genetic segregation from the acute response. J Clin Invest 2002; 110(2):165–175.
69. Martinez FD, Wright AL, Taussig LM, Holberg CJ, Halonen M, Morgan WJ, Group Health Medical Associates. Asthma and wheezing in the first six years of life. N Engl J Med 1995; 332:133–138.
70. Johnson TR, Parker RA, Johnson JE, Graham BS. IL-13 is Sufficient for Respiratory syncytial virus G glycoprotein-induced eosinophilia after respiratory syncytial virus challenge. J Immunol 2003; 170(4):2037–2045.
71. Culley FJ, Pollott J, Openshaw PJ. Age at first viral infection determines the pattern of T-cell-mediated disease during reinfection in adulthood [Comment.]. J Exp Med 2002; 196(10):1381–1386.
72. Tekkanat KK, Maassab HF, Cho DS, Lai JJ, John A, Berlin A, Kaplan MH, Lukacs NW. IL-13-induced airway hyperreactivity during respiratory syncytial virus infection is STAT6 dependent. J Immunol 2001; 166(5):3542–3548.
73. Makela MJ, Tripp R, Dakhama A, Park JW, Ikemura T, Joetham A, Waris M, Anderson LJ, Gelfand EW. Prior airway exposure to allergen increases virus-induced airway hyperresponsiveness. J Allergy Clin Immunol 2003; 112(5):861–869.
74. Castleman WL, Sorkness RL, Lemanske RF Jr., Grasee G, Suyemoto MM. Neonatal viral bronchiolitis and pneumonia induce bronchiolar hypoplasia and alveolar dysplasia in rats. Lab Invest 1988; 59:387–396.
75. Uhl EW, Castleman WL, Sorkness RL, Busse WW, Lemanske RF Jr., McAllister PK. Parainfluenza virus-induced persistence of airway inflammation, fibrosis, and dysfunction associated with TGF-b$_1$ expression in Brown Norway rats. Am J Respir Crit Care Med 1996; 154:1834–1842.
76. Kumar A, Sorkness R, Kaplan MR, Castleman WL, Lemanske RF Jr. Chronic, episodic, reversible airway obstruction after viral bronchiolitis in rats. Am J Respir Crit Care Med 1997; 155:130–134.
77. Sorkness RL, Castleman WL, Kumar A, Kaplan MR, Lemanske RF Jr. Prevention of chronic post-bronchiolitis airway sequelae with interferon-γ treatment in rats. Am J Respir Crit Care Med 1999; 160:705–710.
78. Mikus LD, Rosenthal LA, Sorkness RL, Lemanske RF Jr. Reduced interferon-gamma secretion by natural killer cells from rats susceptible to postviral chronic airway dysfunction. Am J Respir Cell Mol Biol 2001; 24(1):74–82.
79. Bardin PG, Fraenkel DJ, Sanderson G, Dorward M, Lau LCK, Johnston SL, Holgate ST. Amplified rhinovirus colds in atopic subjects. Clin Experiment Allergy 1994; 24:457–464.
80. Sigurs N, Bjarnason R, Sigurbergsson F, Kjellman B, Bjorksten B. Asthma and immunoglobulin E antibodies after respiratory syncytial virus bronchiolitis: A prospective cohort study with matched controls. Pediatric 1995; 95:500–505.

81. Frick WE, German D, Mills J. Development of allergy in children, I. association with virus infection. J All Clin Immunol 1979; 63:228–241.
82. McIntire JJ, Umetsu SE, Macaubas C, Hoyte EG, Cinnioglu C, Cavalli-Sforza LL, Barsh GS, Hallmayer JF, Underhill PA, Risch NJ, Freeman GJ, DeKruyff RH, Umetsu DT. Immunology: hepatitis A virus link to atopic disease. Nature 2003; 425(6958):576.
83. Lemanske RF Jr., Dick EC, Swenson CA, Vrtis RF, Busse WW. Rhinovirus upper respiratory infection increases airway hyperreactivity and late asthmatic reactions. J Clin Invest 1989; 83:1–10.
84. Skoner DP, Doyle WJ, Seroky J, Fireman P. Lower airway responses to influenza A virus in healthy allergic and nonallergic subjects. Am J Respir Crit Care Med 1996; 154:661–664.
85. Calhoun WJ, Dick EC, Schwartz LB, Busse WW. A common cold virus, rhinovirus 16, potentiates airway inflammation after segmental antigen bronchoprovocation in allergic subjects. J Clin Invest 1994; 94:2200–2208.
86. Laing I, Riedel F, Yap PL, Simpson H. Atopy predisposing to acute bronchiolitis during an epidemic of respiratory syncytial virus. Br Med J 1982; 284:1070–1072.
87. Rooney JC, Williams HE. The relationship between proved viral bronchiolitis and subsequent wheezing. J Pediatr 1971; 79:744–747.
88. Zweiman B, Schoenwetter WF, Pappano JE, Tempest B, Hildreth EA. Patterns of allergic respiratory disease in children with a past history of bronchiolitis. J All Clin Immunol 1971; 48:283–289.
89. Pullan CR, Hey EN. Wheezing, asthma, and pulmonary dysfunction 10 years after infection with respiratory syncytial virus in infancy. Br Med J 1982; 284:1665–1669.
90. Murray M, Webb MSC, Ocallaghan C, Swarbrick AS, Milner AD. Respiratory status and allergy after bronchiolitis. Arch Dis Child 1992; 67:482–487.
91. Noma T, Yoshizawa I. Induction of allergen-specific IL-2 responsiveness of lymphocytes after respiratory syncytial virus infection and prediction of onset of recurrent wheezing and bronchial asthma. J All Clin Immunol 1997; 98: 816–826.
92. Welliver RC. Immunologic mechanisms of virus-induced wheezing and asthma. J Pediatr 1999; 135:S14–S20.
93. Sakamoto M, Ida S, Takishima T. Effect of influenza virus infection on allergic sensitization to aerosolized ovalbumin in mice. J Immunol 1984; 132: 2614–2617.
94. Freihorst J, Piedra PA, Okamoto Y, Ogra PL. Effect of respiratory syncytial virus infection on the uptake of and immune response to other inhaled antigens. Proc Soc Exp Biol Med 1988; 188:191–197.
95. Garofalo R, Kimpen JLL, Welliver RC, Ogra PL. Eosinophil degranulation in the respiratory tract during naturally acquired respiratory syncytial virus infection. J Pediatr 1992; 120:28–32.
96. Kimpen JLL, Garofalo R, Welliver RC, Ogra PL. Activation of human eosinophils in vitro by respiratory syncytial virus. Pediatr Res 1992; 32:160–164.

97. Welliver RC, Wong DT, Rijnaldo D, Ogra PL. Predictive value of respiratory syncytial virus-specific IgE responses for recurrent wheezing following bronchiolitis. J Pediatr 1986; 109:776–780.

98. Volovitz B, Welliver RC, De Castro G, Krystofik DA, Ogra PL. The release of leukotrienes in the respiratory tract during infection with respiratory syncytial virus: role in obstructive airway disease. Pediatr Res 1988; 24:504–507.

99. Welliver RC, Wong DT, Sun M, Middleton EJr, Vaughan RS, Ogra PL. The development of respiratory syncytial virus-specific IgE and the release of histamine in nasopharyngeal secretions after infection. N Engl J Med 1981; 305:841–846.

100. Rabatic S, Gagro A, Lokarkolbas R, KrsulovicHresic V, Vrtar Z, PopowKraupp T, Drazenovic V, MlinaricGalinovic G. Increase in CD23(+) B cells in infants with bronchiolitis is accompanied by appearance of IgE and IgG4 antibodies specific for respiratory syncytial virus. J Infect Dis 1997; 175(1):32–37.

101. Patel JA, Kunimoto M, Sim TC, Garofalo R, Eliott T, Baron S, Ruuskanen O, Chonmaitree T, Ogra PL, Schmalstieg F. Interleukin-1α mediates the enhanced expression of intercellular adhesion molecule-1 in pulmonary epithelial cells infected with respiratory syncytial virus. Am J Respir Cell Mol Biol 1995; 13:602–609.

102. van Schaik SM, Tristram DA, Nagpal IS, Hintz KM, Welliver RC, Welliver RC. Increased production of IFN-gamma and cysteinyl leukotrienes in virus-induced wheezing. J All Clin Immunol 1999; 103(4):630–636.

103. McNamara PS, Flanagan BF, Baldwin LM, Newland P, Hart CA, Smyth RL. Interleukin 9 production in the lungs of infants with severe respiratory syncytial virus bronchiolitis. Lancet 2004; 363(9414):1031–1037.

104. Arnold R, König B, Galatti H, Werchau H, König W. Cytokine (IL-8, IL-6, TNF-a) and soluble TNF receptor-I release from human peripheral blood mononuclear cells after respiratory syncytial virus infection. Immunology 1995; 85:364–372.

105. Tsutsumi H, Matsuda K, Sone S, Takeuchi R, Chiba S. Respiratory syncytial virus-induced cytokine production by neonatal macrophages. Clin Exp Immunol 1996; 106(3):442–446.

106. Takeuchi R, Tsutsumi H, Osaki M, Sone S, Imai S, Chiba S. Respiratory syncytial virus infection of neonatal monocytes stimulates synthesis of interferon regulatory factor 1 and interleukin-1b (IL-1b)-converting enzyme and secretion of IL-1b. J Virol 1998; 72:837–840.

107. Olszewska-Pazdrak B, Casola A, Saito T, Alam R, Crowe SE, Mei F, Ogra PL, Garofalo RP. Cell-specific expression of RANTES, MCP-1, and MIP-1α by lower airway epithelial cells and eosinophils infected with respiratory syncytial virus. J Virol 1998; 72(6):4756–4764.

108. Welliver RC, Garofalo RP, Ogra PL. Beta-chemokines, but neither T helper type 1 nor T helper type 2 cytokines, correlate with severity of illness during respiratory syncytial virus infection. Pediatr Infect Dis J 2002; 21(5):457–461.

109. Harrison AM, Bonville CA, Rosenberg HF, Domachowske JB. Respiratory syncytial virus-induced chemokine expression in the lower airways: eosinophil

recruitment and degranulation. Am J Respir Crit Care Med 1999; 159: 1918–1924.

110. van Schaik SM, Tristram DA, Nagpal IS, Hintz KM, Welliver CII, Welliver RC. Increased production of IFN-g and cysteinyl leukotrienes in virus-induced wheezing. J All Clin Immunol 1999; 103:630–636.

111. Comoy EE, Pestel J, Duez C, Stewart GA, Vendeville C, Fournier C, Finkelman F, Capron A, Thyphronitis G. The house dust mite allergen, *Dermatophagoides pteronyssinus*, promotes type 2 responses by modulating the balance between IL-4 and IFN-γ. J Immunol 1998; 160:2456–2462.

112. Calhoun WJ, Swenson CA, Dick EC, Schwartz LB, Lemanske RF Jr., Busse WW. Experimental rhinovirus 16 infection potentiates histamine release after antigen bronchoprovocation in allergic subjects. Am Rev Respir Dis 1991; 144: 1267–1273.

113. Gern JE, Calhoun WJ, Swenson C, Shen G, Busse WW. Rhinovirus infection preferentially increases lower airway responsiveness in allergic subjects. Am J Respir Crit Care Med 1997; 155:1872–1876.

114. Duff AL, Pomeranz ES, Gelber LE, Price HW, Farris H, Hayden FG, Platts-Mills TAE, Heymann PW. Risk factors for acute wheezing in infants in infants and children: viruses, passive smoke, and IgE antibodies to inhalant allergens. Pediatr 1993; 92:535–540.

115. Avila PC, Abisheganaden JA, Wong H, Liu J, Yagi S, Schnurr D, Kishiyama JL, Boushey HA. Effects of allergic inflammation of the nasal mucosa on the severity of rhinovirus 16 cold. J Allergy Clin Immunol 2000; 105(5):923–932.

116. De Kluijver J, Evertse CE, Sont JK, Schrumpf JA, Van Zeijl-Van Der Ham CJ, Dick CR, Rabe KF, Hiemstra PS, Sterk PJ. Are rhinovirus-induced airway responses in asthma aggravated by chronic allergen exposure?. Am J Respir Crit Care Med 2003; 168:1174–1180.

117. Malcolm E, Arruda E, Hayden FG, Kaiser L. Clinical features of patients with acute respiratory illness and rhinovirus in their bronchoalveolar lavages. J Clin Virol 2001; 21(1):9–16.

118. Alwan WH, Record FM, Openshaw PJM. Phenotypic and functional characterization of T-cell lines specific for individual respiratory syncytial virus proteins. J Immunol 1993; 150:5211–5218.

119. Jackson M, Scott R. Different patterns of cytokine induction in cultures of respiratory syncytial (RS) virus-specific human Th-cell lines following stimulation with RS virus and RS virus proteins. J Med Virol 1996; 49(3):161–169.

120. Peebles RS Jr., Sheller JR, Johnson JE, Mitchell DB, Graham BS. Respiratory syncytial virus infection prolongs methacholine-induced airway hyperresponsiveness in ovalbumin-sensitized mice. J Med Virol 1999; 57:186–192.

121. Lukacs NW, Tekkanat KK, Berlin A, Hogaboam CM, Miller A, Evanoff H, Lincoln P, Maassab H. Respiratory syncytial virus predisposes mice to augmented allergic airway responses via il-13-mediated mechanisms. J Immunol 2001; 167(2):1060–1065.

122. Peebles RS, Jr., Sheller JR, Collins RD, Jarzecka AK, Mitchell DB, Parker RA, Graham BS. Respiratory syncytial virus infection does not increase allergen-induced type 2 cytokine production, yet increases airway hyperresponsiveness in mice. J Med Virol 2001; 63(2):178–188.

123. Renzi PM, Turgeon JP, Marcotte JE, Drblik SP, Bérubé D, Gagnon MF, Spier S. Reduced inteferon-γ production in infants with bronchiolitis and asthma. Am J Respir Crit Care Med 1999; 159:1417–1422.

124. Copenhaver CC, Gern JE, Li Z, Shult PA, Rosenthal LA, Mikus LD, Kirk CJ, Roberg KA, Anderson EL, Tisler CJ, DaSilva DF, Heimke HJ, Gentile K, Gangnon RE, Lemanske RF, Jr. Cytokine response patterns, exposure to viruses, and respiratory infections in the first year of life. Am J Respir Crit Care Med 2004; 170:175–180.

125. Parry DE, Busse WW, Sukow KA, Dick CR, Swenson C, Gern JE. Rhinovirus-induced PBMC responses and outcome of experimental infection in allergic subjects. J All Clin Immunol 2000; 105:692–698.

126. Brooks GD, Buchta KA, Swenson CA, Gern JE, Busse WW. Rhinovirus-induced interferon gamma and airway responsiveness in asthma. Am J Respir Crit Care Med 2003; 168:1091–1094.

127. Papadopoulos NG, Stanciu LA, Papi A, Holgate ST, Johnston SL. A defective type 1 response to rhinovirus in atopic asthma. Thorax 2002; 57(4): 328–332.

128. Bont L, Heijnen CJ, Kavelaars A, Van Aalderen WM, Brus F, Draaisma JT, Geelen SM, Kimpen JL. Monocyte IL-10 production during respiratory syncytial virus bronchiolitis is associated with recurrent wheezing in a one-year follow-up study. Am J Respir Crit Care Med 2000; 161(5):1518–1523.

129. Hull J, Thomson A, Kwiatkowski D. Association of respiratory syncytial virus bronchiolitis with the interleukin 8 gene region in UK families. Thorax 2000; 55(12):1023–1027.

130. Hoebee B, Bont L, Rietveld E, van Oosten M, Hodemaekers HM, Nagelkerke NJ, Neijens HJ, Kimpen JL, Kimman TG. Influence of promoter variants of interleukin-10, interleukin-9, and tumor necrosis factor-alpha genes on respiratory syncytial virus bronchiolitis. J Infect Dis 2004; 189(2):239–247.

131. Choi EH, Lee HJ, Yoo T, Chanock SJ. A common haplotype of interleukin-4 gene IL-4 is associated with severe respiratory syncytial virus disease in Korean children. J Infect Dis 2002; 186(9):1207–1211.

132. Hull J, Rowlands K, Lockhart E, Moore C, Sharland M, Kwiatkowski D. Variants of the chemokine receptor CCR5 are associated with severe bronchiolitis caused by respiratory syncytial virus. J Infect Dis 2003; 188(6):904–907.

133. Hoebee B, Rietveld E, Bont L, Oosten M, Hodemaekers HM, Nagelkerke NJ, Neijens HJ, Kimpen JL, Kimman TG. Association of severe respiratory syncytial virus bronchiolitis with interleukin-4 and interleukin-4 receptor alpha polymorphisms. J Infect Dis 2003; 187(1):2–11.

134. Lahti M, Lofgren J, Marttila R, Renko M, Klaavuniemi T, Haataja R, Ramet M, Hallman M. Surfactant protein D gene polymorphism associated with severe respiratory syncytial virus infection. Pediatr Res 2002; 51(6):696–699.

135. Hoffjan S, Ostrovnaja I, Nicolae D, Newman DL, Nicolae R, Gangnon R, Steiner L, Walker K, Reynolds R, Greene D, Mirel D, Gern JE, Lemanske RF, Jr., Ober C. Genetic variation in immunoregulatory pathways and atopic phenotypes in infancy. J Allergy Clin Immunol 2003; 113:511–518.

136. Kellner JD, Ohlsson A, Gadomski AM, Wang EE. Bronchodilators for bronchiolitis. Cochrane Database Syst Rev 2000;(2):CD001266.

137. Garrison MM, Christakis DA, Harvey E, Cummings P, Davis RL. Systemic corticosteroids in infant bronchiolitis: a meta-analysis. Pediatrics 2000; 105(4):E44.

138. Rachelefsky G. Treating exacerbations of asthma in children: the role of systemic corticosteroids. Pediatrics 2003; 112(2):382–397.

139. Bulow SM, Nir M, Levin E, Friis B, Thomsen LL, Nielsen JE, Holm JC, Moller T, Bonde-Hansen ME, Nielsen HE. Prednisolone treatment of respiratory syncytial virus infection: a randomized controlled trial of 147 infants. Pediatrics 1999; 104(6):e77.

140. van Woensel JB, Kimpen JL, Sprikkelman AB, Ouwehand A, Van Aalderen WM. Long-term effects of prednisolone in the acute phase of bronchiolitis caused by respiratory syncytial virus. Pediatr Pulmonol 2000; 30(2):92–96.

141. Cade A, Brownlee KG, Conway SP, Haigh D, Short A, Brown J, Dassu D, Mason SA, Phillips A, Eglin R, Graham M, Chetcuti A, Chatrath M, Hudson N, Thomas A. Randomised placebo controlled trial of nebulised corticosteroids in acute respiratory syncytial viral bronchiolitis. Arch Dis Child 2000; 82(2):126–130.

142. Richter H, Seddon P. Early nebulized budesonide in the treatment of bronchiolitis and the prevention of postbronchiolitic wheezing. J Pediatr 1998; 132(5):849–853.

143. Fox GF, Everard ML, Marsh MJ, Milner AD. Randomized controlled trial of budesonide for the prevention of post-bronchiolitis wheezing. Arch Dis Child 1999; 30:343–347.

144. Reijonen TM, Korppi M. One-year follow-up of young children hospitalized for wheezing: the influence of early anti-inflammatory therapy and risk factors for subsequent wheezing and asthma. Pediatr Pulmonol 1998; 26(2):113–119.

145. Kajosaari M, Syvanen P, Forars M, Juntunen-Backman K. Inhaled corticosteroids during and after respiratory syncytial virus—bronchiolitis may decrease subsequent asthma. Pediatr All Immunol 2000; 11(3):198–202.

146. Carlsen KH, Leegaard J, Larsen S, Orstavik I. Nebulized beclomethasone dipropionate in recurrent obstructive episodes after acute bronchiolitis. Arch Dis Child 1988; 63(12):1428–1433.

147. Reijonen T, Korppi M, Kuikka L, Remes K. Anti-inflammatory therapy reduces wheezing after bronchiolitis. Arch Pediatr Adolesc Med 1996; 150(5):512–517.

148. Rowe BH, Keller JL, Oxman AD. Effectiveness of steroid therapy in acute exacerbations of asthma: a meta-analysis. Am J Emerg Med 1992; 10(4): 301–310.

149. Murphy S, Bleecker ER, Boushey H, Brown C, Buist AS, Busse W, Clark NM, Eigen H, Ford JG, Gergen PJ, Janson S, Kelly HW, Lemanske RF, Jr., Lopez CC, Martinez F, Nelson HS, Nowak R, Petsonk EL, Platts-Mills TAE, Shapiro GG, Stoloff S, Weiss K. Guidelines for the diagnosis and management of asthma. National Asthma Education and Prevention Program, editor. II, 1–150. 1997. Bethesda, MD, National Institutes of Health.

150. Harrison TW, Oborne J, Newton S, Tattersfield AE. Doubling the dose of inhaled corticosteroid to prevent asthma exacerbations: randomized controlled trial. Lancet 2004; 363(9405):271–275.

151. Brunette MG, Lands L, Thibodeau L-P. Childhood asthma: prevention of attacks with short-term corticosteroid treatment of upper respiratory tract infection. Pediatrics 1988; 81:624–628.

152. Tal A, Levy N, Bearman JE. Methylprednisolone therapy for acute asthma in infants and toddlers: a controlled clinical trial. Pediatrics 1990; 86:350–356.

153. Dolan L, Kesarwala HH, Holroyde J, Fischer TJ. Short-term, high-dose, systemic steroids in children with asthma: the effect on the hypothalamic-pituitary-adrenal axis. J All Clin Immunol 1987; 80:81–87.

154. Wilson NM, Silverman M. Treatment of acute, episodic asthma in preschool children using intermittent high dose inhaled steroids at home. Arch Dis Child 1990; 65(4):407–410.

155. Daugbjerg P, Brenoe E, Forchhammer H, Frederiksen B, Glazowski MJ, Ibsen KK, Knabe N, Leth H, Marner B, Pedersen FK. A comparison between nebulized terbutaline, nebulized corticosteroid and systemic corticosteroid for acute wheezing in children up to 18 months of age. Acta Paediatr 1993; 82(6-7):547–551.

156. Connett G, Lenney W. Prevention of viral induced asthma attacks using inhaled budesonide. Arch Dis Child 1993; 68(1):85–87.

157. Svedmyr J, Nyberg E, Asbrink-Nilsson E, Hedlin G. Intermittent treatment with inhaled steroids for deterioration of asthma due to upper respiratory tract infections. Acta Paediatr 1995; 84(8):884–888.

158. Volovitz B, Bentur L, Finkelstein Y, Mansour Y, Shalitin S, Nussinovitch M, Varsano I. Effectiveness and safety of inhaled corticosteroids in controlling acute asthma attacks in children who were treated in the emergency department: a controlled comparative study with oral prednisolone. J Allergy Clin Immunol 1998; 102(4 Pt 1):605–609.

159. Schuh S, Reisman J, Alshehri M, Dupuis A, Corey M, Arseneault R, Alothman G, Tennis O, Canny G. A comparison of inhaled fluticasone and oral prednisone for children with severe acute asthma. N Engl J Med 2000; 343(10):689–694.

160. Krawiec ME, Westcott JY, Chu HW, Balzar S, Trudeau JB, Schwartz LB, Wenzel SE. Persistent wheezing in very young children is associated with lower respiratory inflammation. Am J Respir Crit Care Med 2001; 163(6):1338–1343.

161. Behera AK, Kumar M, Matsuse H, Lockey RF, Mohapatra SS. Respiratory syncytial virus induces the expression of 5-lipoxygenase and endothelin-1 in bronchial epithelial cells. Biochem Biophys Res Commun 1998; 251(3):704–709.

162. Wedde-Beer K, Hu C, Rodriguez MM, Piedimonte G. Leukotrienes mediate neurogenic inflammation in lungs of young rats infected with respiratory syncytial virus. Am J Physiol Lung Cell Mol Physiol 2002; 282(5):L1143–L1150.

163. Bisgaard H. A randomized trial of montelukast in respiratory syncytial virus postbronchiolitis. Am J Respir Crit Care Med 2003; 167(3):379–383.

164. Rotbart HA. Pleconaril treatment of enterovirus and rhinovirus infections. Infect Med 2000; 17(7):488–494.

165. Rotbart HA. Treatment of picornavirus infections. Antiviral Res 2002; 53:83–98.

166. Turner RB, Dutko FJ, Goldstein NH, Lockwood G, Hayden FG. Efficacy of oral WIN 54954 for prophylaxis of experimental rhinovirus infection. Antimicrob Agents Chemother 1993; 37:297–300.

167. Turner RB, Wecker MT, Pohl G, Witek TJ, Mcnally E, St George R, Winther B, Hayden FG. Efficacy of tremacamra, a soluble intercellular adhesion molecule 1, for experimental rhinovirus infection - A randomized clinical trial. Journal of the American Medical Association 1999; 281(19):1797–1804.

168. Zalman LS, Brothers MA, Dragovich PS, Zhou R, Prins TJ, Worland ST, Patick AK. Inhibition of human rhinovirus-induced cytokine production by AG7088, a human rhinovirus 3C protease inhibitor. Antimicrob Agents Chemother 2000; 44(5):1236–1241.

8

Controlling the Environment of Asthmatic Children: Benefits and Limitations

ANDREA J. APTER

Division of Pulmonary, Allergy, Critical Care
   Medicine, Department of Medicine,
   University of Pennsylvania
Philadelphia, Pennsylvania, U.S.A.

PEYTON A. EGGLESTON

Johns Hopkins University School of
   Medicine
Baltimore, Maryland, U.S.A.

I. Introduction

In this chapter we discuss environmental exposures that lead to respiratory morbidity in asthmatic children. Research in this area is difficult to conduct. First, characterizing personal exposures and monitoring important fluctuations over time is challenging. Second, cross-sectional studies are easier to accomplish than longitudinal studies and serve to generate causal hypotheses, but cross-sectional studies cannot draw conclusions about cause and effect (1). Third, important confounders such as family history of atopy or pollutant exposures, or social variables such as access to care may not be available in studies using historical datasets. Finally, randomized intervention trials that might be used to confirm hypotheses are made difficult by the behavioral changes required, such as removal of a pet, laundering bedding, or stopping smoking. Keeping these limitations in mind, we review the most important allergic and nonallergic environmental triggers of asthma in children and then make recommendations for primary and secondary prevention of relevant exposures. We have divided this discussion into what is known about allergic and nonallergic exposures (Table 1).

Table 1 Allergic and Nonallergic Perennial Environmental Exposures Reviewed in this Chapter That Have Been Studied as Risk Factors for Asthma in Children

Allergic	Nonallergic
Animals (e.g., pets)	Environmental tobacco smoke
Insects (mite, cockroach)	Endotoxin
Fungi	Pollutants
	Viral infections
	Social exposures (e.g., poverty, family dysfunction)

II. Allergic Environmental Triggers

For this review we will concentrate on perennial allergens, especially those considered most important in childhood asthma.

A. Animals

Animal allergens are carried on particles that range from less than 1 µ to greater than 20 µ in mean aerodynamic diameter, with at least 15% less than 5 µ in size (2). The particles appear to be very sticky, leading to widespread distribution in the environment both within homes, where they may be found on walls and other surfaces, and on clothing. This stickiness may be responsible for the finding that animal allergen can be found in homes without a pet and in public buildings such as schools (3). At the same time, concentrations of the allergen in settled dust and in air are 10–1000 times higher in homes with a pet (3). The small size of these particles dictates that they remain airborne longer than particles with mite and cockroach allergen (4) and will deposit more extensively in the respiratory track.

Studies in Swedish schools have demonstrated that animal allergens may be found in settled dust (3) and air (5) in buildings that never housed a pet (Fig. 1). Furthermore, these investigators demonstrated that pet allergen could be transferred from the school to the homes of children who did not own a pet. Almqvist and colleagues (3) gave children with and without pets new T-shirts at home and demonstrated that the shirts of the children who owned cats arrived at school with high levels of cat allergen. The shirts of the children without pets had negligible cat allergen when they came to school, but by the time they left, had measurable levels, nearly 100 times the earlier levels (3). Finally, these investigators demonstrated that asthmatic children who did not live with a cat but were sensitized to cat allergen had increased respiratory problems (low PEFR, more symptoms, more β-agonist use, more steroid use) when they returned to school—but only if

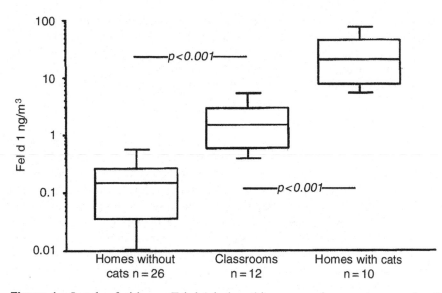

Figure 1 Levels of airborne Fel d 1 in breathing zones of non–cat owners in all classrooms compared with children in homes without cats ($p < 0.001$) and children in homes with cats ($p < 0.001$). *Source*: From Ref. 3.

they attended a classroom with many children who owned a cat (6). These studies demonstrate the difficulty of pet allergen avoidance in a society where many families have pets and where accidental and undetected exposure may occur. Since incidental exposure to low levels of cat allergen can induce symptoms, they also demonstrate the futility of trying to reduce home exposure significantly while the pet is still in the home. Clinically, it is clear that many patients with asthma and cat or dog sensitivity suffer from a more severe form of the disease because of continuous, ongoing exposure to a family pet. At the same time these studies demonstrate that animal allergens are important causes of chronic airway inflammation even in patients without known exposure.

B. Dust Mite

House dust mites are ubiquitous in all but the least humid areas of the world. Their bodies and feces are the sources of indoor allergen (4,7). House dust mites infest fabrics, including mattresses, bedding, rugs, upholstered furniture, and carpets (8). The fact that the allergen is found in the bedroom, especially in the bed, and that most of the allergenic activity is found in large particles, which do not remain airborne for more than a few seconds, dictate that exposure will be limited to close contact. These facts make bedding the logical target for interventions. Having mite allergen assays made it possible to demonstrate that vacuuming the floor or treating bedding and rugs with acaracide or tannic acid did not adequately reduce exposure. Consistently, encasing mattress and pillows with materials capable of excluding small allergen-containing particles has been shown to be effective, usually reducing concentration by 50% or more. Washing the bedding was also helpful, but not without encasing the mattress and pillow.

C. Cockroach

Cockroach allergens are derived from several sources, e.g., saliva, fecal material, secretions, cast skins, debris, and dead bodies. Cockroach allergen levels are highest in the kitchen, which is the primary site of cockroach accumulation. However, somewhat lower allergen levels can also be found in dust samples from sofas, bedding, and bedroom floors (9,10). Approximately 20–48% of homes without visible cockroaches contain detectable cockroach allergen in dust samples (9,11). It is important to note that cockroach sensitization is not found exclusively in low-income homes. In a recent study cockroach allergen was detected in approximately 50% of suburban middle class homes that were investigated (12). Sensitization occurred in 21% of the children from these homes (12).

Cockroach allergen Bla g 1 was detectable in bedding and bedroom floor samples of 85.3% of homes of inner-city children with asthma, and levels of Bla g 1 ≥ 8 U/g of dust, considered high and proposed as a disease-induction threshold, were found in 50.2% of those bedrooms. On the other hand, only 12.6% and 9.7% of the bedrooms had high levels of cat and mite allergens, respectively, indicating that cockroach exposure may be very important in this group of asthmatic children (13). Heavy cockroach infestations in homes may create reservoirs of allergen in carpets and rugs, as well as in inaccessible spaces around appliances and furniture.

D. Indoor Fungi

Although home and school dampness and the presence of fungi are associated with respiratory symptoms in children, evidence of whether fungi contribute to these symptoms as perennial allergens or toxins is scant (14–18). Only a few studies have quantitatively measured fungal allergen in the home (17,18). Douwes and colleagues (18) used an enzyme immunoassay of extracellular polysaccharides (EPS) of *Aspergillus* and *Penicillium* species, in dust as a marker of fungal exposure. They found fungal EPS to be more plentiful in the living room and higher on carpeted floors and correlated with the presence of house dust mites allergens. Levels in the living room were associated with respiratory symptoms in children living in these homes. The EPS levels in the bedroom were inversely associated with respiratory symptoms, but the analysis did not control for other environmental exposures such as pets and mites although mite levels were measured. Chew and colleagues (17) measured culturable fungi in both the dust and air of bedrooms. They found only a weak relationship between culturable fungi in the dust and in the air and recommended sampling by both procedures. Stark et al. (19) measured fungal concentrations as predictors of non-wheezing lower respiratory illnesses (croup, bronchiolitis, and bronchitis) in infants in their first year of life as part of a prospective birth cohort. Whether these children, who are at increased risk of asthma, will develop asthma is not yet known.

III. Nonallergic Environmental Triggers

Nonallergic triggers of asthma exacerbations in children affect both atopic and non-atopic children. We discuss those that have raised the most concern for children: environmental tobacco smoke (ETS), endotoxin, nitrous oxide, and other pollutants, and the implications of the Hygiene Hypothesis. We also discuss another exposure not generally considered with these triggers: the social environment.

A. Environmental Tobacco Smoke (ETS)

ETS is a common indoor exposure, which can be assessed by measuring cotinine, a metabolite of nicotine, in urine or saliva. Thus, this exposure is unique in that there is a feasible, inexpensive means of measuring personal exposure over time. According to a recent Institute of Medicine report, smoking in the home is causally related to exacerbations of asthma in preschool aged children (20). ETS is associated with asthma in older children also (21). Additionally, researchers have theorized that ETS may enhance atopy and have proposed several mechanisms, including promoting increased airway mucosal permeability and directly affecting immune function (22–26). While there is support in animal studies for this theory, more research in humans is necessary to establish a link between ETS and atopy.

The magnitude of the effect of ETS on children's symptoms and lung function has been systematically reviewed by Cook and Strachan (27). These investigators concluded that smoking by either parent, but especially the mother, increases the risk of wheezing in infants and preschool children; the effect is less clear in older children and adults. Maternal smoking during pregnancy increases the risk of asthma during the first seven years of the child's life (28).

B. Hygiene Hypothesis

In developed countries the prevalence of asthma is believed to have increased. The Hygiene Hypothesis was formulated as a possible explanation of this increase (29–31). It states that improved hygiene has led to the underdevelopment of Th-1 immune responses in favor of enhanced Th-2 responses. Thus, factors that diminish the Th-1 response, such as the increased use of antibiotics, should promote atopy and consequently allergic asthma. Alternatively, factors that invoke a Th-1 response, such as exposure to endotoxin or bacterial infections, should protect against the development of atopic diseases. According to this hypothesis, exposure to viral infections such as might occur in day care may also reduce the incidence of atopy and asthma, as opposed to the theories of the previous section on viral infections. While the evidence for viruses as a cause of asthma exacerbations is very clear, as noted below the evidence for the Hygiene Hypothesis is less certain (29,32). Prospective cohort studies are needed (32).

C. Viral Infections

Viruses are the most important cause of acute infection-induced wheezing in infants and children (33–35). In children beyond infancy, viruses associated with episodes of wheezing include RSV, rhinovirus, parainfluenza virus, influenza virus, and coronavirus (36).

Lower respiratory infections early in life have been shown to be inversely associated with asthma later in childhood (37). On the other hand, children with severe viral respiratory infections, particularly RSV infections, are at risk for the development of asthma (33,34,38). Exploration of the role of genetic factors on the immunity of these children in fighting these infections, and hence playing a role in the development of asthma, has begun (39).

D. Day Care

According to the Hygiene Hypothesis, day care with its associated exposures to viral and bacterial infections would be expected to be protective of the development of asthma (40). Indeed, this was the finding of the Tucson Children's Respiratory Study: exposure to day care in the first six months of life was protective against the development of asthma between ages six and 13 months was protective against the development of asthma (39,41). Such children also had more wheezing episodes at year 2, but fewer from years 8 to 13. Celedon et al. (42) conducted a prospective birth cohort study of 453 children with a parental history of atopy. For those children with a maternal history of asthma, day care in the first year of life did not decrease the risk of asthma at age six, although for the whole cohort, day care in the first year was associated with a decreased risk of asthma. Although the study populations, day care environments, and social settings differed somewhat, these interesting and difficult-to-accomplish studies suggest the need for further exploration of causes of asthma in combination with genetic studies to better define populations.

E. Antibiotic Use

At least one study has observed increased exposure to antibiotics associated with a risk of asthma, consistent with the Hygiene Hypothesis. McKeever et al. (43) found four or more courses of antibiotics in the first year of life to be associated with an increased incidence of asthma in their large retrospective cohort study using the West Midlands General Practice Research Database. Celedon and colleagues (44) found a somewhat different result from their birth cohort in which there was a history of atopy in at least one parent. These investigators examined use in the first year of life and searched for the presence of asthma, allergic rhinitis, and eczema at age five. No significant association between antibiotic use in the first year of life and asthma was detected.

F. Endotoxin

Endotoxin, lipopolysaccharide (LPS), is a major component of the outer membrane of gram-negative bacteria. It induces Th-1 activity, including stimulating interleukin-12 (IL-12), and interferon gamma (IFN-γ) production (45). Airborne endotoxin levels are higher in homes with pets, accumulated dust, cool humidifiers, water damage, and tobacco smoke (45,46). Levels are decreased in homes with air conditioners (45,47).

Exposure to endotoxin in infancy is theorized to be protective of the development of allergy and asthma (48–51). In light of endotoxin's Th-1-inducing activity, this theory is consistent with the Hygiene Hypothesis. However, exposure later in life is proposed to increase acute and chronic inflammation (52). From animal studies researchers have postulated that high levels of exposure to endotoxin are protective against sensitization and asthma, while low levels may increase the risk of sensitization and asthma (53). There is some clinical evidence supporting this concept (49,54). Gehring and colleagues (49,54) in cross-sectional surveys found LPS higher levels of endotoxin in house dust associated with lower prevalence of allergic sensitization. However Park et al. (53,55) and Litonjua (56) in longitudinal studies found LPS levels in house dust were positively correlated with wheezing. In persons already sensitized to allergens, conditions expected to enhance exposure to ambient LPS are also associated with asthma symptoms. The presence of a dog is associated with high endotoxin levels, likewise gram-negative bacteria may grow in humidifiers and in damp or water-damaged areas (42,53,55,56). While cross-sectional studies cannot investigate cause and effect, additional prospective longitudinal studies are needed to elucidate the true relationship between endotoxin exposure and the risk of asthma.

G. Farms

Living on a farm is reported to be associated with lower incidence of asthma and atopy (50). It is probable that children living in farm environments have substantial exposure to animal, insect, fungal, and pollen allergens. Thus, the theorized protective effect is consistent with the Hygiene

Hypothesis. Farm homes may have more endotoxin, which is theorized to be protective against asthma (52). The farm environment is a complicated one and likely not homogeneous from farm to farm. The studies supporting the hypothesis that living on a farm is protective are largely cross-sectional and many do not control for family atopy; that is, families that are allergic may be less likely to live on a farm. Finally, farm environments may vary markedly: some having barns attached to the house, some unattached; some raising cattle, others poultry, and others crops. Socioeconomic levels of the farmers may also vary. Thus, this interesting hypothesis needs further exploration. Separating irritant from allergen exposures in farming and non-farming environments deserves investigation. While city-dwellers may have more exposure to car exhaust, farm vehicles also may release substantial exhaust and farm homes may have pollutants from gas and wood stoves. Once again, combining genetic and environmental studies that keep track of the myriad of respiratory exposures are needed.

H. Pollutants

Investigated outdoor pollutants include ozone, sulfur dioxide, particulate matter, and other components of motor vehicle exhaust (46). Hospitalizations for asthma have increased with a rise in ambient ozone, SO_2, and particulate matter (57). A study from London found more acute wheeze in children during higher SO_2 and ozone levels (58,59). More respiratory symptoms have been observed in children during higher ambient ozone levels (60). However, not all studies have found an association (61). Many studies have observed a relationship between asthma hospitalizations and airborne particulate matter (62–65).

There are studies that suggest that pollutants such as nitrogen dioxide may enhance a subsequent allergen-induced asthmatic reaction (61). Nicolai et al. (66) conducted a cross-sectional study of traffic exposure using traffic counts and a model to predict emissions. High traffic counts were associated with current asthma and symptoms, but no pollutant was associated with allergic sensitization. Current asthma or wheeze and current cough were associated with soot, benzene, and nitrogen dioxide (NO_2).

Studies addressing the role of pollutants are difficult and expensive. Longitudinal studies frequently rely on patient report of symptoms as an outcome rather than clinical measures. Measurements of pollutants over a significant time period are costly; surrogate measures like traffic counts may be more feasible than measuring the actual pollutants (66). Also difficult is assessing which among the myriad of possible simultaneously present outdoor inhalants is associated with asthma (66). For example, low-income urban individuals tend to live in less desirable areas, which frequently are regions of high traffic and/or high pollution.

Diesel exhaust is a mixture of organic and inorganic particulate and gaseous compounds, including carcinogens, mutagens, and toxins (67). Animal studies have suggested that diesel exhaust promotes allergic responses (68,69). Diaz-Sanchez et al. (70–73) in a series of studies found an association between diesel exhaust and manifestations of immediate hypersensitivity. However, a study of healthy human cells suggested the effect of diesel organic extracts is more nonspecific in terms of Th-1 and Th-2 effects (74). The effects of specific components of diesel exhaust must be further investigated.

Indoors, gas and wood stoves (NO_2) release nitrogen dioxide and other respiratory irritants. Nitrogen dioxide has been associated with respiratory symptoms in children (75–77), although an Institute of Medicine report evaluating the evidence found it insufficient to determine an association (20). Recently, Chauhan et al. (78) measured personal exposure to NO_2 in a cohort of 114 asthmatic children aged 8 to 11 years weekly for up to 13 months. The investigators found high exposure to NO_2, although at levels within current air quality standards, in the week before the start of a viral respiratory infection associated with an increase in the severity of the resulting asthma exacerbation. Belanger et al. (16) in a cohort of 849 infants with an asthmatic sibling found that among infants of mothers with no asthma history exposure to gas and wood-burning stoves increased the risk of persistent cough. In addition, higher measured nitrogen dioxide levels were associated with this increased risk.

As in studying outdoor exposures, accounting for the many indoor inhalants is a formidable research task. Brugge et al. (79) attempted to characterize indoor respiratory exposures of nine families living in public housing in Boston for insects, fungi, humidity, temperature, and pollutants. They found high levels of nitrogen dioxide from gas stoves, volatile organic compounds, particulate matter from smoking, and variably high levels of cockroach, mouse, pet, and fungal proteins. They concluded that future studies must account for exposures from many sources. Other investigators have attempted to control many of the implicated exposures at once without trying to identify the specific cause (80). Some of these studies are in progress.

I. Social Exposures (SES, Family Size, Family Dysfunction, Stress)

Social setting is associated with asthma. Children from lower socioeconomic households and urban ethnic minorities are at increased risk for the development of asthma and, once developed, it tends to be more severe (13,81). Access to appropriate medication and consistent care are important determinants of asthma health (82,83).

There are a number of psychosocial factors associated with asthma (84). Parental stress and family dysfunction are associated with asthma morbidity in children (85). Exposure to violence may contribute to asthma morbidity (86). Poverty is associated with morbidity (81,82), and the aspects of poverty that are directly responsible require urgent study. Some clues are given by Chen et al. (85) who studied psychosocial factors associated with re-hospitalization in 115 children between the ages of 8 and 18. Re-hospitalizations were associated with caretaker characteristics of lower sense of mastery and being less emotionally bothered by asthma. Family characteristics were family strain and conflict as well as financial strain.

IV. Limiting Exposure to Allergens: Primary and Secondary Prevention of Allergic Asthma

Studies of allergen avoidance can be categorized as primary and secondary prevention studies. By primary prevention, we mean that avoiding exposure prevents the development of allergic asthma. Secondary prevention refers to the avoidance of exposure to allergens in a child who has already developed asthma. Since the evidence for secondary prevention is better studied than for primary prevention we will consider secondary prevention first.

A. Secondary Prevention—The Prevention of Asthma Exacerbations in Already-Sensitized Children

Eliminating Cat Exposure

An asthmatic patient who is sensitized to cat or dog allergen should not live with a pet in their home (4,87). Because the risk of sensitization is great in atopic patients, a patient with allergic airway disease should not bring a pet into their home. This is clearly the correct advice from a medical standpoint and health care providers should not shy away from strenuously recommending it (88). That being said, there are no clinical trials testing the effect of removing a cat or dog from the home of a sensitized asthmatic, but our clinical experiences support this notion.

Once a cat has been removed from the home, it is important to recognize that the clinical benefit may not be seen for a period of at least several months, since allergen levels fall quite slowly after cat removal (89). In most homes, levels in settled dust will have fallen to those seen in homes without cats within four to six months following cat removal. Levels may fall much more quickly if extensive environmental control measures are undertaken, such as removal of carpets, upholstered furniture, and other reservoirs from the home. Thorough and repeated cleaning will be required once the animal has been removed. Since cat allergen may persist in mattresses for years after a cat has been removed from a home (90), the purchase of new bedding or impermeable encasements should also be recommended.

Because so many patients are unwilling to remove their pet, even if they themselves are sensitized, many compromise measures have been suggested. DeBlay et al. (91,92) demonstrated significant reductions in airborne Fel d 1 with a combination of air filtration, cat washing, vacuum cleaning, and removal of furnishings, but these studies could not be confirmed and were shown to produce only a transient decrease in airborne allergen levels. Although tannic acid has been shown to reduce cat allergen levels in carpets (4,88), the effects are modest and short-lived when a cat is present, so this treatment should not be routinely recommended. The notion of creating a clean room from which the cat is excluded and vigorous environmental control measures such as vacuuming, mattress and pillow covers, carpet removal, and room air filters was tested recently. In one study (93) adults with asthma or allergic rhinitis and cat sensitivity were asked to keep their bedroom doors closed, and a combination of a bedroom air cleaner and covers for mattresses and pillows was provided. A control group was provided with nonactive air cleaners. Airborne cat allergen was reduced, but no significant differences were detected between the groups having active or placebo filters in symptom scores, peak flow rates, medication requirements, pulmonary function studies, or methacholine challenges. In the second study (94) children with asthma and sensitivity to either cat or dog were treated with either active or placebo air cleaners in both the bedroom and the living room. The investigators found that the active treatment group in this study had a significant reduction on airway hyperresponsiveness but no change in any other clinical measure. Both of these studies showed that minimal benefit can be expected from compromise measures with the cat remaining in the home (95).

Reducing Exposure to Dust Mite

Studies show dramatic clinical improvement when asthmatic patients moved to mountain residential care centers (96) or into hospitals (97) where mite allergen exposure can be documented to be very low. These studies also establish an important principle in the effects of allergen avoidance on asthma. Despite almost complete elimination of exposure, disease changes occurred gradually, with significant changes only seen after a month or more.

In home settings, it is impossible to achieve this level of allergen avoidance and changes have been even more gradual. When evaluating the efficacy shown in these trials, it is important to critically examine data on the degree to which exposure could be reduced. To date only 32 publications of clinical trial data have appeared and not all have included allergen measures to demonstrate that exposure had changed. Based on the degree of exposure reduction that could be achieved and the effect on disease

Table 2 Measures to Reduce Dust Mite Exposure

1. Cover mattress and pillows with vapor-permeable or fine weave materials
2. Vacuum weekly
3. Encase box-spring in vinyl or plastic
4. Wash bedding weekly in hot (>130°F) water
5. If possible, remove carpets from the bedroom and other rooms
6. Remove stuffed animals from the bed.

activity, these trials have allowed us to prioritize house dust mite avoidance recommendations into first line and second line (Table 2). First line measures are consistently effective and are feasible. Second line measures have inconsistent effects and may be difficult to implement.

At the top of the list of effective interventions is allergen-proof encasings for the mattress and pillow (8). Much progress has been made in materials, and the current products available by mail or in retail stores are breathable, comfortable and nearly 100% exclusive (8). While a number of clinical trials have been published that demonstrate a reduction in mite allergen and a clinical effect (96,98–102), not all trials have reported an effect (103,104), but some had methodologic problems such as short duration or no estimation of mite exposure. However, one of the most successful trials (105) also had these problems and had a successful outcome. The most consistent physiologic outcome is a reduction in bronchial hyperresponsiveness, but most show a clinical outcome as well.

Walshaw and Evans (98) were able to achieve a 99% reduction in mite numbers, and found a clinically important reduction in symptoms, medication use, morning PEFR, and histamine inhalation challenge during the course of the yearlong experiment. Carswell and colleagues (99) tested mattress and pillow encasings together with frequent professional laundering. Mite allergen in bedding was relatively low to begin with, but decreased by an additional 90% in the intervention group. Although the intervention group experienced a reduction in chest symptoms and a comparable degree of decrease in bronchodilator requirement, these changes were of marginal significance. There was a twofold improvement in bronchial hyperresponsiveness. Although Carswell in particular concluded that treatment had a modest effect, these responses compare favorably to treatment with low-dose inhaled corticosteroids or with leukotriene modifiers. A recent study by Busse and colleagues (106) compared fluticasone 88 µg/day and montelukast 10 mg per day in adult asthmatics and found that symptoms scores were reduced 52% and 36%, respectively, and that β-adrenergic use was reduced by 61% and 56%, respectively. In the study by Walshaw and Evans, symptoms were decreased 69% and β-adrenergic use was reduced 67%. These figures are comparable to those of Carswell et al. who reported the number of children who reported any symptoms or who required any β-adrenergic use;

these numbers were reduced by 63% and 72%, respectively; in the actively treated group. Another recent study, a prospective, double-blind, placebo-controlled study of 60 children with asthma and mite allergy by Halken et al. (102) randomized children to mite-impermeable compared with placebo mattress and pillow encasings. After one year the investigators found that of the 47 children remaining in the study 19 out of 26 in the experimental group and 5 out of 21 in the control group could lower their inhaled steroid dose by at least 50%. Thus, successful dust mite intervention can produce clinical improvement comparable to pharmacologic treatment appropriate for mild to moderate asthma and may reduce medication requirements.

Recently, Woodcock and colleagues (104) published the largest randomized trial to date of impermeable bedcovers in adult asthma. Planned as an effectiveness trial, the investigators randomized 1122 adults with asthma recruited from general practitioners' offices to have impermeable mattress and pillow encasings installed by a technician or to have placebo covers installed. Patients in the treatment group had no greater changes in asthma symptoms, peak expiratory flow rates, and medication use over the course of a year than did the control group, leading the authors to conclude that allergen-proof encasings alone were not adequate to reduce allergen-related symptoms. In rebuttal, it should be pointed out that allergen levels in the active group decreased at six months (from 1.03 to 0.58 µg/gm) but increased by 12 months (1.05 µg/gm). In addition, the patients in the study were older (mean age 36–37 years) than in other studies. They were symptomatic despite taking relatively large doses of inhaled steroids (400 µg/d beclomethasone or 1000 µg/d budesonide) and had a relatively high rate of cigarette use (23%). Is it possible that they had irreversible asthma or chronic obstructive pulmonary disease (COPD)? Neither of these questions would invalidate the study, but they might explain why the outcome was negative.

In addition to allergen-proof encasings for the mattress and pillow, other first-line measures include thorough vacuuming which removes bulk dust. Washing all bedding (sheets, blankets, comforters, and bedspreads) in warm water with detergent and with 8 to 10 minutes cycles removes virtually all mite and animal allergen (8), but the procedure must be repeated weekly. Washing sheets, pillowcases, blankets, and mattress pads at least weekly is equally important to reduce bedding exposure. Washing with hot water (55°C or 130°F) kills mites and removes most allergen, but this presents a scalding risk in homes with children, so this may not be practical. Dry cleaning (107) and prolonged tumble-drying (8) effectively kills mites, but is less effective at destroying allergens. Vacuuming reduces the bulk of household dust and reduces the overall burden. Low pile carpeting retains less dust mite allergen (8). Second line measures include relocating the bedroom, application of acaracides such as benzyl benzoate, dehumidification, and removing wall-to-wall carpeting. The support for relocating the bedroom from the basement or ground floor is the consistent association of carpeted slab floors with higher mite infestation (4,7,8). Acaracides are effective in the laboratory but field trials have generally found that carpet dust mite allergen is reduced minimally, probably because it is so difficult to get the material into the deepest areas of the carpet (8,108,109). Removing other fabrics from rooms, whether as carpets or as curtains and furniture, has been shown to produce minimal changes in settled dust allergens or in bedding allergen levels. Steam cleaning has been found to reduce mite allergen levels and when used on beds may reduce levels enough to affect asthma morbidity (110). The evidence supporting the use of dehumidification is conflicting. Trials in England were not able to reduce settled dust allergen levels (111) but a well-done study in the United States (112) and one from Denmark (113,114) were able to achieve significant reduction.

Reducing Cockroach Exposure

Inspection is an important first step in cockroach extermination. Not only can species be identified, but their likely hiding places and travel routes can be identified so that insecticide can be targeted to hiding areas. In addition to seeing living insects, evidence of cockroach habitation should be sought, including body parts, feces (black specks the size of sand grains), and stains from regurgitated digestive juices that appear as brown stains in the edges of cabinets or inside drawers. The inspection should also identify food sources for the insects, including grease and other cooking debris in the kitchen, garbage cans kept inside, pet food, and open snack food containers. To prevent re-infestation, families need to change these practices (115).

A number of effective insecticides (abamectin, fipronil, and hydomethylnon) are currently available that are capable of reducing cockroach populations by 90% and more and are at the same time safe for indoor use. Older pesticides were either less effective (boric acid) or were more toxic (diazinon). Although the pesticides may be applied in almost any form, the preferred method is to use selected placement of gels or baits. The approach of limiting pesticide application in the home and providing advice to remove food, water, and harborages, termed "Integrated Pest Management," has become a widespread practice employed in inhabited buildings to avoid risk from the pesticides (115).

Bait traps have been developed with narrow openings that limit access to the attractant and pesticide; these products are just as effective as gel baits if used properly. One of the important conditions for successful use of enclosed or gel baits is to provide enough coverage for large populations. Be aware that hungry roaches may clean out the traps before the whole population is controlled. Most technicians will recommend a second treatment within a week or two to overcome this problem.

Household cleaning is an essential adjunct to successful allergen removal. Before applying insecticide, a good general cleaning should remove additional food sources so that the insects are more likely to eat the gels or baits. Following the application of insecticides, cleaning should be delayed for a week to avoid removal of the insecticides. Allergen is likely to be left adherent to walls, floors, appliances, countertops, and woodwork; these areas should be scrubbed with water and detergent. Bedding, curtains, and clothing are usually contaminated and should be washed as well.

Clinical Trials of Reducing Exposure to Cockroach

Field trials of allergen reduction methods have shown that extermination is much easier than allergen removal (116–119). The best one can expect is to reduce settled dust allergen concentrations by 95% with repeated cleaning for six months following successful extermination. The only reported clinical trial of the health effects of allergen reduction is the National Cooperative Inner City Asthma Study (80). In this trial, cockroach allergen treatment was only one part of a global intervention. Disease activity was significantly improved, but median cockroach allergen concentration in treated homes was not reduced; therefore the improvement of disease activity could not be attributed to allergen reduction. Other trials are currently underway but outcomes are not yet available.

Controlling Indoor Fungal Exposure

A small number of studies have been published addressing the effectiveness of techniques to reduce exposure to fungal allergens. Garrison et al. (120) conducted extensive cleaning of central air-conditioning systems in several residences. These measures included disassembling and cleaning the condensing unit with glutaraldehyde 0.25%, vacuuming the inside of duct work and all the heating registers in the house, and then treating with a vinyl copolymer fogger. After the cleaning and antifungal treatment, they installed an electrostatic filter in the furnace. They provided data that airborne colony counts in the home fell dramatically after treatment. They identified 2 to 23 spores in open culture plates in the winter and 4 to 500 in the summer before the intervention. These were reduced to 0 to 10 of various species in either season after the treatment (an estimated 91% reduction). They also measured total spores with a Burkard trap and reported a decrease of 83% in the treated homes and a small increase in control homes. They repeated airborne measures for eight weeks and the effect persisted. Unfortunately, they did not provide data regarding health effects. Savilahti et al. (121) described two schools in Finland with severe water damage that included wet foundations, walls, and ceilings that were damaged by roof and plumbing leaks, and mold contamination. One of the schools was repaired (the details are not given) but the second was not and served as a control. Respiratory visits per child in the treated school decreased from an average of 0.81 per year before renovation to

0.55 afterwards, while in the control school the comparable figures were 0.64 before and 0.50 afterward. These differences were statistically significant. Many questions remain from the school study, including exactly what was done in the buildings and what the children were exposed to at home and other places.

Another issue raised by these studies is whether fungi are sources of nonallergic toxins rather than allergens in schools and homes that could cause respiratory symptoms (122). Currently there is no evidence to support this concern, but it is clear that water-damage and moist indoor environments where molds are present are associated with respiratory and other complaints (122–124). Further complicating our understanding of the role of fungi in respiratory disease is one interesting study of *Aspergillus* that found that although *Aspergillus* was present in the dust, it did not get into the indoor air although it was present in outdoor disturbed air (125). Clearly what constitutes a healthy indoor environment needs further study. Much research remains to be accomplished in understanding if fungi either as an allergen or toxin contribute to indoor respiratory problems.

Eliminating ETS

Exposure to ETS is the most potentially modifiable nonallergic exposure, and yet physicians rarely address smoking in parents of children (24,25,27,126). Behavioral interventions to reduce ETS exposure have not been uniformly successful. Hovell et al. (127) conducted a study of the efficacy of coaching families to reduce ETS exposure in asthmatic Latino children, ages 3 to 17 years. The researchers found that family-reported ETS exposure was lower both in the treatment and control groups and that there was a small but statistically significant trend towards more avoidance in the treatment group. Urinary cotinine levels showed small but significant decreases in both groups but the difference was not significant. Unfortunately, they did not include measures of the children's asthma severity during the trial, so it is not known if there was a health effect.

Wilson et al. (128) used feedback of cotinine levels to parents and measured health care utilization of children with asthma in a randomized controlled trial. These predominantly minority children from low-income households were between 3 and 12 years. Feedback combined with asthma education reduced health care utilization in the year following the intervention. However, loss of follow-up of patients was problematic. The reduction in cotinine levels did not reach statistical significance.

B. Primary Prevention—Does Avoiding Exposure Prevent Sensitization?

A very interesting recently proposed theory is that exposure to allergen in infancy is protective against sensitization and the later development to asthma. The research on such primary prevention is incomplete, with many of the studies addressing the question via cross-sectional or historical rather than prospective cohort trials. The results have been inconsistent. A potential limitation of these papers are the difficulties in defining atopy and measuring allergen exposure (32). An important confounder is family history. As an example of the difficulty in measuring family history consider if atopy is measured by questionnaire. Unless a questionnaire is validated it may not accurately include those with true allergic disease. Additionally atopy is not the same as cat allergy, with only a minority of allergic individuals allergic to cats. Thus, if one measures sensitivity to cats in the subject but measures family history more generally as atopy, the analysis may yield misleading results. Another difficulty is taking account of exposure to allergen in public places and homes, where there are no pets.

Prospective cohort studies are in progress and should help address the question of whether exposure is related to sensitization and hence the development of asthma. In the interim our advice is that if there is an atopic history in the family, avoidance of exposures of children to perennial allergens is recommended.

V. Conclusion

We need to understand better the impact of allergens and irritants on susceptible individuals and to define better susceptibility. Until we have more information we must control irritant exposures in all individuals and limit allergen exposure in children from families with a history of atopy.

References

1. Hennekens CH, Buring JE, Mayrent SL. Epidemiology in Medicine. Boston: Little, Brown and Company, 1987:20–21.
2. Luczynska CM, Li Y, Chapman MD, Platts-Mills TA. Airborne concentrations and particle size distribution of allergen derived from domestic cats (Felis domesticus). Measurements using cascade impactor, liquid impinger, and a two-site monoclonal antibody assay for Fel d 1. Am Rev Respir Dis 1990; 141(2):361–367.
3. Almqvist C, Larsson PH, Egmar AC, Hedren M, Malmberg P, Wickman M. School as a risk environment for children allergic to cats and a site for transfer of cat allergen to homes. J Allergy Clin Immunol 1999; 103(6):1012–1017.
4. Platts-Mills TA. Indoor allergens. In: Adkinson NJ, Yunginger J, Busse W, Bochner B, Holgate S, Simons F, eds. Middleton's Allergy: Principles and Practice. Philadelphia: Mosby, 2003:557–572.
5. Munir AK, Einarsson R, Dreborg S. Variability of airborne cat allergen, Fel d l, in a public place. Indoor Air 2003; 13(4):353–358

6. Almqvist C, Wickman M, Perfetti L, Berglind N, Renstrom A, Hedren M, Larsson K, Hedlin G, Malmberg P. Worsening of asthma in children allergic to cats, after indirect exposure to cat at school. Am J Respir Crit Care Med 2001; 163(3 Pt 1):694–698.

7. Eggleston PA, Bush RK. Environmental allergen avoidance: an overview. J Allergy Clin Immunol 2001; 107(3 Suppl):S403–S405.

8. Arlian LG, Platts-Mills TA. The biology of dust mites and the remediation of mite allergens in allergic disease. J Allergy Clin Immunol 2001; 107(3 Suppl): S406–S413.

9. Gelber LE, Seltzer LH, Bouzoukis JK, Pollart SM, Chapman MD, Platts-Mills TA. Sensitization and exposure to indoor allergens as risk factors for asthma among patients presenting to hospital. Am Rev Respir Dis 1993; 147(3):573–578.

10. de Blay F, Sanchez J, Hedelin G, Perez-Infante A, Verot A, Chapman M, Pauli G. Dust and airborne exposure to allergens derived from cockroach (Blattella germanica) in low-cost public housing in Strasbourg (France). J Allergy Clin Immunol 1997; 99(1 Pt 1):107–112.

11. Chew GL, Burge HA, Dockery DW, Muilenberg ML, Weiss ST, Gold DR. Limitations of a home characteristics questionnaire as a predictor of indoor allergen levels. Am J Respir Crit Care Med 1998; 157(5 Pt 1):1536–1541.

12. Matsui EC, Wood RA, Rand C, Kanchanaraksa S, Swartz L, Curtin-Brosnan J, Eggleston PA. Cockroach allergen exposure and sensitization n suburban middle-class children with asthma. J Allergy Clin Immunol 2003; 112(1):87–92.

13. Rosenstreich DL, Eggleston P, Kattan M, Baker D, Slavin RG, Gergen P, Mitchell H, McNiff-Mortimer K, Lynn H, Ownby D, Malveaux F. The role of cockroach allergy and exposure to cockroach allergen in causing morbidity among inner-city children with asthma. N Engl J Med 1997; 336(19):1356–63.

14. Rosenstreich DL, Eggleston P, Kattan M, Baker D, Slavin RG, Gergen P, Mitchell H, McNiff-Mortimer K, Lynn H, Ownby D, Malveaux F. The role of cockroach allergy and exposure to cockroach allergen in causing morbidity among inner-city children with asthma. N Engl J Med 1997; 336(19): 1356–1363.

15. Garrett MH, Rayment PR, Hooper MA, Abramson MJ, Hooper BM. Indoor airborne fungal spores, house dampness and associations with environmental factors and respiratory health in children. Clin Exp Allergy 1998; 28(4): 459–467.

16. Halonen M, Stern DA, Wright AL, Taussig LM, Martinez FD. Alternaria as a major allergen for asthma in children raised in a desert environment. Am J Respir Crit Care Med 1997; 155(4):1356–1361.

17. Belanger K, Beckett W, Triche E, Bracken MB, Holford T, Ren P, McSharry JE, Gold DR, Platts-Mills TA, Leaderer BP. Symptoms of wheeze and persistent cough in the first year of life: associations with indoor allergens, air contaminants, and maternal history of asthma. Am J Epidemiol 2003; 158(3): 195–202.

18. Chew GL, Douwes J, Doekes G, Higgins KM, van Strien R, Spithoven J, Brunekreef B. Fungal extracellular polysaccharides, beta (1→3)-glucans and

culturable fungi in repeated sampling of house dust. Indoor Air 2001; 11(3): 171–178.

19. Douwes J, van der Sluis B, Doekes G, van Leusden F, Wijnands L, van Strien R, Verhoeff A, Brunekreef B. Fungal extracellular polysaccbarides in house dust as a marker for exposure to fungi: relations with culturable fungi, reported home dampness, and respiratory symptoms. J Allergy Clin Immunol 1999; 103(3 Pt 1):494–500.

20. Stark PC, Burge HA, Ryan LM, Milton DK, Gold DR. Fungal levels in the home and lower respiratory tract illnesses in the first year of life. Am J Respir Crit Care Med 2003; 168(2):232–237.

21. Johnston RB Jr, Burge HA, Fisk WJ, Gold DR, Gordis L, Grunstein MM, Kinney PL, Mitchell HE, Ownby DR, Platts-Mills TAE, Sarpong SB,Wilson S. Institute of Medicine Report: Clearing the Air, Asthma and Indoor Air Exposures. Washington, DC: National Academy Press, 2000.

22. Sturm JJ, Yeatts K, Loomis D. Effects of tobacco smoke exposure on asthma prevalence and medical care use in north Carolina middle school children. Am J Public Health 2004; 94(2):308–313.

23. Strachan DP. The role of environmental factors in asthma. Br Med Bull 2000; 56(4):865–882.

24. Sherriff A, Peters TJ, Henderson J, Strachan D. Risk factor associations with wheezing patterns in children followed longitudinally from birth to 3(1/2) years. Int J Epidemiol 2001; 30(6):1473–1484.

25. Cook DG, Strachan DP, Carey IM. Health effects of passive smoking. Thorax 1999; 54(5):469.

26. Cook DG, Strachan DP. Health effects of passive smoking-10: summary of effects of parental smoking on the respiratory health of children and implications for research. Thorax 1999; 54(4):357–366.

27. Cook DG, Strachan DP, Carey IM. Health effects of passive smoking. 9. Parental smoking and spirometric indices in children. Thorax 1998; 53(10): 884–893.

28. Strachan DP, Cook DG. Health effects of passive smoking. 6. Parental smoking and childhood asthma: longitudinal and case-control studies. Thorax 1998; 53(3):204–212.

29. Jaakkola JJ, Gissler M. Maternal smoking in pregnancy, fetal development, and childhood asthma. Am J Public Health 2004; 94(1):136–140.

30. Liu AH, Murphy JR. Hygiene hypothesis: fact or fiction? J Allergy Clin Immunol 2003; 111(3):471–478.

31. Moss M, Gern J, Lemanske RJ. Asthma in infancy and childhood. In: Adkinson NF Jr, Yunginger J, Busse WW, Bochner BS, Holgate ST, Simons F, eds. Middleton's Allergy: Principles and Practie. Philadelphia: Mosby, 2003:1225–1256.

32. Johnston SL, Pattemore PK, Sanderson G, Smith S, Campbell MJ, Josephs LK, Cunningham A, Robinson BS, Myint SH, Ward ME, Tyrrell DA, Holgate ST. The relationship between upper respiratory infections and hospital admissions for asthma: a time-trend analysis. Am J Respir Crit Care Med 1996; 154(3 Pt 1):654–660.

33. Apter AJ. Early exposure to allergen: is this the cat's meow, or are we barking up the wrong tree? J Allergy Clin Immunol 2003; 111(5):938–946.

34. Welliver RC, Sun M, Rinaldo D, Ogra PL. Predictive value of respiratory syncytial virus-specific IgE responses for recurrent wheezing following bronchiolitis. J Pediatr 1986; 109(5):776–780.

35. Stein RT, Sherrill D, Morgan WJ, Holberg CJ, Halonen M, Taussig LM, Wright AL, Martinez FD. Respiratory syncytial virus in early life and risk of wheeze and allergy by age 13 years. Lancet 1999; 354(9178):541–554.

36. Johnston SL, Pattemore PK, Sanderson G, Smith S, Lampe F, Josephs L, Symington P, O'Toole S, Myint SH, Tyrrell DA, Holgate ST. Community study of role of viral infections in exacerbations of asthma in 9–11 year old children. BMJ 1995; 310(6989):1225–1229.

37. Hull J, Thomson A, Kwiatkowski D. Association of respiratory syncytial virus bronchiolitis with the interleukin 8 gene region m UK families. Thorax 2000; 55(12):1023–1027.

38. Castro-Rodriguez JA, Holberg CJ, Wright AL, Halonen M, Taussig LM, Morgan WJ, Martinez FD. Association of radiologically ascertained pneumonia before age 3 yr with asthmalike symptoms and pulmonary function during childhood: a prospective study. Am J Respir Crit Care Med 1999; 159(6): 1891–1897.

39. Martinez FD, Wright AL, Taussig LM, Holberg CJ, Halonen M, Morgan WJ. Asthma and wheezing in the first six years of life. The Group Health Medical Associates. N Engl J Med 1995; 332(3):133–138.

40. Taussig LM, Wright AL, Holberg CJ, Halonen M, Morgan WJ, Martinez FD. Tucson children's respiratory study: 1980 to present. J Allergy Clin Immunol 2003; 111(4):661–675; quiz 76.

41. Svanes C, Jarvis D, Chinn S, Omenaas E, Gulsvik A, Burney P. Early exposure to children in family and day care as related to adult asthma and hay fever: results from the European Community Respiratory Health Survey. Thorax 2002; 57(11):945–950.

42. Ball TM, Castro-Rodriguez JA, Griffith KA, Holberg CJ, Martinez FD, Wright AL. Siblings, day-care attendance, and the risk of asthma and wheezing during childhood. N Engl J Med 2000; 343(8):538–543.

43. Celedon JC, Wright RJ, Litonjua AA, Sredl D, Ryan L, Weiss ST, Gold DR. Day care attendance in early life, maternal history of asthma, and asthma at the age of 6 years. Am J Respir Crit Care Med 2003; 167(9):1239–1243.

44. McKeever TM, Lewis SA, Smith C, Collins J, Heatlie H, Frischer M, Hubbard R. Early exposure to infections and antibiotics and the incidence of allergic disease: a birth cohort study with the West Midlands General Practice Research Database. J Allergy Clin Immunol 2002; 109(1):43–50.

45. Celedon JC, Litonjua AA, Ryan L, Weiss ST, Gold DR. Lack of association between antibiotic use in the first year of life and asthma, allergic rhinitis, or eczema at age 5 years. Am J Respir Crit Care Med 2002; 166(1):72–75.

46. Reed CE, Milton DK. Endotoxin-stimulated innate immunity: a contributing factor for asthma. J Allergy Clin Immunol 2001; 108(2):157–166.

47. Peden DB. Air Pollution: Indoor and Outdoor. In: Adkinson NJ, Yunginger JW, Busse WW, Bochner BS, Holgate ST, Simons FER, eds. Middleton's

Allergy: Principles and Practice e-ditionSixth Edition ed.. Philadelphia: Elsevier, 2003:514–28.

48. Gereda JE, Klinnert MD, Price MR, Leung DY, Liu AH. Metropolitan home living conditions associated with indoor endotoxin levels. J Allergy Clin Immunol 2001; 107(5):790–796.

49. Gereda JE, Leung DY, Thatayatikom A, Streib JE, Price MR, Klinnert MD, Liu AH. Relation between house-dust endotoxin exposure, type 1 T-cell development, and allergen sensitisation in infants at high risk of asthma. Lancet 2000; 355(9216):1680–3.

50. Gehring U, Bischof W, Fahlbusch B, Wichmann HE, Heinrich J. House dust endotoxin and allergic sensitization in children. Am J Respir Crit Care Med 2002; 166(7):939–944.

51. Riedler J, Braun-Fahrlander C, Eder W, Schreuer M, Waser M, Maisch S, Carr D, Schierl R, Nowak D, von Mutius E. Exposure to farming in early life and development of asthma and allergy: a cross-sectional survey. Lancet 2001; 358(9288):1129–33.

52. Braun-Fahrlander C, Riedler J, Herz U, Eder W, Waser M, Grize L, Maisch S, Carr D, Gerlach F, Bufe A, Lauener RP, Schierl R, Renz H, Nowak D, von Mutius E. Environmental exposure to endotoxin and its relation to asthma in school-age children. N Engl J Med 2002; 347(12):869–77.

53. Liu AH. Endotoxin exposure in allergy and asthma: reconciling a paradox. J Allergy Clin Immunol 2002; 109(3):379–392.

54. Park JH, Spiegelman DL, Gold DR, Burge HA, Milton DK. Predictors of airborne endotoxin in the home. Environ Health Perspect 2001; 109(8): 859–864.

55. Gehring U, Bolte G, Borte M, Bischof W, Fahlbusch B, Wichmann HE, Heinrich J. Exposure to endotoxin decreases the risk of atopic eczema in infancy: a cohort study. J Allergy Clin Immunol 2001; 108(5):847–54.

56. Park JH, Gold DR, Spiegelman DL, Burge HA, Milton DK. House dust endotoxin and wheeze in the first year of life. Am J Respir Crit Care Med 2001; 163(2):322–328.

57. Litonjua AA, Milton DK, Celedon JC, Ryan L, Weiss ST, Gold DR. A longitudinal analysis of wheezing in young children: the independent effects of early life exposure to house dust endotoxin, allergens, and pets. J Allergy Clin Immunol 2002; 110(5):736–742.

58. Delfino RJ, Gong H Jr, Linn WS, Pellizzari ED, Hu Y. Asthma symptoms in Hispanic children and daily ambient exposures to toxic and criteria air pollutants. Environ Health Perspect 2003; 111(4):647–656.

59. Buchdahl R, Parker A, Stebbings T, Babiker A. Association between air pollution and acute childhood wheezy episodes: prospective observational study. BMJ 1996; 312(7032):661–665.

60. Nicolai T. Pollution, environmental factors and childhood respiratory allergic disease. Toxicology 2002; 181–182:317–321.

61. Gent JF, Triche EW, Holford TR, Belanger K, Bracken MB, Beckett WS, Leaderer BP. Association of low-level ozone and fine particles with respiratory symptoms in children with asthma. JAMA 2003; 290(14):1859–67.

62. Strand V, Rak S, Svartengren M, Bylin G. Nitrogen dioxide exposure enhances asthmatic reaction to inhaled allergen in subjects with asthma. Am J Respir Crit Care Med 1997; 155(3):881–887.
63. Bates DV, Baker-Anderson M, Sizto R. Asthma attack periodicity: a study of hospital emergency visits in Vancouver. Environ Res 1990; 51(l):51–70.
64. Schwartz J, Slater D, Larson TV, Pierson WE, Koenig JQ. Particulate air pollution and hospital emergency room visits for asthma in Seattle. Am Rev Respir Dis 1993; 147(4):826–831.
65. Atkinson RW, Anderson HR, Sunyer J, Ayres J, Baccini M, Vonk JM, Boumghar A, Forastiere F, Forsberg B, Touloumi G, Schwartz J, Katsouyanni K. Acute effects of particulate air pollution on respiratory admissions: results from APHEA 2 project. Air Pollution and Health: a European Approach. Am J Respir Crit Care Med 2001; 164(10 Pt 1):1860–6.
66. Lin M, Chen Y, Burnett RT, Villeneuve PJ, Krewski D. The influence of ambient coarse particulate matter on asthma hospitalization in children: case-crossover and time-series analyses. Environ Health Perspect 2002; 110(6): 575–581.
67. Nicolai T, Carr D, Weiland SK, Duhme H, von Ehrenstein O, Wagner C, von Mutius E. Urban traffic and pollutant exposure related to respiratory outcomes and atopy in a large sample of children. Eur Respir J 2003; 21(6): 956–63.
68. Kagawa J. Health effects of diesel exhaust emissions—a mixture of air pollutants of worldwide concern. Toxicology 2002; 181–182:349–353.
69. Fahy O, Hammad H, Senechal S, Pestel J, Tonnel AB, Wallaert B, Tsicopoulos A. Synergistic effect of diesel organic extracts and allergen Der p 1 on the release of chemokines by peripheral blood mononuclear cells from allergic subjects: involvement of the map kinase pathway. Am J Respir Cell Mol Biol 2000; 23(2):247–54.
70. Fahy O, Tsicopoulos A, Hammad H, Pestel J, Tonnel AB, Wallaert B. Effects of diesel organic extracts on chemokine production by peripheral blood mononuclear cells. J Allergy Clin Immunol 1999; 103(6):1115–1124.
71. Diaz-Sanchez D, Tsien A, Fleming J, Saxon A. Combined diesel exhaust particulate and ragweed allergen challenge markedly enhances human in vivo nasal ragweed-specific IgE and skews cytokine production to a T helper cell 2-type pattern. J Immunol 1997; 158(5):2406–2413.
72. Diaz-Sanchez D, Dotson AR, Takenaka H, Saxon A. Diesel exhaust particles induce local IgE production in vivo and alter the pattern of IgE messenger RNA isoforms. J Clin Invest 1994; 94(4):1417–1425.
73. Diaz-Sanchez D, Garcia MP, Wang M, Jyrala M, Saxon A. Nasal challenge with diesel exhaust particles can induce sensitization to a neoallergen in the human mucosa. J Allergy Clin Immunol 1999; 104(6):1183–1188.
74. Diaz-Sanchez D, Penichet-Garcia M, Saxon A. Diesel exhaust particles directly induce activated mast cells to degranulate and increase histamine levels and symptom severity. J Allergy Clin Immunol 2000; 106(6):l140–1146.
75. Senechal S, de Nadai P, Ralainirina N, Scherpereel A, Vorng H, Lassalle P, Tonnel AB, Tsicopoulos A, Wallaert B. Effect of diesel on chemokines and

chemokine receptors involved in helper T cell type 1/type 2 recruitment in patients with asthma. Am J Respir Crit Care Med 2003; 168(2):215–21.

76. Brunekreef B, Houthuijs D, Dijkstra L, Boleij JS. Indoor nitrogen dioxide exposure and children's pulmonary function. J Air Waste Manage Assoc 1990; 40(9):1252–1256.

77. Dijkstra L, Houthuijs D, Brunekreef B, Akkerman I, Boleij JS. Respiratory health effects of the indoor environment in a population of Dutch children. Am Rev Respir Dis 1990; 142(5):1172–1178.

78. Neas LM, Dockery DW, Ware JH, Spengler JD, Speizer FE, Ferris BG Jr. Association of indoor nitrogen dioxide with respiratory symptoms and pulmonary function in children. Am J Epidemiol 1991; 134(2):204–219.

79. Chauhan AJ, Inskip HM, Linaker CH, Smith S, Schreiber J, Johnston SL, Holgate ST. Personal exposure to nitrogen dioxide (NO2) and the severity of virus-induced asthma in children. Lancet 2003; 361(9373):1939–44.

80. Brugge D, Vallarino J, Ascolillo L, Osgood ND, Steinbach S, Spengler J. Comparison of multiple environmental factors for asthmatic children in public housing. Indoor Air 2003; 13(l):18–27.

81. Evans R, 3rd, Gergen PJ, Mitchell H, Kattan M, Kercsmar C, Crain E, Anderson J, Eggleston P, Malveaux FJ, Wedner HJ. A randomized clinical trial to reduce asthma morbidity among inner-city children: results of the National Cooperative Inner-City Asthma Study. J Pediatr 1999; 135(3): 332–8.

82. Litonjua AA, Carey VJ, Weiss ST, Gold DR. Race, socioeconomic factors, and area of residence are associated with asthma prevalence. Pediatr Pulmonol 1999; 28(6):394–401.

83. Chen E, Fisher EB, Bacharier LB, Strunk RC. Socioeconomic status, stress, and immune markers in adolescents with asthma. Psychosom Med 2003; 65(6):984–992.

84. Sullivan SD, Weiss KB, Lynn H, Mitchell H, Kattan M, Gergen PJ, Evans R. The cost-effectiveness of an inner-city asthma intervention for children. J Allergy Clin Immunol 2002; 110(4):576–81.

85. Wade S, Weil C, Holden G, Mitchell H, Evans R 3rd, Kruszon-Moran D, Bauman L, Crain E, Eggleston P, Kattan M, Kercsmar C, Leickly F, Malveaux F, Wedner HJ. Psychosocial characteristics of inner-city children with asthma: a description of the NCICAS psychosocial protocol. National Cooperative Inner-City Asthma Study. Pediatr Pulmonol 1997; 24(4):263–76.

86. Chen E, Bloomberg GR, Fisher EB Jr, Strunk RC. Predictors of repeat hospitalizations in children with asthma: the role of psychosocial and socio-environmental factors. Health Psychol 2003; 22(1):12–18.

87. Wright RJ, Steinbach SF. Violence: an unrecognized environmental exposure that may contribute to greater asthma morbidity in high risk inner-city pop-ulations. Environ Health Perspect 2001; 109(10):1085–1089.

88. Eggleston P. Environmental allergen avoidance: an overview. J Allergy Clin Immunol 2001; 107:S403–S405.

89. Chapman MD, Wood RA. The role and remediation of animal allergens in allergic diseases. J Allergy Clin Immunol 2001; 107(3 Suppl):S414–S421.

90. Wood RA, Chapman MD, Adkinson NF Jr, Eggleston PA. The effect of cat removal on allergen content in household-dust samples. J Allergy Clin Immunol 1989; 83(4):730–734.
91. van der Brempt X, Charpin D, Haddi E, da Mata P, Vervloet D. Cat removal and Fel d 1 levels in mattresses. J Allergy Clin Immunol 1991; 87(2):595–596.
92. de Blay F, Spirlet F, Gries P, Casel S, Ott M, Pauli G. Effects of various vacuum cleaners on the airborne content of major cat allergen (Fel d 1). Allergy 1998; 53(4):411–414.
93. de Blay F, Chapman MD, Platts-Mills TA. Airborne cat allergen (Fel d 1). Environmental control with the cat in situ. Am Rev Respir Dis 1991; 143(6): 1334–1339.
94. Wood RA, Johnson EF, van Natta ML, Chen PH, Eggleston PA. A placebo-controlled trial of a HEPA air cleaner in the treatment of cat allergy. Am J Respir Crit Care Med 1998; 158(1):115–120.
95. van der Heide S, van Aalderen WM, Kauffman HF, Dubois AE, de Monchy JG. Clinical effects of air cleaners in homes of asthmatic children sensitized to pet allergens. J Allergy Clin Immunol 1999; 104(2 Pt 1):447–451.
96. Gore RB, Bishop S, Durrell B, Curbishley L, Woodcock A, Custovic A. Air filtration units in homes with cats: can they reduce personal exposure to cat allergen? Clin Exp Allergy 2003; 33(6):765–769.
97. Peroni DG, Boner AL, Vallone G, Antolini I, Warner JO. Effective allergen avoidance at high altitude reduces allergen-induced bronchial hyper responsiveness. Am J Respir Crit Care Med 1994; 149(6):1442–1446.
98. Platts-Mills TA, Tovey ER, Mitchell EB, Moszoro H, Nock P, Wilkins SR. Reduction of bronchial hyperreactivity during prolonged allergen avoidance. Lancet 1982; 2(8300):675–678.
99. Walshaw MJ, Evans CC. Allergen avoidance in house dust mite sensitive adult asthma. Q J Med 1986; 58(226):199–215.
100. Carswell F, Oliver J, Weeks J. Do mite avoidance measures affect mite and cat airborne allergens? Clin Exp Allergy 1999; 29(2):193–200.
101. Htut T, Higenbottam TW, Gill GW, Darwin R, Anderson PB, Syed N. Eradication of house dust mite from homes of atopic asthmatic subjects: a double-blind trial. J Allergy Clin Immunol 2001; 107(l):55–60.
102. Ehnert B, Lau-Schadendorf S, Weber A, Buettner P, Schou C, Wahn U. Reducing domestic exposure to dust mite allergen reduces bronchial hyper-reactivity in sensitive cliildren with asthma. J Allergy Clin Immunol 1992; 90(1):135–138.
103. Halken S, Host A, Niklassen U, Hansen LG, Nielsen F, Pedersen S, Osterballe O, Veggerby C, Poulsen LK. Effect of mattress and pillow encasings on children with asthma and house dust mite allergy. J Allergy Clin Immunol 2003; 111(1):169–76.
104. Terreehorst I, Hak E, Oosting AJ, Tempels-Pavlica Z, de Monchy JG, Bruijnzeel-Koomen CA, Aalberse RC, Gerth van Wijk R. Evaluation of impermeable covers for bedding in patients with allergic rhinitis. N Engl J Med 2003; 349(3):237–46.
105. Woodcock A, Forster L, Matthews E, Martin J, Letley L, Vickers M, Britton J, Strachan D, Howarth P, Altmann D, Frost C, Custovic A. Control of expo-

sure to mite allergen and allergen-impermeable bed covers for adults with asthma. N Engl J Med 2003; 349(3):225–36.

106. Murray AB, Ferguson AC. Dust-free bedrooms in the treatment of asthmatic children with house dust or house dust mite allergy: a controlled trial. Pediatrics 1983; 71(3):418–422.

107. Busse W, Raphael GD, Galant S, Kalberg C, Goode-Sellers S, Srebro S, Edwards L, Rickard K. Low-dose fluticasone propionate compared with montelukast for first-line treatment of persistent asthma: a randomized clinical trial. J Allergy Clin Immunol 2001; 107(3):461–8.

108. Vandenhove T, Soler M, Birnbaum J, Charpin D, Vervloet D. Effect of dry cleaning on mite allergen levels in blankets. Allergy 1993; 48(4):264–266.

109. Lau S, Wahn J, Schulz G, Sommerfeld C, Wahn U. Placebo-controlled study of the mite allergen-reducing effect of tannic acid plus benzyl benzoate on carpets in homes of children with house dust mite sensitization and asthma. Pediatr Allergy Immunol 2002; 13(1):31–36.

110. Kroidl RF, Gobel D, Balzer D, Trendelenburg F, Schwichtenberg U. Clinical effects of benzyl benzoate in the prevention of house-dust-mite allergy. Results of a prospective, double-blind, multicenter study. Allergy 1998; 53(4): 435–440.

111. Colloff MJ, Taylor C, Merrett TG. The use of domestic steam cleaning for the control of house dust mites. Clin Exp Allergy 1995; 25(11):1061–1066.

112. Hyndman SJ, Vickers LM, Htut T, Maunder JW, Peock A, Higenbottam TW. A randomized trial of dehumidification in the control of house dust mite. Clin Exp Allergy 2000; 30(8):1172–1180.

113. Arlian LG, Neal JS, Morgan MS, Vyszenski-Moher DL, Rapp CM, Alexander AK. Reducing relative humidity is a practical way to control dust mites and their allergens in homes in temperate climates. J Allergy Clin Immunol 2001; 107(1):99–104.

114. Harving H, Korsgaard J, Dahl R. Clinical efficacy of reduction in house-dust mite exposure in specially designed, mechanically ventilated "healthy" homes. Allergy 1994; 49(10):866–870.

115. Harving H, Korsgaard J, Dahl R. House-dust mite exposure reduction in specially designed, mechanically ventilated "healthy" homes. Allergy 1994; 49(9):713–718.

116. Eggleston PA, Arruda LK. Ecology and elimination of cockroaches and allergens in the home. J Allergy Clin Immunol 2001; 107(3 Suppl):S422–S429.

117. Arbes SJ, Jr., Sever M, Archer J, Long EH, Gore JC, Schal C, Walter M, Nuebler B, Vaughn B, Mitchell H, Liu E, Collette N, Adler P, Sandel M, Zeldin DC. Abatement of cockroach allergen (Bla g 1) in low-income, urban housing: A randomized controlled trial. J Allergy Clin Immunol 2003; 112(2):339–45.

118. Eggleston PA. Cockroach allergen abatement: the good, the bad, and the ugly. J Allergy Clin Immunol 2003; 112(2):265–267.

119. Eggleston PA, Wood RA, Rand C, Nixon WJ, Chen PH, Lukk P. Removal of cockroach allergen from inner-city homes. J Allergy Clin Immunol 1999; 104(4 Pt 1):842–846.

120. Eggleston PA. Control of environmental allergens as a therapeutic approach. Immunol Allergy Clin North Am 2003; 23(3):533–547, viii–ix.

121. Garrison RA, Robertson LD, Koehn RD, Wynn SR. Effect of heating-ventilation-air conditioning system sanitation on airborne fungal populations in residential environments. Ann Allergy 1993; 71(6):548–556.
122. Savilahti R, Uitti J, Laippala P, Husman T, Roto P. Respiratory morbidity among children following renovation of a water-damaged school. Arch Environ Health 2000; 55(6):405–410.
123. Nordness ME, Zacharisen MC, Fink JN. Toxic and other non-IgE-mediated effects of fungal exposures. Curr Allergy Asthma Rep 2003; 3(5):438–446.
124. Hardin BD, Kelman BJ, Saxon A. Adverse human health effects associated with molds in the indoor environment. J Occup Environ Med 2003; 45(5): 470–478.
125. Meklin T, Husman T, Vepsalainen A, et al. Indoor air microbes and respiratory symptoms of children in moisture damaged and reference schools. Indoor Air 2002; 12(3):175–183.
126. Bush RK, Portnoy JM. The role and abatement of fungal allergens in allergic diseases. J Allergy Clin Immunol 2001; 107(3 Suppl):S430–S440.
127. Winickoff JP, McMillen RC, Carroll BC, Klein JD, Rigotti NA, Tanski SE, Weitzman M. Addressing parental smoking in pediatrics and family practice: a national survey of parents. Pediatrics 2003; 112(5):1146–51.
128. Hovell MF, Meltzer SB, Wahlgren DR, Matt GE, Hofstetter CR, Jones JA, Meltzer EO, Bernert JT, Pirkle JL. Asthma management and environmental tobacco smoke exposure reduction in Latino children: a controlled trial. Pediatrics 2002; 110(5):946–56.
129. Wilson SR, Yamada EG, Sudhakar R, Roberto L, Mannino D, Mejia C, Huss N. A controlled trial of an environmental tobacco smoke reduction intervention in low-income children with asthma. Chest 2001; 120(5):1709–22.

9

Early Pharmacologic Intervention of Asthma: How Early and What Treatment?

SØREN PEDERSEN

Department of Pediatrics, University of Southern Denmark, Kolding Hospital
Kolding, Denmark

I. Introduction

Twenty years ago, the majority of children with asthma received only intermittent anti-asthma treatment in association with exacerbations of the disease. Evolution of treatment since then has included the use of continuous treatment with theophylline, β2-agonists or sodium cromoglycate for children with moderate or severe, persistent asthma. During the 1990s, nedocromil sodium was introduced as an alternative to these drugs and the use of inhaled corticosteroids increased markedly. Initially inhaled corticosteroids were reserved for patients with severe and moderate persistent asthma, who were not controlled on other drugs, but later they became first choice of treatment in these disease severities. Over the last 10 years several studies have reported an often unexpectedly high morbidity and impairment also in patients with mild persistent asthma (1–4). This morbidity has been shown to be markedly reduced by continuous treatment with inhaled corticosteroids (1–3). Therefore, most international guidelines now recommend inhaled corticosteroids as the preferred first-line treatment for patients with mild, moderate, and severe persistent asthma rather than reserving this therapy for the more severe cases. This change in practice is often referred to as *early intervention* with inhaled corticosteroids. However, in the present paper the term early intervention will be used in its original meaning, which is initiation of a treatment *early in the course of the disease*. In contrast, a child who has had symptoms compatible with asthma for years before he/she is diagnosed or given treatment with inhaled corticosteroids as the first choice will be defined as receiving inhaled corticosteroids as first-line treatment.

The distinction between these two definitions may mainly be important when the ability of a treatment to modify the natural course or long-term outcomes is assessed. Finally, only early pharmacologic intervention in established disease will be discussed.

When the potential benefits of an early intervention strategy are assessed it is important first to discuss the research questions, the possible outcomes, relevant patient groups, and then the optimal study designs and interventions. In the following review these issues will be briefly discussed. This will be followed by the main results from studies assessing early pharmacologic intervention in children and to some extent also in adults.

A. Research Questions

There are several theoretical reasons for early pharmacological intervention in children with asthma. The three main ones are:

1. Does early pharmacologic intervention result in achievement of immediate clinical benefits (reduction in the morbidity and impairment caused by untreated disease)?
2. Does early pharmacologic intervention result in achievement of long-term benefits (modification of the natural course of the untreated disease)?
3. Does early pharmacologic intervention produce better short-term or long-term results or a more rapid improvement than later intervention?

B. Outcomes

The outcomes to assess depend on the research question addressed. With regard to the immediate benefits of the intervention the traditional outcomes from clinical trials can be used. The most relevant effects are outcomes that directly reflect patient or societal benefits such as (i) symptoms and/or symptom-free days, (ii) lung-function, (iii) need for rescue medication or other anti-asthma drugs, (iv) frequency and severity of asthma exacerbations, (v) quality of life, (vi) impairment and level of physical activity, (vii) unscheduled visits, emergency room visits, hospitality, and mortality, and (viii) health care costs and cost benefits.

In addition, protective effects on direct or indirect challenges and effects on airway inflammation may sometimes be feasible in such studies.

The traditional outcomes used to assess the immediate clinical benefits of a treatment have generally been well studied and validated–except for daily life impairment, which is normally assessed by questionnaires rather than objective measurements. Preliminary data indicate that in children, questionnaires may underestimate the actual impact of the disease on daily activities, so in the future, objective measurements of the physical activity combined with measurement of quality of life may provide additional information about the immediate benefits.

The best outcomes to assess long-term benefits of an intervention are less well characterized. They must represent and reflect some important features of the natural course of untreated disease. Consequently, their quality and clinical importance are very dependent on accurate knowledge about the long-term course of untreated disease, preferably in individual patients. Such knowledge is difficult or even impossible to obtain since a substantial proportion of patients in a study or a cohort will inevitably receive some kind of intervention because of their disease. Furthermore, this intervention is likely to be dependent on disease severity or the "true" spontaneous course of the disease, i.e., those with progression of the disease are more likely to receive some form of intervention. Therefore, in real life the comparator group of the effect of a pharmacological intervention on long-term benefits will always be patients exposed to varying degrees of other interventions rather than no other interventions at all. That complicates the interpretation of long-term pharmacologic intervention trials and the selection of appropriate outcomes.

With these reservations in mind some potentially useful outcomes would be:

1. Changing the natural course of the disease, including:

    A. reduction in or prevention of progression in disease severity,
    B. increasing periods of remission,
    C. cure.

2. Ensuring normal lung growth and normal growth (later in life normal decline) of lung function.
3. Prevention of airway remodeling and its possible long-term clinical consequences.

Both the short- and long-term outcomes listed above may be used to assess whether early pharmacologic intervention will produce better results than later intervention.

The best way to accurately monitor and assess the possible long-term benefits of an early pharmacologic intervention is more controversial and less well studied and validated. Before the different outcomes are discussed in some detail some general considerations about some potential benefits of early pharmacologic interventions on the *time course* of clinical improvements will be discussed.

After initiation of treatment with inhaled corticosteroids different asthma outcomes improve at different rates; some show marked initial improvements within days to weeks after which small, gradual improvements continue with time. Other outcomes such as bronchial hyper responsiveness or asthma stability and "clinical remission on treatment" may continue to improve for years (2,5). Until now almost all studies have focused on either the generally accepted short-term outcomes used in most clinical trials of three months duration or some very long-term outcomes assessed after several years. However, clinically, the rate of improvement may be equally important (Fig. 1). Even if no differences exist between an early and a late intervention strategy after 10 years, differences in rates of improvement between the two strategies might still be clinically very important and result in marked mediate-term differences (Fig. 1). At present that potentially important outcome of early versus late pharmacologic intervention has not been studied.

C. Changing the Natural Course of the Disease

Progression

There does not seem to be any universally accepted definition of asthma disease progression. One manageable definition could be the development of one or more of the following:

1. Increased frequency or severity of symptoms
2. Development of exacerbations or increase in frequency and/or severity of asthma exacerbations
3. Increased bronchial hyperresponsiveness
4. Increasing medication requirement
5. Increased impairment
6. Increased healthcare costs
7. Development of chest deformities

Although this may seem straightforward, it is not. Asthma is a variable disease and recent studies suggest that patients not receiving any prophylactic treatment spontaneously may change levels of symptoms, exacerbations, and requirement of rescue β2-agonist and health care services over short periods of time; the shifts both going from good to worse and the other way (6). Therefore, there must also be some time period over which these outcomes are assessed otherwise, they will merely reflect changes in the immediate benefit outcomes rather than a long-term disease modifying effect. The optimal duration of this time period is not known. It should probably be several years.

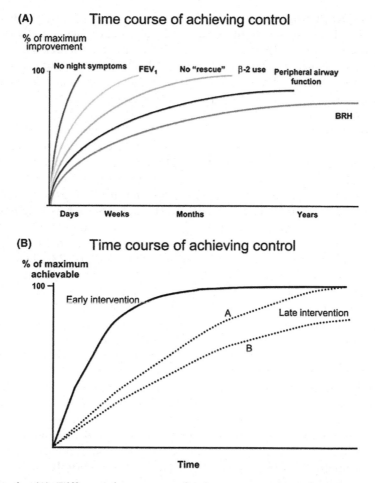

Figure 1 (A) Different time courses for improvement in various outcomes in patients receiving treatment with inhaled corticosteroids. The various curves are not based on specific studies but represent the findings in many different studies. There are important differences in the rate of improvement but not in the maximum achievable improvement between early and late intervention. (B) A theoretical course of the same outcome after initiation of therapy. Important differences in both rate of improvement and maximum achievable improvement between early and late intervention. The scenario emphasizes the importance of repeated measurements when comparing early and late interventions.

Several cross-sectional studies in children and adults have found that in groups of asthma patients long duration of asthma was associated with reduced lung functions, increased bronchial hyperresponsiveness, greater use of rescue medication, and more frequent and severe asthma symptoms (7–9). This could suggest a progression of asthma severity over time. However, this finding could also to some extent be caused by a selection bias if patients with mild disease outgrow their disease more frequently than patients with more severe disease–which seems to be the case. Still, the finding of the association between asthma duration and greater asthma severity also in groups of patients with mild asthma suggests that selection bias may not be the only explanation.

At present mainly cohort studies have followed children for long periods of time, but as mentioned earlier most cohort studies have not been designed so that they can effectively control for all confounders that might influence disease progression, i.e., information about use of asthma drugs is far less reliable than in regular asthma trials. Furthermore, most cohort studies focus on questionnaires and outcomes such as lung function and bronchial hyperresponsiveness.

The findings in cohort studies suggest that there is a marked tracking between asthma severity in childhood and adulthood (10–28). Thus only a minority (15–20%) of children with mild disease during childhood develops more severe disease in adulthood and most patients' with severe asthma continue to have severe asthma later in life (around 60%). So, even if a progression may occur to a significant extent with time in some patients, it does not seem to be the case for all. This complicates accurate assessment of prevention or reduction of disease progression since clinically relevant findings may be missed in trials due to insufficient statistical power unless carefully selected high-risk patients or very big populations are studied. Unfortunately, at present our knowledge is not sufficient for an accurate selection of high-risk patients. Moreover, the larger a trial is the greater the limitation on accurate outcome measurements and careful monitoring. So, considering the heterogeneity of the patient populations and the spontaneous fluctuations in disease severity over short periods of time, it is obvious that unequivocal conclusions about possible interference with long-term disease progression is difficult to obtain. Perhaps the best outcome would be a sort of "asthma stability index," which reflects the spontaneous fluctuations in disease severity seen in untreated disease (6). This might be used to assess how early intervention influences long-term stability of the disease (Fig. 2).

Remission

There is no accepted definition of remission. *Clinical remission* is used to describe patients who have had no symptoms and used no asthma medication for a certain period of time. Due to the fluctuating nature of the disease many children with mild to moderate asthma will undergo a spontaneous clinical remission for short periods of time. The question is how long should the period be before it can be defined as clinical remission? One year has

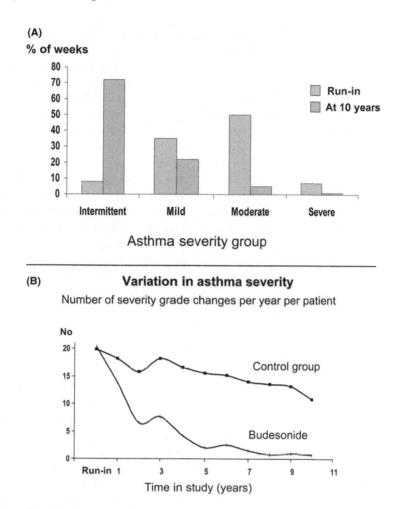

Figure 2 (A) Changes with time in asthma severity during long-term treatment with inhaled budesonide. A marked shift towards milder disease is seen with time. The data are based on four periods of 4 weeks of monitoring each year. (B) Mean number of times per year an individual asthma patient changes severity grading. With continued treatment with inhaled budesonide the asthma becomes more stable. The control group receives combinations of asthma medication, but not inhaled corticosteroids. The study is not randomized and at the end there are only 24 patients left in the control group (62 at entry).

been suggested, but the appropriateness of this has not been validated. Clinical remission can occur at any age, but the greatest likelihood seems to be in late adolescence and early adult lives. This must be remembered when studies are designed to assess the influence of pharmacologic intervention on clinical remission. It is also important to differentiate between clinical remission on treatment and remission after the treatment is stopped. Children with mild persistent asthma who have been treated with inhaled corticosteroids for several years may obtain a state of "clinical remission" while on treatment. This may last for a long period after ICS treatment has been stopped. However, stopping inhaled corticosteroids is usually associated with a deterioration in asthma control and return of bronchial hyperresponsiveness to pretreatment level within weeks to several months, in the majority of patients, though in some the beneficial effects are maintained much longer (29). The studies with the highest and longest remission rates seem to be those which have treated patients with rather mild disease for a period of one year or more (30–32). Discontinuation of inhaled corticosteroids has, however, mainly been evaluated after less than a couple of years of continuous treatment, and never in a group of children in whom the treatment was initiated shortly after the onset of the disease. The question is how long should the treatment-free clinical remission after stoppage of inhaled corticosteroids be to become categorized as a significant treatment-induced remission? We know too little about this and need more information about spontaneous clinical remissions before an accurate definition can be made.

As mentioned earlier, long-term (clinical) remission while on continued treatment might also be an important outcome to assess in pharmacologic intervention trials. This is less ambitious than remission without treatment, but perhaps more realistic and still clinically important for the patient. Airway inflammation is a response, which may be provoked or enhanced by allergic reactions, infections, and other environmental factors and it would be expected that continued or repeated anti-inflammatory therapy would be necessary to maintain remission.

Finally, although a clinical remission can be defined and used as an outcome in a long-term trial, the clinical importance of a remission may be complex since studies have found that individuals in clinical remission may continue to have airway inflammation (airway inflammatory infiltrates and thickening of the reticular basement membrane), lung-function abnormalities, increased bronchial hyperresponsiveness and elevated exhaled nitric oxide levels (33–35). A certain proportion of these patients will have a relapse of their asthma later–if not before, then in adulthood. This makes it difficult to interpret the long-term importance of clinical remission from a disease point of view–though the importance for the patient is obvious. If remission is chosen as an outcome in an intervention trial it would be preferable also to include some objective measures in the definition.

Cure

Cure would be the ultimate outcome for an early pharmacologic intervention. As for "remission" a definition of "cure" is needed. Most consider "cure" to be a long-term remission without need for any asthma treatment or restrictions in lifestyle. The question is should "cure" include objective measurements such as assessment of inflammation and bronchial hyperresponsiveness?

It also needs to be defined when a "remission" can be called a "cure." At present it seems that long-term treatment with inhaled steroids suppresses the underlying mechanisms of asthma and causes "clinical remission" of the condition without "curing" the disease. However, it has not been studied whether early treatment initiated before the disease becomes clinically established will be able to "cure" the disease.

D. Normal Growth of Lung Function and Lung Development

Lung functions have been the main focus of pediatric studies and little systematic information is available about the influence of the asthma disease on structural lung growth and development. Untreated asthma can result in hyper-expansion of the lungs. With time this may lead to marked chest deformities, suggesting that asthma may adversely affect normal lung growth and development in some patients (36). However, more thorough assessments have not been done. This is understandable because at present it is not possible to separate structure from function in real life. Most people assume that growth in lung function is an adequate surrogate marker for structural growth, so if lung growth is abnormal, lung function will be abnormal too. However, this may not necessarily be the case. For instance, the two major variable determinants of maximum expiratory flow at wave speed, airway lumen caliber and wall elastance, could work in opposite directions to permit "normal" flow, despite reduced caliber and increased elastance. Perhaps future improvements in imaging techniques will be of help in assessing structural lung growth and development.

The body of information is therefore about growth of lung function in patients with asthma. Generally, the various studies have used rather crude outcome measures, such as FEV_1 or FVC, which do not reflect smaller airway function or peripheral airway inflammation and which may remain normal even in the presence of marked damage of the smaller airways (37–40).

It is not known whether measurement of other outcomes would be more sensitive in detecting the influence of the asthma disease on the growth of lung functions. A recent study suggests that this may very well be the case (41). Most people agree that postbronchodilator lung-function values are preferable to prebronchodilator values, but this has not been formerly validated. Genetic heterogeneity of bronchodilator response or an increased bronchodilator response with time as a result of remodeling of the airway smooth muscles as reported by some studies (1,41) might complicate the interpretation of postbronchodilator values (Fig. 3). Finally, a substantial part of the information on the normal development of lung

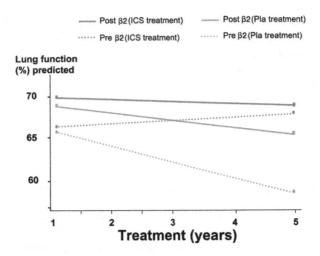

Figure 3 An illustration of the problems of interpreting different measures of decline in lung function. One group of patients receives inhaled corticosteroids and the other placebo. A marked difference is seen in development in prebronchodilator lung function with time. However, due to less bronchodilatation with time in the inhaled corticosteroid treated group and increased bronchodilator response in the placebo group the differences in postbronchodilator values are smaller. Does this mean that inhaled corticosteroids have no effect on decline in lung function? Or does it mean that the decline is modified and that inhaled corticosteroids modify remodeling of the airway smooth muscles?

function comes from cohort studies, the limitations of which have already been discussed. With these reservations in mind some conclusions about growth of lung function with time can be made.

It seems that in groups of patients with asthma the percent predicted lung function declines with time (7,21,42–52). The decline occurs in childhood but may be even steeper in adulthood (8,53–55). In children with asthma, the concern is that maximal lung or airway growth may not occur so that young adults with childhood-onset asthma may be starting out with diminished lung function, and thus at even greater risk of the development of significant airflow obstruction later in life. The data suggest that the influence may be more marked early in the disease (10,56) and that the phenomenon may be more pronounced in patients with more severe disease (48). Furthermore, lung function appears to track with age so that children with low lung functions seem to be more likely to have persistently low lung function later in life (57–63) and increased bronchial reactivity to specific and non-specific agents (64–67) regardless of the presence of asthmatic symptoms. Finally, several studies have reported patients in whom chronic childhood asthma has been suspected of leading to some chronic irreversible airway obstruction to a clinically important extent (9,47,57–61,68).

Some of these data come from cross-sectional studies and some from cohort studies. However, the findings in some controlled, longitudinal studies support the conclusions from these studies. Thus the inhaled steroid treatment as regular therapy in early asthma (START) study, which followed more than 7000 patients aged 5 to 66 years, with mild persistent asthma for three years, found the following three years, declines in postbronchodilator FEV_1: 6- to 10-years group $= 2.3\%$, 11- to 18-years group $= 0.4\%$, and the adult group $= 3.6\%$ in patients treated with placebo. The declines were statistically significant in the younger and older age groups, but not in the 11–18-year-olds. Some smaller randomized, prospective studies also reported significant declines in both pre- and postbronchodilator lung functions in patients, mild and moderate asthma treated with salmeterol (5) and placebo (41). In the latter study the decline seemed more marked in lung-function parameters reflecting the more peripheral airways (41). In contrast to this the CAMP study only found a small, non-significant decline of 1% in postbronchodilator FEV_1 percent predicted and a 1.7% decline in postbronchodilator FEV_1/FVC ratios over four years (69) in 400 patients with mild persistent asthma with a mean age of 9.5 years at study entry. The discrepancy between the findings in CAMP and the findings in the other three prospective studies or the cohort studies is not known. Compared with the findings in START three possible differences may have been important:

(1) *Differences in asthma duration.* All patients in the START study had a very short duration of asthma. This was not the case for the patients in CAMP (mean duration of asthma at study entry was five years). This difference may be important if the decline in lung function is more pronounced early in the disease as suggested by some studies.

(2) *Differences in age.* The mean age at study entry of the patients in the CAMP study (69) was 9.5 years. So agewise their patients resembled the 11–17 years olds in the START study in whom no significant decline in postbronchodilator FEV_1 was seen (1). It is not known why the findings in adolescents should be different from other age groups. However, during puberty the relationship between height and lung functions is more complex than in other periods of life and assessment of FEV_1 percent predicted may not be as suitable a measure as in other ages (70–72). So, more studies are needed in pubertal children before conclusions from these age groups can be generalized to other age groups.

(3) *Assessed by pretreatment lung functions the asthma severity.* There may also have been some differences in asthma severity between the two studies.

The data in the various studies have normally been presented as significant differences in the group mean data. However, the inter-patient variation seems to have been quite marked. Only few studies have looked carefully at individual risk factors so it will be difficult to identify in advance those individuals who are likely to develop these complications to a clinically important extent. It seems, however, that the risk is higher in patients with more severe disease.

E. Prevention of Remodeling and Its Long-Term Clinical Consequences

It has become well established that airway inflammation is present in all patients with asthma, including early asthma as well as patients experiencing symptoms for only a short period or with just mild disease. Airway remodeling, including increases in airway smooth muscle (hyperplasic and hypertrophy), vascular proliferation, increases in bronchial glands, goblet cell hyperplasic, edema formation, and collagen deposition and perhaps epithelial shedding (73–77) is also present in all patients with asthma. Airway remodeling seems to be a result of an ongoing destruction and repair and should not be considered an entirely fixed, irreversible condition (74). The structural changes are believed to transiently or permanently affect the functional properties of the tissues. Inflammation and remodeling seem to be connected to some extent and treatment with inhaled corticosteroids modify both (41,78–81). However, it is not known whether inflammation precedes the remodeling, whether the morphological changes are secondary to the inflammation or some or even all of the structural changes are independent of inflammation. Since airway inflammation may be patchy and fluctuate over time it is almost impossible with the currently available techniques to further elucidate the relationship between airway inflammation and remodeling, so these questions are probably not going to be unequivocally answered until new techniques have been developed.

The questions are if and how inflammation and remodeling and their effect on the functional properties of the tissues are linked to long-term clinical outcomes of asthma such as disturbances of lung function, development of irreversible airway obstruction, clinical disease progression, and increased bronchial responsiveness. This is difficult to assess because we have no good ways of quantifying the degree of remodeling in the small airways or measuring the function of the peripheral airways. Data obtained from the central airways may have little relevance for the disease processes in or function of the more peripheral airways (39,40). The current paradigm is that the structural changes in the airways are to some extent associated with, or linked to, progression of the asthma disease. In agreement with this observation, many studies have demonstrated associations between some structural changes and clinical outcomes linked to asthma severity/progression (41,82–85). Not unexpectedly several other studies have not been able to confirm such an association.

The direct relation of the airway inflammation and remodeling to the course of clinical disease is not only difficult to assess, but also very complex. Though inflammation in itself causes increased bronchial responsiveness or worsens it, bronchial hyperresponsiveness without signs of inflammation has also been reported (78,86,87). Moreover, some elements of responsiveness are amenable to treatment with inhaled steroids and others are not. The question is whether this *resistant* component in some patients represents scarring that might have been prevented by either rigorous early treatment or a different therapeutic approach. In support of this some trials found that late use of inhaled corticosteroids is associated with a smaller effect on bronchial hyperresponsiveness compared with early use (30,88,89). Finally, to add to the complexity the dose-response and time-effect relationships of inhaled corticosteroids on inflammation, remodeling, and bronchial hyperresponsiveness seem to be different. A few weeks, treatment with inhaled corticosteroids may produce marked reductions in inflammation, but little or no effect on remodeling or bronchial hyperresponsiveness, whereas continued long-term treatment with the same dose may modify remodeling and bronchial hyperresponsiveness without any additional effect on inflammation (90) (Fig. 4).

One small study has tried to assess the association between development/progression of asthma, airway inflammation and remodeling (91). It was found that patients with silent bronchial hyperresponsiveness (no asthma symptoms) differed from asthmatics in that their basement membranes only showed areas of patchy fibrosis while continuous thickening was seen in the patients with symptoms of asthma. In addition, the asymptomatic bronchial hyperresponsiveness group had intermediate numbers of mucosal inflammatory cells between those with asthma and the nonasthmatic controls. Over the two-year study period, FEV_1 tended to decline while bronchial hyperresponsiveness increased and serum immunogloblulin E (IgE) levels rose in those with asymptomatic bronchial hyperresponsiveness, and four of the ten subjects with silent bronchial hyperresponsiveness developed asthma.

The bronchial biopsies of these patients showed increased basement membrane thickness and increased numbers of mucosal inflammatory cells. This study suggests that airway inflammation may precede asymptomatic bronchial hyperresponsiveness and that progression of the airway inflammation is associated with increased airway remodeling and asthma development. If this can be confirmed in larger, controlled studies it elicits the hope that very early interventions, which reduce the inflammation, may be able to have long-term modifying effects on asthma development or progression.

Finally, some studies with inhaled corticosteroids indicate that modification of airway inflammation and remodeling may be important for medium-term clinical outcomes in asthma. One prospective study used bronchial hyperresponsiveness as a surrogate marker of airway inflammation in combination with traditional clinical outcomes to adjust the inhaled steroid dose in one group of patients and only traditional clinical outcomes in another group. Inclusion of bronchial hyperresponsiveness in the

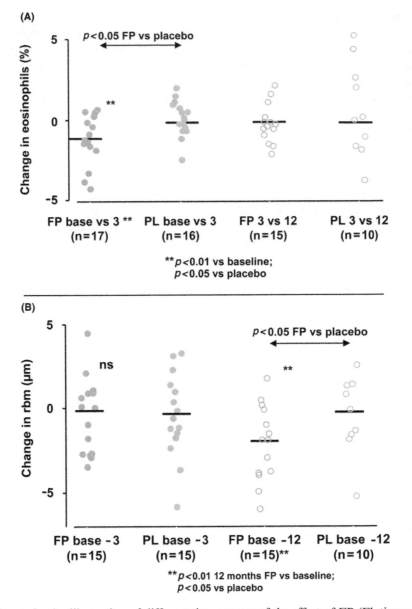

Figure 4 An illustration of different time-courses of the effect of FP (Fluticasone propionate) on different outcomes. *Top:* A statistically significant reduction on airway eosinophils is seen after three months treatment and after this point in time no further reductions are seen with continued treatment. *Bottom:* With respect to thickness of the reticular basal membrane (rbm) no effect is seen after three months treatment whereas significant effects are seen in the fluticasone treated patients after one year. *Source:* From Refs. 24,27.

assessment resulted in a 60% increase in the dose of inhaled corticosteroid as well as significant improvements in both clinical outcomes and airway inflammation and remodeling over the two-year period (41). In agreement with this a similarly designed study found better clinical effects of the same mean corticosteroid dose when sputum eosinophils was used as a marker of airway inflammation in addition to traditional clinical outcomes instead of traditional outcomes alone (92). These and other studies indirectly support a link between airway inflammation and clinical outcomes and perhaps also airway remodeling. However, if inflammation were the most important factor for asthma progression it would be expected that asthma would progress in all patients in whom airway inflammation was not suppressed by treatment. This does not seem to be the case. Several studies have found that asthma only seems to progress in a certain proportion of patients (1,2,93). So, although inflammation and remodeling may play a role for the progression of asthma other factors seem to be at least as important for disease progression. Therefore, more data are needed before airway inflammation and remodeling can be used as surrogate markers in the assessment of the benefits of early pharmacologic intervention in asthma. At present these measures should be used in combination with other outcomes to increase our understanding of asthma management and disease progression.

II. Which Patients?

Little is known about the optimal selection of patients for early pharmacologic intervention trials. There does not seem to be any firm association between the various outcomes that would be relevant to assess (exacerbations, bronchial hyperresponsiveness, decline in lung function, asthma stability, remission, etc.) (1,2) so selection of patients on the basis of risk factors for one important outcome such as decline in postbronchodilator FEV_1 might obtain valid conclusions about that outcome at the expense of missing important information or even be misleading with respect to conclusions about other outcomes reflecting disease progression. So, one approach would be to perform a large study on thousands of patients with recent debut of asthma and then do subgroup analyses after completion of the study. However, such studies are expensive and difficult to do meticulously with sophisticated measurements, so another option would be to select smaller groups at risk of a certain outcome such as accelerated decline in lung function and do careful, sophisticated body box pletysmography, airway inflammation measurements, imaging techniques, and direct and indirect airway challenges at regular intervals at centers experienced in these measurements. This would most likely answer one or two important questions, but the conclusions could not be generalized to the same extent as in the first approach.

Individual asthma patients move between different asthma severities over time (6). During one period the disease may be mild intermittent, during another moderate persistent, etc. In some patients these changes in severity occur frequently and in others only occasionally. Since early intervention should be initiated shortly after the debut of the disease long observation periods are not possible and a reliable disease severity grading will be difficult. At best it might be rather inaccurate, but it might even be wrong or useless. The longer the observation period is before the intervention is initiated the more reliable a disease severity grading would be, but this gain could easily be negated by the delay in intervention.

Asthma can begin at any age during childhood so preferably all ages should be studied. However, in the majority of children the disease starts during the first three years of life (28,94,95). This makes patient selection even more difficult. At that age we do not have a standardized definition of asthma, nor do we have readily available, non-invasive measures of airway inflammation, the presence of atopy or allergy is more difficult to establish, and important outcomes such as reliable lung-function measurements are almost impossible to obtain in large number of patients. Moreover, only a fraction of patients who wheeze at that age have asthma, and although some prediction indices have been developed, conclusions from studies on children with a high risk of asthma (recurrent wheezing and risk factors for persistent asthma such as a parent with asthma or the presence of eczema) may not be applicable to children with a lower risk, who, in spite of a lower risk still do develop asthma–although less frequently. Therefore, studies in these age groups should probably be conducted in both high- and low-risk patients. No matter which selection strategy is used in these children, the chosen intervention will always be applied to a large number of children who will never develop persistent asthma. This may jeopardize the interpretation of the effect of an intervention unless a substantial number of patients are included in the study. With these difficulties it is understandable that so far no early intervention trials have been conducted in these age groups.

III. Which Study Designs?

It has been hypothesized that there may be a "window-opportunity in relation to early pharmacologic intervention in asthma," following which remodeling and lung function changes occur and cannot be reversed so that even the introduction of inhaled steroids may not lead to a total normalization of the pathology (76,91) (Fig. 5). This contention is supported by the findings that airway inflammation and remodeling may be present early in the disease and these phenomena normally precede clinical symptoms. So, the time of first clinical symptoms may actually be late in the course

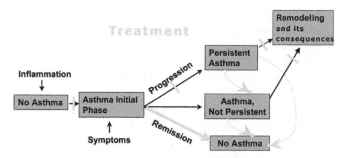

Figure 5 Potential benefits of early pharmacologic interventions. The timing of the intervention may be important for what is achievable. The theory is that the earlier the better, however, more studies are needed to assess whether there is a "window of opportunity" after which it will be too late.

of the disease. Most of the patients included in the various treatment studies have experienced symptoms and persistent asthma for a long time at study entry. When increased bronchial responsiveness is detected the theory is that the opportunity of optimal intervention may have been missed–or perhaps longer treatment with higher doses of drug will be needed. However, this has not been formerly validated. Even if it would be theoretically advantageous to study patients immediately after their first symptoms that would be almost impossible in real life. Here early intervention will almost always be after symptoms have been present for some time–months or even a year. In young children the asthma diagnosis is more difficult and subtle asthma symptoms are often missed. So the delay before the intervention is initiated is likely to be longer in these age groups.

Perhaps a widened view of asthma, taking into account also patients with asthma-like symptoms (inflammation), would improve early detection of symptoms and lead to more effective interventions (96). The same might be the case if the intervention could start as soon as the airway inflammation is present. However, it remains to be seen whether such an approach would have any impact on the pattern of asthma severity or modify the course of the disease.

It requires different study designs to address the three potential arguments for early intervention in recent-onset asthma. Achievement of immediate clinical benefits is the easiest to address since this question can be assessed in traditional prospective, randomized, placebo-controlled trials of relatively short duration measuring standard clinical outcomes.

In contrast it requires very long-term (several years) prospective, controlled clinical studies to study the potential long-term benefits or whether early intervention produces better long-term results than later intervention. This makes true placebo comparisons difficult or impossible unless the disease is and stays very mild throughout the study and then the relevance of the findings for more severe disease may be questioned. The START study is a good example of the problems encountered in long-term trials (1). Even if the patients at study entry were predominantly classified as mild persistent asthmatics, 25% in the placebo group ended up on inhaled corticosteroids during the first three years of the study. In addition, a substantial amount of placebo-treated patients were prescribed other asthma drugs during this period. The need for additional inhaled corticosteroids and other asthma medication was significantly less in patients receiving early intervention with budesonide. Such difference in use of other asthma medication complicate the interpretation of a study. Can the need for additional asthma medication be used as a marker of disease progression? Can it be assumed that the patients receiving additional medication are no different from the patients not receiving any? If not, are the budesonide group and the "true placebo patients" who did not achieve any additional inhaled corticosteroids still comparable after three years? Or are we comparing apples and oranges at that time?

Although sophisticated statistical analyses can be made to reduce the impact of different confounders they cannot completely negate them. These problems will be more pronounced the longer the study is. Prohibiting additional asthma medication does not solve the problem, since this is likely to result in a large number of drop-outs in the placebo arm.

The optimal duration of a long-term study is not known. Different outcomes improve at different rates, some within days to weeks while others such as bronchial hyperresponsiveness or asthma stability and "remission on treatment" may continue to improve for years (97). Therefore, for efficacy reasons the potential long-term effects of an intervention should probably be studied for more than five years, though this has not been formerly assessed.

The studies assessing treatment duration have not been early intervention studies but only first-line treatment trials in which the patients have had clinical asthma symptoms for several years before study entry. When inhaled corticosteroid treatment has been discontinued in such trials after one to four years of treatment, asthma control and bronchial hyperresponsiveness have usually degenerated to pretreatment levels within weeks to months (2,98), though in some patients the beneficial effect is maintained much longer (29). This pattern is also seen when any other anti-asthma medication is withheld. The studies with the highest and longest remission rates seem to be those which have treated patients with rather mild disease for a period of one year or longer (30–32,99). Only CAMP has treated with inhaled corticosteroids for longer periods than two years before cessation of treatment. Although the bronchial hyperresponsiveness after four years of budesonide treatment in CAMP increased after cessation it was still significantly improved as compared with placebo six months after cessation of the treatment (Fig. 6). For the majority of children, then, it seems that once the asthma is fully developed inhaled steroids will mainly suppress the underly-

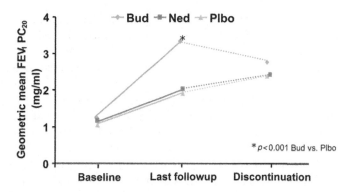

Figure 6 Influence of budesonide, nedocromil, and placebo treatment of bronchial hyper-responsiveness in 1000 children with a mean duration of asthma of five years at study entry (*Baseline*). Only budesonide improved bronchial hyper-responsiveness significantly (*Last follow-up*). After cessation of treatments the bronchial hyper-responsiveness in the budesonide group increased (PC_{20} fell) towards the levels in the other groups. However, six months after cessation of treatment (*Discontinuation*) the differences between budesonide and placebo were still statistically significant, indicating some possible long-term effects on this outcome. *Source*: From Ref. 116.

ing mechanisms of asthma and cause remission of the condition without curing the disease. As mentioned earlier discontinuation of inhaled corticosteroids has, however, never been evaluated in a group of children in whom the treatment was initiated shortly after the onset of the disease. On the other hand, infiltration of inflammatory cells in the lamina propria of the airways has been shown to persist in patients with mild to moderate asthma despite regular treatment with inhaled steroids (100). This indicates a need for regular maintenance anti-inflammatory treatment. Asthmatic inflammation is a response, which is often provoked by allergic reactions, infections, and other common environmental factors; one would expect, then, that continued or repeated anti-inflammatory therapy would be necessary if the treatment had not induced a complete remission of the disease. Clinical data suggest, however, that the dose can be stepped-down over time without loss of asthma control in the majority of patients (8).

In addition to the traditional outcomes used in short-term trials, long-term studies also require other outcomes, including the need for asthma medications other than the study drug, tracking of sophisticated body box pletysmography measurement, bronchial hyperresponsiveness, assessment of asthma stability and remissions, rate of improvement of the various outcomes, and perhaps also some surrogate markers such as assessment of airway inflammation and remodeling.

Studies trying to assess whether early intervention is better than late should at some stage either allow the placebo-treated patients to be switched over to the active treatment arm after a certain period or stop the active treatment to provide direct comparisons of the patients starting early with those starting late or not receiving any treatment at all. Both these approaches have their problems such as ethical considerations, lack of knowledge about the active treatment time before the change should be made or the duration of the period after the change before any conclusions can be made, and which outcomes should be compared.

Undoubtedly, less ambitious study designs may also provide some information about possible beneficial long-term effects, but the information from such studies will be less valid and the interpretation of the findings open to discussion. However, in light of the problems outlined above less controlled studies or studies comparing different treatments will probably also play an important role in the future–even in the days of evidence-based medicine.

IV. Interventions

A. What Medication and Dose Should Be Used?

Our understanding of the effect of various drugs on the different aspects of control of disease is at a very early stage. We know that the *dose* of drug sufficient to normalize one outcome may be quite different from the dose required to control other outcomes. Furthermore, a certain *drug* may produce excellent control of one outcome such as symptoms without having any significant effects upon another such as exacerbations or bronchial hyperresponsiveness (5,101,102). With respect to immediate outcomes we have some understanding of the doses required to produce certain effects. However, when it comes to long-term outcomes, disease modification, or time course of effects our knowledge about dose-response relationships is quite sparse (101). Therefore, ideally, several doses of drug should be studied in order to assess an optimal treatment intervention (Fig. 7). It is possible that a dose of a drug that is clinically useful in short-term trials may not have any disease-modifying effects, whereas a higher dose of the same drug might. The concern therefore is that low doses of inhaled corticosteroid may produce good *subjective control without optimal disease control*, i.e., achieving the short-term aim only. The results of a recent study indirectly supports this assumption since inclusion of bronchial hyperresponsiveness (surrogate marker of inflammation) as an outcome in the daily clinical management led to the use of higher doses of inhaled corticosteroid, improved asthma control, less airway remodeling, and fewer exacerbations (103) (Fig. 8). Further, studies are needed to address this question, particularly because safety issues will become more important when higher doses are used for long periods of time. To overcome this problem trial designs using initially high doses followed by step-down and more variable dosing might be an option (8). However, virtually nothing is known about optimal criteria and/or time for the dose adjustments. At present two ongoing studies in children less than three years of age use different approaches. One uses a

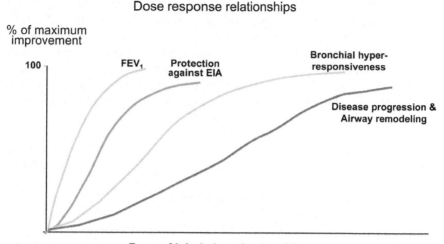

Figure 7 Dose-response relationships of inhaled corticosteroids on various outcome parameters. Different doses may be needed to optimally control different outcomes. Doses that control short-term outcomes such as symptoms may have sub-optimal disease modifying effects. This has not been extensively studied, but several studies indicate that maximum effects on bronchial hyper-responsiveness and airway remodeling may require higher doses than the doses needed to control symptoms.

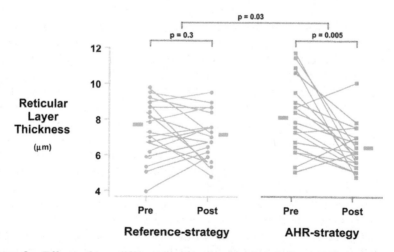

Figure 8 Effects of two different treatment strategies on airway inflammation and remodeling. When control of bronchial hyper-responsiveness was included in the treatment objectives 50% higher doses of inhaled corticosteroid were needed. This was associated with significantly better asthma control, higher lung functions, and greater effects on airway remodeling. *Source*: From Ref. 117.

rather low, fixed dose of inhaled corticosteroids (104), the other initial high doses followed by gradual step-down, so together these studies are likely to provide more information about optimal dosing in these patients (105).

Inhaled corticosteroids modify more outcomes than any other asthma drug in the majority of patients. These drugs are therefore the most likely candidates for early pharmacologic intervention studies. Therefore, it is not surprising that virtually all studies conducted so far have been using inhaled corticosteroids. However, inhaled corticosteroids do not totally control all outcomes, and combinations of treatments such as inhaled corticosteroids plus leukotriene modifiers, long acting β2-agonists or anti-IgE administrations would also be candidates for early intervention trials (106).

V. Studies Addressing Early Intervention

At present only one study (START) has been designed to study early pharmacologic intervention in newly diagnosed asthma (1). In START around 7000 patients aged 6 to 60 years (3000 between 5 and 15 years), from 31 countries, with mild persistent asthma of less than two years, duration were randomized to once-daily treatment with budesonide, 200 μg (<11 years) or 400 μg (≥11 years), or placebo via Turbuhaler® for three years. The double-blind treatment period was followed by a two-year period of open budesonide treatment for all patients. The primary outcome measures were time to the first severe asthma-related event during the first three years of the study, and the change in postbronchodilator FEV_1 from baseline. This would elucidate whether early intervention with inhaled corticosteroids can modify the evolution towards more severe asthma and the accelerated decline in lung function that several studies suggest occurs in asthma. It would also allow an estimate of the impact of three years, delay of inhaled corticosteroid treatment as compared with early use.

As the efficacy of inhaled steroid treatment had been demonstrated in numerous clinical trials, the START study was designed as an effectiveness study in order to make the conclusions applicable for overall asthma control in clinical practice. Therefore, compliance with treatment during the study was not assessed. Furthermore, throughout the study, other asthma medication could be given as judged appropriate by the individual investigators. This would also allow the need for additional asthma medication as a surrogate outcome for asthma progression. The main findings of the first three years of the study can be summarized as follows:

Early use of budesonide reduced the risk of a severe asthma exacerbation by 44% and significantly prolonged the time to the first severe asthma exacerbation. Life-threatening asthma exacerbations were reduced by 63% (nine in budesonide and 24 in placebo), hospital days by 69%, emergency room visits by 67%, and lost days of work or school by 37%. In addition to study treatment, the placebo group, despite a significantly greater use of non-steroid asthma treatments, received more and earlier additional inhaled glucocorticosteroids and oral steroids than the budesonide group.

Postbronchodilator FEV_1 declined significantly over three years in patients not treated early with inhaled corticosteroids (Fig. 9). There seemed to be some differences between the various age groups, the three-year decline in 6- to 11-year-old children being 2.5% and in adults 3.6%, whereas no significant decline was seen in teenagers. Two hundred µg budesonide per day significantly reduced (but did not prevent) the annual decline in postbronchodilator FEV_1 percent predicted by 22% (2.3% in placebo to 1.8% in budesonide) in 2000 young children and 400 µg/day reduced the decline by 42% (3.6% in placebo to 2.1% in budesonide) in adults ($p < 0.001$) (Fig. 9). No treatment effect was seen in the adolescents whose FEV_1 did not decline during placebo treatment. These data supported that accelerated decline in lung function is seen in patients with newly diagnosed mild disease, and that treatment with inhaled corticosteroids can modify this decline–perhaps in a dose-dependent way. However, more studies are needed to assess the optimal inhaled corticosteroid dose and whether the accelerated decline in lung function occurs in all patients or only in subgroups, and which lung-function parameters should be used to best assess this. Budesonide also modified the selected surrogate outcomes for asthma progression. So in this study early intervention with inhaled budesonide clearly resulted in marked achievement of immediate clinical benefits. It also modified some long-term

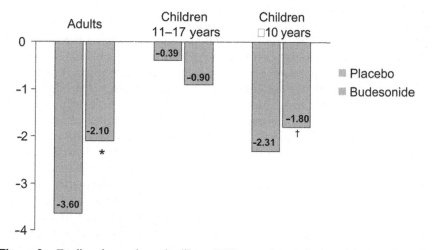

Figure 9 Declines in postbronchodilator FEV_1 over 3 years in recent onset asthma in patients treated with inhaled budesonide or placebo. Significant declines were seen in placebo treated patients in children and adults, whereas no decline was seen in adolescents. Budesonide treatment significantly reduced the decline by 42% in adults, who received 400 µg/day, and by 22% in children who received 200 µg/day. No differences were seen between budesonide and placebo in the adolescent group. *Source*: From Ref. 1.

outcomes (decline in lung function and progression) over the first three years. However, the very long-term consequences of this remain to be shown. Moreover, the question of whether early was better than late intervention was not answered by the first three years of the study.

The results of the START study clearly illustrate why the true long-term benefits of early pharmacologic intervention may never be completely elucidated in a strict, scientific trial. Even if this study was a large, well-designed long-term study lots of unanswered questions remain about the long-term consequences of this early intervention, how the control group would have been doing without any intervention at all, and about the optimal doses of inhaled corticosteroid and treatment duration. Furthermore, a significant decline in postbronchodilator FEV_1 was only seen in a proportion of patients. Therefore, future research must try to define patients at risk for lung function declines and try to establish if these are the same patients who are at risk of progression in other markers of asthma severity. In the START study there was no association between pretreatment lung function, decline in lung function, and progression of other markers of disease severity.

No studies exist on early pharmacologic intervention in preschool children. However, within the next couple of years two studies will provide some information about early intervention with inhaled corticosteroids in children less than three years of age who wheeze. One is a two-year study using low doses of inhaled corticosteroids (107) and the other is a four- to five-years study using initially high and later disease severity-tailored doses of inhaled corticosteroids (105). These two studies seem to be supplementary, but as for START the research questions about very long-term benefits will not be answered by any of these studies unless the early intervention results in remission or cure, which seem most unlikely.

Since our information about early pharmacologic intervention is still limited to one trial, the findings in some randomized, controlled studies on long-term (one year or more) treatment will also be briefly discussed. No such placebo-controlled studies exist with theophylline, sodium chromoglycate, nedocromil sodium, or leukotriene modifiers. Only inhaled corticosteroids have been studied in this way. Furthermore, inhaled corticosteroids have sometimes been compared with other drugs instead of placebo in such trials. In light of the findings in the START study it is unlikely that studies of less than two years, duration will have the power to provide any firm information about decline in FEV_1, unless a substantial number of patients is studied, other lung-function parameters used, or selected groups of patients included in the study.

A. Other Studies Related to Early Pharmacologic Intervention–First-Line Treatment Studies

In this section only studies in children and adolescents will be discussed.

Short-Term Trials

Several studies have found that inhaled corticosteroids have a greater effect upon more asthma outcome parameters than any other anti-asthma drug in patients with asthma regardless of disease severity. Inhaled corticosteroids have been documented in controlled trials in both children and adults to improve day- and nighttime symptoms and lung function; reduce morbidity, mortality, the frequency of acute exacerbations, and the number of hospital admissions; improve bronchial hyperresponsiveness, quality of life and capacity for physical activity; and reduce chronic inflammatory changes in the airways, airway remodeling and restrictions in daily activities (102,108). The percent reduction in hospitalizations, exacerbations, emergency room visits, prednisolone use, nighttime and daytime symptoms, use of rescue-inhaled β2-agonist, and the need for other asthma medication seem to be independent of disease severity. As a consequence of this all international guidelines recommend inhaled corticosteroids as the preferred first-line treatment in all patients with all severities of persistent asthma. So, with respect to achievement of as marked immediate clinical benefits as possible and reducing the frequency and duration of undertreatment the literature strongly supports the use of early intervention with inhaled corticosteroids. Such recommendation is supported by the findings in START in patients with mild asthma (1), but the literature suggests that this will also be true for more severe disease.

Long-Term Studies

The CAMP study is a prospective, randomized, placebo-controlled landmark study, which has provided important information about the management of mainly mild persistent asthma (2,7,109). Since the mean duration of asthma at study entry was around five years CAMP was not an early intervention study. However, it was a well-designed study to assess the most suitable first-line treatment of mild persistent asthma. Around 1000 children with a mean age around 10 at study entry were randomized treatment with budesonide, nedocromil sodium, or placebo for four years. At baseline long duration of asthma was associated with lower lung functions, greater hyperresponsiveness, and more asthma symptoms and rescue β2-agonist use (7). As in other clinical trials budesonide was more effective than both placebo and nedocromil sodium. Budesonide treatment was associated with marked immediate clinical benefits such as reductions in hospitalizations, exacerbations, emergency room visits, prednisolone use, nighttime and daytime symptoms, and use of rescue-inhaled β2-agonist. Moreover, bronchial hyperresponsiveness improved over the whole study period. In contrast, nedocromil sodium only had a significant effect on two out of the many outcomes studied.

Although CAMP was not designed to evaluate reductions in lung function with time or disease progression, post hoc analyses of the data have provided some interesting information about these issues (7,69). With respect to progressive loss of lung function a nonsignificant 0.9% decline in postbronchodilator $FEV_1\%$ predicted over four years was seen for the whole CAMP population and postbronchodilator FEV_1/FVC ratios decreased by 1.7% in the placebo group (2). Due to the lack of a significant decline in postbronchodilator $FEV_1\%$ predicted in the placebo group it was not possible to make firm conclusions on the effects of budesonide on decline in that parameter. As discussed earlier the lack of decline in postbronchodilator $FEV_1\%$ predicted was in agreement with the findings in the 11–18-year-old children in the START study. The only parameter (FEV_1/FVC ratio), which declined to some extent with time in CAMP was also the one that came closest to a treatment effect ($p = 0.08$). Finally, when treatments were stopped after 4.5 years the budesonide-induced improvements in bronchial hyperresponsiveness disappeared within months, suggesting that this marker of progression is only modified as long as the treatment was given. This is in agreement with the findings in other studies. Interestingly, the children in the budesonide group continued to need fewer courses of prednisolone than the other treatment groups even after the treatments had been stopped, suggesting that the four years of treatment had some disease-modifying effects beyond the period of treatment.

Another prospective, randomized, placebo-controlled study on children with mild and moderate asthma compared the effects of two years, treatment with 600 μg budesonide per day with placebo. Budesonide treatment reduced exacerbations, emergency room visits, prednisolone use, nighttime and daytime symptoms, and use of rescue-inhaled β2-agonist, and improved bronchial hyperresponsiveness over the whole study period (97). Thorough body box plethysmography lung-function measurements were made at regular intervals. In addition to FEV_1 a variety of other lung-function parameters were followed, including flows at different percent of TLC. Significant declines in both pre- and postbronchodilator lung functions were seen in the placebo group (41) and the decline seemed more marked in lung-function parameters reflecting the more peripheral airways. Budesonide treatment normalized postbronchodilator lung-function development of central and intermediate airways over two years (41). Small airway caliber was also improved significantly by budesonide treatment, but still remained somewhat reduced. Continuous treatment with inhaled budesonide was associated with a diminished bronchodilator response with time, whereas the bronchodilator response seemed to increase with time in the placebo group. These findings are in agreement with the findings in the START study (1). The question remains whether the increased bronchodilator response with time can be interpreted as a result of remodeling of the airway smooth muscles and that inhaled corticosteroids modified this expression of the remodeling. More studies are needed to elucidate that.

The safety of fluticasone propionate 200 μg/day has been compared with nedocromil sodium in a prospective, randomized study (3). The study was not designed to assess decline in lung functions or efficacy of the treatments. However, compared with nedocromil sodium, fluticasone treatment resulted in statistically significant increases in lung functions, increased number of days with good asthma control, fewer exacerbations, emergency room visits and prednisolone treatments, and less requirement of additional asthma medications, including long-acting β2-agonists. The clinical benefits were maintained over the two-year study period, corroborating the good effects of inhaled corticosteroids reported in other trials on immediate clinical benefits by first-line treatment with inhaled corticosteroids.

Verberne et al. (5) found that one-year treatment with beclomethasone 400 μg/day had significantly better effect than salmeterol 50 μg twice daily on lung function, rate of asthma exacerbations, morning and evening PEF rates, and symptoms in children with asthma. Furthermore, both pre- and postbronchodilator lung functions grew significantly better during treatment with beclomethasone. A significant decrease in lung function over the year ($p = 0.05$) and an increase in bronchial hyperresponsiveness ($p < 0.05$) was seen among the children treated with salmeterol.

A controlled, but open and not randomized, study compared inhaled budesonide in initially high doses (800 μg/day gradually stepped down until minimal effective dose) with treatment combinations of other anti-asthma drugs—β2-agonists, theophylline, and disodium cromoglycate—in 278 children with mainly moderate persistent asthma (some had mild persistent asthma) over a period of three to six years (8). Marked improvements were seen in lung function, peak flow variability, symptoms, and hospitalization rate in the budesonide-treated group. Furthermore, the group treated with budesonide showed significantly increased lung-function growth rates according to age compared with the children not receiving inhaled budesonide, and prebronchodilator FEV_1 in the control group not receiving inhaled steroids showed an annual decline of 1.1%.

The long-term implications of these studies are not known. A study in 181 patients aged 13–44 years, which assessed the chance of improving or even becoming symptom-free over a period of more than 25 years, found that the longer the patients went without treatment after debut of symptoms the less likely they were to show decline in, or normalization of, bronchial hyperresponsiveness (110). The data also indicated that patients who improved or became symptom-free tended to be those who were diagnosed and treated at a younger age or had less severe disease at the time of diagnosis. This corroborates the observation in another study: children who started inhaled corticosteroids early had better lung function at a lower accumulated dose of budesonide after 4.5 years of treatment than children in whom inhaled steroids were not initiated until after more than five years of symptoms (8). Furthermore, the patients in START who had their budesonide treatment delayed for three years required more medication during years 4 to 5 than the patients who received budesonide at study entry (data not published yet). These studies, together with the findings in CAMP that fewer prednisolone courses were needed in the budesonide group after the treatment was stopped, suggest that early treatment or first-line treatment with inhaled corticosteroids may be associated with some long-term beneficial effects. However, the evidence is still weak and further studies are needed.

B. Early Better Than Late

As mentioned earlier, the question about whether early pharmacologic intervention is associated with better short- and long-term effects than later use will probably never be answered in a definite way due to difficulties with appropriate study designs, drop-outs, and selection bias mainly in the group whose treatment is delayed. So suggestions about this are presently based upon sub-optimally designed studies. Since so few studies exist, results from studies in adults also will be briefly mentioned.

In a long-term study in children (8), inhaled budesonide treatment was compared with treatment combinations of other anti-asthma drugs in 278 children over a period of three to six years. Children who started treatment early (within two years) after the debut of symptoms had a more rapid response and obtained significantly greater increases in lung functions than children in whom budesonide was not started until some years after the onset of asthma symptoms (Fig. 10). In addition, the accumulated dose of budesonide taken after 4.5 years of continuous treatment was significantly lower among the children who started budesonide treatment early than in the group of children in whom budesonide treatment was not initiated until after more than five years of continuous symptoms. These findings suggest that in children with mainly moderate asthma early pharmacologic intervention with inhaled corticosteroids may produce better long-term results that delayed treatment.

A study in adults compared two treatment strategies: inhaled corticosteroids as early intervention versus β2-agonist alone (30,31) in patients with asthmatic symptoms of less than a years duration and with no previous history of anti-inflammatory therapy. The two-year treatment with high doses of inhaled budesonide resulted in almost complete clinical recovery and normalization of lung function. Furthermore, inhaled budesonide was clinically superior to β2-agonist treatment. Bronchial biopsies, taken from a subgroup of patients, revealed that the budesonide-treated patients had a significantly greater reduction in the numbers of inflammatory cells than the terbutaline-treated patients (111). The study was continued for a third year to investigate the effects of discontinuation of steroid treatment and

Annual change in percent predicted FEV₁

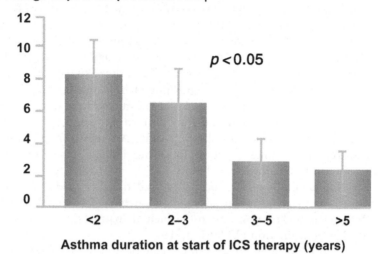

Figure 10 Influence of the duration of asthma on the effect of inhaled budesonide on prebronchodilator FEV_1 in children with mild and moderate persistent asthma. A significantly better effect was seen in children in whom budesonide treatment was initiated early in the course of the disease. *Source*: From Ref. 8.

a delayed introduction of inhaled steroids. Most of the patients who switched from budesonide to placebo showed a gradual and slight decline in lung function, which became significant towards the end of the third year, but 20% did not deteriorate at all (30). Those patients who had received terbutaline for two years before treatment with budesonide was initiated did not reach the same level of lung function or improvement in bronchial hyperresponsiveness as those who were treated with budesonide during the first two years of the disease. This finding suggests that some functional reversibility was lost by delaying the start of inhaled corticosteroid treatment–perhaps due to the failure of a continuous β2-agonist to affect the underlying airway inflammation of asthma.

Overbeek et al. reported similar results in a more heterogeneous group of patients who had already experienced symptoms for several years by study start. The patients, who were on maintenance β2-agonist therapy, were randomized to 2.5 years additional intervention with either inhaled anti-cholinergic, inhaled corticosteroids, or placebo (88). The addition of inhaled corticosteroids, to maintenance treatment with β2-agonists improved symptoms, lung functions, and bronchial responsiveness. The study was continued after the first 2.5 years to investigate the effects of adding 800 μg daily inhaled beclomethasone to the patient groups that had not previously received it. Airway hyperresponsiveness showed no significant change after

60 months in these patients, whereas it had shown significant improvement as early as three months after starting inhaled corticosteroids among the patients who had received beclomethasone during the initial 2.5-year treatment period. Likewise, the increase in lung function was lower when inhaled corticosteroids were started after 2.5 years, delay compared with the early initiation of inhaled corticosteroids. The authors suggested that the use of inhaled steroids should not be postponed in asthmatics with documented airways obstruction. Selroos et al. (112) evaluated the correlation between the response to treatment and the duration of symptoms prior to starting inhaled corticosteroids for the first time. A negative correlation between improvement in lung function following inhaled corticosteroid therapy and duration of asthma was found.

Similar findings have been reported in other studies in children and adults: early introduction of inhaled corticosteroids produced a better effect on lung function and/or bronchial hyperresponsiveness compared with late introduction (30,89,113,110).

Although all of these studies can be criticized for flaws in design, patient selection, or sub-optimal statistics, their abundance and the agreement with the findings in START that patients who had their budesonide treatment delayed required more medication during years four to five than the patients who received budesonide at study entry suggest that early or first-line treatment with inhaled corticosteroids may produce better effects than later treatment. However, this question has not been resolved and more studies are definitely needed.

VI. Summary

- At present only two studies (one in adults only) have been designed to formally assess pharmacologic intervention early in the course of the asthma disease, so the majority of information about these issues comes from other trials with different objectives.
- Airway inflammation is present in early asthma, even in patients with mild disease.
- Airway remodeling seems to take place in all patients with asthma.
- Airway inflammation seems to be linked to airway remodeling to some extent, but to which degree is not known. The two phenomena occur in the same patient but that does not necessarily imply a causal relationship. One study suggests that inflammation may precede remodeling and that progression of inflammation leads to progression of remodeling, but that needs further study.
- The exact clinical consequences of airway inflammation and remodeling are not known. Some studies suggest that control of airway inflammation improves asthma control and reduces airway remodeling.

- Percent predicted FEV_1 shows accelerated decline with time in groups of asthmatics, but marked variations exist and in patients with mild asthma 50–60% of patients show no decline. The decline may be more marked in patients with moderate and severe asthma and in the beginning of the disease.
- Percent predicted FEV_1 may be an insensitive measure of decline in lung function and conclusions about disease progression based solely on this measure should be made with great caution.
- Total gas volume or total lung capacity or other lung-function parameters related to these measures may be more sensitive measures of peripheral airway, inflammation, and changes in lung function over time.
- Early intervention with inhaled corticosteroids reduces the occurrence of undertreatment and improves most immediate term asthma outcomes in the majority of patients to a greater extent than any other anti-asthma treatment.
- Some studies suggest that early use of inhaled corticosteroids may produce a better clinical result than delayed use, but more well-designed studies are needed to confirm this.
- Discontinuation of anti-inflammatory therapy in patients who have had untreated asthma for years prior to the initiation of treatment results in a deterioration in asthma control and bronchial hyperresponsiveness to pretreatment levels in the majority of patients. Discontinuation trials have never been performed in an early intervention trial.

More studies are needed to assess whether early anti-inflammatory treatment may also influence the natural history of the asthma disease, but before this can be done definitions and validation of relevant outcomes must be made.

VII. Discussion

It is obvious that our understanding of how to put early pharmacologic intervention into practice and how to validate this is still at a very early stage. That does not mean that it is not worth implementing early pharmacologic intervention in the daily treatment practice. The well-documented marked immediate clinical effects of early intervention with inhaled corticosteroids in all asthma disease severities is sufficient to recommend that approach in the daily asthma management. In countries where this has been implemented the strategy has been associated with reductions in undertreatment and impairment in daily life and improvements in the quality of life and health care statistics of the asthma population (114,115). In contrast with these well-documented effects of early pharmacologic intervention, the evidence for important long-term benefits is much weaker. This may of course be because there are no substantial long-term benefits, but it may as well be due to the fact that these potential benefits have not been thoroughly studied or because of inappropriate and insensitive outcome selection, study design/duration or drug/dose selection. With respect to the potential long-term benefits we still have a long way to go and unfortunately we walk with very small steps. However, increasing understanding of relevant lung-function parameters and drug dose response relationships on different outcomes together with improved imaging techniques and better perception of asthma progression elicit the hope that one day the question about potential long-term benefits will also be answered with sufficient certainty.

References

1. Pauwels RA, Pedersen S, Busse WW, Tan WC, Chen YZ, Ohlsson SV, Ullman A, Lamm CJ, O'Byrne PM. Early intervention with budesonide in mild persistent asthma: a randomized, double-blind trial. Lancet 2003; 361(9363):1071–1076.
2. Long-term effects of budesonide or nedocromil in children with asthma. The Childhood Asthma Management Program Research Group [see comments]. New Engl J Med 2000; 343:1054–1063.
3. Roux C, Kolta S, Desfougeres JL, Minini P, Bidat E. Long-term safety of fluticasone propionate and nedocromil sodium on bone in children with asthma. Pediatrics 2003; 111(6 Pt 1):e706–e713.
4. Becker JM, Rogers J, Rossini G, Mirchandani H, D'Alonzo GE, Jr. Asthma deaths during sports: report of a 7-year experience. J All Clin Immunol 2004; 113(2):264–267.
5. Verberne AA, Frost C, Roorda RJ, van der Laag H, Kerrebijn K. One year treatment with salmeterol, compared with beclomethasone in children with asthma. Am J Respir Crit Care Med 1997; 156:688–695.
6. Calhoun WJ, Sutton LB, Emmett A, Dorinsky PM. Asthma variability in patients previously treated with β2-agonists alone. J All Clin Immunol 2003; 112(6):1088–1094.
7. Zeiger RS, Dawson C, Weiss S. Relationships between duration of asthma and asthma severity among children in the Childhood Asthma Management Program (CAMP). J All Clin Immunol 1999; 103(3 Pt 1):376–387.
8. Agertoft L, Pedersen S. Effects of long term treatment with an inhaled corticosteroid on growth and pulmonary function in asthmatic children. Respir Med 1994; 88:373–381.
9. Brown PJ, Greville HW, Finucane KE. Asthma and irreversible airflow obstruction. Thorax 1984; 39:131–136.
10. Sears MR, Greene JM, Willan AR, Wiecek EM, Taylor DR, Flannery EM, Cowan JO, Herbison GP, Silva PA, Poulton R. A longitudinal, population-based, cohort study of childhood asthma followed to adulthood. N Engl J Med 2003; 349(15):1414–1422.

11. Oswald H, Phelan PD, Lanigan A, Hibbert M, Bowes G, Olinsky A. Outcome of childhood asthma in mid-adult life. BMJ 1994; 309(6947):95–96.
12. Phelan PD. Asthma in children: epidemiology. BMJ 1994; 308(6944): 1584–1585.
13. Kelly WJ, Hudson I, Phelan PD, Pain MC, Olinsky A. Childhood asthma in adult life: a further study at 28 years of age. Br Med J (Clin Res Ed) 1987; 294(6579):1059–1062.
14. Martinez FD. Links between pediatric and adult asthma. J All Clin Immunol 2001; 107(5 Suppl):S449–S455.
15. Taussig LM, Wright AL, Holberg CJ, Halonen M, Morgan WJ, Martinez FD. Tucson Children's Respiratory Study: 1980 to present. J All Clin Immunol 2003; 111(4):661–675.
16. Ulrik CS, Backer V, Dirksen A, Pedersen M, Koch C. Extrinsic and intrinsic asthma from childhood to adult age: a 10-yr follow-up. Respir Med 1995; 89(8):547–554.
17. Johnstone DE. A study of the natural history of bronchial asthma in children. Am J Dis Child 1968; 115(2):213–216.
18. Ryssing E, Flensborg EW. Prognosis after puberty for 442 asthmatic children examined and treated on specific allergologic principles. Acta Paediatr 1963; 52:97–105.
19. Gerritsen J, Koëter GH, Monchy JGR, Champagne JGL, Knol K. Change in airway responsiveness to inhaled house dust form childhood to adulthood. J All Clin Immunol 1990; 85:1083–1089.
20. Martin AJ, McLennan LA, Landau L, Phelan PD. The natural history of childhood asthma to adult life. BMJ 1980; 280:1397–1400.
21. Kelly WJ, Hudson I, Raven J, Phelan PD, Pain MC, Olinsky A. Childhood asthma and adult lung-function. Am Rev Respir Dis 1988; 138:26–30.
22. Kelly WJ, Hudson I, Phelan PD, Pain MC, Olinsky A. Childhood asthma in adult life: a further study at 28 years of age. BMJ 1987; 294:1059–1062.
23. Buffum WP, Settipane GA. Prognosis of asthma in childhood. Am J Dis Child 1966; 112(3):214–217.
24. Blair H. Natural history of childhood asthma. 20-year follow-up. Arch Dis Child 1977; 52(8):613–619.
25. Rackemann FM, Edwards MC. A follow-up study of 688 patients after an interval of twenty years. N Engl J Med 1952; 246(21):815–823.
26. Kokkonen J, Linna O. The state of childhood asthma in young adulthood. Eur Respir J 1993; 6(5):657–661.
27. Jenkins MA, Hopper JL, Bowes G, Carlin JB, Flander LB, Giles GG. Factors in childhood as predictors of asthma in adult life. BMJ 1994; 309(6947): 90–93.
28. Strachan DP, Butland BK, Anderson HR. Incidence and prognosis of asthma and wheezing illness from early childhood to age 33 in a national British cohort. BMJ 1996; 312(7040):1195–1199.
29. Waalkens HJ, van Essen-Zandvliet E, Hughes MD, Gerritsen J, Duiverman E, Knol K, Kerrebijn K, Quanjer P, Sluiter HJ, Pouw EM, Schoonbrood DF, Roos CM, Jansen HM, Brand PL, Kerstjens HA, De Gooijer A, Postma DS, Van der Mark TW, Gerritsen F. Cessation of Long-term Treatment with inhaled

Corticosteroid (Budesonide) in Children with asthma Results in Deterioration. Am Rev Respir Dis 1993; 148:1252–1257.

30. Haahtela T, Järvinen M, Kava T, Kiviranta K, Koskinen S, Lehtonen K, Nikander K, Persson T, Selroos O, Sovijärvi A, Stenius-Aarniala B, Svahn T, Tammivaara R, Laitinen LA. Effects of reducing or discontinuing inhaled budesonide in patients with mild asthma. New Engl J Med 1994; 331:700–705.

31. Haahtela T, Jarvinen M, Kava T, Kiviranta K, Koskinen S, Lehtonen K, Nikander K, Persson T, Reinikainen K, Selroos O, Sovijärvi A, Stenius-Aarniala B, Svahn T, Tammivaara R, Laitinen LA. Comparison of a β2-agonist, terbutaline, with an inhaled corticosteroid, budesonide, in newly detected asthma. New Engl J Med 1991; 325:388–392.

32. Juniper E, Kline PA, Vanzieleghem MA, Ramsdale H, O'Byrne P, Hargreave F. Effect of long-term treatment with an inhaled corticosteroid (budesonide) on airway hyperresponsiveness and clinical asthma in nonsteroid-dependent asthmatics. Am Rev Respir Dis 1990; 142:832–836.

33. van den Toorn LM, Overbeek SE, Prins JB, Hoogsteden HC, de Jongste JC. Asthma remission: does it exist?. Curr Opin Pulm Med 2003; 9(1):15–20.

34. van den Toorn LM, Overbeek SE, de Jongste JC, Leman K, Hoogsteden HC, Prins JB. Airway inflammation is present during clinical remission of atopic asthma. Am J Respir Crit Care Med 2001; 164(11):2107–2113.

35. van den Toorn LM, Prins JB, Overbeek SE, Hoogsteden HC, de Jongste JC. Adolescents in clinical remission of atopic asthma have elevated exhaled nitric oxide levels and bronchial hyperresponsiveness. Am J Respir Crit Care Med 2000; 162(3 Pt 1):953–957.

36. Gilliam GL, McNicol KN, Willams HE. Chest deformity, residual airways obstruction and hyperinflammation, and growth in children with asthma. Arch Dis Child 1970; 45:789–799.

37. de Jong PA, Nakano Y, Lequin MH, Mayo JR, Woods R, Pare PD, Tiddens HA. Progressive damage on high resolution computed tomography despite stable lung-function in cystic fibrosis. Eur Respir J 2004; 23(1):93–97.

38. Gono H, Fujimoto K, Kawakami S, Kubo K. Evaluation of airway wall thickness and air trapping by HRCT in asymptomatic asthma. Eur Respir J 2003; 22(6):965–971.

39. Hamid Q, Song Y, Kotsimbos TC, Minshall E, Bai TR, Hegele RG, Hogg JC. Inflammation of small airways in asthma. J All Clin Immunol 1997; 100(1):44–51.

40. Sutherland ER, Martin RJ, Bowler RP, Zhang Y, Rex MD, Kraft M. Physiologic correlates of distal lung inflammation in asthma. J All Clin Immunol 2004; 113(6):1046–1050.

41. Merkus PJ, van Pelt W, van Houwelingen JC, van Essen Zandvliet LEM, Duiverman EC, Kerrebijn KF, Quanjer PH. Inhaled corticosteroids and growth of lung-function in asthmatic children. Eur Respir J 2004; 23:861–868.

42. Ulrik CS, Backer V. Nonreversible airflow obstruction in life-long nonsmokers with moderate to severe asthma. Eur Respir J 1999; 14(4):892–896.

43. Ulrik CS, Backer V. Markers of impaired growth of pulmonary function in children and adolescents. Am J Respir Crit Care Med 1999; 160(1):40–44.

44. Ulrik CS. Outcome of asthma: longitudinal changes in lung-function. Eur Respir J 1999; 13(4):904–918.
45. Strachan DP, Griffiths JM, Johnston ID, Anderson HR. Ventilatory function in British adults after asthma or wheezing illness at ages 0–35. Am J Respir Crit Care Med 1996; 154(6 Pt 1):1629–1635.
46. Lange P, Parner J, Vestbo J, Schnohr P, Jensen G. A 15-year follow-up study of ventilatory function in adults with asthma. N Engl J Med 1998; 339:1194–1200.
47. Peat JK, Woolcock A, Cullen K. Rate of decline of lung-function in subjects with asthma. Eur J Respir Dis 1987; 70:171–179.
48. Phelan PD, Robertson CF, Olinsky A. The Melbourne Asthma Study: 1964–1999. J All Clin Immunol 2002; 109(2):189–194.
49. Rasmussen F, Taylor DR, Flannery EM, Cowan JO, Greene JM, Herbison GP, Sears MR. Risk factors for airway remodeling in asthma manifested by a low postbronchodilator FEV1/vital capacity ratio: a longitudinal population study from childhood to adulthood. Am J Respir Crit Care Med 2002; 165(11):1480–1488.
50. Devulapalli CS, Haaland G, Pettersen M, Carlsen KH, Lodrup Carlsen KC. Effect of inhaled steroids on lung-function in young children: a cohort study. Eur Respir J 2004; 23(6):869–875.
51. Cibella F, Cuttitta G, Bellia V, Bucchieri S, D'Anna S, Guerrera D, Bonsignore G. Lung-function decline in bronchial asthma. Chest 2002; 122(6):1944–1948.
52. Wang X, Mensinga TT, Schouten JP, Rijcken B, Weiss ST. Determinants of maximally attained level of pulmonary function. Am J Respir Crit Care Med 2004; 169(8):941–949.
53. Rasmussen F, Taylor DR, Flannery EM, Cowan JO, Greene JM, Herbison GP, Sears MR. Risk factors for airway remodeling in asthma manifested by a low postbronchodilator FEV1/vital capacity ratio: a longitudinal population study from childhood to adulthood. Am J Respir Crit Care Med 2002; 165(11):1480–1488.
54. Roorda RJ, Gerritsen J, van Aalderen WM, Schouten JP, Veltman JC, Weiss ST et al. Follow-up of asthma from childhood to adulthood: influence of potential childhood risk factors on the outcome of pulmonary function and bronchial responsiveness in adulthood. J All Clin Immunol 1994; 93(3):575–584.
55. Apostol GG, Jacobs DR, Jr., Tsai AW, Crow RS, Williams OD, Townsend MC, Beckett WS. Early life factors contribute to the decrease in lung-function between ages 18 and 40: the Coronary Artery Risk Development in Young Adults study. Am J Respir Crit Care Med 2002; 166(2):166–172.
56. Martinez F, Wright AL, Taussig L, Holberg CJ, Halonen M, Morgan WJ. Asthma and wheezing in the first six years of life. New Engl J Med 1995; 332:133–138.
57. Akhter J, Gaspar M, Newcomb RW. Persistent peripheral airway obstruction in children with severe asthma. Ann All 1989; 63:53–58.
58. Martin AJ, Landau L, Phelan PD. Lung-function in young adults who had asthma in childhood. Am Rev Respir Dis 1980; 122:609–617.

59. Blackhall M. Ventilating function in subjects with childhood asthma who have become symptom free. Arch Dis Child 1970; 45:363–366.

60. Friberg S, Bevegard S, Graff-Lonnevig V. Asthma from childhood to adult age. A prospective study of twenty subjects with special reference to the clinical course and pulmonary function. Acta Paediatr Scand 1988; 77:424–431.

61. Kelly WJ, Hudson I, Raven J, Phelan PD, Pain MC, Olinsky A. Childhood asthma and adult lung-function. Am Rev Respir Dis 1988; 138:26–30.

62. Kelly WJ, Hudson I, Phelan PD, Pain MC, Olinsky A. Childhood asthma in adult life: a further study at 28 years of age. BMJ 1987; 294:1059–1062.

63. Gerritsen J, Koeter GH, Postma DS, Schouten JP, Knol K. Prognosis of asthma from childhood to adulthood. Am Rev Respir Dis 1989; 140:1325–1330.

64. Nelson HS, Szefler SJ, Jacobs J, Huss K, Shapiro G, Sternberg AL. The relationships among environmental allergen sensitization, allergen exposure, pulmonary function, and bronchial hyperresponsiveness in the Childhood Asthma Management Program. J All Clin Immunol 1999; 104(4 Pt 1): 775–785.

65. Gerritsen J, Koëter GH, Monchy JGR, Champagne JGL, Knol K. Change in airway responsiveness to inhaled house dust form childhood to adulthood. J All Clin Immunol 1990; 85:1083–1089.

66. Davé NK, Hopp RJ, Biven RE, Degan J, Bewtra AK, Townley RG. Persistence of increased nonspecific bronchial reactivity in allergic children and adolescents. J All Clin Immunol 1990; 86:147–153.

67. Foucard T, Sjöberg O. A prospective 12-year follow-up study of children with wheezy bronchitis. Acta Pædiatr Scand 1984; 73:577–583.

68. Burrows B, Knudson RJ, Lebowitz MD. The relationship of childhood respiratory illness to adult obstructive airway disease. Am Rev Respir Dis 1977; 115:751.

69. Covar RA, Spahn JD, Murphy JR, Szefler SJ. Progression of asthma measured by lung-function in the Childhood Asthma Management Program. Am J Resp Crit Care Med 2004.

70. Merkus PJ, Tiddens HA, de Jongste JC. Annual lung-function changes in young patients with chronic lung disease. Eur Respir J 2002; 19(5):886–891.

71. DeGroodt EG, van Pelt W, Borsboom GJ, Quanjer PH, van Zomeren BC. Growth of lung and thorax dimensions during the pubertal growth spurt. Eur Respir J 1988; 1(2):102–108.

72. DeGroodt EG, Quanjer PH, Wise ME, van Zomeren BC. Changing relationships between stature and lung volumes during puberty. Respir Physiol 1986; 65(2):139–153.

73. Laitinen LA, Laitinen A. Remodeling of asthmatic airways by glucocorticosteroids. J Allergy Clin Immunol 1996; 97(Suppl):153–158.

74. Tiddens H, Silverman M, Bush A. The role of inflammation in airway disease: remodeling. Am J Respir Crit Care Med 2000; 162(2 Pt 2):S7–S10.

75. Haahtela T. Airway remodelling takes place in asthma–what are the clinical implications? Clin Exp Allergy 1997; 27:351–353.

76. Haahtela T. The importance of inflammation in early asthma. Respir Med 1995; 89:461–462.

77. Laitinen LA, Laitinen A, Haahtela T. Airway mucosal inflammation even in patients with newly diagnosed asthma. Am Rev Respir Dis 1993; 147: 697–704.

78. Booth H, Richmond I, Ward C, Gardiner PV, Harkawat R, Walters EH. Effect of high dose inhaled fluticasone propionate on airway inflammation in asthma. Am J Respir Crit Care Med 1995; 152(1):45–52.

79. Chetta A, Marangio E, Olivieri D. Inhaled steroids and airway remodelling in asthma. Acta Biomed Ateneo Parmense 2003; 74(3):121–125.

80. Chetta A, Zanini A, Foresi A, Del Donno M, Castagnaro A, D'Ippolito R, Baraldo S, Testi R, Saetta M, Olivieri D. Vascular component of airway remodeling in asthma is reduced by high dose of fluticasone. Am J Respir Crit Care Med 2003; 167(5):751–757.

81. Olivieri D, Chetta A, Del Donno M, Bertorelli G, Casalini A, Pesci A, Testi R, Foresi A. Effect of short-term treatment with low-dose inhaled fluticasone propionate on airway inflammation and remodeling in mild asthma: a placebo-controlled study. Am J Respir Crit Care Med 1997; 155(6):1864–1871.

82. Chetta A, Foresi A, Del Donno M, Bertorelli G, Pesci A, Olivieri D. Airways remodeling is a distinctive feature of asthma and is related to severity of disease. Chest 1997; 111(4):852–857.

83. Chetta A, Foresi A, Del Donno M, Consigli GF, Bertorelli G, Pesci A, Barbee RA, Olivieri D. Bronchial responsiveness to distilled water and methacholine and its relationship to inflammation and remodeling of the airways in asthma. Am J Respir Crit Care Med 1996; 153(3):910–917.

84. Minshall EM, Leung DY, Martin RJ, Song YL, Cameron L, Ernst P, Hamid Q. Eosinophil-associated TGF-beta1 mRNA expression and airways fibrosis in bronchial asthma. Am J Respir Cell Mol Biol 1997; 17(3):326–333.

85. Laitinen A, Altraja A, Kampe M, Linden M, Virtanen I, Laitinen LA. Tenascin is increased in airway basement membrane of asthmatics and decreased by an inhaled steroid. Am J Respir Crit Care Med 1997; 156(3 Pt 1):951–958.

86. Chapman ID, Foster A, Morley J. The relationship between inflammation and hyperreactivity of the airways in asthma. Clin Exp All 1993; 23:168–171.

87. Reid DW, Johns DP, Feltis B, Ward C, Walters EH. Exhaled nitric oxide continues to reflect airway hyperresponsiveness and disease activity in inhaled corticosteroid-treated adult asthmatic patients. Respirology 2003; 8(4): 479–486.

88. Overbeek SE, Kerstjens HA, Bogaard JM, Mulder P, Postma DS. Is delayed introduction of inhaled corticosteroids harmful in patients with obstructive airways disease (asthma and COPD)? Chest 1996; 1:335–341.

89. Suzuki N, Kobayashi N, Kudu K. Early start of inhaled corticosteroid therapy is important for the improvement of bronchial hyperresponsiveness. J Aer Med 1997; 10(3):277.

90. Ward C, Pais M, Bish R, Reid D, Feltis B, Johns D, Walters EH. Airway inflammation, basement membrane thickening and bronchial hyperresponsiveness in asthma. Thorax 2002; 57(4):309–316.

91. Laprise C, Laviolette M, Boutet M, Boulet LP. Asymptomatic airway hyperresponsiveness: relationships with airway inflammation and remodelling. Eur Respir J 1999; 14(1):63–73.

92. Green RH, Brightling CE, McKenna S, Hargadon B, Parker D, Bradding P, Wardlaw AJ, Pavord ID. Asthma exacerbations and sputum eosinophil counts: a randomised controlled trial. Lancet 2002; 360(9347):1715–1721.

93. Godden DJ, Ross S, Abdalla M, McMurray D, Douglas A, Oldman D, Friend JA, Legge JS, Douglas JG. Outcome of wheeze in childhood. Symptoms and pulmonary function 25 years later. Am J Respir Crit Care Med 1994; 149(1):106–112.

94. Anderson HR, Pottier AC, Strachan DP. Asthma from birth to age 23 incidence and relation to prior and concurrent atopic disease. Thorax 1992; 47:537–542.

95. Silverman M, Taussig L, Martinez F, Wilson N, Burr M, Weiss S, Jeffery P, Martin RJ, Holt P, Larsen G, Stocks J, Marchal F, Tepper R, Busse W, Castleman W, Heymann P, Le Souef P, Price J, Pedersen S, Mellis C, Landau L. Early childhood asthma: what are the questions?. Am J Respir Crit Care Med 1995; 151:S1–S42.

96. Rytila P, Metso T, Heikkinen K, Saarelainen P, Helenius IJ, Haahtela T. Airway inflammation in patients with symptoms suggesting asthma but with normal lung-function. Eur Respir J 2000; 16(5):824–830.

97. van Essen-Zandvliet E, Hughes MD, Waalkens HJ, Duiverman E, Pocock SJ, Kerrebijn K. Effects of 22 months of treatment with inhaled corticosteroids and/or beta-2-agonists on lung-function, airway responsiveness and symptoms in children with asthma. Am Rev Respir Dis 1992; 146:547–554.

98. Sovijarvi AR, Haahtela T, Ekroos HJ, Lindqvist A, Saarinen A, Poussa T, Laitinen LA. Sustained reduction in bronchial hyperresponsiveness with inhaled fluticasone propionate within three days in mild asthma: time course after onset and cessation of treatment. Thorax 2003; 58(6):500–504.

99. Juniper E, Kline PA, Vanzieleghem MA, Hargreave F. Reduction of budesonide after a year of increased use: a randomized controlled trial to evaluate whether improvements in airway responsiveness and clinical asthma are maintained. J All Clin Immunol 1991; 87:483–489.

100. Sont JK, Van Krieken JH, Evertse CE, Hooijer R, Willems LN, Sterk PJ. Relationship between the inflammatory infiltrate in bronchial biopsy specimens and clinical severity of asthma in patients treated with inhaled steroids. Thorax 1996; 51:496–502.

101. Pedersen S. Long-term outcomes in paediatric asthma. Allergy 2002; 57 Suppl 74:58–74.

102. Barnes PJ, Pedersen S, Busse WW. Efficacy and safety of inhaled corticosteroids. New developments. Am J Respir Crit Care Med 1998; 157(3 Pt 2): S1–S53.

103. Sont JK, Willems LN, Evertse CE, Vanderbroucke JP, Sterk PJ. Long-term management of asthma: is it worth to treat bronchial hyperresponsiveness (BHR) beyond clinical symptoms and lung-function. Am J Respir Crit Care Med 1997; 155:A203.

104. Design and implementation of a patient education center for the Childhood Asthma Management Program. Childhood Asthma Management Program Research Group. Ann All Asthma Immunol 1998; 81(6):571–581.

105. Agertoft L, Pedersen S. Inhaled steroid treatment in early wheeze in children younger than three years. Long-term Early Asthma Prevention (LEAP) study. Rationale and design. Control.Clin.Trials. (in press) 2004.
106. Wallin A, Sue-Chu M, Bjermer L, Ward J, Sandstrom T, Lindberg A, Lundback B, Djukanovic R, Holgate S, Wilson S. Effect of inhaled fluticasone with and without salmeterol on airway inflammation in asthma. J All Clin Immunol 2003; 112(1):72–78.
107. Guilbert TW, Morgan WJ, Krawiec M, Lemanske RF, Jr., Sorkness C, Szefler SJ, Larsen G, Spahn JD, Zeiger RS, Heldt G, Strunk RC, Bacharier LB, Bloomberg GR, Chinchilli VM, Boehmer SJ, Mauger EA, Mauger DT, Taussig LM, Mrtinez FD . The Prevention of Early Asthma in Kids study: design, rationale and methods for the Childhood Asthma Research and Education network. Control Clin Trials 2004; 25(3):286–310.
108. Barnes PJ, Pedersen S. Efficacy and safety of inhaled corticosteroids in asthma. Report of a workshop held in Eze, France, October 1992. Am Rev Respir Dis 1993; 148(4 Pt 2):S1–S26.
109. The Childhood Asthma Management Program (CAMP): design, rationale, and methods. Childhood Asthma Management Program Research Group. Control Clin Trials 1999; 20(1):91–120.
110. Panhuysen CI, Vonk JM, Koeter GH, Schouten JP, van Altena R, Bleecker ER, Postma DS. Adult patients may outgrow their asthma: a 25-year follow-up study. Am J Respir Crit Care Med 1997; 155(4):1267–1272.
111. Laitinen LA, Laitinen A, Haahtela T. A comparative study of the effects of an inhaled corticosteroid, budesonide, and of a beta-2-agonist, terbutaline, on airway inflammation in newly diagnosed asthma. J All Clin Immunol 1992; 90:32–42.
112. Selroos O, Pietinalho A, Löfroos AB, Riska H. Effect of early vs. late intervention with inhaled corticosteroids in asthma. Chest 1995; 108:1228–1234.
113. Selroos O, Backman R, Forsen KO, Löfroos AB, Niemistö M, Nyberg P, Nyholm JE, Pietinalho A, Riska H. The effect of inhaled corticosteroids in asthma is related to the duration of pretreatment symptoms. Am J Respir Crit Care Med 1994; 149:A211.
114. Wennergren G, Kristjansson S, Strannegard IL. Decrease in hospitalization for treatment of childhood asthma with increased use of antiinflammatory treatment, despite an increase in the prevalence of asthma. J All Clin Immunol 1996; 97:742–748.
115. Haahtela T, Klaukka T, Koskela K, Erhola M, Laitinen LA. Asthma programme in Finland: a community problem needs community solutions. Thorax 2001; 56(10):806–814.
116. Brand PL, Duiverman EJ, Waalkens HJ, Essen-Zandvliet EE, Kerrebijn KF. Peak flow variation in childhood asthma: correlation with symptoms, airways obstruction, and hyperresponsiveness during long-term treatment with inhaled corticosteroids. Dutch CNSLD Study Group. Thorax 1999; 54(2):103–107.
117. Sont JK, Willems LN, Bel EH, van kriekenj, Vandenbroucke JP, Sterk PJ. Clinical control and histopathologic outcome of asthma when using airway hyperresponsiveness as an additional guide to long-term treatment. Am J Respir Crit Care Med 1999; 159(4 Pt 1):1043–1051.

10

Measuring Pulmonary Function in Young Children

WAYNE MORGAN and THERESA GUILBERT

Arizona Respiratory Center,
University of Arizona
Tucson, Arizona, U.S.A.

GARY L. LARSEN

National Jewish Medical and Research
Center, University of Colorado Health
Sciences Center
Denver, Colorado, U.S.A.

I. Introduction

The assessment of lung function is central to the management of children with recurrent wheezing and asthma (1,2). Forced expiratory flow measurement has played a key role in the characterization of the ontogeny of wheeze in early childhood (3–5) and the long-term response to inhaled corticosteroid therapy (6). At the same time there has been a rapid improvement over the last two decades in our ability to assess lung function in infants and young children (7). These technologies include innovative methods for the assessment of both forced expiratory flow and respiratory resistance. Further, there is also now strong evidence that the majority of young children can accomplish voluntary spirometry before the age of six years (8).

Although clinical outcomes remain core components of clinical trials in young children with asthma, there is a need for the integration of lung function assessment in these studies so that the relationship between symptoms and physiology can be better defined (7). The relationship between the apparent lung dysanapsis that occurs in children who wheeze from infancy through preschool years and biomarkers of atopy and airways inflammation (4,9–11) needs further clarification. We also need to determine whether or not the progression of asthma in early life can be prevented (9).

Age does not need to be a barrier to understanding the impact of asthma on the development of lung function. Although the potential utility of lung function assessments in clinical trials of young children with asthma seems clear, there is little information on the implementation of these techniques in day-to-day asthma management. There is a clear need to begin to integrate the techniques discussed in this chapter into our care of young children with wheeze and asthma and to rigorously assess their contribution to the goal of improving asthma outcomes.

II. Resistance Measurements

The measurement of airway and respiratory system resistance has a long history. Over the last two decades, however, there has been a rapid increase in sophisticated, non-invasive measurement techniques that can be used to assess lung function in young children. Although this development has been worldwide, many European clinical research centers have played a key role in the development of these technologies, particularly in young children. As noted by Goldman (12) in a recent review of the forced oscillation technique, there is a large body of literature in this area and only a limited number of studies can be presented in a single review, and, inevitably, some key contributions unfortunately must be omitted.

The measurement of resistance by the interrupter technique, forced oscillation technique, and plethysmography has the great advantage of requiring limited subject cooperation. Forced oscillation technique also has the added advantage of assessing the reactance of the respiratory system, which at lower frequencies of oscillation may reflect small airway function (13). As compared to spirometry these methods have the disadvantage of somewhat greater intra- and inter-subject variation and, at least theoretically, may be less sensitive to obstruction of the small airways by virtue of including the large resistance of the central airways and compliance of the mouth and upper airway.

They have the theoretical advantage of measuring the respiratory system in the volume range of tidal breathing and thus may be more sensitive to increases in airway resistance by avoiding bronchodilation associated with the deep inspiration required for spirometry (14). These methods have been well described, including published reference values, and have been demonstrated to detect changes in pulmonary function with disease and airway challenge or bronchodilator administration. As such, these methods are beginning to be used in clinical trials of children with asthma.

A. Interrupter Technique

The measurement of airway resistance by the interrupter technique (R_{int}) requires only the willingness of the child to breathe through a mouthpiece-shutter-pneumotachograph system in a regular, relaxed manner. This makes it potentially ideal for the assessment of airway function in children with a limited ability to cooperate. Although this concept has existed for almost 80 years, it has only been applied in the last decade to the assessment of R_{int} in young children (15,16). The physiologic basis of this technique consists of two key concepts. The first is that during tidal breathing the difference between the pressure at the mouth (P_{mo}) and alveolar pressure (P_{alv}) at any instant is the driving pressure for flow through the airways. The second is the assumption that during the rapid, brief interruption of tidal flow by the shutter there is a prompt equilibration of pressure measured at the mouth (P_{int}) with alveolar pressure (P_{alv}). In this case, the difference between P_{mo} prior to the interruption and P_{int} can be related to the flow measured just prior to interruption (V'_{int}) to give the airway resistance ($R_{int} = (P_{int} - P_{mo})/V'_{int}$). The shutter system should close in less than 10 msec and the interruption time should last approximately 100 msec. The timing of closure is commonly programmed to occur at or close to peak inspiratory or expiratory tidal flow to achieve closure at mid-tidal volume.

Digital systems are available that are relatively easy to use, meet these physical standards, and automatically calculate R_{int} (17–19). Figure 1 presents a schematic for the pressure wave measured with the interrupter technique. Following shutter closure there is a rapid rise in pressure with subsequent oscillation. Frey et al. (20) demonstrated that the frequency of these pressure oscillations correlated with thoracic gas volume (TGV) and that the dampening properties were correlated with maximal expiratory flow at 50% of vital capacity (MEF_{50}) in older children and adults. Mathematical models (21) and studies in animals (22) suggest that the early rapid rise in average (non-oscillating) pressure predominantly represents pressure overcoming the resistance of the conducting airways. The later slow rise in pressure is likely due to a combination of delayed pressure equilibration due to ventilation inhomogeneity and the viscoelastic properties of the lung and chest wall. The technical challenges in making this measurement lie in avoiding leaks at the mouthpiece, extreme flexion or extension of the neck, vocal cord closure, irregular breathing, subject movement during shutter closure, or incompletely relaxed breathing (15). A leak at the mouthpiece can be determined by a slow rise in P_{int} follow occlusion or a dampened oscillation phase. Variation due to inconsistent breathing or movement can result in an irregular or kinked pressure wave following the end of oscillation. Theoretical challenges lie in the assumption that P_{int} is reaching equilibration with P_{alv} and that this change in pressure only represents the pressure drop across the conducting airways. As noted above, the rise

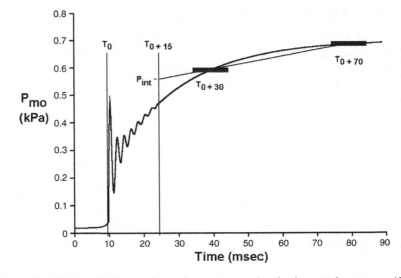

Figure 1 This modeled waveform demonstrates the rise in mouth pressure (P_{mo}) seen following shutter closure in the interrupter technique with a slow rise to plateau as may be seen in obstruction. Pressure has a rapid rise, followed by a period of oscillation, and then a slow asymptotic rise to a near-plateau. The regression line demonstrates the measurement of R_{int} at $T_0 + 15$ msec as described in the text.

in P_{int} does not stabilize instantaneously, but rises asymptotically to reach an apparent plateau. Thus, the algorithm used to estimate P_{int} can have a substantive effect on the calculated R_{int} (15) and use of P_{int} estimated during or near shutter closure can lead to a falsely low R_{int}, particularly in children with airway obstruction (15).

A commonly used algorithm defines the time of shutter closure (T_0) as the point at which 25% of the first rapid change in pressure has occurred. The P_{int} is then determined by back extrapolating linearly through the averages of two 10 msec portions of the pressure wave centered at $T_0 + 30$ msec and $T_0 + 70$ msec to a point at $T_0 + 15$ msec. The pressure at this point on the regression line is then taken as P_{int} (Fig. 1). This method includes both phases of the change in P_{int} and therefore is a lumped assessment of resistance of the conducting airways, ventilation inhomogeneity, and tissue characteristics of the lung and chest wall (16,21,22).

Sly and Lombardi (16) have recently reviewed the theoretical and technical challenges of the interrupter method and have delineated a number of unsettled issues in this technique. They concluded that although the interrupter technique has considerable promise, standard procedures should be developed and then rigorously followed in the conduct of this measurement. In the presence of airway inflammation or bronchospasm, the long time constants of the most obstructed units may preclude their being assessed by this method, thereby underestimating the increase in airway resistance. Similarly, as airway obstruction worsens, the in-series compliance of the extra-thoracic airways and mouth has a greater impact in dampening the early, rapid rise in pressure and can lead to reduced precision in R_{int}. Supporting the cheeks and floor of the mouth can help to reduce this compliance and limit this source of error (23). Measurement of R_{int} can be made in both phases of tidal breathing with expiration demonstrating higher R_{int} than inspiration (23–25), a phenomenon that appears to vary with age (26).

Short-term reproducibility has been assessed in a number of studies with healthy children aged 4 to 16 years demonstrating a 9% intrasubject coefficient of variation (23), and three-year-old children with a history of wheeze a 13% intrasubject coefficient of variation (27).

Variability can theoretically be determined by obtaining several measurements and then taking the median to avoid outliers; however, the mean may suffice as well (24). As expected, older children are more often able to complete the measurement with one study in an ambulatory setting demonstrating success rates of 56%, 81%, and 95% in two to three, three to four, and four to six year old children respectively (28). Long-term repeatability has been assessed in 26 healthy children with a mean of 2.5 months between measurements (29). The mean of the first set of expiratory R_{int} measurements was 1.094 kPa/L sec while the second was 1.060 kPa/L sec with a repeatability of 0.208 kPa/L sec or approximately 20% of expected. This level of repeatability has been confirmed by Chan et al. (18), who demonstrated a repeatability of 20% of expected values both across a short-term administration of a placebo inhaler and over a long-term assessment with three weeks between measurements.

Reference values have been reported for 284 healthy Italian Caucasian children ages 3 to 6.4 years (29). Multivariate regression demonstrated that R_{int} on expiration was inversely related to height and R_{int} on inspiration to a function of age, weight, and height. Gender differences were not apparent. Reference R_{int} values obtained from 54 healthy Dutch Caucasian children ages two to seven years (30) similarly showed an inverse relationship to height and higher expiratory ($R_{int\ exp}$) than inspiratory resistance ($R_{int\ insp}$). In contrast, a multi-center study of 91 healthy French Caucasian children ages 3.5–7.2 years (26) demonstrated that $R_{int\ insp} - R_{int\ exp}$ decreases with age so that three to four year-old children appeared to have higher $R_{int\ insp}$ than $R_{int\ exp}$ and older children the converse. Merkus et al. (31) reported reference values from 208 healthy Dutch Caucasian children ages 3 to 13 and found a curvilinear relationship of R_{int} to height and no gender differences. McKenzie et al. (32) studied 236 healthy children of three ethnic backgrounds (Afro-Caribbean or African, Bangladeshi, and Caucasian British) and found neither ethnic nor gender-related differences and reported predicted values similar to the above referenced data. Thus, multiple studies have demonstrated that height is the major predictor of R_{int} with little variation due to age, gender, weight, or ethnicity once height has been accounted for in the analysis. However, it should be noted that more data are needed in older, post-pubertal children to determine whether the lack of relationship to ethnicity remains valid at older ages when ethnic-related differences in upper to lower segment ratios may be more pronounced following pubertal growth. Figure 2 shows the relatively high degree of comparability of the selected reference values for R_{int} measured during expiration.

Several studies have demonstrated a response to bronchodilator administration in both healthy children (26,33) and children with a history of wheeze or asthma (28,33,34). McKenzie et al. studied children aged from two to five years to assess differences in R_{int} and response to albuterol administration (35). They compared children who had a history of recurrent wheeze and children who had a history of recurrent cough without wheeze with a control group. Median baseline R_{int} was higher in the wheeze group when compared to the cough and control groups (1.16, 0.94, and 0.88 kPa/L sec, respectively) and both the cough and wheeze groups had a greater response to the albuterol than did the controls. Beydon et al. (34) compared baseline $R_{int\ exp}$ and response to bronchodilator in 74 preschool children with a medical diagnosis of asthma to values from 84 healthy control subjects. Again, the asthmatics had a higher mean $R_{int\ exp}$ when

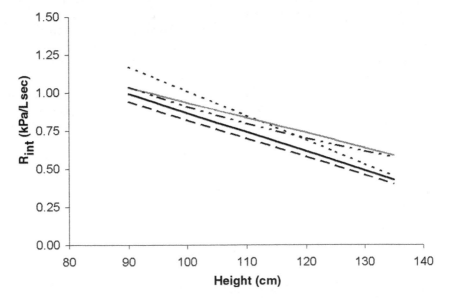

Figure 2 Comparison of predicted values for R_{int} (kPa/L sec) measured in expiration plotted against height (cm) from five different studies of healthy children. Lombardi (29)—solid dark line, Merkus (30)—dotted line, Beydon (26)—dashed line, Merkus (31)—solid grey line, Mckenzie et al. (32)—dash and dotted line.

compared to the controls (0.92 ± 0.22 vs. 0.77 ± 0.20; $p < 0.001$). Response to the administration of albuterol demonstrated substantive overlap between groups. A reduction of $R_{\text{int exp}}$ of 35% or more had a likelihood ratio of three for separating the bronchodilator response for asthmatics from that of the controls with a specificity of 92%.

However, this demanding criterion resulted in a sensitivity of only 24%. It should be noted, though, that this overlap might have more to do with the characteristics of young children's airways than it does with the interrupter technique's limitations per se.

Phagoo et al. (15) used the interrupter technique to demonstrate increases in R_{int} following methacholine in five-year-old children and found that R_{int} was of comparable sensitivity to mechanical properties of resistance (R_{RS}) measured by forced oscillation, but both had less sensitivity than transcutaneous oxygen tension measurement. In a similar study of three-year-olds with a history of wheeze, R_{int} appeared to be even less sensitive to bronchoconstriction than in the older children, but was able to detect bronchodilation following administration of albuterol (27). Frey and Kraemer (36) have demonstrated in older children that analysis of the frequency and dampening characteristics of the rapid oscillation in pressure following shutter closure change systematically with bronchoconstriction and bronchodilation and thus may help to overcome the limitations of R_{int} that can occur in moderate airway obstruction.

B. Forced Oscillation Technique

The assessment of respiratory mechanics (RS) by the forced oscillation technique (FOT) is based upon the concept that the respiratory system has the mechanical properties of resistance (R_{RS}), capacitance or compliance (C_{RS}), and inertance (I_{RS}) (12,37,38). If an oscillating or varying pressure is applied to the airway at the mouth or to the chest wall with the use of a loudspeaker or piston then the flow generated can be related to the forcing pressure to estimate each of these characteristics and their vector sum, the impedance of the respiratory system (Z_{RS}; Fig. 3). The pressure required to overcome R_{RS} is in phase with flow (V') as would be expected because without flow there can be no pressure due to resistance. If R_{RS} were the only mechanical process being acted on, then the pressure signal would be in phase with the flow and Z_{RS} would equal R_{RS}; however, at most frequencies of oscillation, this is not the case. Since the inertance of the system must be overcome and gas accelerated prior to the generation of flow, the pressure acting on the I_{RS} will occur one-quarter of an oscillatory cycle (90°) before flow. In direct contrast, a change in lung volume must be preceded by flow into the system and so the pressure acting on the C_{RS} will occur one-quarter of an oscillatory cycle (90°) after flow and one-half of a cycle (180°) after pressure due to C_{RS}. The vector sum of I_{RS} and C_{RS} is the out of phase component of Z_{RS} and is called the reactance of the respiratory system (X_{RS}). C_{RS} predominates at low frequencies, and the pressure wave due to X_{RS} lags behind flow and has a negative value, whereas at high frequencies I_{RS} predominates and the pressure wave leads flow and has a positive value. The vector sum of the X_{RS} and R_{RS} is then the total impedance, Z_{RS}, of the respiratory system. At the resonant frequency of the system (f_{res}), I_{RS} is equal to C_{RS} and thus their vector sum (X_{RS}) is zero; i.e., they effectively cancel each other out. At this frequency, flow and pressure are completely in phase and Z_{RS} is equal to R_{RS}.

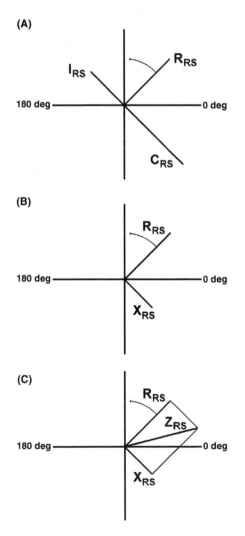

Figure 3 (*Caption on facing page*)

Early measurements attempted in order to adjust a single frequency, forcing function to achieve f_{res} (37), or to graphically or electronically (39) measure the in-phase component of pressure then divide this by flow to calculate R_{RS}. With the development of digital signal processing, however, the use of the Fast Fourier Transform (FFT) has allowed the use of more complex forcing functions containing a broad range of oscillatory frequencies and the assessment of more complex models of the RS that have included different numbers and positions of inertances, resistances, and capacitances. A detailed discussion of these different forcing methods and models, however, is beyond the scope of this article. The main impact of the use of multi-frequency forcing and FFT analysis has been to allow a more sophisticated characterization of the system at multiple frequencies particularly regarding X_{RS}, f_{res}, and the frequency dependence of R_{RS}. Although in a simple system with a limited number of I_{RS}, R_{RS}, and C_{RS} components, the R_{RS} should be constant. The mechanical complexity of the lung, including substantive variation in regional time constants (ventilatory inhomogeneities), leads to an apparent decrease in R_{RS} with increasing frequencies, which is exaggerated in subjects with airway disease. R_{RS} and X_{RS} are commonly reported for frequencies in the range of 4 to 32 cycles per second (Hz), although studies of higher frequencies may also give relevant information (40).

Limitations in the method lie in two main areas. First, even seven element models of the respiratory system are likely too simple to perfectly account for complex regional ventilation inhomogeneities and the viscoelastic properties of the lung and chest wall. However, phenomena that are

---

Figure 3 (*Facing page*) (A) A polar plot schematic of the pressures generated to overcome the three components of respiratory system impedance and cause flow. *Abbreviations*: I_{RS}, inertance; R_{RS}, resistance; C_{RS}, capacitance. One complete cycle at the frequency being measured would represent 360° of rotation on this diagram in the direction of the arrow. The flow wave (not shown) would be in phase with the pressure due to R_{RS} at 45° in this diagram. Note that the pressure due to I_{RS} leads R_{RS} by 90° and the pressure due to C_{RS} lags R_{RS} by the same amount so that they are 180° out of phase with each other. The length of each vector represents the magnitude of each pressure component. (B) The vector sum of I_{RS} and C_{RS} has been calculated to obtain the pressure due to reactance (X_{RS}). Note that the frequency for this polar plot must be below resonant frequency since C_{RS} has predominated and X_{RS} lags behind R_{RS}, i.e., is negative. At resonant frequency C_{RS} would equal I_{RS} and X_{RS} would be zero, while above resonant frequency I_{RS} would predominate and X_{RS} would be leading R_{RS}; i.e., would be positive. (C) In this polar plot, the pressure measured due to respiratory system impedance (Z_{RS}) has been calculated as the vector sum of R_{RS} and X_{RS} and is greater than both, but less than the simple sum of their magnitudes. In the measurement of respiratory system mechanics, the analytical techniques used separate Z_{RS} into R_{RS} and X_{RS} based upon the magnitude of Z_{RS} and the phase relationships between pressure and flow.

counter-intuitive such as a frequency dependence of resistance may represent a useful signal to assess increased regional variation in the lung. The method of linkage of the forcing function to the respiratory system is the second area of concern. The easiest method is to measure input impedance by varying pressure at the mouth. However, when there is increased or increasing Z_{RS}, the capacitance of the mouth and upper airways represents a shunt for pressure, allowing an energy loss that can result in an apparent reduction in Z_{RS} in the face of worsening airway resistance (38). This can be partly limited by supporting the cheeks of the subject, however, another effective if more cumbersome approach is to apply the same pressure, variations around the head as are applied to the airway using a head box or generator (41–43). Transfer impedance measurements avoid the problem of shunt capacitance by generating the forcing pressure at the chest wall (44,45). In this method, the upper airway is not pressurized and thus shunt capacitance is limited, however, the equipment involved is relatively large and somewhat unwieldy resembling a head-out plethysmograph and is not readily available commercially. The European Respiratory Society (14) has recently published a particularly useful statement regarding forced oscillation techniques in children and adults. The authors concluded that forced oscillation is sensitive to environmentally induced impairments in lung function and is reliable in assessing bronchial hyperresponsiveness in adults and children. They further suggested that the limited cooperation required makes it ideal for epidemiologic and field studies.

Similar to the interrupter technique, FOT requires limited subject cooperation and simply requires the subject to breathe quietly through a mouthpiece connected to the measurement system, to tolerate the forcing function, and to avoid blocking the mouthpiece with the tongue while supporting the cheeks. This has made it an attractive option for measuring lung mechanics in young children. Some early studies, however, were less than optimistic regarding the utility of this technique in young children (46–48). Cuijpers et al. (48) studied 1792 children ages 6 to 12 with FOT and a respiratory health questionnaire and found significantly higher R_{RS} at 8 Hz ($R_{RS}8$), more negative $X_{RS}8$, and a greater frequency dependence of R_{RS} in girls with asthma-like symptoms as compared to symptom-free girls. Boys, however, did not demonstrate any differences and receiver operator curve (ROC) analysis of the above measures, as well as more sophisticated analyses, demonstrated a relatively poor diagnostic ability for FOT. The authors concluded that this could potentially represent the lack of measurable functional differences between symptomatic and symptom-free children at this age.

The forced oscillation technique has been applied with multiple different systems and forcing functions and published reference values have been developed for some of these methods. Cuijpers et al. (49) studied 371 healthy Dutch children, aged 5 to 12 years, and demonstrated that negative frequency dependence of R_{RS} was a common finding but became less marked with growth. As expected with increasing height, R_{RS} decreased and X_{RS} increased (became less negative). Some gender differences were found with younger girls demonstrating higher $R_{RS}8$ and more negative $X_{RS}8$ with the converse being the case in older children. Hordvik et al. (50) used a commercial system to study 138 healthy children aged from 2 to 16 years and reported similar reference equations although they modeled these as a quadratic function of height. They estimated that the expected intrasubject coefficient of variation of repeated within-test measurements would be about 10%. However, Z_{RS} parameters from 13 children who had asthma with an FEV_1 less than 80% of predicted fell within the normal range in all but two participants. Within-test and between-test variation were assessed by Malmberg et al. (51) in 131 healthy Finnish schoolchildren ages two to seven years and achieved a success rate of 89% with a within-test coefficient of variation of only 6.2% for $R_{RS}5$ and 5.6% for $Z_{RS}5$ and no significant response in post-albuterol testing. A study of 377 healthy Belgian children between three and 18 years of age by Lebecque et al. (52) demonstrated that children less than six years of age had no trouble with using the forced oscillation technique, but could not demonstrate any relationship to environmental risk factors such as tobacco smoke exposure in either the Z_{RS} parameters or in spirometry.

Klug and Bisgaard (53) used the interrupter technique (R_{int}), forced oscillation (Z_{RS}, X_{RS}, and R_{RS}), and specific airway resistance by plethysmography (sRaw) to study 151 young children aged two to seven years. They obtained data in 121 of these participants (mean age 5.3 ± 1.5 years) and failed in 30 (mean age 3.0 ± 0.9 years). Similar to other studies in this age range, the within-subject coefficients of variation for sRaw, R_{int}, $Z_{RS}5$ and $R_{RS}5$ were 11.1%, 8.1%, 10.8%, and 10.2%, respectively. Significant linear, negative correlations were found between age, height, and weight with R_{int}, $Z_{RS}5$, and $R_{RS}5$ while $X_{RS}5$ was positively correlated to age and body size. As expected, sRaw was not correlated with age or body size and none of the indices varied with gender. Ducharme et al. (54) studied 206 healthy Canadian children of varied ethnicities aged 3 to 17 years. The reference equations from this large study are comparable to those reported above and, similar to R_{int}, height was the best predictor of the Z_{RS} parameters with neither gender nor weight playing a significant role. The head generator technique was used by Mazurek et al. (42) to study 127 healthy children aged 2.8–7.4 years. Again height was the only significant predictor for all Z_{RS} parameters and results were remarkably similar to those reported by Ducharme (54) (Fig. 4). Hellinckx et al. (55) used impulse oscillometry to study baseline lung function and bronchodilator response to albuterol in 281 preschool children aged 2.7–6.6 years old. The participants included 247 healthy children and 34 children with questionnaire-defined asthma. There were no differences seen in FOT parameters between healthy and stable

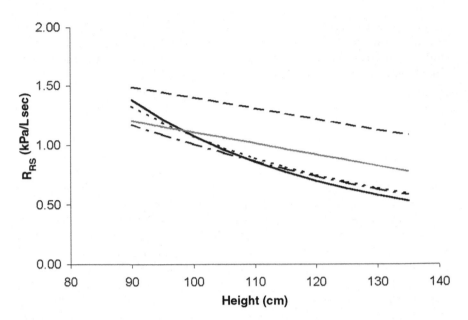

Figure 4 Comparison of predicted values for R_{RS} measured by FOT at low frequencies (5–8 Hz) plotted against height. Ducharme (54)—solid dark line, Mazurek (42)—dotted line, Klug (53)—dashed line, Hellinckx (55)—solid gray line, Hordvik (50)—dash and dotted line.

asthmatic children suggesting that either the physiologic dysfunction was limited or that the method was unable to detect relevant reductions in lung function in the asthmatic group. The former may be the case since grouping children who have been wheezing since early life with those who had a later onset of asthma would tend to reduce any detectable differences (4). Figure 4 presents mean predicted values of R_{RS} measured at low frequencies (5–8 Hz) against height from selected studies demonstrating a remarkable similarity across most.

Within-test and short-term variations in Z_{RS} parameters and spirometry were assessed by Timonen et al. (56) in children ages 7 to 12 years old with symptoms of chronic cough, wheeze, or the physician diagnosis of asthma. Spirometric variables demonstrated low intrasubject coefficients of variation (COV) with FEV_1 demonstrating a 3.2%, 3.0%, and 4.7% within-test, day-to-day, or week-to-week COV, respectively. Intrasubject COV were roughly three times greater for R_{RS} with 9.1%, 16.0%, and 13.2% within-test, day-to-day, or week-to-week COV, respectively, even when within-test reproducibility was required to be within a 0.11 kPa/L sec reliability index. This variation, however, was similar to that seen with isovolume flows and forced expiratory flow $(FEF)_{25-75}$. The authors also conducted exercise challenge testing in 12 of the children and despite the greater variability in FOT parameters, R_{RS} demonstrated the greatest relative change, increasing 1.8 times in the within-test COV as compared to FEV_1, which only decreased 0.9 COV. They concluded that although R_{RS} was the most sensitive parameter in the exercise challenge test, its high degree of variation might limit its utility in longer-term studies.

One potential advantage of FOT over the interrupter technique and plethysmography is that it partitions respiratory system mechanics into resistance and reactance. At any given frequency, the more negative the X_{RS}, the more energy is being used to overcome the apparent elastance of the respiratory system. Decreases in X_{RS} may thus give important information about reductions in small airway conductance and increased lung elastance. This is analogous to assessing reductions in dynamic compliance, but without the necessity of invasive methods to estimate pleural pressure. Bouaziz et al. (57) studied the Z_{RS} response to methacholine in 38 children with asthma aged 6 to 14.5 years using the head-generator FOT and spirometry. Comparing the 23 participants who decreased FEV_1 by at least 20% to the 15 who did not, there were significantly greater increases in R_{RS} and decreases in X_{RS} in those who responded to methacholine. The authors proposed that the optimal diagnostic values for response to methacholine were an increase in R_{RS} of 70% (sensitivity 87%, specificity 67%) and a decrease in X_{RS} of –0.1 kPa/L sec (sensitivity 70%, specificity 80%). They concluded that X_{RS} adds to the specificity of the assessment of airway reactivity and propose that an increase in R_{RS} in the absence of a decrease in X_{RS} may represent an upper airway phenomenon with or without lower airway obstruction. A recent study of twenty-four 10–17-year-old children with asthma used impulse oscillometry and spirometry on three consecutive days to assess within-subject variation by Goldman et al. (13). In addition to reporting $R_{RS}5$, $X_{RS}5$, and f_{res}, Goldman's group described a new parameter, the low frequency reactance area, AX. This is the integral of X_{RS} from $X_{RS}5$ to the resonant frequency where, by definition, X_{RS} is zero. The benefit of AX may be an improved signal-to-noise ratio by virtue of combining multiple X_{RS} values and the value of f_{res} into a single parameter. In this study, impedance parameters were all well correlated with FEV_1 and FEF_{25-75} with r^2 values in the range of 0.35–0.53. Impedance parameters demonstrated within-test COV similar to those found by Timonen et al. (56) and did not appear to be altered by cheek support below 15 Hz. The frequency dependence of resistance ($R_{RS}5 - R_{RS}15$), $R_{RS}5$, and AX all showed significant within-subject day-to-day variability by analysis of variance (ANOVA) when spirometry did not. The authors concluded that the FOT parameters were more sensitive to day-to-day variation in bronchomotor tone than was spirometry. In the absence of longer-term clinical outcome data or other confirmatory physiologic studies, it remains to be seen, however, what proportion of this variability (13,56) is signal and what proportion is noise.

The lack of cooperation needed in FOT also makes it potentially useful in the emergency department management of acutely ill asthmatics of all ages since it does not require the effort of peak flow measurement nor does it risk bronchospasm as can occur with spirometry in this setting. Ducharme and Davis (58) studied 150 children aged 3 to 17 years being treated for acute asthma in a tertiary-care emergency department. Of the 114 children able to complete lung function testing, all were able to reproduce $R_{RS}8$ and 75% "could achieve" $R_{RS}16$, but only 57% were able to perform spirometry. The change in percent of predicted $R_{RS}8$ following bronchodilator therapy was as responsive as either the change in FEV_1 or the four clinical signs most responsive to change (respiratory rate, wheezing, air entry, and suprasternal retraction) in those who could complete spirometry. In the children unable to do spirometry, FOT was comparable to the clinical signs. The authors concluded that R_{RS} measured by FOT was a reproducible and responsive measure of lung function in children with acute asthma either too young or too sick to perform spirometry.

The forced oscillation technique has the potential to assess airway reactivity in young children at risk for asthma. A recent study (59) of children ages four to five years enrolled in the Childhood Asthma Prevention Study (CAPS) demonstrated little difference in baseline FOT parameters or in bronchodilator response between children with and without asthma; however, when atopic children were analyzed, those with asthma demonstrated a significantly greater improvement in $R_{RS}5$, $R_{RS}10$, and $X_{RS}10$ than those without. There were no differences seen in spirometric studies conducted at the same time. Based upon epidemiologic studies of childhood respiratory illness (4,60), the authors argued that the FOT bronchodilator studies effectively elucidated lung dysfunction in those children who were at greater risk for persistent asthma due to the combination of atopy with recurrent wheeze. They also suggested that a decrease of 15–20% in $R_{RS}5$ following albuterol administration represented a significant response. It may well be the case, however, that indirect measures of airway inflammation such as exhaled nitric oxide (FE_{NO}) could offer improved characterization of those children with early-onset asthma. Malmberg et al. (10) recently demonstrated with a receiver operator curve analysis that FE_{NO} provided the greatest power in discriminating between children with probable asthma and healthy controls when compared to baseline and post-bronchodilator FOT parameters. However, they did not present data for bronchodilator response analyzed only in the atopic population, somewhat limiting any comparison with the CAPS (59) report.

C. Whole Body Plethysmography

The measurement of airway resistance by use of the whole body plethysmograph is a standard technique in older children and adults that was originally described almost 50 years ago (61), and the basic concepts of this commonly used method will not be repeated in depth. Several studies have used plethysmography to assess airway resistance in young children and in many cases, plethysmography was compared to other methodologies and these studies will be discussed later in a section on comparison studies.

The measurement of specific airway resistance (sRaw) by plethysmography has been successfully accomplished in young children in the three to six years age group (62). The demands of this technique include the child being willing to sit inside the closed plethysmograph for several minutes, to wear a nose-clip, and to breathe quietly through a mouthpiece pneumotachograph system with a good lip seal and without occluding the mouthpiece. Although the measurement of absolute airway resistance (R_{aw}) requires the subject to breathe against a closed system to allow the measurement of TGV (1), specific airway resistance (sRaw = TGV × Raw) can be assessed during quiet breathing without the need for cooperation with this discomfiting maneuver (62,63). During quiet breathing, flow (V') is plotted against box volume (V_{box}) to give several flow/volume loops and the following equation uses the inverse slope of the flow/volume lot to calculate sRaw: sRaw = $\Delta V_{box}/\Delta V' \times (P_{amb} - PH_2O)$, where P_{amb} is equal to ambient pressure and PH_2O to water vapor pressure at body temperature.

This method also requires an estimate of the volume of the subject to adjust for the actual gas volume of the box and of the expected TGV (64) to adjust for the resistance of the pneumotachograph to correct the sRaw values (62,63). A parent or other adult caregiver can sit inside the plethysmograph with the subject to reassure the child and improve the likelihood of success (62) without significantly changing the results obtained. The adult need simply slowly exhale following a deep inspiration during the measurement of sRaw to avoid generating artifact in the measurement. Klug and Bisgaard (62) used this technique to study 131 children with asthma aged two to eight years of whom 57 accomplished measurements with and without an adult in the plethysmograph. Data were obtained in 83% of children with sRaw values (mean ± SD) of 1.45 ± 0.36 kPa sec and 1.44 ± 0.38 kPa sec with and without adult accompaniment, respectively. The within-subject coefficients of variation with an accompanying adult were comparable to other resistance methodologies with a mean of 8%. The authors also studied eleven older children to assess the efficacy of electronic compensation for body temperature and pressure saturated (BTPS) compensation as compared to using air heated and humidified to BTPS conditions and found that the electronic method overestimated sRaw by 43%. Badier et al. (65) used the sRaw methodology to conduct carbachol challenge in children ages three to six years. They studied 44 children with clinical asthma, 44 children with chronic cough, 38 asymptomatic children with wheezy bronchitis in the first two years of life, and 40 healthy controls. Similar to other studies of resistance measures in this age range, there was no difference between the groups in baseline sRaw and they were within the normal range published by Zapletal et al. (64). However, the asthma, cough, and wheezy bronchitis groups all demonstrated significantly greater reactivity to carbachol than did the controls. The clinical asthma group also demonstrated greater reactivity than the cough or wheezy bronchitis groups while the cough and wheezy bronchitis groups were similar to each other. This finding is suggestive of the phenotypes of early wheeze and cough demonstrated by epidemiologic and hospital-based studies (5,66) where children with asthma appear to be a group that is phenotypically and immunologically distinct from children with early transient wheeze or non-atopic cough and wheeze.

Bisgaard and Nielsen (67) used sRaw to demonstrate that montelukast effectively protected against bronchoconstriction induced by cold (–15°C), dry air challenge (CaCh) in 13 asthmatic children three to five years of age. Baseline sRaw values were significantly higher than the predicted reference values. Following a single step, isocapneic CaCh lasting four minutes, sRaw increased 17% after treatment with montelukast and 45% after placebo. Interestingly, this effect was independent of concurrent treatment with inhaled corticosteroids. In a similar study, Nielsen and Bisgaard (68) characterized the effect of formoterol and albuterol in both bronchodilation and protection against CaCh. Using sRaw they were able to demonstrate significant bronchodilation and bronchoprotection with both medications as compared to placebo. Moreover, they were able to demonstrate that bronchoprotection from formoterol lasted at least eight hours compared to placebo and was greater from four hours onward as compared to albuterol. Thus, sRaw has been able to effectively demonstrate both improvements in airway resistance following administration of a bronchodilator and protection against CaCh conferred by both a leukotriene receptor antagonist and a long-acting bronchodilator. Clearly, the use of this physiologic technique has opened the way for the more sophisticated physiologic assessment of asthma therapies in this insufficiently studied age group.

III. Comparison of Techniques in Young Children

There have been several studies published in the last decade that have compared different measurement techniques in young children. In general, they have used comparisons of healthy controls with children who had asthma or other wheezing illnesses and have commonly used airway challenge methodologies to perturb the respiratory system in order to allow the methods to be compared both at baseline and following alterations in airway tone. Rather than present these under a single methodology section, the results from these comparison studies will be reviewed together.

The inverse of R_{int}, interrupter conductance (G_{int}) was shown by Carter et al. (25) to correlate with baseline FEV_1 with a relatively high

r^2 of 0.59 in a study of 107 children aged 3 to 12 years of whom 21 were healthy, 74 had asthma, and 12 had cystic fibrosis. Seventeen of the children with asthma also had plethysmographic R_{aw} measured along with R_{int} before and after treatment for airway obstruction. Baseline R_{int} was almost double R_{aw} and the two were highly correlated ($r^2 = 0.83$) and demonstrated comparable changes following treatment for airway obstruction.

Methacholine responsiveness has commonly been used to compare different techniques. Wilson et al. (47) conducted an abbreviated methacholine challenge in 30 children aged five years with a history of wheeze and six healthy controls. Auscultation for wheeze, change in transcutaneous oxygen ($P_{tc}O_2$) and FOT (69) ($R_{RS}6$ and $R_{RS}8$) were used to assess changes in lung function during the challenge. They found that both auscultation and FOT were unsatisfactory in detecting changes in lung function at a priori thresholds with a 15% decrease in $P_{tc}O_2$ occurring in 29 of 30 asthmatics and with a 35% increase in $R_{RS}6$ occurring in only 18. They concluded that the $P_{tc}O_2$ method was the most technically reliable for measuring response to bronchoconstriction. A similar study by Beydon et al. (70) used $P_{tc}O_2$ and R_{int} to assess response to methacholine in young children. They found that only 79% of the children who decreased their $P_{tc}O_2$ by at least 20% also increased their R_{int} by at least two intrasubject standard deviations.

In other words, conducting methacholine challenge with R_{int} as the only outcome would have missed significant drops in $P_{tc}O_2$. The authors concluded that although methacholine challenge appears safe with $P_{tc}O_2$ as the outcome measure, their results suggested that this was not the case for R_{int} used alone. In contrast to these two studies, Bisgaard and Klug (71) found that the FOT method was more sensitive than sRaw, $P_{tc}O_2$, FEV_1, and R_{int} in detecting bronchoconstriction due to methacholine in 21 children with asthma aged four to six years. They compared relative responses in these different methods using a standard deviation index (SDI) that was equal to the change in lung function post-diluent administration divided by the within-subject baseline standard deviation for that measure. Reactance at 5 Hz ($X_{RS}5$) demonstrated both the greatest change when analyzed by slope (SDI/methacholine concentration step) and greatest sensitivity when assessed by the provocative concentration required to cause a three SDI change in lung function. The order of sensitivity in this study was $X_{RS}5 > sRaw > P_{tc}O_2 > FEV_1 > R_{RS}5 > R_{int}$. All methods detected improvement from methacholine-induced bronchoconstriction following albuterol administration, however, only FOT, sRaw, and R_{int} demonstrated reductions to levels below baseline values. Spirometry (FEV_1) and $P_{tc}O_2$ did not detect these apparently sub-clinical baseline levels of airway tone that must have been present prior to the challenge. These same authors (72) performed a similar study without spirometry in 20 children with stable asthma only two to four years of age. In this case, the sensitivity ranking for the detection of methacholine induced bronchoconstriction using the SDI was sRaw > $X_{RS}5$ > $P_{tc}O_2$ > R_{int}. Although the sensitivity of sRaw and $X_{RS}5$ were not different from each other, both were significantly more sensitive than either R_{int} or $R_{RS}5$. The authors concluded that all the evaluated techniques reliably reflected short-term changes in lung function in these young children.

Klug and Bisgaard (73) also assessed the repeatability of methacholine challenges carried out on two separate days in 16 asthmatic children with a mean age of 3.75 years. Using a purpose-built, quantitative aerosol delivery system they conducted methacholine challenges in which the minimum acceptable response was an increase of sRaw of at least 40% or a fall in $P_{tc}O_2$ of at least 2.5 kPa (18.75 Torr). They then calculated the provocative dose of methacholine necessary for a pre-determined percent change in each measured parameter ($PD_\%$): sRaw PD_{50}, R_{int} PD_{30}, $R_{RS}5$ PD_{30}, $X_{RS}5$ PD_{80}, and $P_{tc}O_2$ PD_{10}. The repeatabilities of $P_{tc}O_2$ PD_{10}, sRaw PD_{50}, and $X_{RS}5$ PD_{80} were relatively high at 0.5, 0.7, and 0.8 doubling doses, respectively, across the two separate days of measurement. In contrast, R_{int} PD_{30} and $R_{RS}5$ PD_{30} were less reproducible at 1.2 and 1.6 doubling doses. They concluded that methacholine challenges could be successfully conducted in children aged two to four years using sRaw, $X_{RS}5$, and $P_{tc}O_2$ as outcomes, but suggested that R_{int} and $R_{RS}5$ may be less suitable in young children. The utility of response measures, however, may vary with the challenge method employed. Nielsen and Bisgaard (74) assessed response to cold, dry air challenge in 38 asthmatics as compared to 29 control subjects two to five years of age. Participants completed a four-minute, isocapneic hyperpnea challenge with minute ventilation aimed at 1 L/min/kg body weight while breathing air at −15°C containing 5% CO_2. Following cold air challenge, the group of asthmatics demonstrated significant changes expressed as SDI of 9.0, 2.5, 1.8, and 1.4 in sRaw, R_{int}, $X_{RS}5$, and $R_{RS}5$, respectively, with considerable overlap between asthmatic and healthy control subjects in R_{int}, $X_{RS}5$, and $R_{RS}5$. Whole body plethysmography (sRaw) was superior in separating the asthmatic group from the controls with 68% of asthmatics demonstrating a more than three SDI change as compared to only 7% of controls. In contrast, R_{int}, $X_{RS}5$, and $R_{RS}5$ demonstrated this degree of change in only 32%, 24%, and 18% of asthmatics respectively. Thus, sRaw performed well in both methacholine and cold air challenge with $X_{RS}5$ comparable or superior to sRaw only in methacholine testing.

Vink et al. (75) compared FOT with spirometry and peak flow in 19 children with asthma before, during, and after methacholine challenge. Baseline FOT parameters at 5 and 10 Hz correlated with FEV_1 and, during the challenge, increases in R_{RS} appeared to precede decreases in spirometry and peak flow. Receiver operator curve (ROC) analyses demonstrated that, depending upon the magnitude of change to be detected, $R_{RS}5$ was roughly comparable to peak flow in predicting decreases in FEV_1. The relationship between the decline in FEV_1 and increase in $R_{RS}5$ and $R_{RS}10$ was curvilinear with an apparent breakpoint so that after a 12% decline in FEV_1

there was a slower increase in R_{RS}. The authors also noted that FOT parameters from frequencies above 10 Hz did not appear to be as informative as those from 5 to 10 Hz. They concluded that although the FOT parameters do not directly reflect the "gold standard," FEV_1, they might be helpful in characterizing lung function in children unable to perform spirometry due to age or disability.

Bronchodilator response was studied in 25 asthmatic children aged 5 to 15 years by Bridge et al. (76) using spirometry, peak expiratory flow (PEF), R_{int}, and FOT. At baseline, $1/R_{int}$ (G_{int}) was correlated with FEV_1 ($r^2 = 0.70$), PEF ($r^2 = 0.60$), and $R_{RS}6$ ($r^2 = 0.89$). Although the median intrasubject within-test variability was greatest for R_{int} at 11%, the sensitivity to detect change after albuterol administration expressed as SDI was similar between methods. A significant response (SDI > 2) was seen for R_{int} in 88% of subjects and for $R_{RS}6$ in 84% of subjects as compared to only 64% subjects for FEV_1. Delacourt et al. (77) used bronchodilator response to compare the FOT and R_{int} methods with spirometry in 93 children aged 3 to 16 years with asthma or nocturnal cough. They estimated resistance at 0 Hz ($R_{RS}0$) by using linear regression of R_{RS} on frequency from 4 to 16 Hz and then back extrapolating to 0 Hz. Using receiver operator curves, $R_{RS}0$ demonstrated the best discrimination of an $FEV_1 < 80\%$ with 66% sensitivity at a specificity of 80%. This contrasted favorably with R_{int} which yielded only 33% sensitivity at this level of specificity. Results were not as striking when predicting a postbronchodilator change in FEV_1 of at least 10% with $R_{RS}0$ demonstrating 67% sensitivity at a specificity of 80% and R_{int} a sensitivity of 58%. Nielsen and Bisgaard (78) quantified and compared bronchodilator responsiveness to terbutaline inhalation in 55 asthmatic subjects and 37 healthy controls aged two to six years old using sRaw, R_{int}, and FOT ($R_{RS}5$ and $X_{RS}5$). Lung function at baseline was diminished in asthmatic as compared to control subjects by all methods. Healthy subjects improved sRaw, R_{int}, and $R_{RS}5$, but not $X_{RS}5$ following terbutaline as compared to placebo inhalation. Not surprisingly, lung function improved more in asthmatic subjects than in controls by all methods and no significant difference was seen between asthmatic and control subjects in postbronchodilator lung function. Although all methods clearly detected differences in bronchodilator response in the asthmatics, sRaw had the best discriminative ability followed by $R_{RS}5$, R_{int}, and $X_{RS}5$ in that order–an order that, with the exception of sRaw, is reversed in methacholine challenge studies.

Inter-observer variability for FOT, R_{int}, and sRaw were evaluated by Klug et al. (79) with R_{int} demonstrating the greatest random inter-observer variability. Interestingly, the other methods appeared to have lower random variability, but greater systematic differences between observers than did R_{int}. In summary, sRaw seems effective in both methacholine and carbachol challenge and with bronchodilator administration. $X_{RS}5$ seems comparably effective in methacholine challenge in both preschool and school age children, but of less use in assessing bronchodilator response. R_{int} and $R_{RS}5$ are also capable of detecting changes with both bronchoconstriction and bronchodilation, but challenge studies using these methods should include $P_{tc}O_2$.

More epidemiologic and long-term clinical studies need to be conducted with these methods to better understand their role in characterizing pulmonary physiology in young children with recurrent wheeze and asthma. This is particularly the case for long-term clinical trials using a broad range of outcomes to broaden our understanding of early lung disease and so that the outcomes' relative physiologic and clinical relevance can be assessed. The National Asthma Campaign Manchester Asthma and Allergy Study (NACMAAS) (80) is a prospective study of nearly 1000 healthy children who were enrolled antenatally with their parents and who have been followed comprehensively for respiratory health outcomes and risk factors through childhood. Plethysmography was used to characterize the participant's lung function at three years of age and to relate this to respiratory health and atopic status (81). Healthy children demonstrated Raw values similar to those reported by Klug and Bisgaard (53). Children with a history of wheeze in the first three years had significantly higher sRaw than non-wheezers (1.13 kPa sec vs. 1.07 kPa sec^2 $p = 0.002$) with the greatest difference being between those who had wheezed at least twice compared with the never-wheezed group (1.17 kPa sec vs. 1.07 kPa sec^2 $p = 0.001$). Interestingly, non-wheezers who had two parents with atopy demonstrated sRaw values similar to the wheezing group (1.17 kPa sec) and were significantly higher than other non-wheezers who had only one or no parent with atopy. Similarly, non-wheezers who had at least one positive allergen skin test had significantly higher sRaw than non-wheezers who were skin test negative (1.15 kPa sec vs. 1.05 kPa sec^2 $p = 0.002$). In a multivariate model, both parental atopy and personal atopy were independent predictors of sRaw in the non-wheezing group with non-wheezing children who had both a mother with asthma and a positive skin test demonstrating an adjusted geometric mean sRaw of 1.31 kPa sec. The authors concluded that parental and personal atopy contributed to impaired lung function even in the absence of respiratory symptomatology.

Klug and Bisgaard (82) characterized lung function in 110 children aged two to five years old who had a history of at least three or more episodes of wheezing after the first year of life using R_{aw}, R_{int}, and FOT ($X_{RS}5$ and $R_{RS}5$). Measurements were considered indicative of impaired respiratory function if above the 97.5% prediction limit of their reference value (53) for R_{aw}, R_{int}, and $R_{RS}5$ or below the 2.5% prediction limit for $X_{RS}5$. By these criteria R_{int}, sRaw, $X_{RS}5$, and $R_{RS}5$ demonstrated impaired function in 44%, 14%, 11%, and 7.5% of children, respectively, predominantly so in the two to three-years-old. Follow-up data regarding respiratory health were obtained by telephone interview at a mean of 2.9 years (range 1.6–3.9 years). There was no relationship between impairment of respiratory function at baseline and clinical outcome at follow-up. Children whose baseline R_{int} values were within the normal range had comparable symptoms and medication use to those with normal R_{int} values. In contrast, among children with an atopic predisposition there was a greater persistence of symptoms and use of medication at follow-up than in the non-atopic group. These findings support epidemiologic studies, which have found that early in life wheezing and decreased lung function can co-exist in two or more phenotypes (4,5). Early transient wheezers are born with apparently diminished airway function, but show improvement both in symptoms and somewhat in physiology by age six. In contrast, persistent wheezers start with lung function near the mean of the population at birth and then decline by age six showing no improvement in symptoms, along with the development of an atopic phenotype.

The effort to effectively delineate these groups and their physiologic progression through the preschool years requires both large numbers of participants and the integration of lung function with biomarkers and studies of the ontogeny of their immune phenotypes. Indeed, given the importance of atopy and airway inflammation in the pathophysiology of asthma, it is not surprising that exhaled nitric oxide appears to be more useful in identifying early-onset asthma than baseline lung function or measures of bronchodilator response (10). Another inflammatory biomarker, urinary eosinophilic protein-X (U-EPX), has been demonstrated in the NACMAAS epidemiologic cohort to be increased at three years of age in children with either atopy, eczema, or wheeze (11). Although the greatest increase in U-EPX levels was found in atopic children who had a history of both wheezing and eczema, there was no relationship between U-EPX level and lung function in the group as a whole. This supports the concept that although atopy, airway inflammation, and lung function are related, they are not collinear and can contribute both interactively and independently to the phenotype seen by the clinician or epidemiologist.

Specific airway resistance, R_{int}, and FOT have been used effectively in clinical trials of young children with asthma. Nielsen and Bisgaard (83) assessed the efficacy of inhaled budesonide over eight weeks in a randomized, double-blind, parallel group study of 38 children with asthma who were 35–71 months of age at enrollment. At baseline, sRaw and R_{int} were significantly increased compared to reference values while $X_{RS}5$ and $R_{RS}5$ were not. The children responded clinically to budesonide as compared to placebo and demonstrated improved lung function. Significant improvements were seen in R_{int}, $R_{RS}5$ and $X_{RS}5$ in the treatment group as compared to an apparent worsening in the placebo group. Surprisingly, no treatment effect was detectable with sRaw.

All measures detected decreased responsiveness to cold air challenge in the treatment group, however, no difference could be detected in methacholine response.

IV. Spirometry in Young Children

Spirometry depends upon forced expiration at flow limitation generating a maximal expiratory flow at each lung volume ($V'_{max\ V}$) (84) which is theoretically determined by the ratio of lung elastic recoil pressure to characteristics of the intra-thoracic airways (85) and is independent of pleural pressure. Although it does not allow the separation of changes in elastance from those due to airway resistance, spirometry has become the most commonly used method for the assessment of lung function in children and adults. Spirometry in older children and adults has been well standardized (86,87), as have methods for its interpretation (88). Although maximal expiratory flow volume (MEFV) maneuvers can be reliably obtained in sedated infants and toddlers (89), early efforts at obtaining voluntary MEFV maneuvers in awake children aged two to five years demonstrated a relatively low success rate with few curves meeting American Thoracic Society criteria (90). The use of voluntary partial expiratory flow volume maneuvers (PEFV) to assess maximal flow at functional residual capacity ($V'_{max\ FRC}$) has a higher success rate (91,92) and can detect airway obstruction associated with persistent wheezing in early childhood (4) or cold air challenge (93). PEFV maneuvers also may be more sensitive to subtle increases in airway tone (92,94). Compared to MEFV maneuvers, PEFV testing is limited by increased variability, at least part of which may be due to variation in the FRC with a subsequent increase in variability of the isovolume flow $V'_{max\ FRC}$. Also, the software necessary to accomplish this measurement is not readily available on most commercial spirometry systems and the method has not become widely used.

Spirometry in young children clearly requires some different standards than those proposed for adults and children (8,95). Arets et al. (95) studied 446 children experienced in spirometry to evaluate the applicability of American Thoracic Society criteria. They reported on the standards that 90% of children tested could achieve. Based upon these, they proposed a minimum back-extrapolated volume of <0.12 L and a forced expiratory time of at least one second for children under eight years of age, provided the flow-volume curve demonstrated a gradual, asymptotic approach to the volume axis. They also suggested that the reproducibility of forced expiratory volume is one second (FEV_1) and forced vital capacity (FVC) should be less than 5%, however, it should be noted that this study did not focus on young children and different standards will likely be required. Kanengizer and Dozor (90) reported spirometric data from 98 patients aged three to five years. About 98% of all children cooperated in at least six attempts and 95% gave at least one maximal effort with exhalation lasting at least one second. Success rates and reproducibility improved with age. Eigen et al. (8) studied 259 healthy, untrained children in the preschool setting and found that 83% could accomplish successful spirometry during their

Table 1 Eigen Spirometry Criteria

Peak flow should be clearly determined

Effort should not end abruptly. No cessation in flow while flow >25% of peak flow
Forced exhalation should last at least 1 sec
Inhalation should be greater than the end-inspiratory tidal volume
MEFV curves should be consistent in appearance

Source: Modified from Ref. 8.

first testing session with 95% of these having three technically acceptable curves. The testing sessions were limited to 15 minutes per child including training. Five criteria were used to define acceptability (Table 1) and reproducibility and coefficients of variation for FEV_1 and FVC were comparable to spirometry in older children. Prediction equations were developed against the natural logarithm of height and were virtually coincident with predicted spirometric values for older children (96). Using pulsed negative expiratory pressure technique, Jones et al. (97) have demonstrated that young children are capable of reaching flow limitation during spirometry.

Further, the high degree of reproducibility and agreement with prediction equations developed over 30 years ago strongly suggests that the preschoolers in the Eigen study produced valid, flow-limited MEFV maneuvers. Nystad et al. (98) studied 652 preschool children aged three to six years old. They were able to obtain at least two acceptable maneuvers (87) in 92% of children and modeled spirometric parameters with height, weight, and age. Zapletal and Chalupova (99) reported normative data with prediction equations from 173 healthy preschool children for spirometric parameters including isovolume flows at 25%, 50%, and 75% of FVC (MEF_{25}, MEF_{50}, MEF_{75}). Similar again to other studies, they found that age predicted the success rate with an overall success rate of 62% as compared to a 40% success rate in younger children from three to five years of age. Gender did not seem to be related to lung function, and once again, height had the closest relationship to lung function. Figure 5 presents a comparison of predicted values for FEV_1 from Eigen (8), Zapl et al. (99), and Nystad (98) plotted against height.

Obtaining adequate forced expiratory maneuvers in young children is not only dependent upon the child, but also the skill of the individual performing the measurement (8). Young children require enthusiasm, patience, and an ability to help them focus on the task at hand while being coached and praised so that they do not become fearful of the testing device or situation (8). The use of computer-driven incentive programs may aid in testing (100), however the technician needs to ensure that they do not distract the focus of the child (101). Indeed, failure seems to occur more often due to an unwillingness to participate at all or incoordination rather

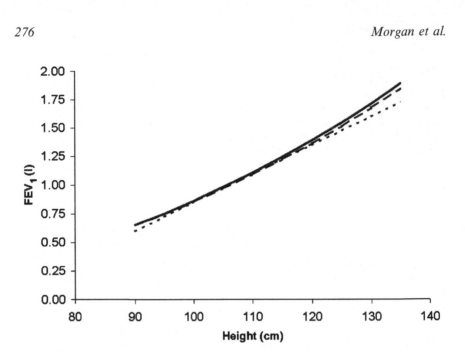

Figure 5   Comparison of predicted values for FEV_1 by spirometry plotted against height. Eigen (8)—solid line, Nystad (98)—dotted line, Zapletal (99)—dashed line.

than lack of motivation in those willing to try the maneuver. The use of noseclips for spirometry has not been addressed in depth for young children, however, Chavasse et al. (102) studied children with asthma or cystic fibrosis at a mean age of 11 years and found no systematic differences between maneuvers with and without the use of noseclips.

One challenge in using MEFV maneuvers in young children is that the time constant of the lung (T = resistance × compliance) is relatively short compared to older children and adults (8,97). Crenesse et al. (103) studied 355 preschool children with pulmonary complaints ages three to six years of age. They found that at least two acceptable maneuvers (104) could be obtained in 52%, 79%, and 79% of three to four, four to five, and five to six years olds, respectively, with 55% of the children being able to perform at least two maneuvers that were reproducible within 0.1 L. FEV_1 and $FEV_{0.75}$ were close to FVC in volume with approximately 21% of children having valid forced expiratory times less than one second. This strongly suggests that, similar to infants (89), $FEV_{0.5}$ and $FEV_{0.75}$ may be more useful parameters of airway function than FEV_1 in young children less than six years of age. Based upon the above studies, spirometry software used in the testing of young children should display a real-time tidal breathing and MEFV trace and be able to report a range of timed volumes (FEV_1, $FEV_{0.75}$, and $FEV_{0.5}$).

More information is needed regarding the changes seen in spirometry with lung disease in young children. Bisgaard and Klug (71) used spirometry to conduct methacholine challenge in 21 children aged four to six years who were suspected of having asthma. They screened 48 children to find 21 capable of performing the multiple steps required in a methacholine challenge. As noted earlier, FOT parameters, sRaw, and $P_{tc}O_2$ appeared to change prior to FEV_1. It was not reported whether other spirometric parameters ($FEV_{0.5}$ and FEF_{25-75}) might have been more sensitive, however, clearly a relevant percentage of young children were able to complete a methacholine challenge. Comparison of their spirometric parameters to healthy children was not reported. Nystad et al. (98) reported on a subset of 476 children in their study for whom they were able to relate parental smoking and personal symptoms of asthma to lung function. Although 30% of children had at least one parent who smoked and 23% had a history of wheeze during the last 12 months, there was no relationship between either of these risk factors and lung function after adjusting for height, weight, and age. Spirometry has been used to assess lung dysfunction in young children with cystic fibrosis (105) by Marostica et al. They studied 38 children aged three to six years of whom 33 were able to perform at least two acceptable MEFV maneuvers. These children had significantly decreased spirometric parameters as compared to normals (8) and demonstrated a moderate correlation of FEV_1 Z-score with a standardized chest roentgenogram score ($r^2 = 0.24$) such that better lung function correlated with a healthier chest roentgenogram. Thus, it appears that somewhere between 50% and 80% of young children can reliably accomplish spirometry and that in diseases with substantive airway inflammation such as cystic fibrosis, spirometry can detect lung dysfunction in preschool children. Although spirometry can be used to assess changes in lung function with methacholine challenge, more studies need to be done early in life with children demonstrating recurrent wheezing and asthma to gain a better understanding of its potential use in research and clinical care. Perhaps the factors that most recommend spirometry are the wide availability of high quality spirometers with software compatible with lung function testing in young children and the breadth and depth of our understanding of spirometry and its relation to health and disease in older children and adults. There is a clear need to implement spirometry in more epidemiologic studies and clinical trials of respiratory health in young children, as well as in the routine clinical assessment and management of children with wheezing respiratory illness. Spirometry can be accomplished in young children with limited training and obtaining successful spirometry in at least 50% of children is still 50% more data than many clinics now have available to guide their management.

V. Summary

In summary, there are a number of well-characterized techniques for the measurement of lung function in young children ages three to six years. Although requiring equipment not commonly found in the clinic setting, measurements of resistance appear to be comparable to spirometry in assessing patients for lung dysfunction and in describing changes with growth (14). They offer the benefit of requiring limited cooperation and having higher success rates than spirometry and may be more sensitive to changes in airway resistance with airway challenge since the bronchodilation seen with full inspiration does not occur. At the same time, young children can accomplish spirometry with success rates approaching 85% in five-year-olds and most clinic and research spirometers can be used for young children without modification. Prediction equations for young children for both resistance methods and spirometry are readily available in the literature. Although a European Respiratory Society working group has addressed the standardization of forced oscillation (14), further work is needed to develop standards for the measurement of sRaw, R_{int}, and spirometry in young children. However, even lacking these standards, there is sufficient information available on these techniques to recommend their implementation more often to assess young children with asthma in both the clinical setting and in epidemiological and clinical trials research.

Abbreviations

AX	Integrated area of reactance from 5 Hz to resonant frequency
BTPS	Body temperature and pressure saturated with water vapor conditions
CaCh	Cold air challenge
CAPS	Childhood Asthma Prevention Study
COV	Coefficient of variation
C_{RS}	Respiratory system capacitance or compliance
exp	Expiration as in $R_{int\ exp}$
FEF_{25-75}	Forced expiratory flow from 25% to 75% of forced vital capacity
FE_{NO}	Fractional concentration of exhaled nitric oxide
FEV_1	Forced expiratory volume in 1 sec
FFT	Fast Fourier Transform
FOT	Forced oscillation technique for the measurement of respiratory system resistance
f_{res}	Resonant frequency
FVC	Forced vital capacity
G_{int}	Airways conductance measured by the interrupter technique equal to $1/R_{int}$
Hz	Hertz (cycles per second)
insp	Inspiration as in $R_{int\ insp}$
I_{RS}	Respiratory system inertance
kPa	Kilopascals
L	Liters
MEF_x	Maximal expiratory flow at "x" percent of vital capacity

(*Continued*)

Abbreviations (*Continued*)

MEFV	Maximal expiratory flow volume maneuver
NACMAAS	National Asthma Campaign Manchester Asthma and Allergy Study
P_{amb}	Ambient or barometric pressure
P_{alv}	Pressure in the alveolus
PD_x	Provocative dose of a challenge agent need to cause "x" percent change in the measured parameter
PEFV	Partial expiratory flow volume maneuver
PH_2O	Pressure of water vapor
P_{int}	Pressure estimated at the time of interruption in the measurement of R_{int}
P_{mo}	Pressure measured at the mouth
R_{aw}	Airways resistance
R_{int}	Airway resistance measured by the interrupter technique
ROC	Receiver operator curve
R_{RS}	Respiratory system resistance
$R_{RS}f$	Respiratory system resistance at frequency f
RS	Respiratory system
sec	Seconds
SDI	Standard deviation index
sRaw	Specific airways resistance
$P_{tc}O_2$	Transcutaneous partial pressure of oxygen
TGV	Thoracic gas volume measured plethysmographically
T_0	Time of shutter closure in the measurement of R_{int}
U-EPX	Urinary eosinophilic protein-X
V'	Flow
V'_{int}	Flow at the time of interruption in the measurement of R_{int}
$V'_{max\ V}$	Maximal flow at volume V
V_{box}	Volume of the plethysmograph
X_{RS}	Respiratory system reactance
$X_{RS}f$	Respiratory system reactance at frequency f
Z_{RS}	Respiratory system impedance

References

1. Anonymous. National asthma education and prevention program expert panel report 2: Guidelines for the Diagn and Manag Asthma. 1997:42–49.
2. Bacharier L, Dawson C, Bloomberg G, Bender B, Wilson L, Strunk R. Hospitalization for asthma: atopic, pulmonary function, and psychological correlates among participants in the childhood asthma management program. Pediatrics 2003; 112:85–92.
3. Martinez F, Morgan W, Wright A, Holberg C, Taussig L. Diminished lung function as a predisposing factor for wheezing respiratory illness in infants. N Engl J Med 1988; 319(17):1112–1117.

4. Martinez F, Wright A, Taussig L, Holberg C, Halonen M, Morgan W. Asthma and wheezing in the first six years of life. N Engl J Med 1995; 332(3):133–138.

5. Stein R, Holberg C, Morgan W, Wright A, Lombardi E, Taussig L, Martinez F. Peak flow variability, methacholine responsiveness and atopy as markers for detecting different wheezing phenotypes in childhood. Thorax 1997; 52: 946–952.

6. The Childhood Asthma Management Program Research Group. Long-term effects of budesonide or nedocromil in children with asthma. N Engl J Med 2000; 343(15):1054–1063.

7. Tepper R, Sly P. Physiological outcomes. Eur Respir J 1996; 21(suppl):12–15.

8. Eigen H, Bieler H, Grant D, Christoph K, Terrill D, Heilman D, Ambrosius W, Tepper R. Spirometric pulmonary function in healthy preschool children. Am J Respir Crit Care Med 2001; 163:619–623.

9. Martinez F. Toward asthma prevention. Does all that really matters happen before we learn to read? N Engl J Med 2003; 349(15):1473–1475.

10. Malmberg L, Pelkonen A, Haahtela T, Turpeinen M. Exhaled nitric oxide rather than lung function distinguishes preschool children with probable asthma. Thorax 2003; 58:494–499.

11. Gore C, Peterson C, Kissen P, Simpson B, Lowe L, Woodcock A, Custovic A. National asthma campaign manchester asthma and allergy study group. Urinary eosinophilic protein x, atopy, and symptoms suggestive of allergic disease at 3 years of age. J Allergy Clin Immunol 2003; 112(4):702–708.

12. Goldman M. Clinical application of forced oscillation. Pulmon Pharmacol Ther 2001; 14(5):341–350.

13. Goldman M, Carter R, Klein R, Fritz G, Carter B, Pachucki P. Within-and between-day variability of respiratory impedance using impulse oscillometry in adolescent asthmatics. Pediatr Pulmonol 2002; 34(4):312–319.

14. Oostveen E, MacLeod D, Lorino H, Farre R, Hantos Z, Desager K, Marchal F. On behalf of the ERS Task Force on Respiratory Impedance Measurements. The forced oscillation technique in clinical practice: methodology, recommendations and future developments. Eur Respir J 2003; 22(6):1026–1041.

15. Phagoo S, Wilson N, Silverman M. Evaluation of the interrupter technique for measuring change in airway resistance in 5-year-old asthmatic children. Pediatr Pulmonol 1995; 20(6):387–395.

16. Sly P, Lombardi E. Measurement of lung function in preschool children using the interrupter technique. Thorax 2003; 58:742–744.

17. Arets H, Brackel H, van der Ent C. Applicability of interrupter resistance measurements using the MicroRint® in daily practice. Respir Med 2003; 97(4):366–374.

18. Chan E, Bridge P, Dundas I, Pao S, Healy M, McKenzie S. Repeatability of airway resistance measurements made using the interrupter technique. Thorax 2003; 58:344–347.

19. Beelen R, Smit H, van Strien R, Koopman L, Brussee J, Brunekreef B, Gerristen J, Merkus P. Short-and-long-term variability of the interrupter technique under field and standardized conditions in 3–6 year-old children. Thorax 2003; 58:761–764.

20. Frey U, Schibler A, Kraemer R. Pressure oscillations after flow interruption in relation to lung mechanics. Respir Physiol 1995; 102(2):225–237.
21. Bates J, Baconnier P, Milic-Emili J. A theoretical analysis of interrupter technique for measuring respiratory mechanics. J Appl Physiol 1988; 64: 2204–2214.
22. Ludwig M, Romero P, Sly P, Fredberg J, Bates J. Interpretation of interrupter resistance after histamine-induced constriction in the dog. J Appl Physiol 1990; 68:1651–1656.
23. Oswald-Mammosser M, Lierena C, Speich J, Donato L, Lonsdorfer J. Measurements of respiratory system resistance by the interrupter technique in healthy and asthmatic children. Pediatr Pulmonol 1997; 24(2):78–85.
24. Bridge P, McKenzie S. Airway resistance measured by the interrupter technique: expiration or inspiration, mean or median? Eur Respir J 2001; 17(3):495–498.
25. Carter E, Stecenko A, Pollock B, Jaeger M. Evaluation of the interrupter technique for the use of assessing airway obstruction in children. Pediatr Pulmonol 1994; 17(4):211–217.
26. Beydon N, Amsallem F, Bellet M, Boule M, Chaussain M, Denjean A, Matran R, Wuyam B, Alberti C, Gaultier C. Pre/postbronchodilator interrupter resistance values in healthy young children. Am J Respir Crit Care Med 2002; 165: 1388–1394.
27. Phagoo S, Wilson N, Silverman M. Evaluation of a new interrupter device for measuring bronchial responsiveness and the response to bronchodilator in 3-year-old children. Eur Respir J 1996; 9(7):1374–1380.
28. Bridge P, Ranganathan S, McKenzie S. Measurement of airway resistance using the interrupter technique in preschool children in the ambulatory setting. Eur Respir J 1999; 13(4):792–796.
29. Lombardi E, Sly P, Concutelli G, Novembre E, Veneruso G, Fromgia G, Bernardini R, Vierucci A. Reference values of interrupter respiratory resistance in healthy preschool white children. Thorax 2001; 56:691–695.
30. Merkus P, Mijnsbergen J, Hop W, de Jongste J. Interrupter resistance in preschool children: measurement characteristics and reference values. Am J Respir Crit Care Med 2001; 163:1350–1355.
31. Merkus P, Artes H, Joosten T, Siero A, Brouha M, Mijnsbergen, J, de Jongste J, van der Ent C. Measurements of interrupter resistance: reference values for children 3–13 years of age. Eur Respir J 2002; 20(4):907–911.
32. McKenzie S, Chan E, Dundas I, Bridge P, Pao C, Mylonopoulou M, Healy M. Airway resistance measured by the interrupter technique: normative data for 2–10 year olds of three ethnicities. Arch Dis Child 2002; 87:248–251.
33. McKenzie S, Mylonopoulou M, Bridge P. Bronchodilator responsiveness and atopy in 5–10 year-old coughers. Eur Respir J 2001; 18(6):977–981.
34. Beydon N, Pin I, Matran R, Chaussain M, Boule M, Alain B, Bellet M, Amsallem F, Alberti C, Denjean A, Gaultier C. Pulmonary function tests in preschool children with asthma. Am J Respir Crit Care Med 2003; 168: 640–644.
35. McKenzie S, Bridge P, Healy M. Airway resistance and atopy in preschool children with wheeze and cough. Eur Respir J 2000; 15(5):833–838.

36. Frey U, Kraemer R. Oscillatory pressure transients after flow interruption during bronchial challenge test in children. Eur Respir J 1997; 10(1):75–81.

37. DuBois A, Brody A, Lewis D, Burgess B Jr. Oscillation mechanics of lungs and chest in man. J Appl Physiol 1955; 8:587–594.

38. MacLeod D, Birch M. Respiratory input impedance measurement: forced oscillation methods. Med Biol Eng Comp 2001; 39(5):505–516.

39. Goldman M, Knudson R, Mead J, Peterson N, Schwaber J, Wohl M. A simplified measurement of respiratory resistance by forced oscillation. J Appl Physiol 1970; 28:113–116.

40. Frey U, Silverman M, Kraemer R, Jackson A. High-frequency respiratory impedance measured by forced-oscillation technique in infants. Am J Respir Crit Care Med 1998; 158:363–370.

41. Marchal F, Mazurek H, Habib M, Duvivier C, Derelle J, Reslin R. Input respiratory impedance to estimate airway hyperreactivity in children: standard method versus head generator. Eur Respir J 1994; 7(3):601–607.

42. Mazurek H, Willim G, Marchal F, Haluszka J, Tomalak W. Input respiratory impedance measured by head generator in preschool children. Pediatr Pulmonol 2000; 30(1):47–55.

43. Marchal F, Loos N, Monin P, Peslin R. Methacholine-induced volume dependence of respiratory resistance in preschool children. Eur Respir J 1999; 14(5):1167–1174.

44. Lutchen K, Sullivan A, Arbogast F, Celli B, Jackson A. Use of transfer impedance measurements for clinical assessment of lung mechanics. Am J Respir Crit Care Med 1998; 157:435–446.

45. Wohl M, Stigol L, Mead J. Resistance of the total respiratory system in healthy infants and infants with bronchiolitis. Pediatrics 1969; 43:495–509.

46. Wilson N, Dore C, Silverman M. Factors relating to the severity of symptoms at 5 years in children with severe wheeze in the first 2 years of life. Eur Respir J 1997; 10(2):346–353.

47. Wilson N, Bridge P, Phagoo S, Silverman M. The measurement of methacholine responsiveness in 5-year-old children: three methods compared. Eur Respir J 1995; 8(3):364–370.

48. Cuijpers CE, Wesseling GJ, Kessels AG, Swaen GM, Mertens PL, de Kok ME, Broer J, Sturmans F, Wouters EF. Low diagnostic value of respiratory impedance measurements in children. Eur Respir J 1997; 10(1):88–93.

49. Cuijpers C, Wesseling G, Swaen G, Wouters E. Frequency dependence of oscillatory resistance in healthy primary school children. Respiration 1993; 60(3):149–154.

50. Hordvik N, Konig P, Morris D, Kreutz C, Pimmel R. Normal values for forced oscillatory respiratory resistance in children. Pediatr Pulmonol 1985; 1(3):145–148.

51. Malmberg L, Pelkonen A, Poussa T, Pohjanpalo A, Haahtela T, Turpeinen M. Determinants of respiratory system input impedance and bronchodilator response in healthy Finnish preschool children. Clin Physiol Funct Imaging 2002; 22(1):64–71.

52. Lebecque P, Desmond K, Swartebroeckx Y, DuBois P, Lulling J, Coates A. Measurement of respiratory system resistance by forced oscillation in normal

children: a comparison with spirometric values. Pediatr Pulmonol 1991; 10(2): 117–122.

53. Klug B, Bisgaard H. Specific airway resistance, interrupter resistance, and respiratory impedance in healthy children aged 2–7 years. Pediatr Pulmonol 1998; 25(5):322–331.

54. Ducharme F, Davis G, Ducharme G. Pediatric reference values for respiratory resistance measured by forced oscillation. CHEST 1998; 113:1322–1328.

55. Hellinckx J, De Boeck K, Bande-Knops J, Van Der Poel M, Demedts M. Bronchodilator response in 3–6.5 years old healthy and stable asthmatic children. Eur Respir J 1998; 12(2):438–443.

56. Timonen K, Randell J, Salonen R, Pekkanen J. Short-term variations in oscillatory and spirometric lung function indices among school children. Eur Respir J 1997; 10(1):82–87.

57. Bouaziz N, Beyaert C, Gauthier R, Monin P, Peslin R, Marchal F. Respiratory system reactance as an indicator of the intrathoracic airway response to methacholine in children. Pediatr Pulmonol 1996; 22(1):7–13.

58. Ducharme F, Davis G. Respiratory resistance in the emergency department: A reproducible and responsive measure of asthma severity. CHEST 1998; 113:1566–1572.

59. Marotta A, Klinnert M, Price M, Larsen G, Liu A. Impulse oscillometry provides an effective measure of lung dysfunction in 4-year-old children at risk for persistent asthma. J Allergy Clin Immunol 2003; 112(2):317–322.

60. Castro-Rodriguez J, Holberg C, Wright A, Martinez F. A clinical index to define risk of asthma in young children with recurrent wheezing. Am J Respir Crit Care Med 2000; 162:1403–1406.

61. DuBois A, Botelho S, Comroe J. A new method for measuring airway resistance in man using a body plethysmograph: values in normal subjects and in patients with respiratory disease. J Clin Invest 1956; 35(3):327–335.

62. Klug B, Bisgaard H. Measurement of the specific airway resistance by plethysmography in young children accompanied by an adult. Eur Respir J 1997; 10(7):1599–1605.

63. Dab I, Alexander F. A simplified approach to the measurement of specific airway resistance. Pediatr Res 1976; 10(12):998–999.

64. Zapletal A. Lung function in children and adolescents. Methods, reference values. In: Bolliger CT, ed. Progress in respiration research. Vol. 22. Prague: Karger, 1987: VIII+220, Figures 59, Tables 283.

65. Badier M, Guillot C, Dubus J. Bronchial challenge with carbachol in 3–6-year-old children: body plethysmography assessments. Pediatr Pulmonol 1999; 27(2):117–123.

66. Wilson N, Phagoo S, Silverman M. Atopy, bronchial responsiveness, and symptoms in wheezy 3-year olds. Arch Dis Child 1992; 67:491–495.

67. Bisgaard H, Nielsen K. Bronchoprotection with a leukotriene receptor antagonist in asthmatic preschool children. Am J Respir Crit Care Med 2000; 162:187–190.

68. Nielsen K, Bisgaard H. Bronchodilation and bronchoprotection in asthmatic preschool children from formoterol administered by mechanically actuated dry-powder inhaler and spacer. Am J Respir Crit Care Med 2001; 164:256–259.

69. Landser F, Nagles J, Demedts M, Billiet L, van de Woestijne K. A new method to determine frequency characteristics of the respiratory system. J Appl Physiol 1976; 41(1):101–106.

70. Beydon N, Trang-Pham H, Bernard A, Gaultier C. Measurements of resistance by the interrupter technique and of transcutaneous partial pressure of oxygen in young children during methacholine challenge. Pediatr Pulmonol 2001; 31(3):238–246.

71. Bisgaard H, Klug B. Lung function measurement in awake young children. Eur Respir J 1995; 8(12):2067–2075.

72. Klug B, Bisgaard H. Measurement of lung function in awake 2–4 year-old asthmatic children during methacholine challenge and acute asthma: a comparison of the impulse oscillation technique, the interrupter technique, and transcutaneous measurement of oxygen versus whole-body plethysmography. Pediatr Pulmonol 1996; 21(5):290–300.

73. Klug B, Bisgaard H. Repeatability of methacholine challenges in 2–4 year-old children with asthma, using a new technique for quantitative delivery of aerosol. Pediatr Pulmonol 1997; 23(4):278–286.

74. Nielsen K, Bisgaard H. Lung function response to cold air challenge in asthmatic and healthy children of 2–5 years of age. Am J Respir Crit Care Med 2000; 161:1805–1809.

75. Vink G, Arets J, van der Laag J, van der Ent C. Impulse oscillometry: a measure for airway obstruction. Pediatr Pulmonol 2003; 35(3):214–219.

76. Bridge P, Lee H, Silverman M. A portable device based on the interrupter technique to measure bronchodilator response in schoolchildren. Eur Respir J 1996; 9(7):1368–1373.

77. Delacourt C, Lorino H, Fuhrman C, Herve-Guillot M, Reinert P, Harf A, Housset B. Comparison of the forced oscillation technique and the interrupter technique for assessing airway obstruction and its reversibility in children. Am J Respir Crit Care Med 2001; 164:965–972.

78. Nielsen K, Bisgaard H. Discriminative capacity of bronchodilator response measured with three different lung function techniques in asthmatic and healthy children aged 2–5 years. Am J Respir Crit Care Med 2001; 164: 554–559.

79. Klug B, Nielsen K, Bisgaard H. Observer variability of lung function measurements in 2–6 year-old children. Eur Respir J 2000; 16(3):472–475.

80. Custovic A, Simpson B, Simpson A, Hallam C, Craven M, Brutsche M, Woodcock A. Manchester Asthma and Allergy Study: low-allergen environment can be achieved and maintained during pregnancy and in early life. J Allergy Clin Immunol 2000; 105(2 Pt 1):252–258.

81. Lowe L, Murray C, Custovic A, Simpson B, Kissen P, Woodcock A. NAC Manchester Asthma and Allergy Study Group. Specific airway resistance in 3-year-old children: a prospective cohort study. Lancet 2002; 359(9321): 1904–1908.

82. Klug B, Bisgaard H. Lung function and short-term outcome in young asthmatic children. Eur Respir J 1999; 14(5):1185–1189.

83. Nielsen K, Bisgaard H. The effect of inhaled budesonide on symptoms, lung function, and cold air and methacholine responsiveness in 2–5-year-old asthmatic children. Am J Respir Crit Care Med 2000; 162:1500–1506.

84. Hyatt R, Schilder D, Fry D. Relationship between maximum expiratory flow and degree of lung inflation. J Appl Physiol 1958; 13:331–336.

85. Dawson S, Elliott E. Wave-speed limitation on expiratory flow-a unifying concept. J Appl Physiol 1977; 43:498–515.

86. Anonymous. Standardization of Spirometry, 1994 Update: American Thoracic Society. Am J Respir Crit Care Med 1995; 152(3):1107–1136.

87. Quanjer P, Tammeling G, Cotes J, Pedersen O, Peslin R, Yernault J. Lung volumes and forced ventilatory flows: Report Working Party Standardization of Lung Function Tests, European Community for Steel and Coal. Official Statement of the European Respiratory Society. Eur Respir J 1993; 16(suppl): 5S–40S.

88. Anonymous. Lung function testing: Selection of reference values and interpretative strategies. Am Rev Respir Dis 1991; 144:1202–1218.

89. Jones M, Castile R, Davis S, Kisling J, Filbrun D, Flucke R, Goldstein A, Emsley C, Ambrosius W, Tepper R. Forced expiratory flows and volumes in infants. Normative data and lung growth. Am J Respir Crit Care Med 2000; 161:353–359.

90. Kanengiser S, Dozor A. Forced expiratory maneuvers in children aged 3–5 years. Pediatr Pulmonol 1994; 18(3):144–149.

91. Taussig L. Maximal expiratory flows at functional residual capacity: a test of lung function for young children. Am Rev Respir Dis 1977; 116(6):1031–1038.

92. Morgan W, Geller D, Tepper R, Taussig L. Partial expiratory flow-volume curves in infants and young children. Pediatr Pulmonol 1988; 5(4):232–243.

93. Lombardi E, Morgan W, Wright A, Stein R, Holberg C, Martinez F. Cold air challenge at age 6 and subsequent incidence of asthma. A longitudinal study. Am J Respir Crit Care Med 1997; 156:1863–1869.

94. Landau L, Morgan W, McCoy K, Taussig L. Gender related differences in airway tone in children. Pediatr Pulmonol 1993; 16(1):31–35.

95. Arets H, Brackel H, van der Ent C. Forced expiratory manoeuvres in children: do they meet ATS and ERS criteria for spirometry? Eur Respir J 2001; 18(4):655–660.

96. Polgar G, Promadhat V. Standard values in pulmonary function testing in children: techniques and standards. Philadelphia: WB Saunders, 1971.

97. Jones M, Davis S, Grant D, Christoph K, Kisling J, Tepper R. Forced expiratory maneuvers in very young children: assessment of flow limitation. Am J Respir Crit Care Med 1999; 159:791–795.

98. Nystad W, Samuelsen S, Nafstad P, Edvardsen E, Stensrud T, Jaakkola J. Feasibility of measuring lung function in preschool children. Thorax 2002; 57:1021–1027.

99. Zapletal A, Chalupova J. Forced expiratory parameters in healthy preschool children (3–6 years of age). Pediatr Pulmonol 2003; 35(3):200–207.

100. Vilozni D, Barker M, Jellousscchek H, Heimann G, Blau H. An interactive computer-animated system (SpiroGame) facilitates spirometry in preschool children. Am J Respir Crit Care Med 2001; 164:2200–2205.

101. Gracchi V, Boel M, van der Laag J, van der Ent C. Spirometry in young children: should computer-animation programs be used during testing? Eur Respir J 2003; 21(5):872–875.
102. Chavasse R, Johnson P, Francis J, Balfour-Lynn I, Rosenthal M, Bush A. To clip or not to clip? Noseclips for spirometry. Eur Respir J 2003; 21(5): 876–878.
103. Crenesse D, Berlioz M, Bourrier T, Albertini M. Spirometry in children aged 3 to 5 years: reliability of forced expiratory maneuvers. Pediatr Pulmonol 2001; 32(1):56–61.
104. Kanner R, Schenker M, Munoz A, Speizer F. Spirometry in children. Methodology for obtaining optimal results for clinical and epidemiologic studies. Am Rev Respir Dis 1983; 127(6):720–724.
105. Marostica P, Weist A, Eigen H, Angelicchio C, Christoph K, Savage J, Grant D, Tepper R. Spirometry in 3–6-year-old children with cystic fibrosis. Am J Respir Crit Care Med 2002; 166:67–71.

11

Inflammatory Mediators of Asthma in Children

PETER G. GIBSON and JODIE L. SIMPSON

Respiratory and Sleep Medicine, Hunter Medical Research Institute,
 John Hunter Hospital
New South Wales, Australia

I. Introduction

Asthma in children is characterized by episodic symptoms, variable expiratory airflow obstruction, airway inflammation, and remodeling of the airway. Effective therapy, when appropriately applied, is able to control symptoms and airflow obstruction in the majority of children. Current treatment for childhood asthma targets the pathophysiological processes of airway inflammation and airway obstruction. These treatments include broncho-dilators for the reversal of airflow obstruction and anti-inflammatory drugs for the management of airway inflammation. The tools currently available to clinicians for asthma management measure symptoms and airflow obstruction. Clinicians commence, monitor, and modify treatment using measures of symptoms and, if possible, airway obstruction. There is a clear discrepancy between asthma treatment targets and the tools used to monitor these treatments. This discrepancy is greatest in the monitoring and treatment of airway inflammation. It is also in this area that the margin for error is lowest because of the side effects of excessive doses of anti-inflammatory therapy in children with asthma.

The consequence of this discrepancy is the imprecise use of treatment, which manifests as both undertreatment and overtreatment of asthma. Undertreatment of asthma occurs when episodic symptoms are not recognized as due to asthma and children fail to receive effective treatment for these symptoms. This can occur when there is a failure to diagnose asthma (underdiagnosis) or when there is ineffective control of symptoms in established asthma. Overtreatment occurs when asthma therapy is applied in doses greater than is needed, when more drug classes are used than are required to control asthma, or when symptoms are not due to asthma and asthma therapy is mistakenly applied to treat these symptoms.

It seems likely that the measurement of inflammation will address this discrepancy and result in improved asthma management. This concept has been formally tested and proven in adults. Green et al. (1) compared the drug therapy of asthma using current best guidelines with an approach based on measurement of airway inflammation with induced sputum. Patients who were managed using induced sputum results to guide therapy in order to suppress sputum eosinophilia had significantly fewer asthma exacerbations (1), yet did not require increased doses of inhaled corticosteroids (ICS). The concept remains to be proven in pediatric asthma; however, it seems likely that the assessment of airway inflammation in asthma will assist in pediatric asthma management. The basis of this approach is the assessment of airway inflammation in asthma. In this chapter, we review available technologies to monitor inflammation in asthma.

II. Key Issues

In assessing the value of new technologies for the management of childhood asthma, several key issues need to be considered. These include the marker itself, the sample collection method, the measurement technique for the proposed marker, and the utility of the results (Table 1).

Sample collection is a crucial aspect relating to the use of new technologies. Each new technology needs to be evaluated for its suitability of use in children, and any age-specific sampling requirements or limitations need to be recognized. Sampling needs to be safe, acceptable to children, parents, and clinicians, and able to be performed on repeated occasions.

Examples of samples being evaluated as markers in asthma care include gases in exhaled breath, the condensate from exhaled breath, induced sputum, blood, and urine. Samples collected directly from the lung (exhaled breath and sputum) have the advantage that they sample the affected organ and should give more specific results, compared with other samples, which only indirectly reflect the inflammatory process in the airway. When formally compared, induced sputum eosinophils had significantly better performance

Table 1 Key Issues for New Monitoring Technologies in Asthma

Sample collection
Safety
Acceptability
Age-specific limitations
Measurements
Sample processing
Personnel requirements
Equipment requirements
Quality control procedures
Utility
Reproducibility
Responsive to change in disease status
Responsive to change in treatment

---

characteristics than blood eosinophils and serum eosinophil cationic protein (ECP) (2).

The measurement process for the proposed marker is also an important issue that will influence the applicability of any technique. Relevant issues include the processing required, the instrumentation required for the assay, the personnel required for the assay, and the quality control requirements for any technique. A point-of-care technique would have wide-ranging applicability in a variety of clinical situations. For this to be successful, it requires a marker where there is minimal sample processing required, no additional personnel, minimal or no instrumentation, and where quality control issues are addressed at the level of the manufacturer. This contrasts with technology that is restricted to a specialist laboratory, either because of the expertise required in processing or measurement, or because specialized equipment is required for assay.

A. Utility of Results

Some properties that would be useful in new technology for asthma care are that the measurement is elevated in asthma compared to non-asthmatics, is related to clinical severity or disease activity, can detect a change in disease status, and is modified by treatment. In addition, the measurement needs to be reproducible in stable children.

Against this background, it is possible to examine the newly emerging technologies for the assessment of asthma in children (Table 2). These technologies include:

- induced sputum,
- exhaled gases,
- exhaled breath condensate.

Table 2 Comparison of Measurement Properties of New Monitoring Technologies

	Induced sputum	Exhaled nitric oxide	Breath condensate
Sample collection			
Age	>6 years	>8 years Possible in younger children with modifications	>4 years
Success (%)	~70%	>90%	100%
Safety	Risk of airway narrowing	Good	Good
Measurement			
Laboratory required	Yes	No	Yes
Equipment	Minimal	Chemiluminescent analyzer	Varies
Time	4 hr	0.5 hr	>8 hr
Point of care	No	Yes	No
Utility			
Reproducible	Yes	?	?
Asthma vs. healthy	Yes	Yes if steroid naïve No if ICS treated	Yes
Asthma severity	Yes	No	?
Responsive to change			
In disease	Yes	Yes	?
Treatment	Yes	?	?
Detects inflammatory pattern	Yes	No	?

III. Induced Sputum

Induced sputum is now well standardized and reproducible protocols are described for use in children (3). Induced sputum is collected by inhalation of nebulized hypertonic saline in stable asthma (4) or with normal saline during exacerbations (5). It may also be collected as part of a combined hypertonic saline challenge (6). The saline is delivered using a mouthpiece and two-way valve connected to an ultrasonic nebulizer. Nebulizers used for sputum induction vary and can be low or high output (3). For sputum induction, bronchodilator medication is given prior to starting the test. Saline is delivered in small amounts, usually not more than five minutes at a time. After each saline dose, airway caliber is assessed and the child is encouraged to cough, clear their throat, and empty the contents of their mouth into a sterile container. If the child's forced expiratory volume (FEV_1) falls below 15% of baseline, further bronchodilator medication is given. The test is normally stopped when an adequate sputum sample is produced or at the end of the full induction protocol, which varies between studies but is usually between 15 and 30 minutes.

A. Tolerability of Sputum Induction

In a study of 53 children who underwent sputum induction, 98% completed the test and 92% were able to produce an adequate sample (Fig. 1). Only one child did not complete the test due to a dislike of the saline taste. The primary side effect noted was a troublesome cough but this did not prevent completion of the test (6).

A combined hypertonic saline challenge/sputum induction was undertaken in 182 children, of whom 90% completed the test. An adequate sample was produced in 70% of children (Fig. 1). The primary reason for an incomplete combined challenge/induction was severe cough (9%) and distress (1%). Some children were able to produce an adequate sample but did not complete the test (4%).

Other side effects include airway obstruction, vomiting, and anxiety. When a sputum induction is performed using pretreatment with β_2-agonist, a fall in lung function of >10% is only observed in 6% of children (3). Pretreatment with bronchodilators improves the success and tolerability of sputum induction in children.

A key issue in sample collection is the delivery of sufficient hypertonic saline to the airway. The nebulizer output and the age of the subject

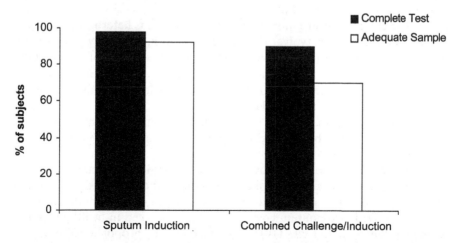

Figure 1 Proportion of children completing tests (*black bar*) and producing adequate samples (*white bar*) for sputum induction and combined saline challenge/sputum induction. *Source*: From Ref. 6.

determine this. High output nebulizers can deliver a greater aerosol dose to the airway in a shorter time period. However, the increased output may be less well tolerated (6). Use of a low output nebulizer is well tolerated in children (3,4).

B. Age-Related Determinants

The age of the child is an important determinant regarding the use of induced sputum. Effectively, this technique is limited to children six years and over because of age-related issues. Hypertonic saline can provoke airflow obstruction in children with asthma. In order to manage this, it is necessary to measure airway caliber during the test. This is usually performed using spirometry, which limits the use of the technique to children who are able to perform spirometry, usually six years and over. The other age-related limitation of induced sputum relates to dose delivery. In children this is dependent on tidal volume, and for hypertonic saline challenge, children aged six and over have sufficient tidal volume to allow the test to be performed in an acceptable time frame (7).

C. Results in Asthma

Children with asthma have increased eosinophil counts in induced sputum compared to healthy children (8,9). The background clinical asthma pattern is also related to the degree of sputum eosinophilia (Fig. 2). Children with persistent asthma have significantly higher eosinophil levels than children with infrequent episodic asthma (10). Sputum inflammatory markers such as ECP have been shown to be superior to systemic measures for monitoring and diagnosis of asthma (8).

The cellular pattern of inflammation in asthma is heterogenous. While many children have a typical eosinophilic pattern, it is now increasingly recognized that children can have asthma in the absence of eosinophilic inflammation, termed non-eosinophilic asthma (11). This heterogeneity has been observed in stable asthma (11), acute severe asthma (12), and in children with a recent onset of asthma-like symptoms (13).

In acute asthma, there is a superimposed neutrophil infiltration (5), which is likely driven by chemokines such as interleukin (IL)-8 (12) induced by viral infection (14).

There is now evidence that sputum eosinophilia predicts a favorable response to corticosteroid treatment (1). One of the advantages of sputum examination is that it can detect this heterogeneity of airway inflammation in asthma. With low sputum eosinophil levels observed in healthy children (ranging from 0.3% to 1.8%) (10) a sputum eosinophil proportion above 1.8% indicates eosinophilia. This may prove to be very important, especially as the response to ICS in childhood asthma is also now known to be heterogenous (15). In adults a heterogenous response is also evident and the presence of

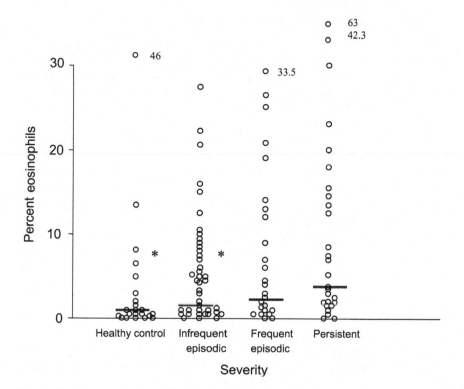

Figure 2 Sputum eosinophils (%) for asthma severity groups. Bars are medians, *p < 0.05 vs. persistent. *Source*: From Ref. 10.

sputum eosinophilia is associated with excellent improvements in airway hyperresponsiveness (16). If the adult studies are replicated in children, then the presence of an elevated sputum eosinophil count will indicate a favorable response to ICS, whereas a normal eosinophil count will indicate that steroids could be reduced.

IV. Exhaled Nitric Oxide

The measurement of exhaled nitric oxide (eNO) is being actively investigated as a marker for use in asthma management. Exogenous NO is derived from L-arginine by the enzyme NO synthase. There are three types of NO synthases: Two are constitutively expressed (NOS1 and nNOS) and the third (NOS2) is inducible. NOS2 has a greater level of activity and is induced by inflammatory cytokines, endotoxin, and viral infections (17). It is thought that the increased levels of NO observed in airway disease are due to induction of NOS2 in response to inflammation.

A. Sample Collection and Measurement

Exhaled NO can be measured using both on-line and off-line testing procedures. A chemiluminescent analyzer is required for analysis. On-line measurement refers to eNO testing with a real-time display of eNO breath profiles. This method requires a chemiluminescent analyzer with a rapid response time. Nitric oxide free air is inhaled to total lung capacity (TLC) and the child then exhales at a constant flow rate. Low flow rates (<0.1 L/sec) amplify the measured NO concentration and are believed to aid in discriminating among subjects. A flow rate of 0.05 L/sec is recommended by current guidelines to be a reasonable compromise between measurement sensitivity and patient comfort. The duration of exhalation must be sufficient to obtain a plateau in the NO versus time profile of at least three seconds [American Thoracic Society (ATS) guidelines].

Off-line testing refers to delayed analysis of breath that is collected into a suitable receptacle. Off-line testing allows the collection of samples from many sites and in the field and also may allow for more efficient use of the analyzer providing some advantage over on-line measurement. However, there are disadvantages that require consideration. These include contamination of the gas from non-airway sources, storage, and sampling errors, and also the inability to have instantaneous results and feedback.

The ATS standardized procedures for the on-line and off-line measurement of exhaled lower respiratory nitric oxide and nasal nitric oxide in adults and children was published in 1999. The basic recommen dations are:

- The child should remain comfortably seated, breathing room temperature air for five minutes before the test to acclimatize to laboratory conditions. The inspired gas should contain <5 ppb NO.
- NO exhaled by children ≥12 years old should be measured by the same technique recommended for adults.
- Subjects inhale to TLC, and then exhale at a constant rate of 50 mL/sec until at least a two-second NO plateau has been achieved and exhalation has lasted for at least four seconds. Repeated exhalations are performed until three NO plateau values agree at the 10% level or two agree at the 5% level. There should be at least a 30 second interval between tests, to allow patients to rest. The mean NO value is then recorded.

The sampling requirements place age-related limitations on eNO testing in children.

About half of children less than eight years old have difficulty performing eNO assessment using the standardized technique of a constant flow. The success of the standardized technique improves in children over eight years of age with 90% of children successfully performing the maneuver.

Success rates in younger children can be increased by the use of a flow regulator. This is an adaptation to the standardized technique that allows the flow to be kept constant by the operator. Ninety-three percent of children under eight years of age and all children over eight years were able to perform a successful eNO maneuver using this adaptation (18).

Tidal breathing maneuvers have been used to assess eNO in infants, however, this method does not show agreement with single breath measures and has several methodological problems (19).

Several variables are known to modify eNO measurements:

Flow Rate

Exhaled NO concentrations are flow-dependent with eNO levels increasing as flow rates decrease (20). The use of constant expiratory flow rates is important in standardized techniques. Many published studies use flow rates that are higher than those recommended by ATS guidelines (50 mL/sec). Lower flow rates have shown to be more useful to discriminate between asthma and healthy controls (21).

Spirometry and Challenges

Nitric oxide analysis should be performed before spirometry or airway challenges as these maneuvers reduce NO levels (22,23). Exhaled NO is reduced immediately after methacholine bronchial provocation challenge (24). It is therefore recommended that eNO be measured before bronchial provocation testing if both tests are to be performed on the same occasion.

Food and Drink

Guidelines recommend that subjects refrain from eating and drinking for one hour before eNO measurements to reduce the risk of food and or drink altering eNO levels. It is also advisable to question patients about recent food intake.

Smoking

Subjects should not smoke in the hour before the test and short- and long-term active and passive smoking history should be recorded.

B. Asthma vs. Normals

Studies consistently demonstrate eNO is elevated in children with asthma when compared to healthy control children. Exhaled NO levels in healthy controls is thought to range from 5 to 20 ppb. Because eNO measurement falls with ICS therapy (25), the elevation of eNO is seen in steroid-naïve asthma (25–29).

The absolute values of eNO that are reported in normals and children with asthma vary widely. This is a reflection of different collection and measurement protocols. This emphasizes the need for standardization in collection procedure and the development of normal values. Until this is done, each laboratory will be required to obtain their own normal values. Recently one analyzer has been approved by the Food and Drug Administration (FDA) for the assessment of eNO in human breath. The Aerocrine NiOX analyzer allows measurement of eNO at ATS-recommended flow rates in adults and children as young as four years of age.

C. Asthma Severity and Disease Status

Few studies have described changes in eNO with asthma severity. In one study Griese et al. (28) examined eNO in 74 children with allergic asthma whose disease was classified using symptoms and lung function according to National Institutes of Health (NIH) guidelines. No relationship was found between eNO and disease severity. In another study of 30 children with asthma, increased eNO levels were found with increasing asthma severity and there was also a correlation between eNO levels, asthma control, and compliance with therapy (30).

Studies that examine this relationship will be confounded by the effect of ICS therapy on eNO. As asthma severity increases, the likelihood that the child will receive ICS will also increase, and this will reduce eNO results. A recent study has demonstrated heterogeneity of eNO levels in children treated with ICS (15). Forty children were selected with stable asthma taking 400 µg budesonide daily. Half of these children had normal eNO and half had raised eNO. Children were randomized to receive 1600 µg budesonide or placebo. In the treatment group 25% of children had increased eNO despite ICS treatment and good clinical control.

Exhaled NO is increased after natural allergen exposure (31) and is reported to be increased in acute asthma (32,33) and after ICS withdrawal in asthma (34).

D. Effect of Therapy

The effect of several asthma therapies on eNO has been examined (35–37). These therapies reduce eNO, and based on reported data, the rank order of effects of treatment on eNO is: corticosteroids (inhaled and oral), omalizumab, leukotriene receptor antagonists, and cromones (Fig. 3). Levels of eNO are correlated with atopy (15,38) and the level of bronchial hyperresponsiveness (3,15).

V. Exhaled Breath Condensate

The measurement of exhaled breath condensate (EBC) is the most recent development in asthma monitoring technologies.

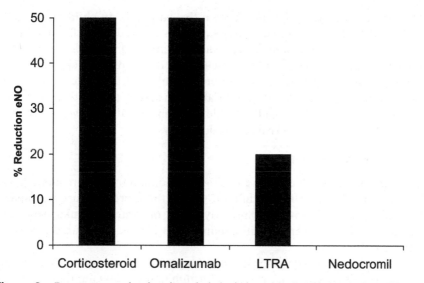

Figure 3 Percentage reduction in exhaled nitric oxide (eNO) levels for different treatments. *Source*: From Refs. 35–37.

A. Sample Collection

Exhaled breath, which contains water vapor along with respiratory droplets and aerosol particles, is condensed by cooling of expired air. These are collected and can then be assessed using conventional assays. The current methods for the collection of EBC vary primarily in the type of condensers that are employed. Simple systems using Teflon® tubing immersed in ice are common, however, the commercially available condensers such as the ECOScreen™ and RTube™ are growing in popularity. The physical surface properties of each condenser system may influence the condensate that is collected. Therefore, it is possible that there may be great variation between systems in terms of the particles collected.

Collection is simple and the main issue concerning collection in children is the ability of the child to use the mouthpiece properly and maintain tidal breathing for the time required to collect a sample (this is often 10–15 min) (39).

B. Reproducibility

The reproducibility of EBC inflammatory markers is controversial. In adults, levels of 8-isoprostane (a measure of oxidative stress produced from free radical peroxidation of arachidonic acid) and H_2O_2 have been shown to have poor reproducibility when samples were collected within the same week (40). However, another report suggests good reproducibility of

H_2O_2 when samples were collected on the same day. In children, repeated H_2O_2 measurements on two consecutive days showed a satisfactory within-subject reproducibility and stored samples remained stable for at least one month at $-20°C$ (41). However, H_2O_2 concentrations are dependent upon expiratory flow rate which is not often controlled in the collection of EBC, and this may explain some of the variability in results (42). Other markers of dilution such as sodium and chloride ion concentration have shown good within-day and between-visits reproducibility (43).

C. Measurements

Oxidative stress can be assessed using the biomarker 8-isoprostane. Levels of 8-isoprostane in EBC in children with asthma are increased compared to healthy controls (44,45). Similarly levels of cysteinyl leukotrienes and leukotriene B_4 are increased in children with asthma compared to healthy children (46).

Levels of exhaled cysteinyl leukotrienes and 8-isoprostane are increased in children during an exacerbation of asthma, and following treatment with oral corticosteroids, 8-isoprostane levels reduce but are still raised compared to healthy children (47).

Levels are no different in children with asthma treated with ICS and those who are steroid-naïve (44). Cysteinyl leukotrienes and 8-isoprostanes in exhaled breath and eosinophils in sputum are reduced after allergen avoidance in children with asthma (48).

VI. Conclusion

Inflammatory markers are needed to help with both diagnosis and treatment of children with asthma. Promising markers include induced sputum, eNO, and EBC. There are advantages and limitations to each marker. Induced sputum gives a measure that relates to disease activity and that predicts treatment response. This technique is limited by collection and measurement issues. Exhaled markers offer simpler collection techniques and the promise of point-of-care testing, however, clinical utility of these techniques remains to be established.

References

1. Green RH, Brightling CE, McKenna S, Hargadon B, Parker D, Bradding P, Wardlaw AJ, Pavord ID. Asthma exacerbations and sputum eosinophil counts: a randomised controlled trial. Lancet 2002; 30:1715–1721.
2. Pizzichini E, Pizzichini MM, Efthimiadis A, Dolovich J, Hargreave FE. Measuring airway inflammation in asthma: eosinophils and eosinophilic cationic protein in induced sputum compared with peripheral blood. J Allergy Clin Immunol 1997; 99:539–544.

3. Gibson PG, Grootendorst DC, Henry RL, Pin I, Rytila PH, Wark P, Wilson N, Djukanovic R. Sputum induction in children. Eur Resp J 2002; 20:44s–46s.

4. Pin I, Radford S, Kolendowicz R, Jennings B, Denburg JA, Hargreave FE, Dolovich J. Airway inflammation in symptomatic and asymptomatic children with methacholine hyperresponsiveness. Eur Resp J 1994; 6:1249–1256.

5. Twaddell SH, Gibson PG, Carty K, Woolley KL, Henry RL. Assessment of airway inflammation in children with acute asthma using induced sputum. Eur Resp J 1996; 9:2104–2108.

6. Jones PD, Hankin R, Simpson J, Gibson PG, Henry RL. The tolerability, safety, and success of sputum induction and combined hypertonic saline challenge in children. Am J Respir Crit Care Med 2001; 164:1146–1149.

7. Riedler J, Robertson CF. Effect of tidal volume on the output and particle size distribution of hypertonic saline from an ultrasonic nebulizer. Eur Respir J 1994; 7:998–1002.

8. Sorva R, Metso T, Turpeinen M, Juntunen-Backman K, Bjorksten F, Haahtela T. Eosinophil cationic protein in induced sputum as a marker of inflammation in asthmatic children. Eur Resp J 1997; 8:45–850.

9. Cai Y, Carty K, Henry RL, Gibson PG. Persistence of sputum eosinophilia in children with controlled asthma when compared with healthy children. Eur Resp J 1998; 11:848–853.

10. Gibson PG, Simpson JL, Hankin R, Powell H, Henry RL. Relationship between induced sputum eosinophils and the clinical pattern of childhood asthma. Thorax 2003; 58:116–121.

11. Douwes J, Gibson P, Pekkanen J, Pearce N. Non-eosinophilic asthma: importance and possible mechanisms. Thorax 2002; 57:643–648.

12. Norzila MZ, Fakes K, Henry RL, Simpson J, Gibson PG. Interleukin-8 and neutrophil recruitment accompanies induced sputum eosinophil activation in children with acute asthma. Am J Respir Crit Care Med 2000; 161:769–774.

13. Gibson PG, Henry RL, Shah S, Powell H, Wang H. Migration to a western country increases asthma symptoms but not eosinophilic airway inflammation. Pediatr Pulmonol 2003; 36:209–215.

14. Wark PA, Johnston SL, Morix I, Simpson JL, Hensley MJ, Gibson PG. Neutrophil degranulation and cell lysis is associated with clinical severity in virus-induced asthma. Eur Resp J 2002; 19:68–75.

15. Buchvald F, Eiberg H, Bisgaard H. Heterogeneity of FeNO response to inhaled steroid in asthmatic children. Clin Exp Allergy 2003; 33:1735–1740.

16. Szefler SJ, Martin RJ, King TS, Boushey HA, Cherniack RM, Chinchilli VM, Craig TJ, Dolovich M, Drazen JM, Fagan JK, Fahy JV, Fish JE, Ford JG, Israel E, Kiley J, Kraft M, Lazarus SC, Lemanske RF Jr, Mauger E, Peters SP, Sorkness CA. Significant variability in response to inhaled corticosteroids for persistent asthma. J Allergy Clin Immunol 2002; 109:410–418.

17. Kharitonov SA, Barnes PJ. Exhaled markers of pulmonary disease. Am J Respir Crit Care Med 2001; 163:1693–1722.

18. Baraldi E, Scollo M, Zaramella C, Zanconato S, Zacchello F. A simple flow-driven method for online measurement of exhaled NO starting at the age of 4–5 years. Am J Respir Crit Care Med 2000; 162:1828–1832.

19. Franklin PJ, Turner SW, Mutch RC, Stick SM. Measuring exhaled nitric oxide in infants during tidal breathing: methodological issues. Pediatr Pulmonol 2004; 37:24–30.

20. Kissoon N, Duckworth LJ, Blake KV, Murphy SP, Taylor CL, Silkoff PE. Fe(NO): relationship to exhalation rates and online versus bag collection in healthy adolescents. Am J Respir Crit Care Med 2000; 162:539–545.

21. Kroesbergen A, Jobsis Q, Bel EH, Hop WC, de Jongste JC. Flow-dependency of exhaled nitric oxide in children with asthma and cystic fibrosis. Eur Resp J 1999; 14:871–875.

22. Deykin A, Halpern O, Massaro AF, Drazen JM, Israel E. Expired nitric oxide after bronchoprovocation and repeated spirometry in patients with asthma. Am J Respir Crit Care Med 1998; 157:769–775.

23. Silkoff PE, Wakita S, Chatkin J, Ansarin K, Gutierrez C, Caramori M, McClean P, Slutsky AS, Zamel N, Chapman KR. Exhaled nitric oxide after β_2-agonist inhalation and spirometry in asthma. Am J Respir Crit Care Med 1999; 159:940–944.

24. Piacentini GL, Bodini A, Peroni DG, Miraglia del Giudice M Jr, Costella S, Boner AL. Reduction in exhaled nitric oxide immediately after methacholine challenge in asthmatic children. Thorax 2002; 57:771–773.

25. Malmberg LP, Pelkonen AS, Haahtela T, Turpeinen M. Exhaled nitric oxide rather than lung function distinguishes preschool children with probable asthma. Thorax 2003; 58:494–499.

26. Narang I, Ersu R, Wilson NM, Bush A. Nitric oxide in chronic airway inflammation in children: diagnostic use and pathophysiological significance. Thorax 2002; 57:586–589.

27. Silvestri M, Spallarossa D, Battistini E, Fregonese B, Rossi GA. How can we best read exhaled nitric oxide flow curves in asthmatic children? Monaldi Arch Chest Dis 2001; 56:384–389.

28. Griese M, Koch M, Latzin P, Beck J. Asthma severity, recommended changes of inhaled therapy and exhaled nitric oxide in children: a prospective, blinded trial. Eur J Med Res 2000; 18:334–340.

29. Bratton DL, Lanz MJ, Miyazawa N, White CW, Silkoff PE. Exhaled nitric oxide before and after montelukast sodium therapy in school-age children with chronic asthma: a preliminary study. Pediatr Pulmonol 1999; 28:402–407.

30. Delago-Corcoran C, Kissoon N, Murphy SP, Duckworth LJ. Exhaled nitric oxide reflects asthma severity and asthma control. Pediatr Crit Care Med 2004; 5:48–52.

31. Piacentini GL, Bodini A, Costella S, Vicentini L, Mazzi P, Suzuki Y, Peroni D, Boner AL. Exhaled nitric oxide in asthmatic children exposed to relevant allergens: effect of flunisolide. Eur Respir J 2000; 15:730–734.

32. Zanconato S, Scollo M, Zaramella C, Landi L, Zacchello F, Baraldi E. Exhaled carbon monoxide levels after a course of oral prednisone in children with asthma exacerbation. J Allergy Clin Immunol 2002; 109:440–445.

33. Tsai YG, Lee MY, Yang KD, Chu DM, Yuh YS, Hung CH. A single dose of nebulized budesonide decreases exhaled nitric oxide in children with acute asthma. J Pediatr 2001; 139:433–437.

34. Silkoff PE, Romero FA, Gupta N, Townley RG, Milgrom H. Exhaled nitric oxide in children with asthma receiving Xolair (omalizumab), a monoclonal anti-immunoglobulin E antibody. Pediatrics 2004; 113:e108–e112.

35. Covar RA, Szefler SJ, Martin RJ, Sundstrom DA, Silkoff PE, Murphy J, Young DA, Spahn JD. Relations between exhaled nitric oxide and measures of disease activity among children with mild-to-moderate asthma. J Pediatr 2003; 142:461–462.

36. Silkoff PE, Romero FA, Gupta N, Townley RG, Milgrom H. Exhaled nitric oxide in children with asthma receiving Xolair (omalizumab), a monoclonal anti-immunoglobulin E antibody. Pediatrics 2004; 113:308–312.

37. Bisgaard H, Loland L, Oj JA. NO in exhaled air of asthmatic children is reduced by the leukotriene receptor antagonist montelukast. Am J Respir Crit Care Med 1999; 160:1227–1231.

38. Strunk RC, Szefler SJ, Phillips BR, Zeiger RS, Chinchilli VM, Larsen G, Hodgdon K, Morgan W, Sorkness CA, Lemanske RF Jr. Relationship of exhaled nitric oxide to clinical and inflammatory markers of persistent asthma in children. J Allergy Clin Immunol 2003; 112:883–892.

39. Rosias PP, Dompeling E, Hendriks HJ, Heijnens JW, Donckerwolcke RA, Jobsis Q. Exhaled breath condensate in children: pearls and pitfalls. Pediatr Allergy Immunol 2004; 15:4–19.

40. Van Hoydonck PG, Wuyts WA, Vanaudenaerde BM, Schouten EG, Dupont LJ, Temme EH. Quantitative analysis of 8-isoprostane and hydrogen peroxide in exhaled breath condensate. Eur Resp J 2004; 23:189–192.

41. Jobsis Q, Raatgeep HC, Schellekens SL, Hop WC, Hermans PW, de Jongste JC. Hydrogen peroxide in exhaled air of healthy children: reference values. Eur Resp J 1998; 12:483–485.

42. Schleiss MB, Holz O, Behnke M, Richter K, Magnussen H, Jores RA. The concentration of hydrogen peroxide in exhaled air depends on expiratory flow rate. Eur Resp J 2000; 16:1115–1118.

43. Zacharasiewicz A, Wilson N, Lex C, Li A, Kemp M, Donovan J, Hooper J, Kharitonov SA, Bush A. Repeatability of sodium and chloride in exhaled breath condensates. Pediatr Pulmonol 2004; 37:273–275.

44. Baraldi E, Ghiro L, Piovan V, Carraro S, Ciabattoni G, Barnes PJ, Montuschi P. Increased exhaled 8-isoprostane in childhood asthma. Chest 2003; 124:25–31.

45. Zanconato S, Carraro S, Corradi M, Alinovi R, Pasquale MF, Piacentini G, Zacchello F, Baraldi E. Leukotrienes and 8-isoprostane in exhaled breath condensate of children with stable and unstable asthma. J Allergy Clin Immunol 2004; 113:257–263.

46. Cap P, Chladek J, Pehal F, Pehal F, Maly M, Petru VV, Barnes PJ, Montuschi P. Gas chromatography/mass spectrometry analysis of exhaled leukotrienes in asthmatic patients. Thorax 2004; 59:465–470.

47. Baraldi E, Carraro S, Alinovi R, Pesci A, Ghiro L, Bodini A, Piacentini G, Zacchello F, Zanconato S. Cysteinyl leukotriens and 8-isoprostanes in exhaled breath condensate of children with asthma exacerbations. Thorax 2003; 58:505–509.

48. Bodini A, Peroni D, Vicentini L, Loiacono A, Baraldi E, Ghiro L, Corradi M, Alinovi R, Boner AL, Piacentini GL. Exhaled breath condensate eicosanoids and sputum eosinophils in asthmatic children: a pilot study. Pediatr Allergy Immunol 2004; 15:26–31.

12

Imaging in Pediatric Asthma

TALISSA A. ALTES

Department of Radiology, Children's
    Hospital of Philadelphia,
Philadelphia, Pennsylvania, and
University of Virginia Health
    Sciences Center
Charlottesville, Virginia, U.S.A.

ALAN S. BRODY

Department of Radiology, Cincinnati
    Children's Hospital Medical Center
Cincinnati, Ohio, U.S.A.

I. Introduction

The clinical role of imaging in asthma is currently limited to the detection of complications of asthma and to the exclusion of alternative diagnoses. However, as imaging techniques are developed and refined, the role of imaging in asthma, particularly in asthma research, may expand. In the following, the technical considerations and clinical applications of the two most common imaging modalities for the evaluation of asthma are discussed. Chest radiography is the most widely used imaging modality in asthma but provides limited information. Chest computed tomography (CT) has the potential to provide more information, but due to the relatively high-radiation dose, should be used judiciously. Although imaging plays a limited role in the clinical management of asthma, the potential role of imaging in asthma research is expanding as existing technologies such as CT are refined and new imaging modalities for the lung are developed.

II. Technical

A. Chest Radiography

Chest radiographs are widely used in the evaluation of children with asthma and have several advantages over other imaging modalities. Chest radiographs are nearly universally available, easily performed, and low in cost. The radiation dose for a chest radiograph is very low, similar to the amount of radiation one is exposed to from background radiation every week.

Accurate image interpretation is dependent on correct positioning and lung inflation. Because cooperation is frequently limited in young children, image quality is highly dependent on the skill and experience of the technologist when imaging children. High-quality frontal and lateral images can be obtained in young children in either the upright or in the supine and decubitus positions. Various holders and positioning aids are available, but these are not required for high-quality images. From the age of five or six years old, conventional imaging techniques using upright postero-anterior and lateral radiographs can be used.

Computed radiography, a technology that provides digital images that are viewed on a computer screen, is replacing conventional film-based chest radiography at many sites. Reusable phosphor plates are exposed to X-rays and then read by a scanning laser. The resulting digital data is then transferred to a picture archiving and communications system (PACS) that stores and displays the image. The system resolution of computed radiography is less than that of film/screen radiography, but the resolution has been shown to be adequate for pediatric chest imaging at all ages (1,2). Image processing capabilities allow the reader to change brightness and contrast when interpreting the chest radiograph. This is useful both to correct an initially sub-optimal image, and to aid in the interpretation of high-quality images. This capability more than offsets the slight loss in resolution.

Even with optimal technique, lung volumes vary widely with chest radiographs. This limits evaluation of air trapping. Air trapping should only be diagnosed if both views show increased lung volumes. Similarly, basilar opacities and prominent lung markings are expected findings when lung volumes are low. These factors and the normal differences in the appearance of the chest radiograph in children of different ages require pediatric imaging expertise in order to avoid errors of interpretation.

B. Computed Tomography

CT uses a rotating fan beam of X-rays to provide a much higher level of anatomic information than can be obtained with chest radiographs. When thin slices are used, the axial sections obtained are similar in appearance to gross pathologic specimens. CT scanning is the imaging method of choice for imaging the airways and the lung parenchyma (3). Airways as small as 1 mm can be measured using current CT techniques (4).

CT scanning technology has improved dramatically in the last decade. Helical techniques move the patient through the X-ray beam in a continuous motion rather than stopping the patient for each section. Multidetector technology uses a thicker fan beam to produce multiple slices during each rotation of the X-ray beam. Together these two advances can decrease scanning time to less than 10 seconds for the entire chest. This technology also allows the use of thinner sections for routine chest imaging with resulting improvement in evaluation of the airways and lung parenchyma as well as improved quality of sagittal, coronal, and three-dimensional reconstructions.

An area of frequent confusion when ordering CT scans is the use of the term high-resolution CT (HRCT). HRCT scanning is a specific technique that typically uses 1–1.5 mm thick sections obtained at 10 mm intervals through the lungs at full inflation. Often expiratory images are obtained as well, usually at wider intervals. No intravenous contrast material is administered. This is a sampling technique that only evaluates a portion of the lung. The technique provides optimal evaluation of the airways and lung parenchyma. Because a thin section is imaged and an adjacent thicker section is not, any pathology that is not included in the thin slice will not be identified. In the case of asthma, this technique is appropriate for the evaluation of bronchiectasis and air trapping, both of which are not expected to be limited to an area small enough to be missed. The technique is not appropriate for the evaluation of suspected tracheal narrowing or a vascular ring, for example, where a crucial area could be missed, and intravenous contrast material should be administered.

Imaging young children requires either cooperation or control of respiration to obtain optimal images. Sedation is used less frequently with the new high-speed CT scanners, but may still be required. Lung volumes are much lower than full inflation in sedated children, which can limit image quality. In addition, expiratory images cannot be obtained which limits the evaluation of air trapping. A specialized technique called controlled ventilation CT has been developed that allows motion-free images at full inflation and at expiration on children from birth to three or four years old (5). This technique uses oral or intravenous sedation and mask ventilation and is currently available at only a few centers. Use of this technique is expected to increase.

An important consideration in using CT is the radiation dose necessary for the study. CT scanning is an important source of radiation exposure to the pediatric population (6). The radiation dose for a chest CT scan is at least 10 times that of a chest radiograph. Children are at a higher risk from radiation than adults, and receive a higher dose from the same amount of radiation due to their smaller size. Increased attention to CT radiation dose has caused many centers to decrease the dose used for the CT of pediatric patients. The radiation dose can be much higher if unnecessarily high-dose CT techniques are used, as when adult imaging techniques are used on young children. These radiation doses can be six times higher than necessary (7).

The amount of risk, if any, of the radiation dose from a CT scan is an area of debate, but most investigators agree that there may be a risk, and therefore measures to decrease radiation dose are appropriate. In addition, the use of CT scanning should be evaluated in terms of risk and benefit. It is widely agreed that the benefit of an indicated CT scan far outweighs the risk. It is incumbent upon all caregivers to be certain that appropriate techniques are used when CT scanning is performed on children and to avoid unnecessary CT scans.

III. Clinical Care

A. Imaging in Asthma

There is currently a limited role for imaging in the clinical care of children with asthma. In a recent volume of the Pediatric Clinics of North America devoted to asthma, there is no mention of imaging (8). There are, however, circumstances when imaging is very helpful in caring for children with wheezing and in those with a diagnosis of asthma. Many experts recommend a chest radiograph at the initial diagnosis of asthma to exclude other pulmonary pathology, but discourage repeat radiographs except when pneumonia is suspected or to exclude complications of asthma such as pneumothorax or pneumomedistinum. The role of CT is even more limited.

B. Mild Asthma

Imaging is not required in the routine care of children with asthma. Asthma care guidelines frequently do not mention the use of imaging (9,10). The typical appearance of the chest radiograph in asthma, with findings including air trapping, peribronchial thickening, and atelectasis, are non-specific (Fig. 1). As discussed previously, air trapping is often difficult to assess on chest radiographs. Chest radiographs are poor indicators of the severity of asthma, and can be completely normal in children with severe asthma requiring hospitalization. In a study of 371 children presenting with an initial episode of wheezing the chest radiographs were normal or consistent with uncomplicated asthma in 94% (11). In 20 of the 21 remaining children, the abnormality was pneumonia or atelectasis and one child had a pneumomediastinum.

If the diagnosis of asthma is questionable, or if the child does not respond to treatment, imaging may be helpful. In this case the primary use of imaging is to exclude other abnormalities that may present with symptoms of asthma. Figure 2 shows an example of a child with an esophageal foreign body who was seen several times for "asthma" before a chest radiograph was obtained.

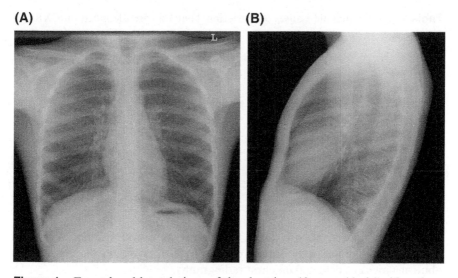

Figure 1 Frontal and lateral views of the chest in a 12-year-old girl with asthma show symmetrical hyperinflation and peribronchial thickening.

Table 1 lists some of the causes of wheezing seen on chest radiograph that can simulate asthma. Chest radiographs can also be helpful in evaluating complications of asthma including pneumomediastinum, pneumothorax, and severe

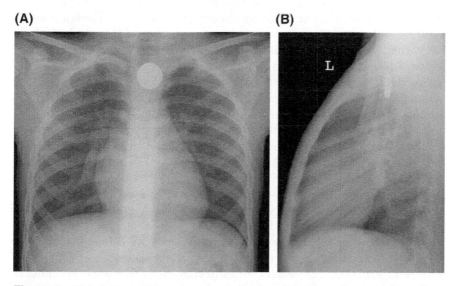

Figure 2 This 3-year-old boy was seen twice for wheezing and treated for asthma before this radiograph was obtained. Three coins were removed from the esophagus endoscopically.

Table 1 Non-asthmatic Causes of Wheezing That Can Be Identified on CXR

Extrinsic	Airway	Lung	Other
Esophageal foreign body	Croup	Pneumonia	Congestive heart failure
Vascular ring or sling	Tracheomalacia	Lobar emphysema	Cystic fibrosis
Mediastinal mass	Tracheal stenosis	Bronchogenic cyst	Immotile cilia syndrome
Neck mass	Airway foreign body	Bronchiolitis obliterans	Chronic lung disease of prematurity

atelectasis. There is no role for CT scanning as a first evaluation in mild asthma. CT scanning may be appropriate to further assess the chest when abnormalities are detected on chest radiographs.

C. Severe or Atypical Asthma

In severe or atypical asthma, the role of chest radiographs is more limited, while CT scanning assumes a greater role. While in many cases CT scanning will be appropriate whether the chest radiograph is normal or abnormal, chest radiographs are usually obtained prior to CT scans. The chest radiograph may identify an unexpected abnormality such as a foreign body or congestive heart failure that would not require a CT scan. If findings suggesting atelectasis or pneumonia are identified, CT scanning is usually better deferred until the acute abnormality has resolved. There are no clear guidelines for CT scanning, but a normal chest radiograph does not exclude abnormality on CT. In the case of a normal chest radiograph, HRCT is usually most appropriate.

The most common HRCT findings in adults with severe asthma include airway wall thickening, expiratory air trapping, inspiratory decreased attenuation, and bronchial luminal narrowing (12,13). Similar findings have been reported in children. Increased bronchial wall thickening in children with difficult-to-treat asthma was shown by Marchac and colleagues who measured the visible peripheral airways on three HRCT sections in the upper, mid, and lower lungs (14). In a study of children with chronic persistent asthma, low attenuation areas were found after three months of fluticasone treatment in 30% despite normalization of FEV_1 (15).

CT scanning can detect unsuspected bronchiectasis in children presenting with symptoms of asthma. Asthma was the most common presenting complaint in a retrospective review of 93 children with non-cystic fibrosis bronchiectasis (16). Chest radiographs were available in 87% and of these 76% of the chest radiographs did not suggest bronchiectasis. An etiology for the bronchiectasis other than asthma was identified in 82%.

A specific use of CT scanning is in the evaluation of patients with asthma and suspected allergic bronchopulmonary aspergillosis (ABPA). It has been suggested that ABPA is extremely rare in children except in cystic fibrosis (17). However, children as young as 12 years old have been diagnosed with ABPA, and it has been suggested that early treatment is important to decrease long-term damage (18). Central bronchiectasis is strongly suggestive of ABPA (19). Other findings include mucoid impaction and centrilobular nodules, both of which can be seen in uncomplicated asthma, but far less frequently than in ABPA (20). This is one of the few situations in which both conventional CT and HRCT may be needed to detect central bronchiectasis and centrilobular nodules, respectively.

Another disease process that can mimic asthma is bronchiolitis oblitterans (21). Except as a complication of therapy, bronchiolitis oblitterans in children is seen most often in the setting of Swyer-James syndrome. This postinfectious bronchiolitis oblitterans often shows a regional localization and is easily distinguished from severe asthma. In diffuse cases of bronchiolitis oblitterans the presence of mosaic attenuation and expiratory air trapping are much more often seen in bronchiolitis oblitterans than asthma (12), although the two diseases may be difficult to distinguish by CT scanning (22).

IV. Research Applications and Future Directions

Since findings on chest radiography are neither sensitive nor specific for distinguishing asthmatic from normal patients or for evaluating the severity of asthma, little research is being done with chest radiography in asthma. Chest CT provides an exquisite depiction of the structural details of the lung and can detect structural changes associated with asthma. There have been number of studies looking at the CT findings in asthma and their correlation with clinical parameters. An intriguing and as yet unproven hypothesis is that airway wall thickening on CT is related to airway remodeling. The use of computer-based image analysis algorithms with chest CT may provide new insights. While CT provides excellent structural detail, abnormalities of lung ventilation are typically inferred indirectly by assessing for areas of hyper-lucency or air trapping. On the horizon are two imaging techniques that directly provide functional information about the lung: positron emission tomography (PET) lung imaging with nitrogen-13 and hyperpolarized gas MR lung imaging. Neither are currently used clinically, but both show promise for the evaluation of lung ventilation and/or perfusion in asthma.

A. Computed Tomography

Clinically, CT is used primarily to evaluate for complications of asthma such as ABPA or to detect alternative diagnoses such as vascular rings or retained foreign body (Fig. 3). However, CT can be used to image the underlying disease process of asthma with the most common CT findings in childhood asthma being airway wall thickening, focal air trapping, and alterations in bronchial caliber. Other findings that have been observed in adult asthmatics, including mucoid impaction, emphysema, bronchiectasis, and linear scars, were not found in a study of 27 pediatric patients with difficult-to-treat asthma and may be the sequelae of long-standing asthma (14).

Airway wall thickening is a common finding in pediatric asthmatics (23) and was the only CT finding that correlated with asthma severity in a study of 39 asthmatics and 14 normal subjects (13). Further, airway wall thickness increased with increasing asthma severity in a study of adult asthmatics with a history of a near-fatal asthma attack as compared with mild and moderate asthmatics and normal subjects (24). Since patients with a history of a near-fatal asthma attack are thought to be at increased risk for airway remodeling, this suggests the airway wall thickening on CT may be related to airway remodeling. In a recent study, 45 steroid-naïve, asthmatic adults were imaged before and after a 12-week treatment with

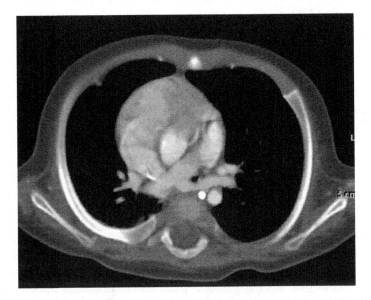

Figure 3 Axial contrast enhanced CT shows aberrant origin of the left pulmonary artery from the right pulmonary artery, a pulmonary sling. The left pulmonary artery courses between the narrowed distal trachea and the esophagus, which contains a NG tube.

beclomethasone. The airway wall thickness decreased 11% following treatment, but remained greater than that of 28 normal control subjects (25). Such studies have led to the postulate that airway wall thickening on CT, or perhaps persistent airway wall thickening, is related to airway remodeling.

At present, CT cannot distinguish among the many processes that could cause airway wall thickening including airway remodeling, airway edema, smooth muscle hypertrophy, smooth muscle contraction, and increased mucus on the mucosal surface of the airway. Some studies suggest that the apparent airway wall thickness is dynamic and changes following treatment with methacholine (26). In addition, the apparent airway wall thickness on CT depends upon the degree on inspiration. Thus further work is required to elucidate the relationship between airway wall thickness on CT and airway remodeling, but it seems likely that a relationship exists.

One of the difficulties with CT is that the imaging findings in asthma can be subtle and asthmatics can be difficult to distinguish from normal subjects (13,22). The above studies were performed with human reader scoring of the CT images. Quantitative chest CT, with computer-based image analysis algorithms, may be able to elucidate more information from the CT images than can human readers (27). In patients with emphysema, areas of low attenuation on CT (black areas) have been shown to correspond to emphysematous change within the lung (28). Quantitative CT has been used to measure the percent of emphysematous lung by computing the percent of lung pixels which have an attenuation value below a given threshold with the threshold selected as lower limit of normal lung attenuation.

Similar image analysis techniques have been applied in asthma, and asthmatics have been found to have more low attenuation pixels than normal subjects (29). Following methacholine challenge, the median CT lung attenuation decreased in 15 asthmatic subjects but not in normal subjects and returned to baseline following the administration of albuterol (30). This implies that the decreased lung attenuation in asthmatics is a dynamic process and is most likely related to changes in lung ventilation. Thus in asthmatics, particularly pediatric asthmatics, CT low attenuation areas are more likely the result of regional lung hyperinflation than tissue destruction as in emphysema. However, regional hyperinflation may not be the sole contributor to low attenuation regions. Areas of the lung that are hypoventilated may undergo compensatory vasoconstriction thus reducing the volume of blood per CT pixel. Since much of the attenuation of the lung on CT is due to blood, hypoperfused regions will also appear hypodense. Thus both hypoperfused regions and areas of focal air trapping will appear hypoattenuating.

Other more sophisticated CT image analysis algorithms are being developed. Some assess the regional texture of the lung, and these algorithms may bring new insights into the etiology of these low attenuation regions. Another promising area of development is automated segmentation of the tracheobronchial tree (31). This may permit a much more sophisticated assessment of bronchial diameter and airway wall thickness since the automated algorithm can analyze the entire portion of the tracheobronchial tree that is visible on CT. In addition to permitting a far more extensive evaluation of the tracheobronchial tree than is possible with human readers, such algorithms will likely produce more accurate results (32). It is expected that such algorithms will be useful in the elucidation of the relationship between airway wall thickening on CT and airway remodeling.

The radiation dose from a typical chest CT is as much as one year or more of background radiation. Since children are more radiation-sensitive than adults, it is problematic to use chest CT in research in pediatric asthmatics, particularly in protocols that require repeated chest CT scans. In a study of 203 children and young adults, little or no difference in radiologist reader image quality scores were found between high-resolution CT images obtained with the conventional high-radiation dose technique as compared with a low-radiation dose technique (33). Although image artifacts were not significantly increased at the lower radiation dose, image noise, which is known to be inversely proportional to radiation dose, increases. While human readers can read through image noise, the quantitative algorithms are more likely to be affected. The relatively high-radiation dose associated with CT will likely limit the research applications in pediatric asthma unless lower radiation dose techniques can be adopted.

B. Nuclear Medicine

Nuclear medicine techniques have historically been used to evaluate the regional drug deposition of inhaled medications. Conventional nuclear medicine ventilation perfusion scans have found little application in the clinical evaluation of asthma or in asthma research. A relatively new technique using nitrogen-13 as a radiotracer and PET scanning may be able to assess the regional ventilation–perfusion ratio (34,35). N_2 (^{13}NN) in a saline solution is intravenously injected and consecutive PET images of the lung are acquired during a breath hold (up to 60 sec). Since nitrogen has a low solubility in the blood, most of the radiotracer rapidly diffuses from the blood into the airspaces of the lung in a concentration that is proportional to regional perfusion, providing PET images of lung perfusion. Next, breathing resumes and additional images are acquired to assess the kinetics of radiotracer washout from the lungs. Regional ventilation can be computed from the rate of radiotracer washout. Combining the information, the regional ventilation–perfusion ratio can be computed. Preliminary studies in healthy volunteers demonstrate the feasibility of this technique in human subjects (36). Since abnormalities of ventilation and the associated abnormalities of perfusion are integral to the pathophysiology of asthma, a technique to non-invasively measure the regional ventilation–perfusion ratio may provide significant new insights into the disease process. However, due to the very short half-life of ^{13}N ($\sim$10 min), this technique will likely remain limited to major academic centers that have a cyclotron on site with which to produce the ^{13}N. Nevertheless, this is a promising technique, which may find application in asthma research.

C. Hyperpolarized Gas MRI

With conventional MR, the MR signal is approximately proportional to the physical density of the hydrogen protons in structure being imaged. Since the lung contains a large amount of air, it has a very low physical density relative to solid tissues and is, thus, much more difficult to image than solid tissues. On conventional proton MR images, the lung typically appears almost black because of the low signal generated by it. However, a new MR contrast agent, hyperpolarized noble gas, produces a large MR signal despite a low physical density. When a hyperpolarized gas is inhaled, areas of the lung that are well-ventilated contain a high concentration of the hyperpolarized gas and appear bright, whereas areas that are poorly ventilated contain little hyperpolarized gas and appear dark. Thus MR imaging following the inhalation of hyperpolarized gas produces MR images of lung ventilation. These images have much higher spatial and temporal resolution than conventional nuclear medicine ventilation images, and thus have the potential to provide more detailed information about lung ventilation (37).

Although hyperpolarized gas MR imaging is a relatively new field, the preliminary results in asthmatics are intriguing. Ventilation defects have been found in asymptomatic asthmatics with normal spirometry, and the number of ventilation defects correlates with increasing asthma severity as measured by spirometry or the National Asthma Education and Prevention Program of the National Institutes of Health (NIH) severity classification system (38–40). The number of ventilation defects increases following methacholine and decreases following albuterol treatment (Fig. 4) (41). Consequently, hyperpolarized gas MR imaging appears to be directly detecting the reversible airway obstruction that characterizes asthma.

Other mechanisms of MR contrast are possible with hyperpolarized gas including techniques that measure the size of the distal airspaces in the lung and that measure the regional ventilation–perfusion ratio (42). Very little work has been done applying these techniques to asthma. However, at least in theory, ventilation–perfusion ratio imaging with hyperpolarized gas MR may provide information similar to ^{13}N PET imaging. One advantage of hyperpolarized gas imaging is that there is no ionizing radiation. Currently, however, the technology to produce hyperpolarized gas is found at only a limited number of academic medical centers. If clinical or research

(A)   **(B)**

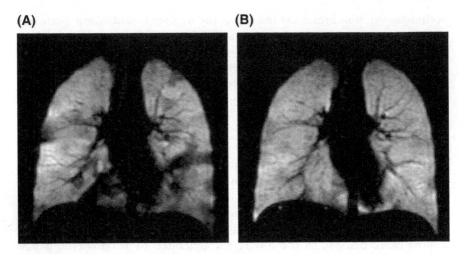

Figure 4 Coronal hyperpolarized helium-3 MR images from an asthmatic (A) before and (B) after treatment with albuterol. Multiple ventilation defects are present on the baseline image, which decrease in size and number following treatment.

applications for this technology were found, the cost of a gas polarizer is relatively low so this technology could become more widely available.

Further work is required to determine whether hyperpolarized gas MRI will find a role in the clinical care of asthmatics or in asthma research. However, the lack of ionizing radiation and the functional information provided make hyperpolarized gas MR imaging a promising modality for imaging pediatric asthma.

V. Summary

Chest radiography and chest CT are the mainstays of clinical imaging in pediatric asthma, but their role is primarily limited to the detection of alternative diagnoses or complications of asthma. The role of CT in asthma research may expand as improved methods for extracting information from CT scans are developed, and this may, in turn, lead to the expansion of the clinical utility of CT. Both chest radiography and chest CT provide information about lung structure, and typically lung function is inferred indirectly from secondary signs such as air trapping. Two new imaging modalities for the lung, ^{13}N PET scanning and hyperpolarized gas MRI, show promise for non-invasively providing functional information about the lung including regional ventilation and ventilation–perfusion ratio. This information may be useful in research to elucidate the underlying pathophysiology of asthma and to understand the response to treatment.

References

1. Kogutt MS, Jones JP, Perkins DD. Low-dose digital computed radiography in pediatric chest imaging. AJR Am J Roentgenol 1988; 151:775–779.
2. Tarver RD, Cohen M, Broderick NJ, Conces DJ, Jr. Pediatric digital chest imaging. J Thorac Imaging 1990; 5:31–35.
3. Teel GS, Engeler CE, Tashijian JH, duCret RP. Imaging of small airways disease. Radiographics 1996; 16:27–41.
4. Long FR, Williams RS, Castile RG. Structural airway abnormalities in infants and young children with cystic fibrosis. J Pediatr 2004; 144:154–161.
5. Long FR, Castile RG, Brody AS, Hogan MJ, Flucke RL, Filbrun DA, McCoy KS. Lungs in infants and young children: improved thin-section CT with a noninvasive controlled-ventilation technique—initial experience 1999; 212: 588–593.
6. Mettler FA, Wiest PW, Locken JA, Kelsey CA. CT scanning: patterns of use and dose. J Radiol Prot 2000; 20:353–359.
7. Paterson A, Frush DP, Donnelly LF. Helical CT of the Body: are Settings Adjusted for Pediatric Patients? AJR Am J Roentgenol 2001; 176:297–301.
8. Stempel DA, Spahn JD. The Pediatric Clinics of North America: Pediatric Asthma. 50. Philadelphia: W. B. Saunders, 32003:523–731.
9. Roy SR, Milgrom H. Management of the acute exacerbation of asthma. J Asthma 2003; 40:593–604.
10. Randolph C. A review of asthma care guidelines in the United States. Minerva Pediatr 2003; 55:297–301.
11. Gershel JC, Goldman HS, Stein RE, Shelov SP, Ziprkowski M. The usefulness of chest radiographs in first asthma attacks. N Engl J Med 1983; 309:336–339.
12. Jensen SP, Lynch DA, Brown KK, Wenzel SE, Newell JD. High-resolution CT features of severe asthma and bronchiolitis obliterans. Clin Radiol 2002; 57:1078–1085.
13. Park CS, Muller NL, Worthy SA, Kim JS, Awadh N, Fitzgerald M. Airway obstruction in asthmatic and healthy individuals: inspiratory and expiratory thin-section CT findings. Radiology 1997; 203:361–367.
14. Marchac V, Emond S, Mamou-Mani T, Le Bihan-Benjamin C, le Bourgeosis M, de Blic J, Scheinmann P, Brunelle F. Thoracic CT in Pediatric Patients with Difficult-to-Treat Asthma. Am J Reontgen Ray 2002; 179:1245–1252.
15. Pifferi M, Caramella D, Ragazzo V, Pietrobelli A, Boner AL. Low-density areas on high-resolution computed tomograms in chronic pediatric asthma. J Pediatr 2002; 141:104–108.
16. Eastham KM, Fall AJ, Mitchell L, Spencer DA. The need to redefine noncystic fibrosis bronchiectasis in childhood. Thorax 2004; 59:324–327.
17. Bremont F, Rittie JL, Rance F, Juchet A, Recco P, Linas MD, Dutau G. Allergic bronchopulmonary aspergillosis in children. Arch Pediatr 1999; 6:87S–93S.
18. Kumar R. Mild, moderate, and severe forms of allergic bronchopulmonary aspergillosis: a clinical and serologic evaluation. Chest 2003; 124:890–892.
19. Eaton T, Garrett J, Milne D, Frankel A, Wells AU. Allergic bronchopulmonary aspergillosis in the asthma clinic. A prospective evaluation of CT in the diagnostic algorithm. Chest 2000; 118:66–72.

20. Ward S, Heyneman L, Lee MJ, Leung AN, Hansell DM, Muller NL. Accuracy of CT in the diagnosis of allergic bronchopulmonary aspergillosis in asthmatic patients. AJR Am J Roentgenol 1999; 173:937–942.
21. Laohaburanakit P, Chan A, Allen RP. Bronchiolitis obliterans. Clin Rev Allergy Immunol 2003; 25:259–274.
22. Copley SJ, Wells AU, Muller NL, Rubens MB, Hollings NP, Cleverley JR, Milne DG, Hansell DM. Thin-section CT in obstructive pulmonary disease: discriminatory value. Radiology 2002; 223:812–819.
23. Ketai L, Coutsias C, Williamson S, Coutsias V. Thin-section CT evidence of bronchial thickening in children with stable asthma: bronchoconstriction or airway remodeling? Acad Radiol 2001; 8:257–264.
24. Awadh N, Müller NL, Park CS, Abboud RT, FitzGerald JM. Airway wall thickness in patients with near fatal asthma and control groups: assessment with high-resolution computed tomographic scanning. Thorax 1998; 53:248–253.
25. Niimi A, Matsumoto H, Amitani R, Nakano Y, Sakai H, Takemura M, Ueda T, Chin K, Itoh H, Ingenito EP, Mishima M. Effect of short-term treatment with inhaled corticosteroid on airway wall thickening in asthma. Am J Med 2004; 116:775–777.
26. Okazawa M, Muller N, McNamara AE, Child S, Verburgt L, Pare PD. Human airway narrowing measured using high-resolution computed tomography. Am J Respir Crit Care Med 1996; 154:1557–1562.
27. Bankier AA, De Maertelaer V, Keyzer C, Gevenois PA. Pulmonary Emphysema: Subjective Visual Grading versus Objective Quantification with Macroscopic Morphometry and Thin-Section CT Densitometry. Radiology 1999; 211: 851–858.
28. Muller NL, Staples CA, Miller RR, Abboud RT. "Density mask". An objective method to quantitate emphysema using computed tomography. Chest 1988; 94:782–787.
29. Newman KB, Lynch DA, Newman LS, Ellegood D, Newell JD Jr. Quantitative computed tomography detects air trapping due to asthma. Chest 1994; 106: 105–109.
30. Goldin JG, McNitt-Gray MF, Sorenson SM, Johnson TD, Dauphinee B, Kleerup EC, Tashkin DP, Aberle DR. Airway hyperreactivity: assessment with helical thin-section CT. Radiology 1998; 208:321–329.
31. Aykac D, Hoffman EA, McLennan G, Reinhardt JM. Segmentation and analysis of the human airway tree from three-dimensional X-ray CT images. IEEE Trans Med Imaging 2003; 22:940–950.
32. Saba OI, Hoffman EA, Reinhardt JM. Maximizing quantitative accuracy of lung airway lumen and wall measures obtained from X-ray CT imaging. J Appl Physiol 2003; 95:1063–1075.
33. Lucaya J, Piqueras J, Garcia-Pena P, Enriquez G, Garcia-Macias M, Sotil J. Low-dose high-resolution CT of the chest in children and young adults: dose, cooperation, artifact incidence, and image quality. AJR 2000; 175:985–992.
34. Rhodes CG, Valind SO, Brudin LH, Wollmer PE, Jones T, Hughes JM. Quantification of regional V/Q ratios in humans by use of PET. I. Theory. J Appl Physiol 1989; 66:1896–1904.

35. Vidal Melo MF, Layfield D, Harris RS, O'Neill K, Musch G, Richter T, Winkler T, Fischman AJ, Venegas JG. Quantification of regional ventilation-perfusion ratios with PET. J Nucl Med 2003; 44:1982–1991.
36. Musch G, Layfield JD, Harris RS, Melo MF, Winkler T, Callahan RJ, Fischman AJ, Venegas JG. Topographical distribution of pulmonary perfusion and ventilation, assessed by PET in supine and prone humans. J Appl Physiol 2002; 93:1841–1851.
37. Altes TA, Rehm PK, Harrell F, Salerno M, Daniel TM, de Lange EE. Ventilation imaging of the lung: comparison of hyperpolarized helium-3 MR imaging with Xe-133 scintigraphy. Academic Radiol 2004; July 11:729–734.
38. National Asthma Education and Prevention Program Expert Panel Report 2: Guidelines for the Diagnosis and Management of Asthma, National Institutes of Health, National Heart, Lung, and Blood Institute. NIH Publication 1997: 4051.
39. Altes TA, Powers PL, Knight-Scott J, Rakes G, Platts-Mills TAE, de Lange EE, Alford BA, Mugler JP, Brookeman JR. Hyperpolarized 3He lung ventilation imaging in asthmatics: preliminary results. J Magn Reson Imaging 2001; 13: 378–384.
40. de Lange EE, Altes TA, Alford BA, Mugler JP. Hyperpolarized helium-3 MR imaging of the lung in asthmatics: correlation of imaging findings with clinical symptoms and spirometry. European Society of Thoracic Imaging, Lausanne, Switzerland, June 14–18, 2003.
41. Samee S, Altes TA, Powers P, Knight-Scott J, Rakes G, Mugler, J, Ciambotti J, Alford B, Brookeman J, de Lange EE, Platts-Mills TAE. Imaging the lungs in asthmatics using hyperpolarized helium-3 MR: Assessment of response to methacholine exercise challenge. J Allergy and Clin Immun 2003; 111:1205–1211.
42. Altes TA, de Lange EE. Applications of hyperpolarized helium-3 gas MR imaging in pediatric lung disease. Top Magn Reson Imaging 2003; 14:231–236.

13

Pharmacogenetics: Will It Have a Place in Managing Childhood Asthma?

SCOTT T. WEISS, KELAN G. TANTISIRA, ERIC SILVERMAN, EDWIN K. SILVERMAN, STEPHEN LAKE, BRENT RICHTER, and ROSS LAZARUS

Channing Laboratory, Pulmonary and Critical Care Medicine,
   Brigham and Women's Hospital
Boston, Massachusetts, U.S.A.

I. Introduction

The purpose of this chapter is to describe the application of pharmacogenetics to asthma treatment in children. The essential principles that are necessary for clinicians to understand and apply existing pharmacogenetic data will be briefly reviewed. There have been a number of recent reviews on this subject that provide a more comprehensive coverage of this topic (1–4).

II. What Is Pharmacogenetics?

Pharmacogenetics can be defined as the study of the role of inheritance in individual variation in drug treatment response. The goal is to identify the optimal drug at the optimal dose for an individual patient. The underlying basis of pharmacogenetics is that there is a substantial inter-person (between person) variation in drug treatment response that is caused by genetic factors. In Figure 1, the distribution of children's lung function in response to inhaled steroids in the Childhood Asthma Management Program's (CAMP) long-term study of steroid effects on lung and somatic growth is shown. There are

10-15% of Asthmatics on Inhaled Steroids
Do Not Respond to Treatment

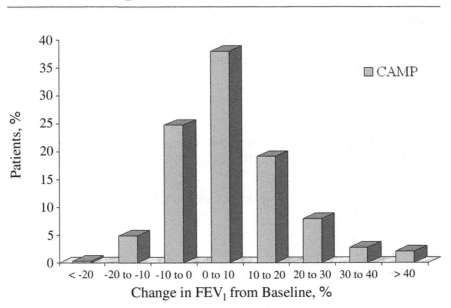

Figure 1   Frequency distribution of numbers of CAMP subjects by change in FEV_1 from baseline to 8 weeks of follow-up. Distribution shows the individual variation in treatment response to inhaled steroids.

individual children in this study that have significant improvement in response to inhaled corticosteroids while others do not. Some individuals appear to have had deterioration in lung function with inhaled corticosteroids. This heterogeneous response to drugs is typical of most therapeutic drug trials of asthma as well as most other genetically complex diseases. The major pharmacogenetics questions are: (a) how much of this inter-person variation in drug treatment response is due to inherited factors and (b) whether or not these factors can be identified and used to better treat asthmatics.

There are a variety of reasons for the observed between-person variation in Figure 1. The most common reason is non-compliance with medication use; however, a variety of environmental factors such as cigarette smoking, use of other drugs, presence or absence of disease, and intrinsic non-genetic characteristics of subjects, such as their age and gender, potentially contribute to between-person variations. Genetics remains an important individual factor in determining drug treatment response. It has been difficult, in the absence of family data, to determine what percentage of between-person variation can be considered due to genetics. At least one study suggests that up to 80% of between-person variation and treatment response in Caucasian individuals has a genetic basis (5). There are some data to suggest that components of endogenous glucocorticoid levels are heritable (6) but little data to suggest that asthmatic responses to exogenous glucocorticoids are heritable. More work must be performed to determine heritability of drug treatment responses in asthma.

There are three main pharmacogenetic mechanisms by which genetic variation influences response to medications: metabolism, adverse events, and pharmacodynamics. Genetic variation can be associated with some change in drug metabolism, i.e., altered uptake, distribution, or degradation of the administered drug. This is one of the classic mechanisms in pharmacogenetics (7), although no specific genes have been identified that influence asthma pharmacogenetics via this mechanism. An obvious asthma drug that likely has pharmacokinetic correlates is theophylline. Theophylline is metabolized by the liver and, hence, susceptible to degradation by liver enzymes, particularly the cytochrome P450 system. Obase et al. have suggested that promoter polymorphisms in the *CYP1A2* gene may affect theophylline clearance in Japanese asthmatics (8).

A second major pharmacogenetic mechanism is adverse drug treatment response. Genetic variants may predict which individuals are resistant to, or more susceptible to, the adverse side effects of a given drug. This mechanism is particularly important in cancer chemotherapy and, again, few studies of the side effects of asthma treatments have been established to have a genetic basis (8). Since the long-term use of high doses of inhaled corticosteroids may result in cataracts, decreased height growth, and reduced bone mineral density, it is interesting to speculate that there may be genetic susceptibility to these steroid side effects. To date, no data link any genes to adverse asthma medication effects.

A third mechanism by which pharmacogenetics may influence drug effects is through pharmacodynamics or the effects of genetic variation to altered drug efficacy or different expression in a particular drug response phenotype (i.e., the drug target itself). In asthma, the bulk of the work in pharmacogenetics performed falls into this category.

III. How Does One Determine Pharmacogenetic Effects in a Clinical Trial?

The standard approach to determining a pharmacogenetic effect in a human population is to perform a genetic association study within the context of a clinical trial. Data from a discrete arm of a clinical trial, given a single dose of a medication, for example, an inhaled corticosteroid, can be analyzed in two ways. The first approach is to examine genetic variation as a continuous linear predictor of outcome, for example, FEV_1 across all subjects in the trial arm as part of a continuous response distribution. This is a form of a cohort analysis. The second approach would be to compare large responders (those at the extreme right of Fig. 1) with those individuals who did not respond at all (the group to the left in Fig. 1) and ascertain which genetic variants are over-represented in one group or the other. This is a standard case-control study nested within an arm of a clinical trial. For asthma trials, the bulk of the studies performed focus on some measure of lung function as the primary outcome, either FEV_1 or peak flow. Alternative outcomes are quality of life assessment, functional status, symptoms, or health care utilization. All of these possible outcomes could be affected by genetic loci of pharmacogenetic importance, but for the most part they have not been examined in asthma pharmacogenetic studies.

In a genetic association study, some type of genetic variation, usually a single nucleotide polymorphism (SNP) is related to a drug response phenotype. SNPs are the most common cause of genetic variation in the human genome and are ubiquitous being found in exons, introns, promoters, and intergenic regions. There are thought to be over three million SNPs in the human genome and they occur in approximately one out of every 1000 base pairs, although this varies by the evolutionary history of self-designated ethnic groups. Their large number, relative ease at which they can be genotyped, and the ability to determine their association with other SNPs makes them ideal for genetic association studies. Other types of genetic polymorphisms, such as insertions, deletions, and repeats can also be genotyped and may be associated with altered therapeutic response; however, they are much less common.

IV. Methodologic Issues in Pharmacogenetic Association Studies

There are a variety of methodologic concerns about pharmacogenetic association studies and some are listed in Table 1. One of the major concerns in pharmacogenetic studies is that clinical trials tend to have restricted enrollment. By restricting to a subset of asthma patients, one may be more likely to demonstrate a significant pharmacogenetic effect; however, one may have difficulty in attempting to generalize these results to other outbred

Table 1 Issues in Pharmacogenetic Association Studies

Generalizability
Population stratification
Hardy–Weinberg equilibrium
Linkage disequilibrium
Sample size/power

populations not included in the clinical trial. Population stratification is the second major concern. This is simply different allele frequencies in the cases and controls as a result of genetic differences between the groups unrelated to drug treatment (i.e., different allele frequencies due to different evolutionary histories or different ethnicities in the cases and controls) rather than a true association between drug treatment response and genotype (9). Basically, this can be considered a form of confounding. To prevent against population stratification it is essential to have cases and controls that are well matched with regard to ethnicity and evolutionary history. Genotyping random SNPs across the genome in the cases and controls can ensure the investigator that the populations are genetically similar. A variety of methods using this form of genomic control have been developed to assess population stratification and, if necessary, to test correctly for association in its presence (10–12).

Hardy–Weinberg equilibrium predicts allele frequencies in a population under random mating. Testing for Hardy–Weinberg equilibrium among the control subjects gives some assurance that genotyping error does not account for an association or lack thereof and provides an independent check on genotype quality in the absence of family data. A recent study suggests that the majority of investigators do not routinely perform this helpful testing (10). Linkage disequilibrium is always a potential cause of a positive genetic association. Linkage disequilibrium occurs when two SNPs close together on a chromosome travel through evolutionary history together and during the process of recombination, these markers will tend to stay together as opposed to migrating to another region of the genome. Because of linkage disequilibrium, any observed association may not be due to that particular SNP or gene but to one that is nearby. This may be less likely to be true when one is looking at genes in a particular pathway as opposed to candidates in a linked region. Nevertheless, there is non-random association of alleles across the genome and this is a function of evolutionary history and genetic distance. Finally, and most importantly for asthma pharmacogenetics, is the issue of sample size. Table 2, drawn from a previous paper by Palmer and coworkers, shows the required sample size for cases needed to detect a true odds ratio or effect size of 1.5 with 80% power and type 1 error probability (α) of 0.05 (11). Relatively large sample sizes of upwards of 300 cases and as many controls would be necessary in assuming a dominant genetic model, as can be seen from this table. In cases where a recessive genetic model is most appropriate an even larger sample size is required to achieve significance. Ninety percent of all asthma clinical trials have less than 200 subjects per treatment arm. Thus, it is clear that sample size is a major issue in asthma pharmacogenetics. Because of all these methodologic concerns, replication of any positive result is critical to allow one to be confident that it is real.

Table 2 Sample Size Requirements for Case-Control Analyses of SNPs (Two Controls per Case; Detectable Difference of OR ≥ 1.5; Power = 80%)

Allele frequency[a] (%)	Dominant model[c]			Recessive model[d]		
	Exposure[b] (%)	No. cases required		Exposure[b] (%)	No. cases required	
		$\alpha = 0.05$	$\alpha = 0.005$		$\alpha = 0.05$	$\alpha = 0.005$
10	19	430	711	1	6,113	10,070
20	36	311	516	4	1,600	2,637
30	51	308	512	9	769	1,269
40	64	354	590	16	485	802
50	75	456	762	25	363	602
60	84	661	1,107	36	311	516

[a]Allele frequency in controls.
[b]Exposure (=prevalence) in controls assuming a diallelic locus with a dominant or recessive allele at Hardy–Weinberg equilibrium.
[c]OR of 1.5 between cases and controls for possession of at least one copy of disease-associated SNP by case.
[d]OR of 1.5 between cases and controls for possession of two copies of disease-associated SNP by case.
Reprinted from Palmer, L. J., and W. O. C. M. Cookson. 2001. Using single nucleotide polymorphisms (SNPs) as a means to understanding the pathophysiology of asthma. Respir Res 2:102–112.

V. Particular Issues in Asthma Pharmacogenetics Relating to Children

There are at least two issues relating to pharmacogenetics in children that are different from those seen in adult studies. The first is the issue of development. Lung development is under active hormonal control with corticosteroids, androgens, and other hormones playing important roles (13,14). Corticosteroids enhance the maturation of the lung in utero but may also function as growth inhibitors (15). Androgens tend to promote lung growth but may also inhibit lung maturation by antagonizing and inhibiting some of the effects of glucocorticoids (16). In addition, the lung continues to develop, making alveoli and growing in size in postnatal life (17). The full complement of alveoli is not reached until age eight or nine. Thus, the lung developmental process may be modulated by environmental events including drugs and must be considered. For example, both endogenous β-agonists and glucocorticoids, which are also the most common drugs used to treat asthma, influence this growth and developmental process in the lung. It is conceivable that insight into asthma and lung development could come from greater knowledge of pharmacogenetics because pharmacogenetic determinants may also affect asthma susceptibility and lung development.

A second issue of importance in asthma pharmacogenetics pertaining to children is that the vast majority of clinical trials occur in adults. Thus, if one is taking a genotype to phenotype approach, testing a variety of candidate genes in childhood asthma, the number and size of clinical trials is a serious limitation. This has the potential to inhibit the advancement of pharmacogenetics as a field. Finally, the distribution of asthma severity and type is different in children than in adults and it may be that factors relating to severe asthma may be more difficult to discern in populations of children because of the rare occurrence of severe childhood asthma. Alternatively since the prevalence of other allergic diseases such as eczema and hay fever are higher in childhood asthmatics than they are in adult asthmatics, factors relating to improvement in allergy may be more readily ascertained in studies of childhood asthma.

VI. Do Asthma Susceptibility Genes Have Pharmacogenetic Effects?

To date, there are four genes identified as asthma susceptibility genes by the use of positional cloning. Positional cloning is a technique where family based data is utilized to first perform linkage to localize a region of the genome that contains a gene that may be related to an asthma phenotype, and then, by adding additional markers, identify the susceptibility gene. This is time-intensive and laborious work; however, it has the advantage of identifying genes that are novel and may be unrelated to known asthma pathobiology. The first of the four genes identified is ADAM33, which is located on chromosome 20p13 (18). The associated phenotypes for ADAM33 are asthma and airway hyperresponsiveness. Three IgE-related genes, PHF11, located on chromosome 13q14 (19), DPP10, located on chromosome 2q14 (20), and GPRA, located on chromosome 7p (21) have also been identified and all relate to asthma and elevated total serum IgE level. None of these four genes have been assessed for their potential to influence pharmacogenetic treatment response phenotypes. Of these four, it appears that GPRA, located on chromosome 7p, appears to have the greatest likelihood of having a pharmacogenetic effect as this gene is a G protein coupled receptor similar to CRHR1 and the β2-adrenergic receptor. Assessment of these genes for pharmacogenetic effects is an important priority.

VII. Previous Studies of Asthma Pharmacogenetics in Children

A. Pharmacogenetics of β-Agonists in Childhood Asthma

β-agonists, either short-acting, such as albuterol, or long-acting, such as salmeterol or fenoterol, are the most commonly prescribed asthma medications. In addition, repeated mini epidemics of asthma mortality have been related to the use of this class of drugs. Thus, identification of genetic variants that could ultimately be used to predict treatment response or adverse effects would have immense clinical value. The molecular genetics of the β2-adrenergic receptor (β2-AR) gene and its molecular biology have recently been reviewed (22). β-agonists act by binding to the β2-AR, a cell surface G protein coupled receptor located on 5q31–32, and causing airway smooth muscle to relax. Linkage studies, which are those investigations that utilize family inheritance to attempt to localize chromosomal regions most likely to be associated with a disease trait, have implicated chromosome 5q31 as a region with an asthma linkage peak. Genes such as the β2-AR located within such a region are called positional candidate genes. This is a region of linkage for asthma so that it makes this particular gene a positional asthma candidate. The gene has been sequenced and a total of 13 polymorphisms and its translational regulator, β-upstream peptide, which regulates translation of the receptor, have been identified (23). Two coding polymorphisms at amino acid position 16 and the other at amino acid position 27, have been extensively studied. The Gly16 polymorphism exhibits enhanced down-regulation in vitro after agonist exposure (23). In contrast, the Arg16 polymorphism is more resistant to down-regulation and, because of linkage disequilibrium within the gene, individuals who are homozygous Arg Arg at position 16 are more likely to be Glu Glu at position 27. Individuals who are Gly Gly at position 16 are more likely to be Gln Gln at position 27. The position 27 genotypes influence but do not abolish the position 16 polymorphism's effect on down-regulation phenotypes in vitro (23). Israel and coworkers have shown that individuals who are Arg Arg and receive regular albuterol have reduced peak flows that continue beyond drug treatment (24). The magnitude of this effect in a population sense is relatively small. Arg Arg individuals represent 15% of the population and this variant explains approximately 5% of the variation in peak flow. In a random population sample, Martinez and coworkers studied acute bronchodilator response to a single dose of albuterol (25). The study group consisted of 191 normal children and 78 children with a history of wheezing, 37 of whom (47%) had a diagnosis of asthma. Children, normal and asthmatic, that were β-agonist-naïve showed a significantly greater bronchodilator response if they were homozygous Arg Arg. This is consistent with Liggett's conjecture that Gly Gly individuals are already down-regulated as a result of exposure to endogenous catecholamines and, thus, tachyphylaxis caused by recurrent exogenous exposure to β-agonist would be more apparent in the Arg Arg patients (23).

To date, in examination of these polymorphisms, there has been no large study of the effect of β-agonist in children. Recently, Silverman and coworkers studied β2-AR polymorphisms in the CAMP participants (26). The strongest associations were observed for the Arg 16 polymorphism with postbronchodilator FEV_1 either as a qualitative or a quantitative

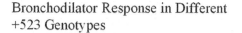

Bronchodilator Response in Different
+523 Genotypes

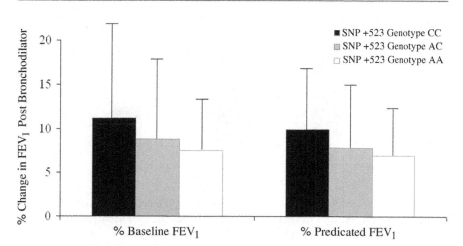

Figure 2 Percent change in FEV_1 postbronchodilator as a function of percent baseline FEV_1 (*left*) as percent predicted (*right*). Results are stratified by SNP genotype at position 523. CC genotype has the greatest response. AA genotype has the smallest response. *Source*: From Ref. 26.

phenotype. However, bronchodilator response was not determined by the polymorphism at position 16 but by a-SNP at +523 (relative to ATG start site) near the 3' untranslated region of the gene. Significant relationships were found for bronchodilator response expressed as a percent of baseline or percent of predicted FEV_1 (Fig. 2). This is significant since the 3' untranslated region of the β2-AR has not been sequenced for polymorphisms. Variation at this end of the gene may be significant with regard to bronchodilator response because it may influence mRNA levels by altering mRNA processing or translation. The CAMP data suggests that the 16 polymorphism is associated with lung function level; however, the 523 polymorphism is actually the variant important for bronchodilator response. The molecular mechanisms responsible for the association of polymorphisms in the β2-AR gene with asthma phenotypes are still unclear and more work needs to be performed to follow up these findings.

B. Inhaled Corticosteroids

Inhaled corticosteroids are the most common anti-inflammatory treatment used for asthma. Tantisira and coworkers recently performed a study of 131 SNPs from 14 steroid pathway candidate genes in asthma (27). The study design was to test these SNPs in an adult asthma study and replicate these

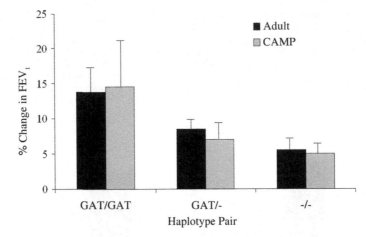

Figure 3 Percent change in FEV$_1$ at 8 weeks of inhaled corticosteroids in two clinical trials (Adult and CAMP). Results are presented by haplotype for *CRHR1* gene. Note that individuals in both trials who are homozygous for the GAT haplotype have a larger steroids treatment response. *Source*: From Ref. 27.

findings in the CAMP population of asthmatic children. Initial associations were seen with five genes but only one gene, corticotropin releasing hormone receptor 1 (CRHR1), was shown to have significant effects in both the adult and the childhood populations. CRHR1 is a G protein coupled receptor expressed in the anterior pituitary gland and is known to modulate endogenous glucocorticoid production by the adrenal gland. Thus, this gene could have two independent effects. Centrally, it could act to set endogenous steroid levels by regulating ACTH release. Peripherally, it could be involved in influencing inflammation in target tissues such as lung. Investigators focused on a three SNP haplotype in the gene, and have found that children who were homozygous for this haplotype had an improvement in pulmonary function of 21.8% at eight weeks of treatment, while children who are homozygous negative for the haplotype improved only 7.4% (Fig. 3). Work is ongoing to determine if other genes in this pathway contain sequence variants that alter response to asthma drugs. For example, corticotropin releasing hormone (CRH), corticotropin binding protein, CRHR2, urocortin 1 and 2, and stressocopin are genes related to CRHR1. Sequencing and genotyping of these genes are currently underway as part of the Pharmacogenetics of Asthma Treatment (PHAT) project.

VIII. Summary

At the present time, pharmacogenetics is in its infancy. It appears that pharmacogenetics does hold promise for issues related to childhood asthma.

In particular, the issue of steroid non-responsiveness is one that can be readily addressed with pharmacogenetics. However, the field is hampered by relatively small clinical trials and the absence of large effects due to any one gene or variant. It seems likely that continued methodologic advances will be necessary to allow for the elucidation of multilocus interaction of variants in several genes in a pathway, as opposed to one individual gene, or the interaction of multiple pathways (e.g., glucocorticoid and β-agonists) to be fully appreciated. In any case, existing data are certainly encouraging and further work will, hopefully, benefit patients.

References

1. Silverman ES, Liggett SB, Gelfand EW, Rosenwasser LJ, Baron RM, Bolk S, Weiss ST, Drazen JM. The pharmacogenetics of asthma: a candidate gene approach. Pharmacogenomics J 2001; 1(1):27–37.
2. Weiss ST, Silverman EK, Palmer LJ. Case-control association studies in pharmacogenetics. Pharmacogenomics J 2001; 1:157–158.
3. Palmer LJ, Silverman ES, Drazen JM, Weiss ST. Pharmacogenomics: the search for individualized therapies. In: Licinio J, Wong ML, eds. Pharmacogenomics of Asthma Treatment. Germany: Wiley-VCH, 2002:215–229.
4. Palmer LJ, Silverman ES, Drazen JM, Weiss ST. Pharmacogenetics of asthma. Am J Respir Crit Care Med 2002; 165:861–866.
5. Drazen JM, Silverman EK, Lee TH. Heterogeneity of therapeutic responses in asthma. British Med Bul 2000; 56:1054–1070.
6. Kirschbaum C, Wust S, Faig H-G, Hellhammer DH. Heritability of cortisol responses to human corticotropin-releasing hormone, ergometry, and psychological stress in humans. J Clin Endocrinol Metab 1992; 75:1526–1530.
7. Weinshilbaum R. Inheritance and drug response. New Engl J Med 2003; 348:529–537.
8. Obase Y, Shimoda T, Kawano T, Saeki S, Tomari SY, Mitsuta–Izaki K, Matsuse H, Kinoshita M, Kohno S. Polymorphisms in the CYP1A2 gene and theophylline metabolism in patients with asthma. Clin Pharmacol Ther 2003; 73(5):468–474.
9. Cardon LR, Palmer LJ. Population stratification and spurious allelic association. Lancet 2003; 361:598–604.
10. Pritchard JK, Stephens M, Rosenberg NA, Donnelly P. Association mapping in structured populations. Am J Hum Genet 2000; 67:170–181.
11. Reich DE, Goldstein DB. Detecting association in a case-control study while correcting for population stratification. Genet Epidemiol 2001; 20:4–16.
12. Long AD, Langley CH. The power of association studies to detect the contribution of candidate genetic loci to variation in complex traits. Genome Res 1999; 9:720–731.
13. Johnson JW, MItzner W, Beck JC, London WT, Sly DL, Lee PA, Khouzami VA, Cavalieri RL. Long-term effects of betamethasone on fetal development. Am J Obstet Gynecol 1981; 141(8):1053–1064.

14. Divers WA, Jr, Wilkes MM, Babaknia A, Yen SS. An increase in catecholamines and metabolites in the amniotic fluid compartment from middle to late gestation. Am J Obstet Gynecol 1981; 139:483–436.
15. Robinson BG, Emanuel RL, Frim DM, Majzoub JA. Glucocorticoid stimulates expression of corticotropin-releasing hormone gene in human placenta. Proc Natl Acad Sci USA 1988; 85:5244–5248.
16. McMillan EM, King GM, Adamson IY. Sex hormones influence growth and surfactant production in fetal lung explants. Exp Lung Res 1989; 15:167–179.
17. Reid LM. Lung growth in health and disease. Br J Dis Chest 1984; 78:113–134.
18. Van Eerdewegh P, Little RD, Dupuis J, Del Mastro RG, Falls K, Simon J, Torrey D, Pandit S, McKenny J, Braunschweiger K, Walsh A, Liu Z, Hayward B, Folz C, Manning SP, Bawa A, Saracino L, Thackston M, Benchekroun Y, Capparell N, Wang M, Adair R, Feng Y, Dubois J, FitzGerald MG, Huang H, Gibson R, Allen KM, Pedan A, Danzig MR, Umland SP, Egan RW, Cuss FM, Rorke S, Clough JB, Holloway JW, Holgate ST, Keith TP. Association of the ADAM33 gene with asthma and bronchial hyperresponsiveness. Nature 2002; 418(6896):426–430.
19. Zhang Y, Leaves NI, Anderson GG, Ponting CP, Broxholme J, Holt R, Edser P, Bhattacharyya S, Dunham A, Adcock IM, Pulleyn L, Barnes PJ, Harper JI, Abecasis G, Cardon L, White M, Burton J, Matthews L, Mott R, Ross M, Cox R, Moffatt MF, Cookson WO. Positional cloning of a quantitative trait locus on chromosome 13q14 that influences immunoglobulin E levels and asthma. Nat Genet 2003; 34(2):181–186.
20. Allen M, Heinzmann A, Noguchi E, Abecasis G, Broxholme J, Ponting CP, Bhattacharyya S, Tinsley J, Zhang Y, Holt R, Jones EY, Lench N, Carey A, Jones H, Dickens NJ, Dimon C, Nicholls R, Baker C, Xue L, Townsend E, Kabesch M, Weiland SK, Carr D, von Mutius E, Adcock IM, Barnes PJ, Lathrop GM, Edwards M, Moffatt MF, Cookson WO. Positional cloning of a novel gene influencing asthma from chromosome 2q14. Nat Genet 2003; 35(3):258–263.
21. Laitinen T, Polvi A, Rydman P, Vendelin J, Pulkkinen V, Salmikangas P, Makela S, Rehn M, Pirskanen A, Rautanen A, Zucchelli M, Gullsten H, Leino M, Alenius H, Petays T, Haahtela T, Laitinen A, Laprise C, Hudson TJ, Laitinen LA, Kere J. Characterization of a common susceptibility locus for asthma-related traits. Science 2004; 304(5668):300–304.
22. Raby B, Weiss ST. Beta-2 adrenergic receptor genetics. Curr Opin Mol Ther 2001; 3:554–566.
23. Liggett SB. The pharmacogenetics of β2-adrenergic receptors: relevance to asthma. J Allergy Clin Immunol 2000; 105:S487–S492.
24. Israel E, Drazen JM, Liggett SB, Boushey HA, Cherniack RM, Chinchilli VM, Cooper DM, Fahy JV, Fish JE, Ford JG, Kraft M, Kunselman S, Lazarus SC, Lemanske RF Jr, Martin RJ, McLean DE, Peters SP, Silverman EK, Sorkness CA, Szefler SJ, Weiss ST, Yandava CN; National Heart, Lung, and Blood Institute's Asthma Clinical Research Network. Effect of polymorphism of the beta(2)–adrenergic receptor on response to regular use of albuterol in asthma. Int Arch Allergy Immunol 2001; 124(1–3):183–186.

25. Martinez FD, Graves PE, Baldini M, Solomon S, Erickson R. Association between genetic polymorphisms of the beta2-adrenoceptor and response to albuterol in children with and without a history of wheezing. J Clin Invest 1997; 100:3184–3188.
26. Silverman EK, Kwiatkowski DJ, Sylvia JS, Lazarus R, Drazen JM, Lange C, Laird NM, Weiss ST. Family–based association analysis of beta2–adrenergic receptor polymorphisms in the childhood asthma management program. J Allergy Clin Immunol 2003; 112(5):870–876.
27. Tantisira KG, Lake S, Silverman ES, Palmer LJ, Lazarus R, Silverman EK, Liggett SB, Gelfand EW, Rosenwasser LJ, Richter B, Israel E, Wechsler M, Gabriel S, Altshuler D, Lander E, Drazen J, Weiss ST. Corticosteroid pharmacogenetics: association of sequence variants in CRHR1 with improved lung function in asthmatics treated with inhaled corticosteroids. Hum Mol Genet 2004; 13(13):1353–1359.

14

Asthma Education: Translating Knowledge into Action

JAMES Y. PATON

Department of Child Health, University of Glasgow
Glasgow, Scotland, U.K.

I. Introduction

Childhood asthma presents a paradox (1). While there have been striking advances in our basic understanding of the disease and in the development of effective clinical treatments (2–4), there has also been a substantial increase in the burden of childhood asthma (5) at a time when the prevalence and morbidity associated with many other childhood illnesses has been decreasing. Although recent years have seen a fall in hospital admissions and a decline in acute asthma consultations that may reflect improved treatment, asthma control remains unsatisfactory for many (6) (Table 1) and the negative impact on patients, their families, and societies remains enormous (7).

One conclusion has been that either clinicians are not delivering state-of-the-art care or patients are not following recommended therapies (8). This disparity between clinicians' knowledge and performance and patients' behaviors has been labeled the "asthma knowledge gap" (8). Asthma is not unique in modern medicine in having a large gap between what is known and what is done—a "know-do" gap. Indeed, it has been suggested that, overall, too much emphasis is placed on biomedical research and not

Table 1 The Global Initiative for Asthma (GINA) Recommended Goals of Asthma Management and Data from the Asthma Insights and Reality in Europe (AIRE Results) Study Showing the Results Actually Reported in 753 Children

GINA recommendation	AIRE result	Symptoms in children (%)
Minimal chronic symptoms	Daytime symptoms once a week	38.2
	Sleep disturbances at least once a week	28.0
Minimal episodes	Reported episodes of coughing, wheezing, chest tightness or shortness of breath in the last month	51.5
No emergency visits	Unscheduled urgent care visits during last year	36.0
	Emergency visits during last year	18
Minimal need for β2-agonists	Used as-required β2-agonists during the last month	61.0
No limitations on activities	Limitation of activities	
	Sports	29.5
	Normal physical activity	19.1
	Choice of jobs/career	–
	Social activities	13.8
	Sleep	31.2
	Lifestyle	18.6
	Housekeeping chores	10.9
	School/work absence	42.7
Normal or near normal lung function	Never had a lung function test	60.5

Source: From Ref. 6.

enough on translating what is already known into actions that improve people's health (9).

Education is of central importance, because it is a key process in bridging this "know-do" gap and in translating medical knowledge and understanding into action. For this reason, education has been moving to center stage in the management of many chronic diseases, including asthma (3,10).

II. Asthma Management Is a Complex Behavior

Since there is no known cure for childhood asthma, the current focus of asthma management is on disease control—controlling symptom, restoring function, improving quality of life and social functionings and providing optimal treatment with minimal side effects (2).

Achieving effective asthma control requires children and their parents to successfully carry out a number of tasks. These include using prescribed drugs correctly to control or prevent symptoms, identifying and, if possible, avoiding asthma trigger factors, developing necessary family or social supports and communicating effectively with health care workers (8). The frequent failure of clinicians to recognize and address the fact that these are all behavioral tasks is one of the main reasons put forward for the persistence of the asthma "know-do" gap.

Managing asthma is made more complex because asthma and its consequences change over time. Children and their families are most aware of these variations, and have to cope with them. In addition, children and their families have information, individual preferences, and beliefs that are complementary to the clinicians. It is clearly impossible for clinicians to provide direction for every contingency or individual circumstance that families might meet. It has become increasingly clear that in order to be able to respond to these variations, children and their caregivers must be able to alter their treatment in response to their own unique and varying circumstances.

All patients have had to self-manage their asthma to some extent, for example, by using reliever medication when necessary, but there has been a progressive move toward involving patients more in their asthma management. This has included involving them in self-monitoring of asthma and in self-adjustment of therapy in response to changes in severity. Such "self-management" is not the same as self-treatment. In self-management, the patient or family provides the individual context, while the clinician provides the general medical backdrop. Both are necessary for effective disease management (11). Ideally, an agreed, cooperative approach to asthma management should involve children, their families, and the health care team. This collaborative approach has been labeled "guided self-management."

In the past, clinicians often failed to recognize that asthma management was primarily a behavioral process. Asthma education frequently focused on transmitting knowledge rather than on changing behaviors. While changes in knowledge may be required before changes in behavior can occur, it is clear that knowledge alone does not result in behavioral change. Indeed, good health behaviors can occur without detailed knowledge (1,12,13). Consequently, patient education has gradually shifted from an emphasis on simply learning facts about the illness or practising skills, toward recognizing and facilitating the patient's central role in managing the disease.

The three most distinctive features of the guided self-management model are: (a) dealing with the consequences of the illness and not just the patho-physiological processes of the disease; (b) being concerned with problem solving, decision making and patient confidence rather than simply prescription and adherence; and (c) placing patients and health professionals in partnership relationships (14).

Self-management education complements traditional patient education in supporting patients to achieve the best possible quality of life with their chronic condition. Whereas traditional patient education offers information

Table 2   Self-management: Tasks and Skills for the Patient

Tasks
   Medical management
   Role management
   Emotional management
Skills
   Problem solving
   Decision making
   Resource utilization
   Formation of a patient-provider partnership
   Action planning
   Self-tailoring

Source: From Ref. 16.

and technical skills, self-management education promotes problem-solving skills (Table 2). A central concept in self-management is self-efficacy—confidence to carry out a behavior and reach a desired goal. Self-efficacy is enhanced when patients succeed in solving patient-identified problems (15). Accordingly, education to facilitate this self-management role must not only assist in gaining skills and the necessary knowledge, attitudes, and beliefs, but also develop the patient's confidence to apply these skills on a day-to-day basis (Table 3) (16). Programs for promoting self-management have been shown to improve health status and decrease health care costs in a variety of chronic diseases (17). The shift to self-management has reached its most developed form in the concept of the "expert patient," defined as one who has the confidence, skills information, and knowledge to play a central role in the management of his or her life with a chronic disease (18).

Children and their parents are not the sole target for asthma management education. There are many other professional groups with important roles in asthma care who require education and training. Indeed, preparing health professionals is turning out to be just as important as preparing the child or family. In the partnership necessary to deliver asthma care, both patients and clinicians must be adequately educated and effectively organized (19).

Table 3   Self-efficacy—Roles for the Teacher

Modeling or demonstration
Setting a clear goal or image of the desired outcome
Providing basic knowledge and skills needed as foundation for the task
Providing guided practice with corrective feedback
Giving students the opportunity to reflect on what they have learned

---

Source: From Ref. 28.

III. Does Asthma Education Work?—Evidence of Effectiveness

The importance of asthma education is now widely acknowledged (2,3,10). Asthma education, whether it be simple training in the use of inhaler devices or more extended programs, is now highlighted as a routine part of asthma care and is emphasized in published guidelines (2,3,10). But what evidence is there that asthma education makes any difference to the patient's experience of the disease or improves relevant health outcomes?

In adults with asthma, education limited to the transfer of information about asthma, its causes, and its treatment, without an action plan, self-monitoring, or regular review has been found to improve knowledge, but not to influence health outcomes (13). By contrast, more extended programs that include self-monitoring, of either peak flow or symptoms, coupled with regular medical review and a written asthma action plan, do improve relevant outcomes (20). These have included substantial reductions in hospitalizations, emergency room visits, unscheduled doctor visits, days off work or school, improvements in nocturnal asthma, and in quality of life. However, lung function was little changed (21). Training programs that enabled people to adjust their medication using a written action plan appeared to be more effective than other forms of asthma self-management. There is also evidence that the use of asthma self-management programs is cost-effective (22,23).

Whether such health outcomes can also be achieved in children has been less clear. A 1995 meta-analysis reviewing the impact of 11 randomized clinical trials of self-management teaching programs, published between 1970 and 1991 and evaluated as of adequate quality, concluded that self-management teaching programs did not reduce school absenteeism, asthma attacks, hospitalizations, hospital days, or emergency visits for asthma (24).

Since 1991 a large number of studies of self-management education in children and adolescents with asthma have been published. Wolf et al. revisited the question of effectiveness in 2002 in a Cochrane systematic review (25,26). By then, they were able to identify 32 randomized trials of adequate design involving 3706 children aged 2 to 16 years. Self-management education programs, when compared to usual care, were associated with modest improvements in: lung function, self-efficacy, reduced days off school and days of restricted activity, and fewer visits to the emergency department.

Subgroup analyses brought out a number of important additional points. Beneficial effects on lung function were seen within six months of starting the programs, but improvements in morbidity, self-efficacy and health care utilization were more evident after 7 to 12 months. While there were no direct comparisons between peak flow and symptom-based strategies, programs based on one or the other led to improvements in self-efficacy scales and reductions in emergency department visits. However, peak flow based strategies demonstrated greater improvements in lung function, and greater reductions in morbidity and health care utilization.

Group or individualized approaches had similar benefits on lung function, self-efficacy, and emergency department visits compared to usual care. Effects on morbidity measures were more marked in trials pooled for individual interventions, while programs targeted at groups had the greatest reduction on hospitalizations. Both single and multiple session interventions were associated with similar improvements in measures of lung function, exacerbations and days of school absence.

Finally, although there were no studies directly comparing subjects with different asthma severities, those programs targeted at subjects with moderate to severe asthma were associated with greater reductions in morbidity, health care utilizations and hospitalizations than those targeted at mild to moderate asthma.

Nevertheless, there were similar improvements in lung function and similar reductions in exacerbations between mild/moderate and moderate/severe subjects so that the effects of education were not confined to those with more severe asthma.

Thus, although there are still deficiencies, there is a substantial body of evidence demonstrating that asthma education has a significant impact on important outcomes in children with asthma. This evidence underpins and supports the central role of asthma education in published guidelines.

IV. Lessons from Research

Over the last two decades, a number of important lessons have emerged from research.

A. The Importance of a Theoretical Framework

Asthma education has frequently been based on an ad hoc set of messages and skills that health professionals believe patients need to know (8). Usually, these messages have been derived from an individual clinician's intuitions, traditions, or habits, and often the messages have been delivered using overly-didactic teaching methods. It is perhaps hardly surprising that there has been debate about whether asthma education works in practice. What has been required is a set of guiding principles based on evidence, or at the very least on successful practice (27,28).

The last two decades have seen the development of a substantial body of theory about health behaviors, how they are learned and how they should be taught. An important stimulus to their development was evidence that patients often fail to follow a wide range of prescribed treatment regimes (29). Initially, efforts were directed to understanding why patients did not comply with treatments, but over time the scope has been widened to include a range of activities that patients must undertake to manage their health problems effectively. Many theoretical models have been developed—theories such as the health belief model, stages of change theory, self-regulation theory, and social learning theory [see Clark and Becker for a brief review (30)]. All these theories try to understand the mechanisms that lead to behavior change. Their application to asthma reflects the growing appreciation that controlling asthma is not just about taking effective drug regimens but is also about the ability to manage the social and behavioral dimensions of the disease.

Clark and Valerio have noted that there is often haziness in the discussions of behavioral theories applicable to the control of respiratory disease (31). They have helpfully grouped theories into three categories.

Theories of Behavior

In this category, Clark and Valerio included theories that attempt to predict or explain why people behave as they do in relation to their health. Clark and Valerio included in this category theories focusing on psychological factors such as the health belief model (32) or the locus of control model (33) and also theories that address the interaction between psychological, behavioral and/or social factors such as the social cognitive theory (34) and self-regulation.

Conceptual Frameworks for Practice

In a second category, Clark and Valerio placed theories that provide conceptual frameworks for practice. These describe conditions within which interventions can be made to be effective. Examples include the transtheoretical (stages of change) model (35), Precede–Proceed (36), the social ecological model (37), and empowerment (38).

Theoretical Principles

In their final category, Clark and Valerio placed theoretical principles derived from successful programs. Successful theories often share a number of common elements. These elements can be distilled into core principles of "behavior change and health education," which can then be used to inform the design and evaluation of any asthma education program (Table 4) (27).

As successful interventions should be targeted on factors that cause behavior, the capacity of a theory to explain behaviors is important. One theory that has proved particularly relevant to the management of chronic illnesses such as asthma is social cognitive theory and its associated construct of self-regulation (34). This theory proposes that an individual's behaviors and perceptions influence and are, in turn, influenced by the surrounding social and physical environment. People make conscious judgments about their own ability to deal with different situations, and these judgments then influence what the person does, how much effort they invest in the task, how long they persist, and whether they approach the task

Table 4 Educational Principles That Should Be Included in an "Ideal" Asthma Education Program

Educational Principle	
Educational diagnosis	Involves identification of the causes of the behavior
Hierarchical approach	States that there is a natural order in the sequence of factors influencing behavior
Cumulative learning	Experiences must be planned in a sequence that takes into account the patient's past learning and his or her present learning opportunities
Participation or ownership	Behavior changes will be greater if the patients have identified their own needs for change and have actively selected a method or approach
Situational specificity	The effectiveness of any educational program depends on the individual circumstances and characteristics of the patient and the educator ("right audience, right time, in right way")
Use of multiple methods	A comprehensive behavior change program should employ different methods to take account of patient or situation specific factors
Individualization	Tailoring education allows interventions that are both patient and situation relevant
Relevance	The more relevant the content and methods to the learner's circumstances, the more likely learning and behavior will be successful
Feedback	Providing feedback allows the patient to adapt learning and response to his or her own situation or pace
Reinforcement	Behavior that is rewarded tends to be repeated
Facilitation	An intervention should provide the means to take action or to reduce the barriers to action

Source: From Ref. 27.

anxiously or with confidence. The motivation to change behavior arises from a judgment that undertaking an action will lead to a desired goal (outcome expectancy) combined with a judgment about an individual's ability to act (efficacy expectancy or "self-efficacy"). These judgments are suggested to arise from four main sources of information set out below in decreasing order of importance:

- personal mastery of a task or behavior (performance attainments),
- observation of other people (role models),
- verbal persuasion (from credible persuaders),
- physiological states (e.g., anxiety and stress associated with anticipating failure).

Successes raise a person's self-efficacy, while failures, especially if they occur early in the learning process and are not due to lack of effort or particularly difficult situations, lower it. Observing other people performing successfully in similar situations can strengthen a person's belief that they can perform a similar task. Verbal persuasion from a credible source can also help. These expectations and performances are not generalizable to all aspects of a patient's life, but relate to particular tasks.

Self-Regulation as a Key Health Behavior for Asthma Management

Clark and colleagues have drawn from both the social learning theory and self-regulation to develop a model particularly applicable to asthma management (8,30,39). Their model is based on three assumptions (Fig. 1). First, several factors predispose a person to manage a disease. Second, patient management arises from a conscious use of strategies in order to manipulate situations to reduce the impact of the disease on daily life. Third, illness management is not an end in itself but, from the patient's viewpoint, is simply the means to an end, such as the reduction of symptoms in a particular situation. Families can use self-regulation processes to observe how the disease prevents them from achieving their specific goals, to judge what type of action might help the situation, to experiment with behaviors, and to draw conclusions or react to the effects of those behaviors. Such an approach is clearly relevant to asthma where there is no definitive formula for optimum management, and where families often have to make their own decisions about changing treatments without immediate advice from health professionals.

Any educational program based on this model would not simply provide information about the disease but would focus on developing the subject's capacity to observe, to make sensible judgments, to feel confident, and to recognize good asthma outcomes (8). In this way, the theoretical

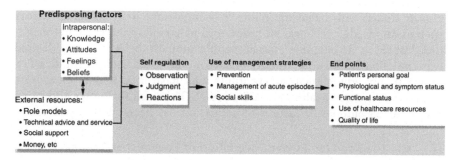

Figure 1 Model of patient management of chronic lung disease. *Source*: From Ref. 8.

model helps define both the aims and the curriculum for an educational intervention.

"There Is Nothing More Practical than a Good Theory" (28)

Increasingly, such theories have underpinned health educational interventions for asthma. Whatever the strengths or weaknesses of a particular theory, the use of a theoretical framework has a number of advantages. First, a good theory can help explain the mechanisms by which changes in a particular behavior come about. Consequently, it provides a basis for optimizing that behavior. When designing interventions, it helps focus on those factors that are likely to lead to the desired behavioral change. Second, if an intervention fails, the theory provides a framework for understanding why failure occurred and how it might be avoided in the future (8). Unfortunately, clinicians are often unaware of this body of theoretical work, and do not appreciate its relevance to their day-to-day clinical practice (40).

B. Measuring Effect—What Are the Outcomes?

Evaluating the impact of an educational intervention should be an integral part of any program. Such evaluation can be as simple as checking that a parent can use an inhaler after instruction by asking them to demonstrate the action, or even checking that education in the use of a device has actually been given.

If asthma management involves behavior, then, ideally, it is the behavior—what the patient or family actually does—that should be measured. Outcomes commonly measured are often either upstream or far downstream of the behavior that the educational intervention is intended to induce. Commonly used outcomes have included: lung function; measures of morbidity and functional status; measures of self-perception, such as self-efficacy and asthma severity scores; and measures of health care utilization (25).

Upstream measures such as tests of knowledge, attitudes, and feelings have frequently been used as proxies for behavior. However, none of these is closely linked with behavior. While it is important to understand factors such as knowledge, feelings, attitudes, and behavior, in the end what makes the difference in outcome is that people actually behave in the desired way, not that they know how to behave or hold particular attitudes (1). Downstream, educational interventions may have little impact on factors such as emergency health care utilizations. The need for better and more standardized outcome measures of education has been emphasized.

C. The Need for a Clear Description of Educational Programs

Surprisingly, what is meant by "asthma education" is not always clear. Many asthma education programs have been poorly documented making replication of the programs difficult or impossible. Furthermore, it may be difficult to identify the components within a program that which have been most effective in changing behavior. The need for a clear description of any program has been emphasized (25,41). Such descriptions should include the theoretical basis, a list of objectives, and a detailed account of what was done.

V. Translating Research into Practice

There are a number of key stages involved in translating research evidence into clinical practice (Table 5).

A. Planning the Intervention

For educational interventions to be successful, two elements seem to be necessary. The first element, the importance of basing the intervention on a sound theoretical base, has already been highlighted. The second element is the need for a systematic approach to the development of the intervention (27).

Increasingly, educational interventions draw on expert knowledge from a range of disciplines, such as behavioral psychology, health education, and teaching. While detailed knowledge of asthma and practical experience in dealing with children and their families are important. It is often helpful to have experts with the appropriate range of expertise contributing to the development of any intervention from an early stage.

There is now a wealth of material, both in primary literature and in more practical manuals, to help clinicians develop educational interventions (for example, Refs. 14, 27, 36, and 42–46). In the following section, only the key steps will be outlined.

Table 5 Key Steps in Translating Research into Practice

Plan the intervention
Perform a needs assessment and an educational diagnosis
Identify goals and define objectives
Detailed practical planning
   Select teaching methods
   Choose the setting and timing
   Who should be educated?
   Who should educate?
   Train the trainers
Successful implementation
   Anticipate and address barriers to successful implementation
   Evaluate outcome

Needs Assessment and Educational Diagnosis

The first step in any educational intervention should be a diagnostic one.

Performing an educational diagnosis does not need to be complicated. Methods such as interviewing families and reviewing local critical incident reports have been used to gain information about the needs of the target population (45,47–49). Frameworks such as "Precede-Proceed" provide extensive health education planning frameworks, and illustrate the preparatory work that may be required to identify health priorities and set objectives (36).

The logic of an approach in which diagnosis precedes intervention will be familiar to all clinicians. Nevertheless, the content of educational interventions has all too often been based on health professionals' preset agendas, without careful assessment of what patients needed or wanted to know. Lists of proposed topics to be included in educational interventions can be found in published guidelines (2,10). Although such lists reflect the accumulated experience of previous successful programs, they should not be implemented uncritically. It is not sensible, for example, to teach inhaler skills if such skills have already been acquired by the target audience (46). A diagnostic approach allows programs to be tailored to needs.

Identifying Goals and Defining Objectives

Educational goals should flow from educational diagnosis, and should define clearly and specifically what the intervention is supposed to address. The objectives represent the steps required to meet the goals, and can serve as useful headings around which to build up learning activities and lessons.

The importance of basing any intervention on a sound theory has already been mentioned. Once the theoretical base is clear, the focus can become more practical. An appropriate methodology can be chosen (27).

Detailed Practical Planning

Selecting Teaching Methods

Careful consideration should be given to the way in which the education will be delivered. Teaching can be carried out either individually or in small groups (50). Neither method has been shown to be superior but one approach may be more appropriate at particular times or for particular individuals. Wilson suggests that individual and group education may have different roles to play at different stages in a "continuum of education" (51).

Regardless of method, the emphasis should be on active learning with ample opportunity for practicing skills and receiving feedback.

Choosing the Setting and Timing

Individual teaching fits more comfortably into a clinic setting and more easily accommodates tailoring education to a particular individual's needs.

Return visits provide a good opportunity to reinforce the messages over time and to ensure that skills are maintained (52). Group teaching methods may be well suited for schools or for the peer group approaches used with adolescents. If successful, group approaches may be more cost-effective.

Timing of education can be another important factor. For example, education following an acute attack, particularly one of sufficient severity to necessitate admission to hospital, has proved particularly effective (53,54).

Who Should Be Educated?

Parents or caregivers have usually been the main target of asthma education. Often children and their parents are treated as though they were identical. In fact, when asked, children and their caregivers have different concerns about asthma: caregivers worry about acute attacks, while their children focus on the effects of asthma on everyday aspects of their lives (55). Gender differences may also be important, as there is evidence that boys and girls differ in how they incorporate asthma and its treatment into their developing social and personal identities (56).

Lewis and Lewis found two principal barriers to involving children in their care. First, some physicians were reluctant to share power with parents, let alone children, and second, some parents felt their role was threatened by sharing responsibility for management with their child (57). Simple interventions may help here. A brief video shown to children in the waiting room improved the rapport between the physician and the child, and encouraged the children to take a more active role in their own management (58).

If children are to be directly involved in asthma education then it is important that the education is developmentally appropriate and takes account of children's different learning styles. Peer-led approaches have been notably successful with adolescents (59). Involvement in asthma management education may actually have wider benefits for the child, with one study finding better performance and higher grades in children receiving asthma education than in controls (60).

Who Should Educate?

Asthma education has been delivered by a wide variety of people. In a hospital or clinic, it is usually a doctor or nurse. In a group setting, studies have used a behavioral therapist (42) or asthma educator. More recent work has used children's peers. Indeed, peer-led approaches appear among the most promising approaches for reaching teenagers (59,61). Recent research in patients with arthritis has shown that patients themselves can make very good lay educators (62). Whether such approaches will work in asthma is currently being studied.

The Importance of Training the Trainers

In a chronic disease such as asthma, the relationship between the patient or parent on the one hand and the health care professional on the other is recognized to be of central importance. Recent work has suggested that clinicians do not acquire the necessary skills in education and communication without training. Specific training for pediatricians in communication skills and asthma education led to significant improvement in prescribing and communications behavior, more favorable patient responses to the doctor's actions, patient–physician encounters that were actually of shorter duration, and reduced use of health care resources (63). Training for clinic staff improved the staff's ability to identify children with asthma, involve them in continuing care, and provide them with state-of-the-art care for asthma (64).

The combination of appropriate education, skillful trained professional input, and the use of anti-inflammatory medicine appears to be a powerful one in controlling symptoms and in reducing the use of health care resources.

Successful Implementation

Educational interventions have to be implemented effectively to be successful. What works on paper does not always work in practice. A number of key points can be highlighted.

Anticipate and Address Barriers to Successful Implementation

It is particularly important to try and anticipate barriers that may hinder implementation of the educational interventions. For patients, such barriers have included failure to recognize the range of social and environmental influences on patients trying to manage their disease, failure to assist patients in developing their self-regulation skills, lack of attention to the patients' asthma management goals (as opposed to clinician's objectives), and overlooking signs that indicate follow-up education is needed (65). Clinicians also face barriers either internal such as lack of awareness, familiarity, or agreement, or external arising out of environmental, guideline, or patient factors (66).

Early piloting can help identify many potential barriers. Formal monitoring procedures may be required if the intervention is to be implemented by other staff (46). Failure to identify and address barriers early can result in much effort being wasted and poor outcomes being achieved.

Evaluate Outcomes

A final, often overlooked part of any educational intervention is the need for evaluation. Evaluation should assess whether the processes planned were completed successfully, whether the desired behavior changes occurred, and, finally, whether desired outcomes were achieved. Only with proper evaluation can judgments be reached about whether the intervention's goals have been achieved.

VI. Educational Materials

Asthma education does not always rely solely upon direct contact with a health professional. Materials such as information booklets are commonly used—sometimes, without any other form of patient education, and at other times, to complement other types of patient education. The range of materials used has been wide—from a simple handwritten plan to the most sophisticated multi-media software programs.

There are huge and increasing demands from patients for medical information to supplement what health professionals tell them (67). At the same time, there has been a remarkable growth in the range of media available for delivering information, such as the World Wide Web and mobile phones able to receive short message service (SMS) text messages (68).

While materials may vary widely in sophistication and complexity, they are ultimately of value only if they achieve what they are produced to accomplish. Unfortunately, the quality of educational materials has been variable, and much is inappropriately targeted and poorly constructed. One study found faults in both the readability and accuracy of information leaflets used in a general practice: nearly half did not follow current U.K. asthma guidelines and the majority of leaflets were at least six years old (69).

To assist in compiling materials of real value to patients, a number of key questions should be considered (14,67).

A. Is It the Information the Patient Wants?

As in other areas of patient education, health professionals often assume that they already know what information families want. In fact, patients have clear but often different views. They want "life impact information" and information about "what to do when." Such information enhances their feeling of control over their lives, and is as important to them as more traditional information about diagnosis and treatment (70,71). Kai reported that parents of preschool children with acute illness wanted to know about the likely cause of the illness, any implications arising from the illness, its treatment, and the potential for prevention. Parents had positive suggestions for information that would be useful, particularly for inexperienced parents, for example, learning from other parents' experiences when dealing with the illness. Although parents wanted jargon-free information, they were keen that it should not omit important technical information that would facilitate understanding (72).

B. Does It Contain the Information the Patient Needs?

Again, health professionals usually assume they know what patients need. As a result, materials are often pitched at the wrong level, usually with too much detail. Practical information important for the patient may be omitted. The only sensible approach is to make sure that a careful needs analysis is conducted before any materials are developed, and that material is carefully piloted with patients before it is finalized.

C. Is the Information of Adequate Quality?

The variable quality of Internet websites has raised more general concerns about the quality of patient information (73). Information is not always of good quality, nor is it necessarily based on sound evidence. As a minimum, materials should include the date of preparation, the sources used, the qualifications of the author, and the sponsors of the information. That basic list gives the user some assessment of the likely accuracy of the information and some assurance of its credibility. Quality checklists are being developed, particularly for online materials (74). Unfortunately, such tools are not yet widely used, and few currently available materials satisfy the proposed standard.

D. Can the Patient Understand the Materials as Presented?

If educational materials are to be useful, they have to be understandable. Many adults have poor reading and comprehension skills. For example, it has been estimated that around one-quarter of the U.S. population are functionally illiterate, i.e., below fifth grade (approximately 10 years old) reading level, while another 25% have marginal reading skills (sixth to ninth grade reading level, 11–14 years). Poor reading skills are also associated with poorer health and greater use of health services (75). Many of the available pamphlets and information sheets about asthma are written at too sophisticated a level, well beyond the reading and comprehension abilities of most of the target population (76). When written communication is essential, material should be pitched at no higher than the sixth grade. In general, adults at all reading levels prefer, remember better, and learn faster from easy-to-read instruction (14).

E. Is the Material Presented in an Appropriate Format to Be Accessible to Its Target Audience?

A final point is whether the information is accessible to its target group. This is particularly relevant for children and for disadvantaged and minority groups. For minority populations, information will often have to be translated into languages other than English. In fact, minority groups are often particularly poorly catered for, and have to cope with material that is both difficult to read and culturally inappropriate. For children and many low-literacy populations, very simple brochures or comics are more likely to be understood. Information presented in alternative ways may be necessary, for example, audiotape or videotape for those with limited reading skills, large print for those with visual impairment or Braille for blind people (77).

With the development of digital technologies, rapid changes are occurring in the ways in which information can be delivered. Computer systems may facilitate tailoring information for the individual (78). Studies have already shown that supplementing conventional asthma care with multimedia education can reduce the burden of childhood asthma (79,80). However, the effectiveness of computer-based education (compared to more traditional means) needs robust evaluation, and newer methods will not always be better or cheaper (81). One randomized trial compared uptake and understanding about fetal anomaly scanning where some antenatal patients were given a touch-screen system while others were given a well-designed printed leaflet. The touch screen seemed to confer no better understanding of the tests and only a 7% increase in information uptake (82).

F. Developing Educational Materials—Simple Rules

It is clear that developing good materials requires a systematic approach. This includes:

- careful identification of the needs of the target audience,
- sensible limits being set on the educational objectives,
- a clear focus on desired behaviors,
- careful piloting.

In the end, there is no substitute for asking the patients whether the materials are "fit for purpose" (83). Thus, a key step in the preparation of any materials is careful field testing of the material with the target audience, to ensure that it is understandable and appropriate before it is finalized.

VII. Conclusion

There is now clear evidence that asthma education can be effective in providing children and their families with understanding, skills, and behaviors that allow them to control asthma more effectively, and to reduce associated morbidity. Education can also help patients and their parents gain the confidence to put these skills into practice. Consequently, asthma education is rightly recognized as having a central role in changing behavior in a way that ultimately leads to more effective asthma management.

The gap between "high technology" skills and "high touch" skills in asthma management has been noted, and may explain why childhood asthma morbidity has not improved more substantially despite advances in both diagnosis and treatment (27). Effective asthma education potentially provides a vital bridge between these two positions.

In the long term, better education is likely to bring substantial benefits to children with asthma and their families. The challenge now is to adapt and implement programs of proven effectiveness in clinical practice.

References

1. Clark NM, Starr Schneidkraut NJ. Management of asthma by patients and families. Am J Respir Crit Care Med 1994; 149:S54–S66.
2. Guidelines for the Diagnosis and Management of Asthma. National Asthma Education Program Expert Panel Report 2. National Asthma Education Program, Office of Prevention, Education and Control, National Heart, Lung and Blood Institute. Bethesda, MD: National Institutes of Health, 1997. Report No: NIH Publication No. 974051.
3. National Asthma Education and Prevention Program. Expert panel report: guidelines for the diagnosis and management of asthma update on selected topics—2002. J Allergy Clin Immunol 2002; 110(5 suppl):S141–S219.
4. The British Thoracic Society, Scottish Intercollegiate Guidelines Network. British guideline on the management of asthma. Thorax 2003; 58:1–94.
5. Akinbami LJ, Schoendorf KC. Trends in childhood asthma: prevalence, health care utilization and mortality. Pediatrics 2002; 110(2):315–322.
6. Rabe KF, Vermeire PA, Soriano JB, Maier WC. Clinical management of asthma in 1999: the Asthma Insights and Reality in Europe (AIRE) study. Eur Respir J 2000; 16(5):802–807.
7. Lenney W. The burden of pediatric asthma. Pediatr Pulmonol Suppl 1997; 15:13–16.
8. Clark NM, Gong M. Management of chronic disease by practitioners and patients: are we teaching the wrong things? BMJ 2000; 320:572–575.
9. Pang T. Filling the gap between knowing and doing. Nature 2003; 426:383.
10. British guideline on the management of asthma. Thorax 2003; 58 (suppl 1): 11–94.
11. Holman H, Lorig K. Patients as partners in managing chronic disease. BMJ 2000; 320:527–528.
12. McQuaid EL, Kopel SJ, Klein RB, Fritz GK. Medication adherence in pediatric asthma: reasoning, responsibility, and behavior. J Pediatr Psychol 2003; 28(5):323–333.
13. Gibson PG, Powell H, Coughlan J, Wilson AJ, Hensley MJ, Abramson M, Bauman A, Walters EH. Limited (information only) patient education programs for adults with asthma. Cochrane Database Syst Rev 2002; (2):CD001005.
14. Lorig K. Patient Education—a Practical Approach. 3rd ed. Thousand Oaks: Sage Publications, Inc. 2001.
15. Bodenheimer T, Lorig K, Holman H, Grumbach K. Patient self-management of chronic disease in primary care. JAMA 2002; 288(19):2469–2475.
16. Lorig KR, Holman H. Self-management education: history, definition, outcomes, and mechanisms. Ann Behav Med 2003; 26(1):1–7.

17. Lorig KR, Ritter P, Stewart AL, Sobel DS, Brown BW Jr, Bandura A, Gonzalez VM, Laurent DD, Holman HR. Chronic disease self-management program: 2-year health status and health care utilization outcomes. Med Care 2001; 39(11):1217–1223.

18. Department of Health. The Expert Patient: A New Approach to Chronic Disease Managemnt in the 21st Century. London: Stationary Office, 2001.

19. Sterk PJ, Buist SA, Woolcock AJ, Marks SB, Platts-Mills TAE, von Mutius E, Bousquet J, Frew AJ, Pauwels RA, Ait-Khaled N, Hill SL, Partridge MR. The message from the World Asthma Meeting. Eur Respir J 1999; 14:1435–1453.

20. Gibson PG, Powell H. Written action plans for asthma: an evidence-based review of the key components. Thorax 2004; 59(2):94–99.

21. Gibson PG, Powell H, Coughlan J, Wilson AJ, Abramson M, Haywood P, Bauman A, Hensley MJ, Walter EH. Self-management education and regular practitioner review for adults with asthma. Cochrane Database Syst Rev 2003; (1):CD001117.

22. Lahdensuo A, Haahtela T, Herrala J, Kava T, Kiviranta K, Kuusisto P, Pekurinen M, Peramaki E, Saarelainen S, Svahn T, Liljas B. Randomised comparison of cost effectiveness of guided self management and traditional treatment of asthma in Finland. BMJ 1998; 316(7138):1138–1139.

23. Liljas B, Lahdensuo A. Is asthma self-management cost-effective? Patient Educ Couns 1997; 32(1 suppl):S97–S104.

24. Bernard-Bonnin AC, Stachenko S, Bonin D, Charette C, Rousseau E. Self-management teaching programs and morbidity of pediatric asthma: a meta-analysis. J Allergy Clin Immunol 1995; 95(1 pt 1):34–41.

25. Wolf FM, Guevara JP, Grum CM, Clark NM, Cates CJ. Educational interventions for asthma in children. Cochrane Database Syst Rev 2003; (1):CD000326.

26. Guevara JP, Wolf FM, Grum CM, Clark NM. Effects of educational interventions for self management of asthma in children and adolescents: systematic review and meta-analysis. BMJ 2003; 326(7402):1308–1309.

27. Green LW, Frankish CJ. Theories and principles of health education applied to asthma. Chest 1994; 108:220S–229S.

28. Kaufman DM. Applying educational theory in practice. BMJ 2003; 326(7382): 213–216.

29. Sackett DL, Haynes RB. Compliance with Therapeutic Regimens. Baltimore & London: John Hopkins University Press, 1976.

30. Clark NM, Becker MH. Theoretical models and strategies for improving adherence and disease managment. In: Shumaker SA, Schron EB, Ockene JK, McBee WL, eds. Handbook of Health Behavior Change. 2nd ed. New York: Springer Publishing, 1998:5–31.

31. Clark NM, Valerio MA. The role of behavioral theories in educational interventions for paediatric asthma. Paediatr Respir Rev 2003; 4:325–333.

32. Janz NK, Becker MH. THe Health Belief Model: a decade later. Health Educ Q 1984; 11(1):1–47.

33. Wallston BD, Wallston KA. Locus of control and health: a review of the literature. Health Educ Monogr 1978; 6(2):107–117.

34. Bandura A. Social Foundations of Thought and Action: a Social Cognitive Theory. Eaglewood Cliffs, NJ: Prentice-Hall, 1986.

35. Prochaska JO, Johnson S, Lee P. The transtheoretical model of behaviour change. In: Shumaker SA, Schron EB, Okene JK, McBee WL, eds. The Handbook of Health Behaviour Change. New York: Springer, 1998; 59–84.
36. Green LW, Kreuter MW. Health Promotion Planning: an Educational and Ecological Approach. Palo Alto: Mayfield, 1991.
37. McLeroy KR, Bihean D, Steckler A, Glanz K. An ecological perspective on health promotion programs. Health Educ Q 1988; 15(4):351–377.
38. Stokols D. Establishing and maintaing healthy environments. Toward a socail ecology of health promotion. Am Psychol 1992; 47(1):6–22.
39. Clark NM, Evans D, Zimmerman BJ, Levison MJ, Mellins RB. Patient and family management of asthma: theory-based techniques for the clinician. J Asthma 1994; 31(6):427–435.
40. Hochbaum GM, Sorenson JR, Lorig K. Theory in health education practice. Health Educ Q 1992; 19(3):295–313.
41. Sudre P, Jacquemet J, Uldry C, Perneger TV. Objectives, methods and content of patient education programmes for adults with asthma: systematic review of studies published between 1979 and 1998. Thorax 1999; 54:681–687.
42. Colland VT. Learning to cope with asthma: a behavioural self-management program for children. Patient Educ Couns 1993; 22(3):141–152.
43. Howell JH, Flaim T, Lung CL. Patient education. Pediatr Clin North Am 1992; 39(6):1343–1361.
44. Kohler CL, Davies SL, Bailey WC. How to implement an asthma education program. Clin Chest Med 1995; 16(4):557–565.
45. Kohler CL, Dolce JJ, Manzella BA, Higgins D, Brooks CM, Richards JM Jr, Bailey WC. Use of focus group methodology to develop an asthma self-management program useful for community-based medical practices. Health Educ Q 1993; 20(3):421–429.
46. Madge P, Paton JY. Developing educational interventions for paediatric respiratory disease: from theory to practice. Paediatr Respir Rev 2004; 5(1): 52–58.
47. Mesters I, Meertens R, Kok G, Parcel GS. Effectiveness of a multidisciplinary education protocol in children with asthma (0–4 years) in primary health care. J Asthma 1994; 31(5):347–359.
48. Clark NM, Feldman CH, Freudenberg N, Millman EJ, Wasilewski Y, Valle I. Developing education for children with asthma through study of self-management behavior. Health Educ Q 1980; 7:278–297.
49. Wilson SR. Patient and physician behavior models related to asthma care. Med Care 1993; 31:MS49–MS60.
50. Wilson SR, Scamagas P, German DF, Hughes GW, Lulla S, Coss S, Chardon L, Thomas RG, Starr-Schneidkraut N, Stancavage FB. A controlled trial of two forms of self-management education for adults with asthma [see comments]. Am J Med 1993; 94(6):564–576.
51. Wilson SR. Individual versus group education: Is one better? Patient Educ Counseling 1997; 32:S67–S75
52. Gebert N, Hummelink R, Konning J, Staab D, Schmidt S, Szczepanski R, Runde B, Wahn U. Efficacy of a self-management program for childhood

asthma—a prospective controlled study. Patient Educ Couns 1998; 35(3):213–220.

53. Madge P, McColl JH, Paton JY. Impact of a nurse-led home-management training programme in children admitted to hospital with acute asthma: a randomised controlled trial. Thorax 1997; 52:223–228.

54. Wesseldine LJ, McCarthy P, Silverman M. Structured discharge procedure for children admitted to hospital with acute asthma: a randomised controlled trial of nursing practice. Arch Dis Child 1999; 80:110–114.

55. Callery P, Milnes L, Verduyn C, Couriel J. Qualitative study of young people's and parents' beliefs about childhood asthma. Br J Gen Pract 2003; 53(3): 185–190.

56. Williams C. Doing health, doing gender: teenagers, diabetes and asthma. Soc Sci Med 2000; 50(3):387–396.

57. Lewis M, Lewis C. Consequences of empowering children to care for themselves. Pediatrician 1990; 17:63–67.

58. Lewis CC, Pantell RH, Sharp L. Increasing patient knowledge, satisfaction, and involvement: randomized trial of a communication intervention. Pediatrics 1991; 88(2):351–358.

59. Shah S, Peat JK, Mazurski EJ, Wang H, Sindhusake D, Bruce C, Henry RL, Gibson PG. Effect of peer led programme for asthma education in adolescents: cluster randomised controlled trial. BMJ 2001; 322(7286):583–585.

60. Clark NM, Feldman CH, Evans D, Wasilewski Y, Levison MJ. Changes in children's school performance as a result of education for family management of asthma. J Sch Health 1984; 54:143–145.

61. Gibson PG, Shah S, Mamoon HA. Peer-led asthma education for adolescents: impact evaluation. J Adolesc Health 1998; 22(1):66–72.

62. Lorig K, Feigenbaum P, Regan C, Ung E, Chastain RL, Holman HR. A comparison of lay-taught and professional-taught arthritis self-management courses. J Rheumatol 1986; 13(4):763–767.

63. Clark NM, Gong M, Schork MA, Evans D, Roloff D, Hurwitz M, Maiman L, Mellins RB. Impact of education for physicians on patient outcomes. Pediatrics 1998; 101(5):831–836.

64. Evans D, Mellins R, Lobach K, Ramos-Bonoan C, Pinkett-Heller M, Wiesemann S, et al. Improving care for minority children with asthma: professional education in public health clinics [see comments]. Pediatrics 1997; 99(2):157–164.

65. Clark NM, Partridge MR. Strengthening asthma education to enhance disease control. Chest 2002; 121(5):1661–1669.

66. Cabana MD, Rand CS, Becher OJ, Rubin HR. Reasons for pediatrician nonadherence to asthma guidelines. Arch Pediatr Adolesc Med 2001; 155(9): 1057–1062.

67. Partridge MR, Hill SR. Enhancing care for people with asthma: the role of communication, education, training and self-management. 1998 World Asthma Meeting Education and Delivery of Care Working Group. Eur Respir J 2000; 16(2):333–348.

68. Neville R, Greene A, McLeod J, Tracy A, Surie J. Mobile phone text messaging can help young people manage asthma. BMJ 2002; 325(7364):600.

69. Smith H, Gooding S, Brown R, Frew A. Evaluation of readability and accuracy of information leaflets in general practice for patients with asthma. BMJ 1998; 317(7153):264–265.
70. Dennis KE. Patients' control and the information imperative: clarification and confirmation. Nursing Res 1990; 39:162–166.
71. Clark CR. Creating information messages for health care procedures. Patient Educ Couns 1997; 30:162–166.
72. Kai J. Parents' difficulties and information needs in coping with acute illness in preschool children: a qualitative study. BMJ 1996; 313:987–990.
73. Jadad AR, Gagliardi A. Rating health information on the internet; navigating to knowledge or babel? JAMA 1998; 279:611–614.
74. Charnock D, Shepperd S. DISCERN Online—quality criteria for consumer health information. http://www discern org uk/1999 OctoberAvailable from: URL: http://www.discern.org.uk/
75. Communicating with patients who have limited literacy skills. Report of the National Work Group on Literacy and Health. J Fam Pract 1998; 46(2): 168–176.
76. Davis TC, Mayeaux EJ, Fredrickson D, Bocchini JAJ, Jackson RH, Murphy PW. Reading ability of parents compared with reading level of pediatric patient education materials. Pediatrics 1994; 93(3):460–468.
77. Raynor DK, Yerassimou N. Medicines information—leaving blind people behind? BMJ 1997; 315(7103):268
78. Osman LM, Abdalla MI, Beattie JA, Ross SJ, Russell IT, Friend JA, Legge JS, Douglas JG. Reducing hospital admission through computer supported education for asthma patients. Grampian Asthma Study of Integrated Care (GRASSIC) [see comments]. BMJ 1994; 308(6928):568–571.
79. Krishna S, Francisco BD, Balas EA, Konig P, Graff GR, Madsen RW. Internet-enabled interactive multimedia asthma education program: a randomized trial. Pediatrics 2003; 111(3):503–510.
80. Guendelman S, Meade K, Benson M, Chen YQ, Samuels S. Improving asthma outcomes and self-management behaviors of inner-city children: a randomized trial of the Health Buddy interactive device and an asthma diary. Arch Pediatr Adolesc Med 2002; 156(2):114–120.
81. Homer C, Susskind O, Alpert HR, Owusu M, Schneider L, Rappaport LA, Rubin DH. An evaluation of an innovative multimedia educational software program for asthma management: report of a randomized, controlled trial. Pediatrics 2000; 106(1 pt 2):210–215.
82. Graham W, Smith P, Kamal A, Fitzmaurice A, Smith N, Hamilton N. Randomised controlled trial comparing effectiveness of touch screen system with leaflet for providing women with information on prenatal tests. BMJ 2000; 320(7228):155–160.
83. Wyatt JC. Information for patients. J R Soc Med 2000; 93(9):467–471.

15

Managing Childhood Asthma: Evolving Guidelines

ALLAN BECKER

Section of Allergy and Clinical Immunology, Department of Pediatrics and
  Child Health, University of Manitoba
Winnipeg, Manitoba, Canada

I. Introduction

Over the past few decades asthma has become an increasing public health problem (1,2). An increased prevalence of asthma was particularly apparent in children in many high-income countries, including Canada (2), the United Kingdom (3), and the United States (4). Through the 1970s and 1980s, increasing numbers of children required admission to hospital for asthma, suggesting that not only had the prevalence of asthma increased but also that the severity of asthma was increasing (5,6). Of major concern, deaths due to asthma, even among children, also appeared to be increasing during this time (7,8). The change in asthma prevalence, morbidity, and mortality increased awareness in the growing community of asthma specialists of the need for a more systematic approach to diagnosis and management of this common disease.

In parallel with the increasing prevalence, morbidity, and mortality of asthma, researchers began to better define the importance of airway inflammation and allergy in asthma. Thus began the "asthma paradox"; that is, as we were better able to understand the disease process and the underlying pathophysiology of asthma, morbidity and mortality from asthma continued to increase in spite of the availability of better therapeutic management options. This conundrum provided the impetus for specialists in asthma to convene expert consensus meetings from which a series of recommendations arose resulting in a number of publications focused on the assessment and treatment of asthma (9–13). These publications were presented as guidelines and were recognized as standards of treatment for asthma by the early 1990s.

Among these original publications, one (10) had a substantive focus on the issues of asthma in childhood and within a few years was already updated (14). This chapter considers factors important in the evolution of guidelines for the diagnosis and management of asthma focused on issues of importance to physicians and other health care professionals who deal with children and their families.

The past few decades have provided a great deal of rationale for development of guidelines and specifically for development of guidelines focused on asthma in children. There are a number of factors to consider in the evolution of guidelines development. These factors include, but are not limited to, the following:

- improved understanding of the pathophysiology of asthma,
- increased awareness of the heterogeneity of asthma, particularly in childhood,
- increased awareness of the onset of asthma in early childhood,
- new medications and approach to pharmacological management of asthma,
- evolving concepts of guidelines,
- dissemination and implementation of guideline recommendations.

Many of these factors are dealt with in much greater depth elsewhere in this publication. However, specific issues that have been instrumental in shaping our understanding of asthma and the subsequent development and evolution of guidelines will be considered.

A. Improved Understanding of the Pathophysiology of Asthma

It is now almost 50 years since the first "expert group" defined asthma as a clinical disease process characterized by airway obstruction that is reversible either spontaneously or with treatment (15). In 1980, an editorial by Nicholas Gross entitled "What is this thing called love?—Or, defining asthma (16)," pointed out the importance of recognizing the heterogeneity of a disease wherein the physiologist, pathologist and clinician each has his own focus of the disease process.

As subsequent research began to better identify the importance of chronic airway inflammation an updated working definition of asthma recognized that: "asthma is a lung disease with the following characteristics:

(1) airway obstruction is reversible either spontaneously or with treatment, (2) airway inflammation, and (3) increased airway responsiveness to a variety of stimuli (13)." More recent definitions, including those from the International Consensus Report (17) and the Global Initiative for Asthma (GINA) (18), further specified the important role of mast cells, eosinophils, and T-lymphocytes in the inflammatory process.

Recognition of the importance of chronic inflammation in asthma lead to a shift in principles of asthma management away from the use of short acting symptom relief medication and toward control of disease by attempts to control airway inflammation. This is exemplified by an early publication from Hargreave et al. of recommendations in a conference report (11), which resulted from a meeting of asthma experts from around the world. They stated that disease control could be accomplished by avoidance of potentially harmful factors, including allergens and irritants, and the appropriate use of anti-inflammatory medication (11). They also specifically stressed the need for treatment to be outcome-oriented in order to achieve and maintain control of asthma. The authors listed parameters they believed important to define control of asthma (Table 1) that were similar to a subsequent publication, which listed the "Goals of therapy" defined by the National Asthma Education Program Expert Panel Report (13). A modified version of the asthma control parameters (Table 2) was published in the 1996 update of the Canadian Asthma Consensus Report (19) and formed the basis of the "Asthma in Canada" study (20). This telephone survey of 1001 adults with asthma or parents of children with asthma used six of the control parameters, which could be questioned by telephone. The survey noted that although 91% of patients thought they had good asthma control, 57% had poor control defined as failing two or more of these parameters for acceptable control. This survey demonstrated that those patients who experienced poor control were significantly more likely to require urgent care or hospitalization in the past

Table 1 Definition of Control of Asthma

1. Minimal symptoms and ideally none
2. Normal activities of daily living (work, school, and recreational exercise)
3. Inhaled β-agonist needed not more than twice daily and ideally none
4. Airflow rates normal or near normal at rest
5. Airflow rates normal after inhaled β-agonist
6. Daily variation of PEFR[a] <20% and ideally <10%
7. Minimal side effects from medications

Abbreviation: PEFR, Peak expiratory flow rate.
Source: From Ref. 11.

Table 2 Criteria for Asthma Control

Parameters	Good control	Acceptable control
Daytime symptoms	None	<3 days/week
Nighttime symptoms	Not awakened	<1 night/week
Physical activity	Normal	Normal
Exacerbations	None	Mild and infrequent
Absenteeism	None	None
Need for prn β_2-agonist	None[a]	<3 doses/week
FEV_1; FEV_1/FVC	Normal	90% personal best
PEF	Normal	90% personal best
PEF variability	<10% diurnal variation[b] 5 days/week	<15% diurnal variation 5 days/week

[a]May use one dose per day for prevention of exercise-induced symptoms.
[b]Diurnal variation is calculated as the highest minus the lowest divided by the highest PEF multiplied by 100.
Abbreviations: FEV_1, Forced expiratory volume in 1s; FVC, Forces vital capacity obtained by spirometry; PEF, peak expiratory flow obtained with a portable peak flow meter.
Source: From Ref. 19.

year and to miss school, work or social engagements because of the asthma (21). This was the first time that a set of control parameters for asthma had been validated. As such, it demonstrated that responses to a simple set of questions can define asthma control and provide guidance to practitioners who care for patients with asthma. Such control concepts have become an integral component of asthma guidelines.

B. Increased Awareness of the Heterogeneity of Asthma, Particularly in Childhood

Asthma in childhood is considered to be a disease predominantly associated with wheezing. However, as noted in the initial international guidelines (10), "In children under five years we can be neither so confident that wheezing is equivalent to asthma, nor that there is a homogeneous underlying pathogenesis... (10)." The issue of the heterogeneity of wheezing illnesses was considered in the Tucson Children's Respiratory Survey, which enrolled 1246 newborns from a general population birth cohort. Over 800 of these children were assessed both at infancy and at six years. Martinez et al. demonstrated that almost half of these children had wheezing in the first six years of life (22). Transient wheezing, that is wheezing before age three, but no longer present by age six, occurred in almost 20% of children. Persistent wheezers were those who had wheezing beginning in the first few years of life and continued to wheeze into their school age (14%). Later wheezing, beginning after age three, occurred in 15% of these children. The authors noted "the majority of infants with wheezing have transient conditions associated with diminished airway function at birth and do not have increased risks of asthma or allergies later in life. In a substantial minority of infants, however, wheezing episodes are probably related to a predisposition to asthma (22)."

In that study, transient wheezing was associated with maternal smoking whereas persistent wheezing was associated with children whose mother had a history of asthma and where the child frequently had a personal history of eczema and/or rhinitis (22,23). Recently there has been an increased tendency for physicians to use a diagnostic descriptor of "reactive airways disease" for wheezing and chronic cough, especially in children. As noted by Fahy and O'Byrne (24) "the problem is that the term may provide physicians with a false sense of diagnostic security." In common practice, this term now appears to be applied to a broad spectrum of respiratory symptoms particularly in young children. Application of "reactive airway disease" as a diagnosis may actually be harmful given the issues that follow. An increased focus on the early diagnosis of asthma in children has become an integral component of guidelines as well exemplified by the 1998 update of the GINA guidelines (25).

C. Increased Awareness of the Onset of Asthma in Early Childhood

Over the past decade there has been an increased awareness that asthma usually begins in childhood. Data from the Rochester epidemiology project used predetermined diagnostic criteria and identified over 3600 incident cases of asthma in their population from 1964 through 1983. The median age of onset of asthma was three years for males and eight years for females. In that analysis, over 80% of all asthma ever diagnosed was initially diagnosed in the preschool child (26) (Fig. 1) supporting the concept that asthma begins in childhood.

The Melbourne asthma study provides the longest, community based, longitudinal data from children with a history of wheezing in childhood (27). Although relatively small numbers of children were enrolled in the study, 87% of the original study groups have been followed to 42 years of age.

Quite striking is the fact that there was early loss of lung function with asthma but even in those children with severe asthma the early life loss in lung function did not progress with worsening into adult life (27). This suggests that remodeling the airways may occur quite early after the onset of asthma in childhood. When considering remodeling of the airway wall, Payne et al. obtained endobronchial biopsies from children with "difficult" asthma, children without asthma, and adults including mild and severe asthma (28). As a measure of remodeling, reticular basement membrane "thickness in the children with asthma was found to be similar to that in adults with either mild or life-threatening asthma."

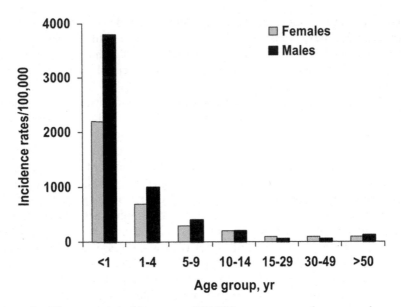

Figure 1 The annual incident rates/100,000 person-years by sex and age for definite plus probably asthma cases among Rochester residents, 1964 through 1983. *Source*: From Ref. 26.

The recognition that most asthma that ever occurs begins in childhood and that remodeling is an early feature of asthma, increased the sense of urgency to have guidelines which specifically focus on young children. The demonstration of changes in early life for pulmonary function and structural abnormalities greatly enhanced the importance of focusing greater interest in developing guidelines for the recognition and treatment of asthma in childhood. This was well recognized by the revision of the British asthma guidelines in 1995 with the development of a section on childhood asthma (29). In that revised guidelines for asthma management, children under five years old were dealt with as a distinct group. As one outcome of that review the committee noted that a number of research questions remained to be resolved relating to both diagnostic and management issues.

D. Development of New Medications and Research on Pharmacological Management of Asthma

Much of our therapeutic approach to the management of asthma in children remains based an extrapolation from studies in adolescents and adults. Many questions exist for which there are no data or for which studies have either recently been completed or are in progress.

Critical studies such as the Childhood Asthma Management Program (30) begin to offer important data on the management of asthma in the school-age child. Very limited data are available for the management of asthma in the preschool child both in terms of efficacy and safety. Although national and international guidelines will continue to be revised, there is an increasing focus in modifying guidelines to consider individual topics for which substantive or pivotal new data become available. This is well-exemplified by the recent Guidelines for the diagnosis and management of asthma—Update on selected topics, 2002 from the National Asthma Education and Prevention Program (NAEPP) expert panel report (31) which specifically focused on a limited number of topics including "long-term management of asthma in children: effectiveness of inhaled corticosteroids compared to other medications (31)." The authors stated that "the NAEPP recognizes the need for continual appraisal of the benefits and potential risks of asthma medications in children." The panel undertook a systematic review of available literature upon which to base their conclusions. They gave special consideration to the management of asthma in infants and very young children recognizing the difficulty in diagnosing asthma in infants. They note the paucity of data available for pharmacotherapy in children younger than three years of age. A major outcome from this review is a series of recommendations for future research. This included the need to compare safety and efficacy of LTRAs and inhaled corticosteroids; consideration of adherence to medication regimens and outcomes; the best approach to adjunctive therapy in children not adequately controlled using inhaled corticosteroids alone; issues of drug delivery and, importantly, they asked "Can early recognition and treatment of an infant or young child at high risk of developing asthma prevent development of persistent asthma"? (31).

II. Evolving Concepts of Guidelines

Initial guidelines evolved from the opinions of physician's expert in the area of asthma. Since the mid 1990s guidelines have become increasingly "evidence based." Recommendations to evaluate the available evidence for inclusion in guidelines became an integral component in development of the more recently updated publications. Most national and international guidelines have now been updated using evidence-based methodology. However, in the area of pediatric asthma the levels of evidence and grades of recommendation often remain based in large part on expert opinion because of the lack of a critical mass of data available to address a number of important questions. Inclusion of a more broadly based core of stakeholders beyond the specialist physician has enhanced the potential value of guideline documents for health care professionals (and even patients and families) to whom guidelines are directed. An additional benefit of the guidelines process has been the formulation of a large number of questions which arise from these reviews and which serve to direct new research approaches.

Recent guideline updates have adopted a new approach in order to ensure that asthma guidelines are both a "dynamic and timely guideline for practicing clinicians (31)." In the United Kingdom, the British Thoracic Society (BTS) and the Scottish Intercollegiate Guidelines Network (SIGN) continued to update guidelines focusing on evidence-based methodology and covering all aspects of asthma care. The recently published "British guideline on the management of asthma" (32) provides a comprehensive overview, which is developed using SIGN methodology (33). The levels of evidence for the data reviewed are translated into grades of recommendation relating to the strength of the evidence (34). "The aim of the guideline is to provide comprehensive advice on asthma management for patients of all ages in both primary and secondary care that will be of use to all health professionals involved in the care of people with asthma."

The guideline development committee has further focused on issues of dissemination and implementation of the guideline (see below). The GINA Program initial report of 1995 (18) was also completely revised in 2002 based on research published through 2000 (35). A 2003 update focused on the review of publications from October 2000 through December 2002 with an intent to provide yearly updated reports on the GINA website (www.ginasthma.com). The GINA strategy will be to completely revise the document every five years. The yearly updates will be focused on research identified to have an impact on the GINA recommendations that will further support or modify the current document (35).

A focused approach has also been taken by the NAEPP in the United States (31). The NAEPP Science Base Committee had the responsibility to monitor the scientific literature and identify topics for review. The current update "has focused on a few of the more pressing asthma issues rather than updating all topics at once (31)." The current update has focused on issues of medications, particularly in children, as well as monitoring and prevention of asthma. The issues of asthma prevention particularly focus on the effects of early treatment on the progression of asthma (31). This review has a strong component of pediatric issues recognizing the availability of improved data to address important questions raised by previous reviews. Unfortunately, recommendations continue to be based on consensus judgment where "the provision of some guidance was deemed valuable, but the clinical literature was insufficient (31,36)." The NAEPP (31) and GINA (35) Guidelines continue to use the previously introduced stepwise approach which was initially adopted for asthma in adults (13) (Table 3). A rather different approach was considered when updating the Canadian Asthma Guidelines in 1999 (37) which recognized asthma as a disease which changes over time and which may better reflect the course of asthma in childhood (Fig. 2).

Table 3 The Stepwise Approach to Asthma Management and Recommended Medications by Level of Severity for Children Under 5 Years of Age

Level of severity	Daily controller medications	Other treatment options
Step 1 Intermittent asthma	None necessary	
Step 2 Mild persistent asthma	Low-dose inhaled glucocorticosteroid	Sustained-release theophylline Cromone Leukotriene modifier
Step 3 Moderate persistent asthma	Medium-dose inhaled glucocorticosteroid	Medium-dose inhaled glucocorticosteroid plus sustained-release theophylline Medium-dose inhaled glucocorticosteroid plus long-acting oral β2-agonist High-dose inhaled glucocorticosteroid Medium-dose inhaled glucocorticosteroid plus leukotriene modifier
Step 4 Severe persistent asthma	High-dose inhaled glucocorticosteroid plus long-acting inhaled β2-agonist, plus one or more of the following, if needed: Sustained-release theophylline Leukotriene modifier Long-acting oral β2-agonist Oral glucocorticosteroid	

All Levels: In addition to regular daily controller therapy, rapid-acting inhaled β2-agonist should be taken as needed to relieve symptoms, but should not be taken more than three to four times a day. Patient education is essential at every level. Once control of asthma is achieved and maintained for at least 3 months, a gradual reduction of the maintenance therapy should be tried in order to identify the minimum therapy required to maintain control
Source: From Ref. 35.

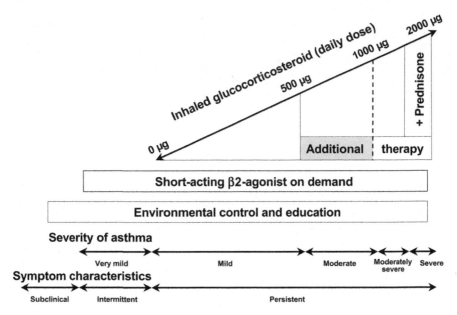

Figure 2 The continuum of asthma management. Severity of asthma is ideally assessed by medication required to maintain asthma control. Environmental control and education should be instituted for all asthma patients. Very mild asthma is treated with short-acting β2-agonists, taken as needed. If β2-agonists are needed more than three times per week (excluding 1 dose/day before exercise), then inhaled glucocorticosteroids should be added at the minimum daily dose required to control the asthma. If asthma is not adequately controlled by moderate doses (500–1000 µg/day of beclomethasone or equivalent), additional therapy (including long-acting β2-agonists, leukotriene antagonists or, less often, other medications) should be considered. Severe asthma may require additional treatment with Prednisone.*Source*: From Ref. 37.

III. Dissemination and Implementation of Guideline Recommendations

National and international guidelines are increasingly seen as evidence based and scientifically sound. Recently, approaches have been adopted to address specific issues and revise components of the guidelines in a timely manner in order to deal with new data, and, in many cases, to address changes that have already occurred in community practice. These approaches have resulted in several recent revisions of national and international guidelines. The ideal is to ensure that updated issues can be rapidly disseminated and implemented within the various heath care communities. However, there appears to be a communications gap between guidelines development, community practice, and control of asthma. The Canadian Asthma Consensus Conference in 1995 produced a set of recommendations published in 1996 (19) which were one of the first developed using evidence-based medicine. Three years later, a random digit dialing telephone survey was undertaken to identify a representative sample of individuals with asthma. A total of 801 adults and 200 parents of children were interviewed over the telephone. Using asthma control as defined in the guidelines in the 1996 guideline publication, 57% of patients failed to meet two or more of the six control criteria and were considered poorly controlled. One-half of the patients with poorly controlled asthma who used inhaled steroids did not understand the role of inhaled steroids and 1/3 of patients with poorly controlled asthma who used symptom relief medication did not understand the role of fast-acting relievers in the management of their asthma (20,21).

Dissemination of the guidelines to health care professionals has been thought to be reasonably successful. However, in a survey of New Zealand general practitioners two weeks after broad dissemination of updated guidelines in 2002, almost 1/3 of the GPs had no recollection of receiving the document (38). The authors note that "the results of this survey may reflect the administrative workload of GPs which results in time constraints, or may indicate that some are in a situation of 'guideline burn out' implementation of the recommendations for the diagnosis and treatment of adult asthma as detailed in guideline may be impaired by the method of dissemination and/or lack of acceptance of guidelines by doctors (38)."

While the gap between guidelines and clinical practice may be shrinking (39) studies have determined that prescribing for children with asthma does not conform to national guidelines (40,41). For example, among children seen in the Emergency Department of Children's Hospital of Philadelphia with an asthma exacerbation, 71% did not have a written action plan for management of worsening asthma (41). One year after introduction of the first NAEPP guidelines (13), Crain et al. surveyed Emergency Department Directors of all U.S. children's hospitals and a sample of public and private or community hospitals (42). Less than half had heard of the guidelines; 24% had read the guidelines and 6% thought that the guidelines would be adopted in their emergency departments. Dr. DeAngelis stated in the editor's note appended to the survey of Pediatric Asthma Care in US Emergency Departments "this article provides interesting data, especially in light of the national movement toward clinical protocols as encouraged by managed care. Three questions come to my mind: Can managed care administrators herd cats? Should cats be herded? If cats are herded, who gets hurt? (42)"

A major issue relating to appreciation of guidelines recommendations is the basis upon which these recommendations have been created. Grading of recommendations may be reasonably straightforward as are those from the NAEPP (31) and GINA (35) (Table 4). The BTS/SIGN levels of

Table 4 Descriptions Levels of Evidence

Evidence category	Sources of evidence	Definition
A	Randomized controlled trials (RCTs). Rich body of data	Evidence is from endpoints of well-designed RCTs that provide a consistent pattern of findings in the population for which the recommendation is made. Category A requires substantial numbers of studies involving substantial numbers of participants
B	Randomized controlled trials (RCTs). Limited body of data	Evidence is from endpoints of intervention studies that include only a limited number of patients, post hoc or subgroup analysis of RCTs, or meta-analysis of RCTs. In general, Category B pertains when few randomized trials exit, they are small in size, they were undertaken in a population that differs from the target population of the commendation, or the results are somewhat inconsistent
C	Nonrandomized trails. Observational studies	Evidence is from outcomes of uncontrolled or non-randomized trials or from observational studies
D	Panel consensus judgment	This category is used only in cases where the provision of some guidance was deemed valuable but the clinical literature addressing the subject was insufficient to justify placement in one of the other categories. The Panel consensus is based on clinical experience or knowledge that does not meet the above-listed criteria

Source: From Ref. 35.

Table 5 Key to Evidence Statements and Grades of Recommendations

Levels of evidence

1++	High quality meta-analyses, systematic reviews of randomized controlled trials (RCTs), or RCTs with a very low risk of bias
1+	Well-conducted meta-analyses, systematic reviews, or RCTs with a low risk of bias
1−	Meta-analyses, systematic reviews, or RCTs with a high risk of bias
2++	High quality systematic reviews of case control or cohort studies High quality case control or cohort studies with a very how risk of confounding or bias and a high probability that the relationship is causal
2+	Well-conducted case control or cohort studies with a low risk of confounding or bias and a moderate probability that the relationship is causal
2−	Case control or cohort studies with a high risk of confounding or bias and a significant risk that the relationship is not casual
3	Non-analytical studies, e.g., case reports and case series
4	Expert opinion

Grades of recommendation

A	At least one meta-analysis, systematic review, or RCT rated as 1++, and directly applicable to the target population A body of evidence consisting principally of studies rated as 1+, directly applicable to the target population, and demonstrating overall consistency of results
B	A body of evidence including studies rated as 2++, directly applicable to the target population, and demonstrating overall consistency of results Extrapolated evidence from studies rated as 1++ or 1+
C	A body of evidence including studies rated as 2+, directly applicable to the target population and demonstrating overall consistency of results Extrapolated evidence from studies rated as 2++
D	Evidence level 3 or 4 Extrapolated evidence from studies rated as 2+

Good practice points
Recommended best practice based on the clinical experience of the guideline development group BTS/SIGN (32)

evidence are more complicated but similarly lead to grades of recommendation (Table 5) (32).

However, even if grades of recommendation are presented in a simplistic manner the data available for childhood asthma frequently do not have the high quality meta-analysis or systemic reviews of randomized control trials recommended as the highest level of evidence leading to the best grade for a recommendation.

A survey of pediatricians showed that fewer than half of those who responded were following the GINA guidelines (43). It may be argued that asthma guidelines are not easily adopted in large part because they may not have been seen to be user friendly for physicians (44). Thus the step from production and dissemination of guidelines to the implementation, which occurs through knowledge transfer remains a major problem. This may relate to the issue of the complexity of levels of evidence leading to grades of recommendation (44). It is also argued that simply the size of the documents creates an issue where "None of the guidelines are exactly light reading nor can these be easily carried in a pocket (44)."

Even simple issues remain an important concern. It is noted that many children are given prescriptions for inhalers that they cannot efficiently or effectively use (45,46). Guidelines do emphasize the importance of choosing an inhaler appropriate for children of varying ages. A recent study in the United Kingdom revealed that a quarter of children did not use a spacer device with a pressurized metered dose inhaler (47). However, guidelines have positively impacted a change in standard practice from using nebulizers to the use of spacers with metered dose inhaler in some settings (47). A recent study using a multi-faceted implementation approach noted increased uptake of guidelines in both the intervention and the control groups suggesting that community pressures and awareness may be the most important component in implementation of guidelines (48). Broad dissemination of the guidelines in a variety of formats will be critical to enhance uptake of guidelines issues by health care professionals.

At least as important will be the need to include not only physicians but all allied health care personnel including nurses, respiratory therapists, and educators in this process. The GINA has established a Dissemination Committee and "GINA will make a worldwide effort to bring the messages of the GINA guidelines in all its documentation to the level of the primary care physician and the patient" (www.ginasthma.com). In addition, each country will have an appointed GINA advisor to supervise implementation of the GINA Guidelines. It is clearly critical to ensure that the knowledge brought together in guidelines is not only disseminated but implemented. These "knowledge translation" activities will require a variety of educational and public relation processes if they are to effectively change behavior of health care professionals as well as patients with asthma and their families (www.ginasthma.com).

One important component of current guidelines is provision of a written self-management (action) plan for patients and their families. A recent qualitative study of asthma nurses, general practitioners and adult patients and teenagers should raise a great deal of concern (49). Using focus groups held separately, the researchers found that health care professionals and patients were aware of guided self-management plans, but made little use of them. Of even more concern, in spite of feedback between the groups, there was little enthusiasm about the value of standardized self-management plans. "All but one of the patients agreed that self-management plans might be of use to other patients but, for differing reasons, were not relevant for them (49)." Research into the value of written asthma action plans for children and their families is urgently required. Expert consensus strongly encourages the use of a written asthma self-management plan for every patient with asthma.

It is increasingly clear that there remains a communication gap between and among health care professionals and between health care professionals and patients with asthma and their families. Dissemination of guidelines is a critical step in ensuring their acceptance by all of the stakeholders in this process, but recognition of the broad range of social factors pertinent to physicians and families is critical to ensure that implementation of the guidelines can take place. The gulf between currently recognized best practice and community practice ensures that we must more effectively "market" guidelines to effect the knowledge transfer critical to improve care for our young patients and their families.

References

1. Centers for Disease Control. Asthma—United States, 1980–1987. MMWR 1990; 39:493–497.
2. Manfreda J, Becker AB, Wang PZ, Roos LL, Anthonisen NR. Trends in physician diagnosed asthma prevalence in Manitoba between 1980 and 1990. Chest 1993; 103:151–157.
3. Burney PGJ, Chinn S, Rona RJ. Has the prevalence of asthma changed? Evidence from the national study of health and growth 1973–1986. Br Med J 1990; 300:1306–1310.
4. Gergen PJ, Mullally DI, Evans R. National survey of prevalence of asthma among children in the United States, 1976–1980. Pediatrics 1988; 81:1–7.
5. Anderson HR. Increase in hospital admissions for childhood asthma: trends in referral, severity, and readmissions from 1970 to 1985 in a health region of the United Kingdom. Thorax 1989; 44:614–619.
6. Anderson HR. Increase in hospitalization for childhood asthma. Arch Dis Cild 1978; 53:295–300.
7. Burney PGJ. Asthma mortality in England and Wales: evidence for a further increase, 1974–1984. Lancet 1988; 2:323–326.
8. Mao Y, Semenciw R, Morrison H, MacWilliam L, Davies J, Wigle D. Increased rates of illness and death from asthma in Canada. Can Med Assoc J 1987; 137:620–624.

9. Woolcock AJ, Rubinfeld AR, Seale JP, et al. Asthma management plan, 1989. Med J Aust 1989; 151:650–653.
10. Warner JO, Gotz M, Landau LI, Levison H, Milner AO, Petersen S, Silverman. Management of asthma: a consensus statement. Arch Dis Child 1989; 64: 1065–1079.
11. Hargreave FE, Dolovich J, Newhouse MT (eds). The assessment and treatment of asthma; a conference report. J Allergy Clin Immunol 1990; 85:1098–1111.
12. British Thoracic Society, Research Unit of the Royal College of Physicians of London, King's Fund Center, National Asthma Campaign. Guidelines for management of asthma I-chronic persistent asthma and II-acute severe asthma. Br Med J 1990; 301:651–653.
13. National Asthma Education Program & Expert Panel Report. Guidelines for the diagnosis and management of asthma. National Institutes of Health. Publication No 91–3042, 1991.
14. International Pediatric Consensus Group. Asthma: a follow-up statement from an International Consensus Group. Arch Dis Child 1992; 67:240–248.
15. CIBA Foundation Guest Symposium. Terminology, definitions, and classifications of chronic pulmonary emphysema and related conditions. Thorax 1959; 14:286–299.
16. Gross NJ. What is this thing called love?—or, defining asthma. Am Rev Respir Dis 1980; 121:203–204.
17. International Report. International Consensus Report on Diagnosis and Treatment of Asthma, National Heart, Lung, and Blood Institute. NIH publication No 92–3091, 1992.
18. Global Initiative for Asthma. Global strategy for asthma management and prevention NHLBI/WHO workshop report. NIH publication No 95–3659, 1995.
19. Ernst P, FitzGerald JM, Spier S, et al. Canadian asthma consensus conference: summary of recommendations. Can Respir J 1996; 2:89–100.
20. GlaxoWelcome Inc., Asthma In Canada: A Landmark Survey, 2000.
21. Chapman KR, Ernst P, Grenville A, Dewland P, Zimmerman. Control of asthma in Canada: failure to achieve guideline targets. Can Respir J Suppl A 2001; 8:35A–40A.
22. Martinez FD, Wright AL, Taussig LM, Holberg CJ, Halonen M, Morgan WJ. Asthma and wheezing in the first six years of life. New Engl J Med 1995; 3: 133–138.
23. Castro-Rodriguez JA, Holberg CJ, Wright AL, Martinez FD. A clinical index to define risk of asthma in young children with recurrent wheezing. Am J Respir Crit Care Med 2000; 162:1403–1406.
24. Fahy JV, O'Byrne PM. Reactive airways disease. Am J Respir Crit Care Med 2001; 163:822–823.
25. Global Initiative for Asthma. Pocket guide for asthma management and prevention, Revised 1998. National Heart, Lung, and Blood Institute NIH Publication 96–3659B, 1998.
26. Yunginger JW, Reed CE, O'Connell EJ, Melton LJ, O'Fallon WM, Silverstein MD. A community-based study of the epidemiology of asthma. Am Rev Respir Dis 1992; 146:888–894.

27. Phelan PD, Robertson CF, Olinsky A. The melbourne asthma study: 1964–1999. J Allergy Clin Immunol 2002; 2:189–194.

28. Payne DNR, Rogers AV, Adelroth E, Bandi V, Guntupalli KK, Bush A, Jeffery PK. Early thickening of the reticular basement membrane in children with difficult asthma. Am J Respir Crit Care Med 2003; 167:78–82.

29. British Asthma Guidelines Co-ordinating Committee. The British guidelines on asthma management 1995 review and position statement. Thorax 1997; 52:S1–24.

30. The Childhood Asthma Management Program Research Group. Long-term effects of budesonide or nedocromil in children with asthma. The childhood asthma management program research group. N Engl J Med 2000; 343:1054–1063.

31. National Asthma Education and Prevention Program. Guidelines for the diagnosis and management of asthma. Update on selected topics 2002. J Allergy Clin Immunol 2002; 110:S142–S219.

32. British Thoracic Society, Scottish Intercollegiate Guidelines Network. British guideline on the management of asthma: a national clinical guideline. Thorax 2003; 58:1–94.

33. Scottish Intercollegiate Guidelines Network (SIGN). SIGN 50: a guideline developers' handbook. SIGN publication No. 50. Edinburgh: SIGN, 2002.

34. Harbour R, Miller J. A new system for grading recommendations in evidence based guidelines. BMJ 2001; 323:334–336.

35. Global Strategy for Asthma Management and Prevention NIH Publication No 02–3659, 1995 (updated 2002, 2003) www.ginasthma.com.

36. Jadad AR, Moher M, Browman GP, Booker L, Sigouin C, Fuentes M, Stevens R. Systemic reviews and meta-analyses on treatment of asthma: critical evaluation. BMJ 2000; 320:537–540.

37. Boulet LP, Becker A, Berube D, Beveridge R, Ernst P. Canadian asthma consensus report, 1999. CMAJ 1999; 191(suppl 11):S1–S62.

38. Martin R, Reid JJ. Dissemination of guidelines on medical practice. N Z Med J 2003; 116:ISSN 1175–8716 (http://www.nzma.org.nz/journal/116–1168/312).

39. Stafford RS, Ma J, Finkelstein SN, Haver K, Cockburn I. National trends in asthma visits and asthma pharmacotherapy 1978–2002. J Allergy Clin Immunol 2003; 111:729–735.

40. Dashash NA, Mukhtar SH. Prescribing for asthmatic children in primary care: are we following guidelines? Saudi Med J 2003; 24:507–511.

41. Scarfone RJ, Zorc JJ, Capraro GA. Patient self-management of acute asthma: adherence to national guidelines a decade later. Pediatrics 2001; 108:1332–1338.

42. Crain EF, Weiss KB, Fagan MJ. Pediatric asthma care in US emergency departments: current practice in the context of national institutes of health guidelines. Arch Pediatr Adolesc Med 1995; 149:893–901.

43. Cabana MD, Rand CS, Becher OF, Rubin HR. Reasons for pediatrician nonadherence to asthma guidelines. Arch Pediatr Adolesc Med 2001; 155:1057–1062.

44. Godfrey S. Asthma guidelines for children—are they useful?—no! pediatric pulmonol 2004; (suppl 26):47–48.

45. Becker AB, Benoit T, Gillespie CA, Simons FER. Terbutaline by metered-dose inhaler: conventional inhaler versus tube spacer for children with asthma. Ann Allergy 1985; 55:724–729.

46. Child F, Davies S, Clayton S, Fryer AA, Lenney W. Inhaler devices for asthma: do we follow the guidelines? Arch Dis Child 2002; 86:176–179.
47. Gazarian M, Henry RL, Wales SR, Micallef BE, Rood EM, O'Meara MW, Numa AH. Evaluating the effectiveness of evidence-based guidelines for the use of spacer devices in children with acute asthma. Med J Aust 2001; 174:394–397.
48. Wright J, Warren E, Reeves J, Bibby J, Harrison S, Dowswell G, et al. Effectiveness of multifaceted implementation of guidelines in primary care. J Health Serv Res Policy 2003; 8:142–148.
49. Jones A, Pill R, Adams S. Qualitative study of views of health professionals and patients on guided self management plans for asthma. BMJ 2000; 321: 1507–1510.

16

Choosing the Appropriate Asthma Medication Delivery Device

MYRNA B. DOLOVICH

Department of Medicine, Faculty of Health Sciences, McMaster University
Hamilton, Ontario, Canada

I. Introduction

Pediatric asthma is a common childhood disease, affecting both infants and children of all ages. The incidence of asthma appears to be increasing worldwide, despite the improvements in treatment approaches and available therapies. There are a number of published pediatric guidelines outlining steps for implementing various therapeutic regimens based on asthma symptoms and disease severity (1,2). Symptoms, however, often go unrecognized, resulting in inadequate treatment for the child (3). Recommendations, based on evidence from the literature, may be included in the various guidelines for using one inhalation device versus another and these may be dependent on the setting and age of the child and the drug being prescribed. The use of self-management devices for older children can improve asthma control, but whether these tools address the proper handling of the inhalation device being used is not clear (4).

In children, as in adults, the success of therapy using aerosolized medications depends upon the ability to deliver sufficient drug to appropriate sites in the lung with few side effects. Children who require inhaled therapy for the treatment of their asthma represent a patient population with considerations that are different from adults', particularly when selecting a delivery device for administering their medication. Differences in lung geometry, ventilatory parameters and competence or ability to inhale correctly from many of the currently available devices (5) are just a few of the considerations that need to be recognized and addressed for this age group.

Education of the child, the child's parents or health care provider, older siblings and, if necessary, the child's school nurse in the use of the delivery device is one of the keys to successful therapy.

Other criteria need to be followed when selecting a device for children's use. The device must be sturdy, easy to use and assemble, not only for the older pediatric patient but also for the caregiver. The delivery system should generate sufficient therapeutic aerosol within the appropriate particle-size range for effective deposition in the pediatric lung, minimize oropharyngeal deposition to reduce side effects and ensure reliable and reproducible device performance over time and with multiple use. With infants and young children, the breathing parameters are a prime influence in determining how much aerosol is inhaled past the lips and what portion of this dose is subsequently lost to the oropharynx and larynx and unavailable as useful therapy (6). Depositing aerosol in the lung involves not only generating sufficient quantities of respirable particles or droplets but also administering the aerosol with minimal losses between the system and the patient. Delivery systems that can accommodate to the pediatric patient should result in beneficial therapy.

This chapter will discuss the variety of aerosol delivery systems available and attempt to provide a means of selecting a system that would provide optimal treatment.

II. Factors Affecting Delivery of Aerosol to Children

Delivering aerosolized medications to the lung combines drug formulation properties with delivery system characteristics. These factors, along with the inhalation technique adopted by the patient [inspiratory flow rate (IFR), inspiratory volume, and breath-holding time] determine the dose of drug from the inhaler used that would be deposited in the lung. The degree of airway narrowing, which varies with the type and severity of the lung disease additionally influences the distribution of aerosolized drug within the lung.

The influence of the above parameters when delivering aerosolized medication to infants and children needs to be recognized (7–11).

Children have lower tidal volumes than adults and this typically translates into reduced delivery of aerosol to the lung (12,13). In addition, pediatric breathing patterns can vary considerably (14) IRFs' ranging from near 0 to approximately 40 lpm are observed while airway size and geometry change significantly through childhood. Furthermore, a crying child will have a higher IFR, with the result that decreased amounts of drug are inhaled into the lung and what drug is inhaled tends to be deposited on more proximal airways (15,16). Inhaling aerosol through the nose or nasal breathing in addition to mouth breathing during treatment also reduces the dose to the lung (17). Similar to the adult patient, infants and toddlers with airways disease will deposit aerosolized medication on proximal rather than distal airways (18,19).

Inhalation of fine particle or droplet aerosols using low IFR helps promote drug delivery to the more peripheral airways. Inhalers can be designed to provide low velocity, fine aerosols as well as including features that limit the patient's breathing rate, all advantages for targeting drug to the lower rather than the upper respiratory tract (20). These key elements along with ease of use, portability and patient compliance monitors, such as dose counters and integrated electronic management systems to track treatments and treatment schedules, drive the current innovations in inhaler design. Inhaler devices are designed generally with the adult patient in mind. A few device companies produce aerosol systems for use in pediatrics, but they typically adapt the standard adult device with add-ons, such as mouthpieces, valves, facemasks designed for children, and chambers for containing the aerosol and that make the device more 'kid-friendly' (21,22).

III. Types of Aerosol Delivery Devices

Systems used to provide unit doses of therapeutic aerosols are the pressurized metered dose inhaler (pMDI) with or without an attached spacer device, and dry powder inhalers (DPIs). Continuous or intermittent generation of aqueous aerosols are provided by pneumatic (jet) and ultrasonic nebulizers. Within these three categories are a variety of devices producing aerosols with somewhat similar characteristics but with a range of fine particle lung delivery efficiencies. What distinguishes the different devices are the means used to produce and dispense the aerosols and the interface to the patient, an important design feature for the pediatric patient.

IV. pMDI + Spacer/Holding Chamber

Synchronization of actuation with inhalation of the pressurized aerosol is difficult for about 30% of adult patients, the elderly and all children. The use of holding chamber devices or tube spacers with pMDIs can eliminate some of these problems. General features of spacers/holding chambers (S-HC) are given in Table 1. These devices effect a reduction in mass

Table 1 Spacers for pMDIs

Three designs	Open tube (OT), valved holding chamber (VHC), and reverse flow (RF) ± facemasks ± flow aids
Materials of manufacture	Plastic, metal, paper, and non-electrostatic plastic
Volumes	15–750 mL
Population	Adults, children, and infants
Setting	Ambulatory, ambulance, and in-hospital (ER, ward, ICU, ICU-MV, and NICU)
Drugs	All pMDIs

median aerodynamic diameter (MMAD) of the original spray through evaporation and impaction of the larger particles on the walls or valves of the S-HC. This results in a 10–15-fold lower oropharyngeal dose from the pMDI and thus a decrease in the total body dose, an important consideration when prescribing steroid aerosols to children. With the retention of the larger droplets in a holding chamber device, the 'cold propellant (Freon®)' effect which causes many children to stop inhaling is eliminated, as is the foul taste associated with some drug aerosols. An in vitro/in vivo study designed to assess the ability of children of varying ages to use a pMDI with holding chamber or a dry powder inhaler clearly showed that infants and children under six years of age should take their aerosol medication using a pMDI with holding chamber (23). Children older than six years were able to successfully use the DPI and receive a consistent dose over the test period. When drug on the filters was corrected for an estimated loss to the oropharynx, the data showed that the dose available to the lung was similar.

Open tube spacers are not recommended for children, as without a built-in valve, actuation of the canister and inhalation of the aerosol must be coordinated, a task many youngsters cannot master. Additionally, the inhalation valve in the holding chamber must have sufficiently low resistance to open readily at the low inspiratory flows of infants and young children (24).

Lung deposition of aerosol inhaled from plastic S-HC devices is reduced due to the electrostatic charge on the spacer walls (25). Priming with extra doses is costly but does reduce retention of drug particles on the plastic, thereby increasing the availability of drug to the lung. Manufacturers now recommend washing their plastic spacers in a mild detergent and air-drying, particularly prior to initial use (26).

A. Non-metallic Spacers

Medical-grade plastics are typically the materials used to manufacture spacers. As mentioned above, plastic spacers carry an electrostatic charge, which attracts the charged drug particles within the pMDI spray, reducing the output of drug from the spacer (27,28). Metal spacers are not susceptible to static charges and their delivery of pMDI drugs is somewhat greater and more consistent than an unwashed plastic spacer.

A number of in vitro studies have shown that using a metal spacer (29) or washing the plastic spacer periodically can overcome the loss of drug, with noticeable benefit to the patient. After being washed, the plastic spacer should be allowed to dry without wiping to minimize reintroducing the electrostatic charge onto the plastic. With use, the interior walls of the plastic spacer will become coated with a thin layer of surfactant and drug, which acts to reduce the charge effect. There is some evidence to suggest that the electrostatic issue is a non-issue for HFA aerosols and that drug available from the plastic spacer is not as dependent on spacer volume as has been the case for CFC aerosols (30). Three non-electrostatic spacers are currently marketed in North America and Europe, two manufactured from thin-walled stainless steel and one of plastic that contains a non-electrostatic material. Wildhaber et al. found both in an in vitro model (31) and an in vivo study that using detergent-coated spacers, a pretreatment that effectively reduces the static charge on the plastic spacer walls caused a greater emitted dose to be available from the spacer with an increased lung deposition for radiolabeled CFC pMDI salbutamol (32). Despite these findings, it has recently been demonstrated in a crossover study in children that clinical effects are not markedly improved when using static-free spacers. Salbutamol was inhaled from plastic spacers holding an electrostic charge and then from the same spacers with their charge removed. A further comparison was made to the Nebuchamber®, the metal spacer from Astra-Zeneca (AstraZeneca, Sweden). No significant difference in peak flow was noted between the metal and plastic static and static-free spacers or to the metal spacer (33). However, given the dose of albuterol used in this study, it is likely that discrimination between treatments using the various spacers was lost as these children, aged four to eight years, had reached their maximal bronchodilatory response, even at the lower dose of 100 µg.

A useful alternative to the S-HC is the AutoHaler. This breath-actuated (BA) device can be used for administering specific pMDIs to children but is currently marketed with only one formulation, pirbuterol (3M Pharmaceuticals Inc., USA). The AutoHaler contains a mechanism for triggering actuation of the pMDI when the patient starts to inhale. While this is a definite advantage in terms of assuring inhalation of the spray, the dose of aerosol to the oropharynx is as high as when using the pMDI alone (34). A recent pharmacokinetic study (35) in 10–14-year-old children confirmed the superior dosing to the lung of HFA beclomethasone using the AutoHaler as the delivery device, compared to its CFC formulation delivered from the Volumatic holding chamber. The data also showed that 18% of the systemically available dose was absorbed from the gastrointestinal tract, i.e., drug deposited in the oropharynx and larynx and swallowed. Thus, were it possible to use this device for administration of HFA steroids, it would still be advantageous to use a holding chamber to reduce the total body dose to the minimum level possible.

B. Spacer Volume/Tidal Volume

One of the main factors affecting the dose delivered from spacers and holding chambers used with pMDIs is the patient's tidal volume. Of necessity, very young children and infants obtain their medication by tidal breathing through a valved holding chamber, similar to when using a nebulizer (36). This inhalation method is easier to perform, and of practical use, particularly when the volume of the spacer device is greater than the inspiratory capacity of the child. It may also be a useful practice in the emergency room for older children and adults, when breathing rates are increased due to acute shortness of breath (37). Despite the loss of aerosol to the walls of the spacer resulting from sedimentation due to gravity, which will occur between tidal breaths, sufficient drug can be obtained to provide a bronchodilator effect. However, the emptying time for large holding chambers may be too long at very low tidal volumes (50 mL). Thus, it would be preferable to use a small volume valved spacer, particularly for infants, that will initially provide a more concentrated aerosol and allow a greater mass of drug to be inhaled with each breath (38–40). Using a large (41) volume holding chamber means a less concentrated aerosol initially and a lower dose with each subsequent inspiratory breath as the particles settle under gravity during the time taken for expiration. Treatment with an increased number of doses may be required to get full benefit from the therapy (42).

C. Face Masks and Valves for Spacers/Holding Chambers

Face masks used with spacers and valved holding chambers have proven useful in treating patients of all ages in the emergency room and also when at home. Points to consider when evaluating a particular facemask are listed in Table 2. If children cannot manage the mouthpiece of the spacer or holding chamber, the facemask packaged with the S-HC should be used. Face Masks with minimal deadspace and low resistance inspiratory and expiratory valves should be selected, particularly with for use with the very young child and infant. However, in a study in non-ventilated, oxygen-dependent neonates with very low tidal volumes (43), Fok et al. found that aerosol delivery was significantly greater when the inspiratory valves were removed from the two holding chambers tested, namely the neonatal Aerochamber® and the Babyhaler®, resulting in improved pulmonary function and mechanics in these infants (44). Facemasks should be positioned securely on the face and a good seal to the cheeks should be made. If not, air will

Table 2 Spacer Issues—Face Mask and Valve Design

Face mask design is critical for young children and infants
    Dead space—should be minimal and ≪tidal volume of child
    Seal to face—should conform to cheeks and preferably have a soft edge
    Air entrainment—should be through S-HC
Face mask expiratory valve: and spacer inspiratory valve
    Design (center cut vs. duck bill vs. side opening)
    Low resistance to open at low flow
    Placement close to mouth
    Durability

---

be entrained around the facemask and this will prevent the drug from being inhaled from the valved spacer into the lung (43,45).

The requirement for low resistance valves also applies to the facemask exhalation valve. Too high a resistance may prevent the valve from opening, contributing to a rebreathing of aerosol accumulated in the facemask area. The dead space of the facemask should also be kept to a minimum for similar reasons. The patient must also be able to easily exhale through the exhalation valve of the facemask; this becomes important if a child is tidal breathing through the spacer—one doesn't have to remove the facemask for exhalation to take place.

The facemask provided with the S-HC product must provide a proper seal to the child's cheeks to avoid loss of dose, an important consideration whether they are inhaling either pMDI aerosols (46) or aerosols from nebulizers (47). Holding the facemask away from the struggling child, termed "blow-by," will not provide effective therapy, demonstrated in both in vitro models of drug delivery (48) and in vivo studies (49,50). The aerosol will just disperse into the atmosphere if an open-tube spacer is used and if a valved holding chamber, will eventually settle onto the device walls. There is some debate as to whether administering aerosol to the sleeping child is more effective than trying to cope with a crying, struggling infant or young child. An early study by Murikami et al. (51) demonstrated improved lung deposition to a sleeping child compared to one awake and crying. However, a recent study from the Netherlands demonstrated that in their study, the majority of sleeping children wake up and fight the facemask, resulting in parents not being able to administer treatment (52).

A number of studies comparing delivery of therapy to infant and children of school age using the pMDI and spacer with facemask compared to nebulizer, have all demonstrated equivalent or better response with the use of valved spacers, including reduced cough and wheeze and days absent from school (53–55). In intubated neonates with RDS or early bronchopulmonary dysplasia, and older infants with recurrent wheeze, lung function and symptoms improved and rates of extubation increased (56,57) when treated with a pMDI and valved holding chambers.

D. Replacement Propellant pMDIs

The HFA pMDIs are replacing the current CFC pMDIs. Two albuterol bronchodilators, AiroMir (3M Pharma, UK) and Ventolin HFA (GlaxoSmithKline, Ware, UK) are available and can be substituted for salbutamol pMDI products (58). In vitro measurements of output from several plastic spacers of different volumes as well as a metal spacer, indicate the same, or enhanced delivery compared to the pMDI alone. Changes to the coarse/fine particle doses available for inhalation from the spacers tested have also been demonstrated compared to the pMDI alone. Moreover, the output appears to be independent of spacer volume (30).

There are several corticosteroid HFA formulations available and several more in development (59). Some CFC propellant formulations have transitioned to HFA solution steroids (HFA beclomethasone dipropionate (QVAR), IVAX Pharmaceuticals, USA; HFA Ciclesonide, Altana Pharma, Germany), while others remain as suspensions (HFA Ventolin, Glaxo-SmithKline, USA; Proventil HFA, Schering-Plough, NJ, USA; HFA Fluticasone, GlaxoSmithKline, USA). The aerosol characteristics of the HFA solution pMDIs are quite different to the original CFC pMDIs in that the aerosol particle size is submicronic or extra-fine in terms of aerosol median diameter. Lung deposition of these extra-fine aerosols is two to threefold greater to the lung and on more distal airways with a markedly reduced oropharyngeal dose (60). Use of a holding chamber with these submicronic aerosols further reduces the oropharyngeal dose fivefold and as such, should be the preferred way to deliver these aerosols to infants and children. Both simulation of delivery (61) and in vivo deposition studies have been carried out with HFA beclomethasone dipropionate solution steroid (QVAR, 3M Pharma Inc., USA), with and without a holding chamber. Delivery is similar to adults, namely approximately 50% of the emitted dose to the lung and reduced dose to the oropharynx (62). As with other deposition studies in children, the dose deposited in the lung is a function of age (63,64). A recent multicenter clinical trial (START study) of approximately 2900 children between the ages of 5 and 15 years, showed no apparent impairment of growth or other systemic effects after five years of treatment using 200–400 μm of QVAR daily (65).

V. Nebulizers

Nebulizers seem to be the preferred way to deliver aerosols to infants and small children. In general, this is an easier method for the child and caregiver, although a crying, squirming infant will receive little, if any, benefit from the treatment (12). And the young child must also be compliant, willing to sit with a facemask kept against the face for the 5–10 minutes needed to complete the treatment. As mentioned above for spacers and holding chambers, the facemask seal is critical for effective therapy. Substitution of the pMDI and valved spacer, or DPI for the child older than five or six years of age (23,66,67), can achieve the same goal more efficiently, provided the drugs are available in a pMDI. A recent meta-analysis of RCTs comparing clinical responses to the same drug given from different inhaler devices and in a variety of patient settings, showed comparable outcomes for both bronchodilators and corticosteroids for adult and pediatric patients (68).

Choices of systems for delivering a liquid solution or suspension are based on a number of factors (e.g., ease of use, convenience, aerosol properties, dose delivery, and drug deposition), the combination of which will impact on the single most important factor, clinical benefit (69,70). Because of cost differences, most home and hospital treatments are performed using conventional, disposable jet nebulizers. The stimulus for developing highly efficient nebulizers with good dosing reliability is mainly to accommodate new chemical entities being evaluated for delivery via the aerosol route. These drugs are most often initially formulated in liquid form and are usually aqueous-based solutions. Insulin to be administered as an aerosol is one such recent example where highly efficient and reliable systems are required to maintain good therapeutic control (71,72).

There are many nebulizer designs available and they vary widely in their ability to generate small-particle aerosols (73). Droplet size ranges from <1 to >6 μm for some older designs of ultrasonic nebulizers. Output of useful aerosol is primarily a function of breathing pattern and particle size produced from the specific nebulizer design. Patient-related factors influencing aerosol delivery from nebulizers to children are shown in Table 3. Simulating aerosol delivery from nebulizers using breath simulators provides a useful way of determining performance and dose of aerosol that would be available to the patient at the mouth (74–77). These types of

Table 3 Patient-Related Factors Confounding Drug Delivery to Children via Nebulizer

Face mask seal
Nasal breathing
Low-tidal volume, inspiratory flow, and pressure
Entrainment
Resistance of inspiratory (nebulizer entrainment)/expiratory (facemask or nebulizer) valves
Irregular breathing
Poor compliance (patient and/or caregiver)

measurements though are only useful when they are performed incorporating testing parameters that are as close as possible to actual conditions of use (78,79).

Currently, the last several years have seen new features and novel designs of nebulizers. These devices can broadly be divided into three main classes: (i) adaptive aerosol delivery devices, (ii) metered dose liquid inhalers (MDLIs), and (iii) BA nebulizers. The most commonly used jet nebulizer is the constant output design, with supplemental air drawn in across the top of the nebulizer, diluting the aerosol produced within the nebulizer as it exits towards the patient. Aerosol is generated continuously and depending on the fill volume, approximately 30–50% of nominal dose can be trapped in the nebulizer, with >60% of the emitted dose wasted to atmosphere. Further refinements to the basic nebulizer design are the BA and breath-enhanced (BE) features. In the former, the flow of air to the jet is curtailed or eliminated by internal valving within the nebulizer until the patient starts to inhale (80), while the latter directs auxiliary air though the nebulizer and across the venturi, sweeping out more of the available aerosol and providing an increased output of drug. The length of time aerosol is delivered during inspiration significantly influences the dose inhaled in children (81), while the use of a properly sealed facemask and breath-actuation can improve delivery in children by 2–10% (47,82). Treatment times are usually prolonged with BA and BE design which may result in children becoming restless during the treatment and potentially refusing to comply.

Treatment times with high frequency ultrasonic nebulizers, vibrating mesh designs, and electronic micropump devices are usually shorter than for conventional jet nebulizers and thus, possibly a more cost-effective way to deliver therapy to children. They are also typically more efficient than conventional pneumatic nebulizers, with three- to eightfold greater lung deposition (83). A recent study compared the efficacy and safety of ipratropium bromide/fenoterol hydrobromide (Berodual®, Boehringer Ingelheim, Germany) delivered via the Respimat® Soft Mist™ Inhaler, a multidose liquid inhaler to a conventional pMDI + Aerochamber in asthmatic children aged 6–15 years. Half the nominal dose of Berodual inhaled via the Respimat was required to give the equivalent response as that from the pMDI + Aerochamber (84). This would enable a reduction in the nominal dose compared to what would be required for administration by pMD + Aerochamber. Clinical responses can vary with the devices tested. A comparison of ultrasonic delivery of salbutamol to jet nebulizer delivery indicated a similar response from both systems in children ages 7–16 years with acute asthma (85). Delivery of surfactant by jet vs. ultrasonic nebulization to an animal model of neonatal respiratory distress showed no clinical benefit even using an ultrasonic system (86).

Only one corticosteroid is currently available as a nebulizer therapy in North America. Budesonide (Pulmicort) suspension, used in Europe and

Canada for several years and recently approved in the United States, has been effective in treating children and adults with asthma (87,88). Because it is a liquid suspension, many jet nebulizers and older designs of ultrasonic nebulizers have been unsuccessful in generating a clinically effective aerosol (89). Newer technologies, such as AeroGen's (AeroGen, Mountain View, CA, USA) micropump design, and other vibrating mesh ultrasonics, devices to use for easily treating children, are all able to effectively aerosolize Pulmicort (73) suspension. Most of the supporting clinical data for this microsuspension of budesonide have been collected using Pari jet nebulizers or the Halolite™ jet nebulizer.

Increasing drug output by air entrainment through, rather than across the nebulizer and decreasing drug wastage by reducing or eliminating aerosol generation during the patient's expiratory phase are two design features developed over the last five years and incorporated into a number of newer nebulizers. Breath-actuation and 'smart' nebulizers have features that help control breathing parameters during inhalation of the drug dose. The MDLIs, for example, newer versions of the AeroDose™ and the Respimat™, produce low velocity sprays, making it easier for patients, both adult and pediatric, to inhale the spray (84). The Halolite was designed to utilize the patient's breathing pattern to calculate an amount of drug to be aerosolized and inhaled per breath. This nebulizer is preprogrammed to automatically stop when the total prescribed dose has been administered and has been tested with Pulmicort suspension and tobramycin (90). Electronic features have been incorporated into several of the MDLI designs, enabling patient compliance, and, also management of the patient's treatment schedule, to be monitored. These features are, however, only beneficial for the older child (>4 years) (91). Lung deposition appears to be greater for all the new technology devices, ranging from 40% to 80% of the emitted dose (83). However, increased deposition, leading to potentially greater improvements in pulmonary function, may also be accompanied by an increased incidence of side effects, perhaps requiring an adjustment of the prescribed dose when these devices are prescribed.

VI. Dry Powder Inhalers

In contrast to pMDIs, DPIs do not require propellants; they are breath-actuated, eliminating the need for synchronization of inhalation with actuation. The DPIs are classified according to their means of storing and providing the drug, that is, as single capsules, in a bulk reservoir or as multi-single unit dose devices (Table 4). The latter can take the form of blisters, blister tape, capsules, or multi-chambered cassettes (92). The DPIs may allow greater formulation flexibility and do not require the same physical and chemical stability of drug, compared with suspension- or

Table 4 Dry Powder Inhalers: Dose Storage

Dose storage	Dry powder inhaler	Number of doses per storage unit
Single capsule	Spiriva (Boehringer-Ingelheim, Ingelheim, Germany)[a]	1
	Aerolizer (Novartis, Surrey, UK)[a]	1
Reservoir	Turbuhaler (Astra Draco, Lund, Sweden)[a]	200
	Easyhaler (Orion Farmos, Kuopio, Finland)[a]	200
	Clickhaler (ML Laboratories, St. Albans, UK)[a]	200
	Taifun (Leiras, Kuopio, Finland)[a]	200
	Pulvinal (Chiesi, Parma, Italy)[a]	200
	Ultrahaler (Aventis, Loughborough, UK)	200
Multi-unit dose		
Blister	Diskhaler (GlaxoSmithKline, Ware, UK)[a]	4–8
Blister/tape	Diskus (GlaxoSmithKline, Ware, UK)[a]	60
Capsule	Inhalator (Boehringer Ingelheim, Ingelheim, Germany)[a]	2

[a]Marketed in Europe, Canada, and/or the United States.

solution-based pMDIs (93). However, gelatine capsules and some drug powders are affected by humidity, necessitating some means of protection from the environment, for example, being foil-wrapped, until the patient is ready to take a dose. With all types of DPIs, some drug remains in the storage medium following dosing (94). Whether this is a greater percentage of the emitted dose when children are dosed compared to adults is not known. The amount of drug available per actuation should account for this loss and be sufficient to achieve a clinical response. With the exception of budesonide and terbutaline sulphate in the Turbuhaler (AstraZeneca, Sweden), most powder devices require a lactose carrier to allow the powder dose to flow out of the inhaler (95). Once inhaled, the drug particles separate from the carrier or are deagglomerated by the inspired airflow; each DPI has its own optimal IFR, determined primarily by the specific resistance of the particular DPI design. Table 5 shows the specific resistances for various DPIs available in North America and Europe. Low resistant devices require less effort to dispense the powder from the device and may be suitable for young children. However, the child would need to be able to inhale from the device with an IFR of at least 60 lpm and this maneuver may not be easily manageable. There are a number of clinical studies in the literature supporting the use of high resistant devices in children more than six years of age.

Adverse effects from inhaling lactose are not common. However, a recent report of such an event occurred in a child with severe milk allergy and persistent asthma, a result of milk protein contamination in lactose of

Table 5 Specific Resistance of Some Available DPIs

Range	Resistance	DPI
>0.1	High	Turbuhaler
		Clickhaler
		EasyHaler
		HandiHaler
0.05–0.1	Medium	Pulvinal
		Diskus
		Diskhaler
<0.05	Low	Spinhaler
		Rotahaler
		Aerolizer

the specific DPI lot used (96). The authors stressed the need to use caution when prescribing DPIs with lactose-based formulations to similar type patients. Alternative choices for delivery systems would be nebulization of a corticosteroid suspension formulation or a pMDI with valved holding chamber. A guide to design and performance characteristics of several multi-dose reservoir or multi-single unit dose DPIs, not all currently available in the United States, allows one to review some physical features of these selected inhalers that may influence selection for pediatric patients, such as whether an asthmatic child can achieve the targeted IFR for the specific DPI (97). The In-Check Dial is a peak inspiratory flow rate (PIF) meter that tests what peak flow rate a patient can achieve when inhaling against the resistance of the prescribed DPI (98). Amirav et al tested children both experienced and inexperienced in the use of DPIs and found that only 88% the experienced users could generate a PIF of 60 LPM through the Turbuhaler, while children older thatn 9 years of age and unfamiliar with DPIs were more likely to be able to achieve this PIF (99).

The DPIs that rely on the patient's inspiratory effort to dispense the dose are often referred to as passive or patient-driven devices as opposed to power-assisted or active DPIs. The advantage of passive devices are that they are breath-actuated and do not require an energy source to generate the aerosol, such as propellants in the pMDI, electrical energy or compressed air. However, because they are dependent on the patient's IFR to dispense the drug powder, there can be differences in lung delivery efficiencies within and between DPIs and, ultimately, clinical response (100). Active or powered devices which are designed to be independent of patient effort require a holding chamber to contain the powder released from the device, and, as with pMDI S-HC, this results in some drug being lost in the chamber.

Because they are breath-actuated, DPIs are not recommended for children less than four to six years old and are definitely not an option for infants. However, releasing the powder into a chamber, independent of the patient and from which the young child can tidal breathe, may lead to a useful delivery system (101,102). Inhalation of insulin powder from a dry powder inhaler with an integrated holding chamber has been developed in the USA and is currently undergoing clinical trials. These types of powder delivery systems, similar in principle to firing a pMDI and containing the dispensed aerosol in a valved holding chamber, may provide an alternative for treating very young children.

Deposition from the Turbuhaler was recently measured in children with cystic fibrosis (CF), ages 3–16 years of age using radiolabeled budesonide (103). Not surprisingly, deposition was unreliable in the youngest group, and increased with age and IFR. Values obtained for the deposited lung dose, corrected for body weight, were within or greater than adult levels, supporting the effectiveness of the Turbuhaler for delivering therapy in young children. Numerous clinical trials have successfully demonstrated that the Turbuhaler can be used to treat children with asthma and recent studies with salmeterol delivered from the Diskus DPI (GlaxoSmithKline, UK) indicate similar outcomes (104).

VII. Measuring In Vitro Drug Delivery from Aerosol Devices: Simulating Pediatric and Adult Use

Careful in vitro assessment of aerosol delivery devices using realistic breathing patterns can be advantageous in choosing an efficient and efficacious delivery system for infants and children. These modeling investigations become more important in assessing delivery to the very young patient, more so if the treatment is not as successful as anticipated. In the past several years simulators have become more sophisticated in design, allowing a range of tidal volumes and flow rates to be programmed and also to drive a delivery system to determine aerosol (drug) output. Additionally, there are devices that capture breath patterns from patients, interface to the simulator, thereby providing a means of determining delivery with in vivo breathing conditions. These measurements provide an indication of aerosol delivery past the lips; estimations of dose deposited in the oropharynx would need to be made to determine what would potentially be deposited in the lung.

In evaluating systems for delivery of aerosols to children, simulated breathing patterns should be used to provide a more accurate estimate of the doses provided, with correlations to clinical outcomes and deposition studies when possible. Measurements of nebulizer output and the output from one dose of Ventolin pMDI used with several spacers have been made at volumes ranging from 50–800 mL (simulating a 7 kg infant to a >70 kg adult) and inspiratory times varying from 0.3 to 1.5 sec. The results showed a linear output from the Pari LC Star with increasing tidal volume (Fig. 1). Output from the spacers was similarly reduced at the low tidal volumes, but also lowest with large versus small volume spacers and the infant breathing pattern. These data paralleled deposition studies in spontaneously breathing, intubated rabbits, showed reduced delivery with the Babyhaler (GlaxoSmithKline, UK) compared to the Nebuchamber (Astra Pharma, Sweden) and Aerochamber (Trudell Medical Group, Canada) (105). Earlier in vitro measurements of output for the above spacers, made at constant flows of 28.3 lpm, did not differentiate drug output between them (106); these in vitro results would then only apply to delivery to adults and pediatric patients whose tidal volumes equalled or exceeded the spacer volume.

A variety of S-HC are available commercially, yet there is little published data to support claims of performance, safety, and efficacy, other than the information required for approval by the regulatory agencies. While many published laboratory studies with S-HCs exist, there are few randomized controlled trials comparing S-HC with the same pMDI formulation. A recent Canadian standard for judging performance under rigorously standardized conditions has been published that outlines a

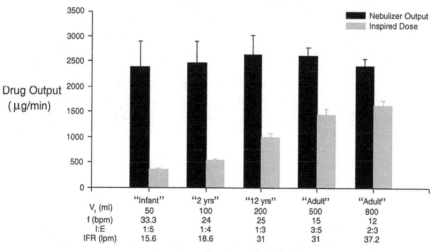

Figure 1 In vitro measurement of the dose of cromolyn sodium available via the Pari LC Star for infant, child and adult breathing patterns. The amount of drug delivered to a filter per minute of nebulization time increases with tidal volume and IFR, approaching the per minute output of the nebulizer when driven continuously, but only for the adult breathing parameters. *Abbreviations*: VT, tidal volume; BF, breathing frequency; I:E, inspiratory/expiratory ratio; IFR, inspiratory flow rate.

number of in vitro test procedures to be performed by the S-HC manufacturer. The aim is to provide data on medication delivery (emitted dose and aerosol size) to patients, physicians and health care workers under various conditions of S-HC use by infants, children and adults (107).

In vitro sampling of aerosols from holding chambers at a constant flow rate may not reveal the limitations of the device when used with infants and very young children. The use of simulation models with realistic variable flow rate patterns can provide this information, measuring drug delivered at low flow rates (108) and also under conditions where patients might delay taking an inhalation from the holding chamber (109). Janssens et al. developed a model of the upper airway (110) and have tested delivery for a number of pMDI formulations under simulated breathing conditions, confirming that in children as in adults, lung dose decreases with increasing inspiratory flow, tidal volume or respiratory rate, due to increased impaction in the upper airways. In addition, they found that deposition was greater for extra-fine aerosols and that reducing electrostatic charge by washing plastic spacers improved aerosol delivery to the lung (111,112).

Simulation techniques have also been used to assess nebulizer performance at flow rates and breathing patterns indicative of children (77) and also DPIs using recorded breathing patterns from children (113). Both these in vitro studies showed, not surprisingly, that delivery was dependent on the pediatric breathing pattern.

While laboratory simulations of drug delivery are extremely useful for understanding factors that affect drug availability to the mouth, there are limitations in what these studies can include as test variables. Most simulations are done under ambient conditions and the effects of airway disease are difficult to incorporate into the existing models. Radiolabeled deposition studies are not always possible to perform in children (114) and clinical trials to correlate outcomes with the in vitro results are rarely done.

VIII. Measuring Drug Delivery from Aerosol Devices: In Vivo Measurements of Lung Deposition

While deposition measurements are felt to be of use in determining the influence of various factors on topical drug delivery to children (113), there are in fact, relatively few studies measuring in vivo deposition of aerosol in children using radiotracers. An early study in children with CF showed that lung deposition was patchy, increased in the central airways and varied with the severity of the disease (44,116). Total deposition was greater in the older CF children, a finding confirmed by Chua et al. (117). The rationale for using adult doses in pediatric patients becomes obvious when in vivo measurements such as those obtained from an early study from Salmon et al. (118)

demonstrate how little drug is deposited in the lungs of young children. These investigators showed that less than 1% of sodium cromoglycate aerosol generated either by nebulizer or metered dose inhaler was deposited in the lungs of 9- to 36-month-old asthmatic children. Onhoj et al. (119) using pharmacokinetic methods, calculated the dose of budesonide delivered via pMDI and metal spacer to children ranging in age from two to six years, comparing their results to a group of adults undergoing the same protocol. The same dose of budesonide was administered to both children and adults. Plasma concentrations were found to be the same for all ages, leading the investigators to conclude that children, with a lower deposition of drug to the lung could be prescribed the same nominal dose of budesonide via Nebuchamber without an increased risk of systemic exposure, Aerosol therapy applied to newborns whether spontaneously breathing or mechanically ventilated is more complex. A deposition study in babies with broncho-pulmonary dysplasia showed that <2% of salbutamol nebulizer solution or pMDI aerosol was deposited in the lungs and that delivery correlated with body weight for the nebulizer but not the pMDI plus Aerochamber (Fig. 2) (19,121). Similar deposition values have been reported in the older child (18).

Radiolabeled deposition studies have demonstrated improved drug delivery in adults when the pMDI is used with a spacer; between 13% and 32% of the dose from CFC pMDIs with a valved holding chamber reaches the lungs, 5–10% is deposited in the mouth and throat, with the balance of the dose remaining in the valved spacer.

Using the Aerochamber[™] with QVAR in both children and adults maintains the lung dose at approximately 53%, but reduces the oropharyngeal dose from 29% with the HFA pMDI alone to 5% with the valved holding chamber, clearly of benefit to the patient being treated with inhaled corticosteroids (60,122). As mentioned earlier in this chapter, this deposition differential, favoring increased deposition of the finer aerosol was confirmed using pharmacokinetic methods to estimate lung deposition (35). These methods have been used by these same investigators to evaluate deposition in children from different DPIs and nebulizers. A recent pharmacokinetic study in children aged 8–14 years, comparing the Turbuhaler to the Diskus showed lung deposition four times higher in children after inhalation of budesonide from the Turbuhaler 29.6%) than after inhalation of fluticasone (7.6%) from the Diskus (123). However, in younger children aged three to six years, delivery of nebulized budesonide from a Pari LC Jet+ nebulizer proved to be less efficient, namely a systemic availability of 6% of the nominal dose (124).

While these comparisons give the clinician a means to compare delivery of drug from the various devices, nevertheless, one has to consider the clinical response data to fully judge the device performance. Manufacturers promote their delivery devices in terms of delivery efficiency. Published values from numerous investigations range from 5 to 80% for all three categories, namely pMDIs +/− S-HCs, DPIs and nebulizers and provide a useful guide for comparing inhalers. However, the information becomes more meaningful when related either to the nominal dose or the emitted dose of drug from the device (125). The simple calculation of Efficiency × Nominal Dose or Efficiency × Emitted Dose gives the microgram quantity of drug deposited in the lung or available for inhalation at the mouth and allows a comparison of the therapeutic index of different corticosteroids to be made. Figure 3 is an illustration of the advantage in knowing the absolute microgram quantity deposited in the lung. While the deposition expressed as a percent of the nominal dose is twofold greater for the pMDI with holding chamber, only 10% more salbutamol in absolute terms (micrograms) was deposited in the lung (120).

IX. Summary

Children between the ages of 5 and 12 commonly have difficulty in using pMDIs properly, particularly children between four and five years of age.

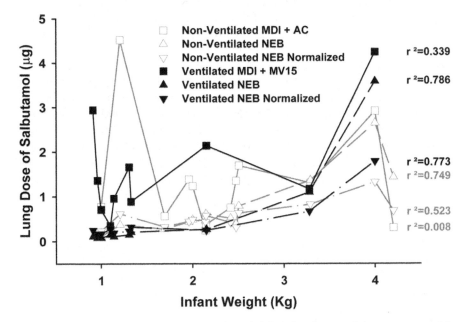

Figure 2 In vivo lung deposition of radiolabeled salbutamol in neonates with bronchopulmonary dysplasia vs. infant weight. The nebulizer delivery, but not the metered dose inhaler, increased with increased weight for both spontaneously breathing infants and intubated infants and when normalized for dose. *Abbreviations*: MDI, metered dose inhaler; AC, aerochamber; NEB, nebulizer; MV15, Aerochamber MV15®. *Source*: From Ref. 121.

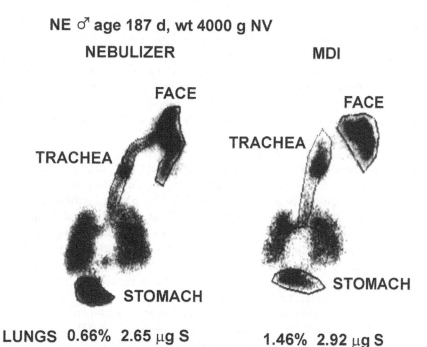

NE ♂ age 187 d, wt 4000 g NV

NEBULIZER   **MDI**

FACE

FACE

TRACHEA

TRACHEA

STOMACH

STOMACH

LUNGS 0.66% 2.65 μg S   **1.46% 2.92 μg S**

Figure 3 Images of radiolabeled salbutamol in an infant with bronchopulmonary dysplasia. The drug deposited in the lung in this 187-day-old infant, weighing 4000 g was similar for both delivery systems when expressed as a microgram dose of salbutamol. *Abbreviations*: NV, non-ventilated; S, salbutamol; MDI, metered dose inhaler. *Source*: From Ref. 19.

They usually can effectively use pMDIs with valved holding chambers, BA pMDIs and DPIs. If a young child can suck on a straw, there is a reasonable chance that he or she can manage to inhale from a DPI, although the IFR may not be the optimal one for the particular DPI. These three options are preferred over nebulizers for this age group because of their portability and a treatment time measured in seconds rather than minutes. The pMDI with holding chamber has the additional advantage of decreasing drug deposition in the back of the throat. The net effect is that holding chambers increase the proportion of drug that reaches the lungs relative to the proportion deposited in the mouth, where it is clinically ineffective. For corticosteroids in particular, this can reduce the unpleasant taste from some formulations, minimize the risk of oral candidiasis and decrease the amount of drug available for systemic absorption via the gut.

    Children over the age of 12 are candidates for the same array of devices that are considered in adults. Children of this age group are usually as capable as adults at learning correct pMDI and DPI technique. Consequently, these devices are widely preferred over nebulizers for use in the outpatient setting.

The substantial oropharyngeal drug deposition associated with DPIs and pMDIs, even when they are used correctly, remains a concern for adolescent patients. An additional problem arising in this age group is that of proper use; DPIs and pMDIs with or without S-HCs require different patient inhalation techniques (fast and forceful vs. slow and steady, with precise timing of the pMDI actuation with inhalation directly into the mouth or through the S-HC). When a DPI corticosteroid is prescribed, a short-acting beta agonist is also prescribed. If this latter inhaler selected for the beta agonist is a pMDI or AutoHaler pMDI, patient education may be more difficult and confusing since two different inhalation techniques must be taught. It would be preferable to use only one type of inhaler for all prescribed drugs for a particular patient; but this may not always be possible. A recent study however, in 112 children, aged 6–16 years presenting to the emergency department with acute asthma, demonstrated equivalent responses to a bronchodilator inhaled either from a DPI or pMDI with large volume spacer (126). The problems associated with using both a DPI and pMDI are largely absent when the pMDI with a valved-holding chamber or a DPI is available for both reliever and controller medications. When choosing among these devices for a specific patient, the lower oropharyngeal deposition for the corticosteroid and more user-friendly nature of the pMDI with holding chamber must be weighed against the greater convenience and portability of the DPI and of the pMDI without holding chamber.

The choices in devices to use for inhalant therapy is increasing and physicians and patients should have a good understanding of the functional differences between them and some of the factors influencing their device selection (Table 6). Despite improved technology, the varying breathing patterns and differences in oropharyngeal and airway geometries cause variations in the inhaled dose between infants, children, adults, and elderly

Table 6 Device Selection

Device	Convenience	Use in Children	Inhalation Techniques	Lung (%)	Mouth and Throat (%)
Nebulizer	±	+	Tidal breathing	1–10	2–5
pMDI ± S-HC	+	With S-HC	IC breath; tidal breathing	10–25; 25–38 with S-HC	60–70; 4–10 with S-HC
DPI	+	>4 years	IC breath	6–32	60–70

patients, factors which will continue to lead to altered clinical responses between patient populations (127).

When selecting an inhaler device, the following points should be considered:

- availability of drug and dosages,
- age of patient,
- competence of patient,
- severity of disease,
- need to provide effective therapy without side effects,
- inhalation technique required,
- all prescribed drugs for the patient available in the same device or same type of device,
- quality of the aerosol–high respirable fraction,
- frequency of dosing for required treatment,
- ease of use and maintenance,
- portability,
- device durability,
- cost, and
- reimbursement by third-party payers.

Patient and caregiver education on device use is key for managing the proper inhalation technique and this should occur with each clinic or office visit. Physicians and patients should understand that for whatever reason, if one device is not providing effective therapy, there are other inhaler devices that can be tried that might meet with success.

References

1. British Guideline on the Management of Asthma . Thorax 2003; 58(I):i1–i94.
2. National Asthma Education and Prevention Program. Expert panel report 2: guidelines for diagnosis and treatment of asthma. Publication No 97–405 1997.
3. Halterman JS, Yoos HL, Kaczorowski JM, McConnochie K, Holzhauer RJ, Conn KM, Lauver S, Szilagyl PG. Providers underestimate symptom severity among urban children with asthma. Arch Pediatr Adolesc Med 2002; 156(2):141–146.
4. Guendelman S, Meade K, Benson M, Chen YQ, Samuels S. Improving asthma outcomes and self-management behaviors of inner-city children: a randomized trial of the health buddy interactive device and an asthma diary. Arch Pediatr Adolesc Med 2002; 156(2):114–120.
5. Everard ML. Inhaler devices in infants and children: challenges and solutions. J Aerosol Med 2004; 17(2):186–195.
6. Rubin BK, Fink JB. Aerosol therapy for children. Respir Care Clin N Am 2001; 7(2):175–213.

7. Chua HL, Collis GG, Newbury AM, Chan K, Bower GD, Sly PD, Le Souef PN. The influence of age on aerosol deposition in children with cystic fibrosis. Eur Respir J 1994; 7(12):2185–2191.
8. Knight V, Yu CP, Gilbert BE, Divine GW. Estimating the dosage of ribavirin aerosol according to age and other variables. J Infect Dis 1988; 158(2): 443–448.
9. Schiller-Scotland C, Hlawa R, Gebhart J. Experimental data for total deposition in the respiratory tract of children. Toxicol Lett 1994; 72:137–144.
10. Hofmann W, Martonen T, Graham R. Predicted deposition of nonhygroscopic aerosols in the human lung as a function of subject age. J Aerosol Med 1989; 2:49–68.
11. Xu J, Yu CP. The effects of age on deposition of inhaled aerosols in the human lung. Aerosol Sci Technol 1986; 5:349–357.
12. Everard ML. Inhalation therapy for infants. Adv Drug Deliv Rev 2003; 55(7):869–878.
13. Collis GG, Cole CH, Le Souef PN. Dilution of nebulised aerosols by air entrainment in children. Lancet 1990; 336(8711):341–343.
14. Bisgaard H. Delivery of inhaled medication to children. J Asthma 1997; 34(6):443–467.
15. Mallol J, Rattray S, Walker G, Cook D, Robertson CF. Aerosol deposition in infants with cystic fibrosis. Pediatr Pulmonol 1996; 21(5):276–281.
16. Everard ML. Aerosol delivery in infants and young children. J Aerosol Med 1996; 9(1):71–77.
17. Everard ML, HardyJG, Milner AD. Comparison of nebulised aerosol deposition in the lungs of healthy adults following oral and nasal inhalation. Thorax 1993; 48(10):1045–1046.
18. Tal A, Golan H, Grauer N, Aviram M, Albin D, Quastel MR. Deposition pattern of radiolabeled salbutamol inhaled from a metered-dose inhaler by means of a spacer with mask in young children with airway obstruction. J Pediatr 1996; 128(4):479–484.
19. Fok TF, Monkman S, Dolovich M, Gray S, Coates G, Paes B, Rashid F, Newhouse M, Kirpalani H. Efficiency of aerosol medication delivery from a metered dose inhaler versus jet nebulizer in infants with bronchopulmonary dysplasia. Pediatr Pulmonol 1996; 21(5):301–309.
20. Dolovich MB. Influence of inspiratory flow rate, particle size, and airway caliber on aerosolized drug delivery to the lung. Respir Care 2000; 45(6): 597–608.
21. Watt PM, Clements B, Devadason SG, Chaney GM. Funhaler spacer: improving adherence without compromising delivery. Arch Dis Child 2003; 88(7):579–581.
22. Hayden MJ, Wildhaber JH, Eber E, Devadason SG. The Chocuhaler: sweet deliverance in asthma management. Med J Aust 1995; 163(11–12): 587–588.
23. Agertoft L, Pedersen S, Nikander K. Drug delivery from the Turbuhaler and Nebuhaler pressurized metered dose inhaler to various age groups of children with asthma. J Aerosol Med 1999; 12(3):161–169.

24. Sennhauser FH, Sly PD. Pressure flow characteristics of the valve in spacer devices. Arch Dis Child 1989; 64:1305–1307.

25. Kenyon CJ, Thorsson L, Borgstrom L, Newman SP. The effects of static charge in spacer devices on glucocorticosteroid aerosol deposition in asthmatic patients. Eur Respir J 1998; 11(3):606–610.

26. Pierart F, Wildhaber JH, Vrancken I, Devadason SG, Le Souef PN. Washing plastic spacers in household detergent reduces electrostatic charge and greatly improves delivery. Eur Respir J 1999; 13(3):673–678.

27. O'Callaghan C. In vitro performance of plastic spacer devices. J Aerosol Med 1997; 10(suppl 1):S31–S35.

28. Clark DJ, Lipworth BJ. Effect of multiple actuations, delayed inhalation and antistatic treatment on the lung bioavailability of salbutamol via a spacer device. Thorax 1996; 51:981–984.

29. Bisgaard H. A metal aerosol holding chamber devised for young children with asthma. Eur Respir J 1995; 8(5):856–860.

30. Katz IM, Martonen TB. Three-dimensional fluid particle trajectories in the human larynx and trachea. J Aerosol Med 1996; 9(4):513–520.

31. Wildhaber JH, Devadason SG, Hayden MJ, James R, Dufty AP, Fox RA, Summers QA, Le Souef PN. Electrostatic charge on a plastic spacer device influences the delivery of salbutamol. Eur Respir J 1996; 9(9):1943–1946.

32. Wildhaber JH, Janssens HM, Pierart F, Dore ND, Devadason SG, LeSouef PN. High-percentage lung delivery in children from detergent-treated spacers. Pediatr Pulmonol 2000; 29(5):389–393.

33. Dompeling E, Oudesluys-Murphy AM, Janssens HM, Hop W, Brinkman JG, Sukhai RN, De Jongste JC. Randomised controlled study of clinical efficacy of spacer therapy in asthma with regard to electrostatic charge. Arch Dis Child 2001; 84(2):178–182.

34. Newman SP, Weisz AW, Talaee N, Clarke SW. Improvement of drug delivery with a breath actuated pressurised aerosol for patients with poor inhaler technique. Thorax 1991; 46(10):712–716.

35. Agertoft L, Laulund LW, Harrison LI, Pedersen S. Influence of particle size on lung deposition and pharmacokinetics of beclomethasone dipropionate in children. Pediatr Pulmonol 2003; 35(3):192–199.

36. Gervais A, Begin P. Bronchodilatation with a metered-dose inhaler plus an extension, using tidal breathing vs jet nebulization. Chest 1987; 92(5):822–824.

37. Gleeson JG, Price JF. Nebuhaler technique. Br J Dis Chest 1988; 82(2):172–174.

38. Mitchell JP, Nagel MW, Dolovich M. Comparative performance of small volume plastic- and metal-bodied holding chambers for pediatric use at low tidal volume. Eur Respir J 1996; 8(suppl 23):S433.

39. Singh M, Kumar L. Randomized comparison of a dry powder inhaler and metered dose inhaler with spacer in management of children with asthma. Indian Pediatr 2001; 38(1):24–28.

40. Kraemer R. Babyhaler—a new paediatric aerosol device. J Aerosol Med 1995; 8(suppl 2):S19–S26.

41. Agertoft L, Pedersen S. Influence of spacer device on drug delivery to young children with asthma. Arch Dis Child 1994; 71(3):217–219.

42. Kraemer R, Frey U, WirzSommer C, Russi E. Short-term effect of albuterol delivered by an auxiliary device in wheezy infants: a double-blind placebo-controlled study. Am J Respir Crit Care Med 1991; 144:347–351.

43. Esposito-Festen JE, Ates B, van Vliet FJ, Verbraak AF, De Jongste JC, Tiddens HA. Effect of a facemask leak on aerosol delivery from a pMDI-spacer system. J Aerosol Med 2004; 17(1):1–6.

44. Fok TF, Lam K, Chan CK, Ng PC, Zhuang H, Wong W, Cheung KL. Aerosol delivery to non-ventilated infants by metered dose inhaler: should a valved spacer be used?. Pediatr Pulmonol 1993; 24(3):204–212.

45. Sangwan S, Gurses BK, Smaldone GC. Face Masks and facial deposition of aerosols. Pediatr Pulmonol 2004; 37(5):447–452.

46. Janssens HM, Heijnen EM, de Jong VM, Hop WC, Holland WP, De Jongste JC, Tiddens HA. Aerosol delivery from spacers in wheezy infants: a daily life study. Eur Respir J 2000; 16(5):850–856.

47. Nikander K, Agertoft L, Pedersen S. Breath-synchronized nebulization diminishes the impact of patient-device interfaces (facemask or mouthpiece) on the inhaled mass of nebulized budesonide. J Asthma 2000; 37(5):451–459.

48. Everard ML, Clark AR, Milner AD. Drug delivery from jet nebulisers. Arch Dis Child 1992; 67(5):586–591.

49. Iles R, Lister P, Edmunds AT. Crying significantly reduces absorption of aerosolised drug in infants. Arch Dis Child 1999; 81(2):163–165.

50. Everard ML. Trying to deliver aerosols to upset children is a thankless task. Arch Dis Child 2000; 82(5):428.

51. Murakami G, Igarashi T, Adachi Y. Measurement of bronchial hyperreactivity in infants and preschool children using a new method. Ann Allergy 1990; 64:383–387.

52. Esposito-Festen JE, Meijers-IJsselstein H, Hop WCJ, van Vliet F, De Jongste JC, Tiddens H. Aerosol therapy in sleeping young children: is it an option? Eur Respir J 2004; 24(suppl 48):S212.

53. Cunningham SJ, Crain EF. Reduction of morbidity in asthmatic children given a spacer device. Chest 1994; 106(3):753–757.

54. Lin YZ, Hsieh KH. Metered dose inhaler and nebuliser in acute asthma. Arch Dis Child 1995; 72(3):214–218.

55. Parkin PC, Saunders NR, Diamond SA, Winders PM, Macarthur C. Randomised trial spacer v nebuliser for acute asthma. Arch Dis Child 1995; 72(3): 239–240.

56. Giep T, Raibble P, Zuerlein T, Schwartz ID. Trial of beclomethasone dipropionate by metered-dose inhaler in ventilator-dependent neonates less than 1500 grams. Am J Perinatol 1996; 13(1):5–9.

57. Williams JR, Bothner JP, Swanton RD. Delivery of albuterol in a pediatric emergency department. Pediatr Emerg Care 1996; 12(4):263–267.

58. Shapiro G, Bronsky E, Murray A, Barnhart F, Vandermeer A, Reisner C. Clinical comparability of ventolin formulated with hydrofluoroalkane or conventional chlorofluorocarbon propellants in children with asthma. Arch Pediatr Adolesc Med 2000; 154(12):1219–1225.

59. Zeidler M, Corren J. Hydrofluoroalkane formulations of inhaled corticosteroids for the treatment of asthma. Treat Respir Med 2004; 3(1):35–44.
60. Dolovich M, Leach C. Drug delivery devices and propellants. In: Busse WW, Holgate ST, eds. Asthma & Rhinitis. UK: Blackwell Science, 2000:1719–1731.
61. Cole CH, Mitchell JP, Foley MP, Nagel MW. Hydrofluoroalkane-beclomethasone versus chlorofluorocarbon-beclomethasone delivery in neonatal models. Arch Dis Child Fetal Neonatal Ed 2004; 89(5):F417–F418.
62. Devadason SG, Huang T, Walker S, Troedson R, Le Souef PN. Distribution of technetium-99m-labelled QVAR delivered using an Autohaler device in children. Eur Respir J 2003; 21(6):1007–1011.
63. Schuepp KG, Straub D, Moller A, Wildhaber JH. Deposition of aerosols in infants and children. J Aerosol Med 2004; 17(2):153–156.
64. Malozowski S, Purucker M. Growth as a biological marker of inhaled corticosteroid activity. Curr Ther Res Clin Exp 2001; 62(11):796–802.
65. Pedersen S, Warner J, Wahn U, Staab D, Le Bourgeois M, Essen-Zandvliet E, Arora S, Szefler SJ. Growth, systemic safety, and efficacy during 1 year of asthma treatment with different beclomethasone dipropionate formulations: an open-label, randomized comparison of extrafine and conventional aerosols in children. Pediatrics 2002; 109(6):e92.
66. British Guideline on the Management of Asthma. Thorax 2003; 58(suppl 1): i1–i83.
67. Buxton LJ, Baldwin JH, Berry JA, Mandleco BL. The efficacy of metered-dose inhalers with a spacer device in the pediatric setting. J Am Acad Nurse Pract 2002; 14(9):390–397.
68. Dolovich M, Ahrens R, Hess DR, Anderson PJ, Dhand R, Rau JL, Smaldone GC, Guyatt G. Device selection and outcomes of aerosol therapy: American College of Chest Physicians/American College of Asthma, Allergy and Immunology evidence-based guidelines. Chest 2005; 127:335–371.
69. Hess DR. Nebulizers: principles and performance. Respir Care 2000; 45: 609–622.
70. Hvizdos KM, Jarvis B. Budesonide inhalation suspension: a review of its use in infants, children and adults with inflammatory respiratory disorders. Drugs 2000; 60:1141–1178.
71. Laube BL, Benedict GW, Dobs AS. The lung as an alternative route of delivery for insulin in controlling postprandial glucose levels in patients with diabetes [see comments]. Chest 1998; 114(6):1734–1739.
72. Kim D, Mudaliar S, Chinnapongse S, Chu N, Boies SM, Davis T, Perera AD, Fishman RS, Shapiro DA, Henry R. Dose-response relationships of inhaled insulin delivered via the Aerodose insulin inhaler and subcutaneously injected insulin in patients with type 2 diabetes. Diab Care 2003; 26(10):2842–2847.
73. Dolovich MB, Fink JB. Aerosols and devices. Respir Care Clin N Am 2001; 7(2):131–73.
74. Roth AP, Lange CF, Finlay WH. The effect of breathing pattern on nebulizer drug delivery. J Aerosol Med 2003; 16(3):325–339.
75. Barry PW, O'Callaghan C. Drug output from nebulizers is dependent on the method of measurement. Eur Respir J 1998; 12(2):463–466.

76. Nikander K, Denyer J, Smith N, Wollmer P. Breathing patterns and aerosol delivery: impact of regular human patterns, and sine and square waveforms on rate of delivery. J Aerosol Med 2001; 14(3):327–333.

77. O'Callaghan C, White J, Jackson J, Barry P, Kantar A. The output of flunisolide from different nebulisers. J Pharm Pharmacol 2002; 54(4):565–569.

78. Smaldone GC. Drug delivery by nebulization: "reality testing" [editorial]. J Aerosol Med 1994; 7(3):213–216.

79. Bosco A, Dolovich M. In vitro estimations of in vivo jet nebulizer efficiency using actual and simulated tidal breathing patterns. J Aerosol Med 2004. In Press.

80. Newnham DM, Lipworth BJ. Nebuliser performance, pharmacokinetics, airways and systemic effects of salbutamol given via a novel nebuliser delivery system ("Ventstream"). Thorax 1994; 49(8):762–770.

81. Nikander K, Turpeinen M, Wollmer P. Evaluation of pulsed and breath-synchronized nebulization of budesonide as a means of reducing nebulizer wastage of drug. Pediatr Pulmonol 2000; 29(2):120–126.

82. Nikander K, Bisgaard H. Impact of constant and breath-synchronized nebulization on inhaled mass of nebulized budesonide in infants and children. Pediatr Pulmonol 1999; 28(3):187–193.

83. Dolovich M. New propellant-free technologies under investigation. J Aerosol Med 1999; 12(suppl 1):S9–S17.

84. von Berg A, Jeena PM, Soemantri PA, Vertruyen A, Schmidt P, Gerken F, Razzouk H. Efficacy and safety of ipratropium bromide plus fenoterol inhaled via Respimat Soft Mist Inhaler vs. a conventional metered dose inhaler plus spacer in children with asthma. Pediatr Pulmonol 2004; 37(3):264–272.

85. Nakanishi AK, Lamb BM, Foster C, Rubin BK. Ultrasonic nebulization of albuterol is no more effective than jet nebulization for the treatment of acute asthma in children. Chest 1997; 97(6):1505–1508.

86. Fok TF, Al Essa M, Dolovich M, Rasid F, Kirpalani H. Nebulisation of surfactants in an animal model of neonatal respiratory distress. Arch Dis Child Fetal Neonatal Ed 1998; 78(1):F3–F9.

87. Shapiro G, Mendelson L, Kraemer MJ, Cruz-Rivera M, Walton-Bowen K, Smith JA. Efficacy and safety of budesonide inhalation suspension (Pulmicort Respules) in young children with inhaled steroid–dependent, persistent asthma [see comments]. J Allergy Clin Immunol 1998; 102(5):789–796.

88. Shapiro G. Once-daily inhaled corticosteroids in children with asthma: nebulisation. Drugs 1999; 58(suppl 4):43–49; discussion 53:43–49.

89. Smaldone GC. In vitro determination of inhaled mass and particle distribution for Budesonide nebulizing suspension. J Aerosol Med 1998; 11: 113–125.

90. Leung K, Louca E, Coates AL. Comparison of breath-enhanced to breath-actuated nebulizers for rate, consistency, and efficiency. Chest 2004; 126(5): 1619–1627.

91. Denyer J. Adaptive aerosol delivery in practice. Eur Respir Rev 1997; 7(51): 388–389.

92. Dolovich M. Changing delivery methods for obstructive lung diseases. [Review] [112 Refs.]. Curr Opin Pulm Med 1997; 97(3):177–189.

93. Moren F. Aerosol dosage forms and formulation. In: Moren F, Dolovich MB, Newhouse MT, Newman S, eds. Aerosols in Medicine: Principles, Diagnosis and Therapy. Amsterdam: Elsevier, 1993:321–350.
94. Hindle M, Byron P. Dose emissions from marketed dry powder inhalers. Int J Pharm 1995; 116:169–177.
95. Ganderton D. The generation of respirable clouds from coarse powder aggregates. J Biopharm Sci 1992; 3:101–105.
96. Nowak-Wegrzyn A, Shapiro GG, Beyer K, Bardina L, Sampson HA. Contamination of dry powder inhalers for asthma with milk proteins containing lactose. J Allergy Clin Immunol 2004; 113(3):558–560.
97. Smith IJ, Parry-Billings M. The inhalers of the future? A review of dry powder devices on the market today. Pulm Pharmacol Ther 2003; 16(2): 79–95.
98. Chrystyn H. Is inhalation rate important for a dry powder inhaler? Using the In-check Dial to identify these rates. Respir Med 2003; 97:181–187.
99. Amirav I, Newhouse MT, Mansour Y. Measurement of peak respiratory flow with in-check dial device to stimulate low-resistance (Diskus) and high resistance (Turbohaler) dry powder inhalers in children with asthma. Pediatr Pulmonol 2005; 39:447–451.
100. Nielsen KG, Skov M, Klug B, Ifversen M, Bisgaard H. Flow-dependent effect of formoterol dry-powder inhaled from the Aerolizer. Eur Respir J 1997; 10(9):2105–2109.
101. Bisgaard H. Delivery of inhaled medication to children. J Asthma 1997; 34(6): 443–467.
102. Bisgaard H. Automatic actuation of a dry powder inhaler into a nonelectrostatic spacer. Am J Respir Crit Care Med 1998; 157(2):518–521.
103. Devadason SG, Everard ML, MacEarlan C, Roller C, Summers QA, Swift P, et al. Lung deposition from the Turbuhaler in children with cystic fibrosis. Eur Respir J 1997; 10(9):2023–2028.
104. Nielsen KG, Auk IL, Bojsen K, Ifversen M, Klug B, Bisgaard H. Clinical effect of Diskus dry-powder inhaler at low and high inspiratory flow-rates in asthmatic children. Eur Respir J 1998; 11(2):350–354.
105. Dubus JC, Rhem R, Monkman S, Dolovich M. Delivery of salbutamol pressurized metered-dose inhaler administered via small-volume spacer devices in intubated, spontaneously breathing rabbits. Pediatr Res 2001; 50(3):384–389.
106. Dubus JC, Dolovich M. Emitted doses of salbutamol pressurized metered-dose inhaler from five different plastic spacer devices. Fundam Clin Pharmacol 2000; 14(3):219–224.
107. Dolovich MB, Mitchell JP. Canadian Standards Association standard CAN/CSA/Z264.1–02:2002: a new voluntary standard for spacers and holding chambers used with pressurized metered-dose inhalers. Can Respir J 2004; 11(7):489–495.
108. Mitchell JP, Nagel MW. In vitro performance testing of three small volume-holding chambers under conditions that correspond with use by infants and small children. J Aerosol Med 1997; 10(4):341–349.

109. Barry PW, O'Callaghan C. The effect of delay, multiple actuations and spacer static charge on the in vitro delivery of budesonide from the Nebuhaler. Br J Clin Pharmacol 1995; 40(1):76–78.

110. Janssens HM, De Jongste JC, Fokkens WJ, Robben SG, Wouters K, Tiddens HA. The Sophia Anatomical Infant Nose-Throat (Saint) model: a valuable tool to study aerosol deposition in infants. J Aerosol Med 2001; 14(4):433–441.

111. Janssens HM, De Jongste JC, Hop WC, Tiddens HA. Extra-fine particles improve lung delivery of inhaled steroids in infants: a study in an upper airway model. Chest 2003; 123(6):2083–2088.

112. Janssens HM, Krijgsman A, Verbraak TF, Hop WC, De Jongste JC, Tiddens HA. Determining factors of aerosol deposition for four pMDI-spacer combinations in an infant upper airway model. J Aerosol Med 2004; 17(1): 51–61.

113. Finlay WH, Gehmlich MG. Inertial sizing of aerosol inhaled from two dry powder inhalers with realistic breath patterns versus constant flow rates. Int J Pharm 2000; 210(1–2):83–95.

114. Everard ML. The use of radiolabelled aerosols for research purposes in paediatric patients: ethical and practical aspects. Thorax 1994; 49(12): 1259–1266.

115. Thomas SH, Batchelor S, O'Doherty MJ. Therapeutic aerosols in children. BMJ 1993; 307(6898):245–247.

116. Alderson P, Secker-Walker R, Strominger D. Pulmonary deposition of aerosols in children with cystic fibrosis. J Pediatr 1974; 84:479–484.

117. Chua H, Collis G, Newbury A. The influence of age on aerosol deposition in children with cystic fibrosis. Eur Respir J 1994; 7:2185–2191.

118. Salmon B, Wilson NM, Silverman M. How much aerosol reaches the lungs of wheezy infants and toddlers? Arch Dis Child 1990; 65(4):401–403.

119. Onhoj J, Thorsson L, Bisgaard H. Lung deposition of inhaled drugs increases with age. Am J Respir Crit Care Med 2000; 162(5):1819–1822.

120. Fok TF, Monkman S, Dolovich M, Gray S, Coates G, Paes B, et al. Efficiency of aerosol medication delivery from a metered dose inhaler versus jet nebulizer in infants with bronchopulmonary dysplasia. Pediatr Pulmonol 1996; 21(5):301–309.

121. Dolovich M, Fok TF, Monkman S, Gray S, Rashid F, Paes B, Newhouse M, Kirpalani H. Relationship between infant weight and lung deposition of aerosol. Eur Respir J 1995; 8(suppl 19):S201.

122. Dolovich M, Conway J, LeSouef PN, Leach C. Lung deposition >50% consistently demonstrated for HFA-beclomethasone dipropionate (BDP) extrafine aerosol. Ann Allergy Asthma Immunol 2000. Ref Type: Abstract.

123. Agertoft L, Pedersen S. Lung deposition and systemic availability of fluticasone diskus and budesonide turbuhaler in children. Am J Respir Crit Care Med 2003; 168(7):779–782.

124. Agertoft L, Andersen A, Weibull E, Pedersen S. Systemic availability and pharmacokinetics of nebulised budesonide in preschool children. Arch Dis Child 1999; 80(3):241–247.

125. Parameswaran K, Leigh R, O'Byrne PM, Kelly MM, Goldsmith CH, Hargreave FE, Dolorich M. Clinical models to compare the safety and

efficacy of inhaled corticosteroids in patients with asthma. Can Respir J 2003; 10(1):27–34.

126. Drblik S, Lapierre G, Thivierge R, Turgeon J, Gaudreault P, Cummins-McManus B, Verdy I, Haddon J, Lee J, Spior S. Comparative efficacy of terbutaline sulphate delivered by Turbuhaler dry powder inhaler or pressurised metered dose inhaler with Nebuhaler spacer in children during an acute asthmatic episode. Arch Dis Child 2003; 88(4):319.

127. Bisgaard H. Future options for aerosol delivery to children. Allergy 1999; 54(suppl 49):97–103.

17

Anticipating and Managing Variable Response to Asthma Therapy

STANLEY J. SZEFLER

Department of Pediatrics and
   Pharmacology, Divisions of Clinical
   Pharmacology and Allergy and
   Immunology, Helen Wohlberg and
   Herman Lambert Chair in
   Pharmacokinetics, National Jewish
   Medical and Research Center, University
   of Colorado Health Sciences Center,
Denver, Colorado, U.S.A.

GLENN WHELAN

Department of Pediatrics,
   Associate Clinical Pharmacologist,
   Clinical Coordinator, National Jewish
   Medical and Research Center
Denver, Colorado, U.S.A.

I. Introduction

The trend of increasing asthma mortality and morbidity has fortunately reached a plateau over the last several years (1). Perhaps a more pro-active approach that facilitates the identification of patients at risk for developing persistent asthma and for a favorable response to selected interventions will be successful in reducing asthma morbidity as well as mortality. This may be made possible by focusing attention on altering the natural history of asthma and also developing new techniques to facilitate an individualized approach for selecting the appropriate intervention.

Inhaled glucocorticoids are now considered the cornerstone for managing persistent asthma, even in children less than five years of age (2–4). New medications and delivery systems have been introduced, including a nebulized inhaled glucocorticoid and a leukotriene antagonist for asthma therapy in children down to one year of age (5,6). These initiatives have made it feasible to intervene at a very early age and thus improve the overall management of childhood asthma (7,8).

New directions in the management of childhood asthma include early diagnosis and intervention with either environmental control in allergen-sensitized patients or administration of long-term control therapy (9,10). Further advances could result in improved methods to make the diagnosis of asthma and to identify methods to effectively intervene in the natural history of asthma. Although inhaled glucocorticoid therapy improves asthma control, it is not clear whether this treatment can prevent all long-term outcomes, especially those related to asthma progression and airway remodeling (Table 1) (11,12).

This review will summarize the currently applied approaches to asthma management in children and the population of patients that could benefit from early intervention with anti-inflammatory therapy. New information related to the variable response to asthma treatment will be discussed since understanding mechanisms for this variability in response could lead to even better methods to tailor therapy for individual patients based on their unique asthma presentation.

II. Managing Asthma in Children Five Years of Age and Older

Current guidelines for asthma management place emphasis on the identification of asthma triggers, environmental control, pulmonary function

Table 1 Risks Related to the Under-Treatment of Asthma

Mortality
Respiratory arrest
Hospitalization
Acute exacerbation
  Emergency department visit
  Course of systemic glucocorticoid therapy
Nocturnal symptoms
Breakthrough symptoms—spontaneous or activity induced
Variability in pulmonary function due to airway sensitivity
School absence
Reduced quality of life, for example
  reduced activity level
  poor self-image
Progression as indicated by
  loss of pulmonary function
  increasing symptoms
  increasing medication requirements
Persistent inflammation
Airway remodeling and irrecoverable loss of pulmonary function
Adverse effects related to overuse of rescue therapy, for example bronchodilators
  and systemic glucocorticoids

---

monitoring, education, and therapeutic intervention (2–4). Asthma is now categorized as intermittent, mild persistent, moderate persistent, and severe persistent based on the frequency of daytime and nighttime symptoms and level and variability of pulmonary function.

The recently updated NAEPP guidelines address the needs of childhood asthma through a careful evidence-based review of critical issues such as the time of intervention, the safety and limitations of inhaled glucocorticoids, and the preferred medication for additive therapy to inhaled glucocorticoids (3,4).

Inhaled glucocorticoids are the preferred first-line treatment in both children and adults (2,3). The preferred additive therapy for inadequate control with low-medium dose inhaled glucocorticoid is a long-acting β-adrenergic agonist (3). Leukotriene antagonists, as well as cromolyn, nedocromil, and theophylline, are considered alternative first-line therapy to inhaled glucocorticoids and alternative additive therapy to long-acting β2-adrenergic agonists once inhaled glucocorticoids have been initiated (3).

Several recent studies solidify the role of inhaled glucocorticoids as first-line therapy in the management of persistent asthma and also identify some limitations in the efficacy of inhaled glucocorticoids, such as a failure to eradicate acute exacerbations and to completely prevent loss in pulmonary function (8,12). Treatment strategies must address the limitations of inhaled glucocorticoids in preventing asthma progression and reversing pulmonary function in longstanding poorly controlled asthma.

The long-term outcome study from the National Heart, Lung and Blood Institute Childhood Asthma Management Program (CAMP) Research Group established the efficacy of inhaled glucocorticoids as first-line long-term control therapy in children 5–12 years of age with mild to moderate persistent asthma (12). The CAMP clinical trial was initiated in 1991 to determine whether continuous long-term treatment with either an inhaled glucocorticoid (budesonide) or an inhaled non-steroid (nedocromil) control medication could improve lung growth safely over a four- to six-year treatment period as compared to placebo (treatment based only on the management of symptoms with albuterol and oral prednisone as needed).

For clinical outcomes examined in the CAMP study, the most significant treatment effect was observed with the inhaled glucocorticoid treatment arm as compared to placebo. The number of acute exacerbations as indicated by hospitalizations, urgent care visits and prednisone courses were all reduced by approximately 45% in the inhaled budesonide group as compared to the placebo group. The inhaled budesonide group also had better asthma control as indicated by significantly lower symptom scores, higher number of episode free days per month, and less albuterol inhalations per week as compared to the placebo group. For the inhaled nedocromil group, only a reduction in urgent care visits and prednisone courses when compared to the placebo group was observed. There were no differences in the other clinical outcome measures when the inhaled nedocromil group was compared to the placebo group.

The time to the first significant asthma exacerbation that required systemic glucocorticoid (prednisone) therapy and the time for adding supplementary inhaled glucocorticoid therapy also was longer for the inhaled budesonide group as compared to the placebo group, with no difference noted for this indicator when the nedocromil group was compared to the placebo group (Fig. 1, Panel D). The proportion of patients necessitating intervention with oral prednisone or supplementary inhaled glucocorticoid therapy was much lower in the inhaled budesonide group as compared to placebo, while the inhaled nedocromil group was once again comparable to the placebo group for this measure of control.

The primary measure of lung growth selected for this study was postbronchodilator-FEV_1% predicted, because it reflects maximal lung capacity. The CAMP trial showed that the inhaled glucocorticoid treatment increased postbronchodilator FEV_1% predicted from a mean 103.2% predicted to 106.8% predicted within the first two months; however, postbronchodilator FEV_1% predicted gradually diminished to 103.8% predicted by the end of the treatment period (Fig. 1, Panel A), and surprisingly it was comparable to that which occurred in the placebo and nedocromil groups. Postbronchodilator FEV_1% predicted in the nedocromil group was similar to that measured in the placebo group throughout the study period indicating that this treatment had no significant effect on lung growth.

The finding that neither budesonide nor nedocromil provided significant benefit over placebo for the postbronchodilator-percent-predicted FEV_1 was an unexpected result compared to data reported from an earlier study by Agertoft and Pedersen (13). This study reported that early intervention with inhaled glucocorticoids in childhood asthma could prevent irrecoverable loss in pulmonary function. However, this study did not specifically examine postbronchodilator FEV_1 as an outcome measure and it was not conducted in a randomized, placebo-controlled design. Because a decline in FEV_1%-predicted did not occur in the placebo group, the CAMP study results raise questions whether airway remodeling is actually occurring in this population of mild to moderate persistent asthma and/or whether inhaled glucocorticoids have any effect on preventing this alteration in airway pathology. The decline in postbronchodilator FEV_1%-predicted noted in the budesonide treatment arm along with the evolving requirement for supplementary therapy in the CAMP study population suggest that asthma may be progressing despite continuous therapy. Ongoing analysis in the CAMP study population has determined that a reduction in postbronchodilator FEV_1%-predicted occurs in a subset of patients and future research will determine the etiology and significance of this pattern (14).

Since a decline in postbronchodilator FEV_1% predicted was not observed in the placebo group of the CAMP study, questions have been

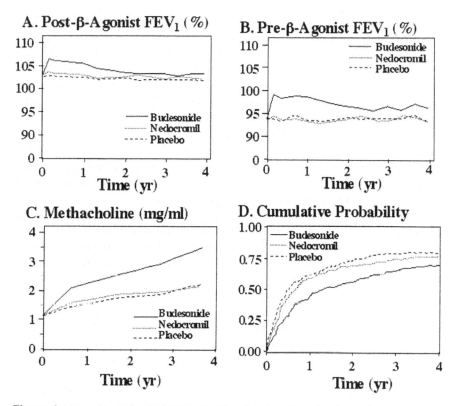

Figure 1 Results of the CAMP Study: Panel A describes the change in postbronchodilator FEV$_1$ during the duration of the study. There was an initial improvement in postronchodilator FEV$_1$ in patients receiving budesonide, but by the end of the study, there were no differences between the three treatment groups. Panel B describes the change in prebronchodilator therapy. Budesonide resulted in a modest, yet statistically significant improvement in prebronchodilator FEV$_1$ throughout the treatment period compared to placebo. Panel C describes the change in methacholine responsiveness over time. Note that all subjects had improvement in bronchial hyperresponsiveness (BHR) as indicated by the increase in methacholine PC$_{20}$ values over the 4–6 years of the trial. Patients randomized to budesonide had a significantly greater reduction in BHR compared to the placebo treated patients. Panel D is a Kaplan–Meier curve describing the cumulative probability of a first course of prednisone during 4 years of followup in the budesonide, nedocromil, and placebo treated children. *Source*: Reprinted from N Engl J Med 2000; 343:1054–63.

raised on whether airway remodeling is occurring in this patient population. It is possible that FEV$_1$%-predictedmay not be sufficiently sensitive to detect the process of airway remodeling. It is also possible that the study did not include patients that are the most susceptible to airway remodeling since patients with severe asthma were excluded. Therefore, those patients who are potentially most susceptible to a progressive loss in $FEV_1\%$ predicted may have been excluded from this study. It is also possible that the most significant effect on FEV_1 decline occurred prior to entering the study as indicated in two previous long-term studies on the natural history of asthma (15,16). Indeed, the mean duration of asthma in the CAMP participants was five years and it is conceivable that the most significant effect on airway structure occurred shortly after the onset of the disease; thus, significant irrecoverable loss in pulmonary function was already established. If these early events are indeed critical, then early diagnosis and prompt effective intervention would be necessary to prevent airway remodeling and the long term consequences of airway inflammation, such as impairment in lung growth or airway hyperresponsiveness.

Other measures of postbronchodilator pulmonary function were not significantly different upon completion of the treatment phase of CAMP. In contrast, in the treatment group, several measurements of pulmonary function obtained prior to bronchodilator administration were different from placebo. The difference in prebronchodilator $FEV_1\%$ predicted following inhaled budesonide treatment as compared to baseline exceeded that in the placebo group (2.9 vs. 0.9, $p = 0.02$) (Fig. 1 Panel B). This observation could possibly be an indicator that the functional airway caliber in the budesonide group was greater than that detected in the placebo group. Although the difference was indeed statistically significant, the magnitude of effect was small.

For inhaled budesonide, the only difference in any measure of pulmonary function when compared to the placebo group was prebronchodilator FEV_1 (liters). Of significant interest was the observation that all of the pulmonary function values were similar for all of the treatment groups four months after the active study medication was discontinued. This important observation suggests that any beneficial effect observed on pulmonary function outcome measures due to active treatment is lost in only a short time following treatment cessation. Moreover, these results indicate that inhaled glucocorticoids do not have a long-term effect on altering the natural history of asthma if administered too late in the course of the disease. Taken together, these CAMP results reinforce the need to perform very early intervention studies to determine if long-term efficacy can be accomplished through early intervention.

The most remarkable effect of inhaled glucocorticoid treatment on a measure of pulmonary function in CAMP was the significant reduction in airway hyperresponsiveness that persisted throughout the treatment period (Fig. 1, Panel C). There was no effect of inhaled nedocromil on airway hyperresponsiveness when compared to placebo. Although inhaled budesonide-reduced airways hyperresponsiveness during treatment, all three groups had similar methacholine PC_{20} after study medication was discontinued. These results further reinforce the concept that long-term outcomes of asthma may not be altered by even the current best treatment option. However, continued prospective evaluation of CAMP participants is ongoing to evaluate the effect of intense long-term treatment courses with anti-inflammatory therapy on maximal lung function and airway hyperresponsiveness as these children approach adulthood.

The CAMP results support the effects of inhaled glucocorticoids on reducing asthma morbidity (12); however, they differ significantly from observations obtained from studies of shorter duration, for example a year or less, particularly in measures of pulmonary function and body growth. The CAMP study showed that the only detectable adverse effect of long-term treatment with inhaled budesonide was a transient reduction in growth velocity that was limited to 1 cm in the first year of treatment that was persistent but not progressive. Based on an estimation of final growth evaluated by bone age and height at the end of the treatment period, the height projected in all three treatment groups would be similar once the participants reached final adult height. Agertoft and Pedersen confirmed this estimate with a report of follow-up in young adults who had received inhaled glucocorticoid therapy during childhood (17). However, long-term follow-up in a prospective study population such as CAMP will still be necessary to relieve the lingering concerns regarding persistent effects of inhaled glucocorticoid therapy on final height.

Importantly, the medications that were studied in the CAMP trial did not completely eliminate the morbidity associated with asthma, such as hospitalization and urgent care visits, and thus there is a need for improvement in overall asthma management. While the CAMP study alleviated some concerns regarding the long-term effect of inhaled glucocorticoid therapy on linear growth, it still raised questions regarding the effect of inhaled glucocorticoids on the natural history of asthma. A greater effect in reducing exacerbations could conceivably be achieved through the use of combination therapy with available medications such as long-acting β2-adrenergic agonists as observed in adults (18), through the introduction of new medications such as the immunomodulators (19), or through earlier intervention with available medications such as inhaled glucocorticoids or even leukotriene antagonist (6,8,20). Some of these various therapeutic alternatives are currently being evaluated in prospective clinical trials.

III. Managing Asthma in Young Children

Studies related to the appropriate time to intervene with anti-inflammatory therapy and the efficacy of such treatments are currently in progress. In this regard, several medications are now labeled and approved for use in young children, specifically nebulized budesonide and montelukast, both approved for use in children as young as one year of age (5,6). Several key pivotal studies substantiate the efficacy of nebulized budesonide in children less than five years of age (5). The approval for montelukast in young children has been based primarily on safety data along with pharmacokinetic data demonstrating that the formulations indicated for use in children provide blood levels comparable to those derived from formulations used in adults. Specific parameters for evaluating the efficacy of montelukast remain to be defined for young children. Currently there is no long-acting β-adrenergic agonist with specific labeling for use in children less than four years old.

Since current treatment plans are based on the assumption that chronic inflammation is a core feature of asthma, and that persistent asthma can occur early in life, there is considerable interest in identifying reliable methods for earlier diagnosis as well as earlier intervention. It remains to be seen whether these strategies for early recognition and early treatment will indeed alter the natural history of asthma and prevent irrecoverable loss of pulmonary function and persistent symptoms. As indicated in the recent update to the NAEPP asthma guidelines, this question calls for the design of prospective, randomized controlled intervention studies with environmental control, pharmacotherapy, immune modulation, or a combination of these alternatives (3).

Currently, asthma management in young children is based primarily on experience derived from studies conducted in older children and adults (2,3,10,20). These limitations are primarily due to challenges related to the diagnosis of early onset asthma and the assessment of asthma control in young children. Although challenging, measurements of pulmonary function in young children are possible, albeit restricted predominantly to research settings in which these types of assessments are routinely performed.

Pharmacotherapy in young children can be further complicated due to the difficulties in properly administering inhaled medication and the dependence of this administration on the caregiver (20). Information regarding the appropriate dose of medications for children less than five years of age is available for some, but not all, medications. The updated asthma guidelines suggest that first-line therapy can start with low-dose inhaled glucocorticoid via nebulizer or alternatively a spacer/holding chamber and face mask (3). As indicated previously, a nebulized budesonide preparation is now approved for use in children as young as one year of age with dosage guidelines for this age group (5). Other alternatives include the use of montelukast that is now available in a granule formulation that can be administered to children as young as one year of age. Comparative studies are needed to determine whether an inhaled glucocorticoid administered by pressurized metered dose inhaler along with a spacer and face-mask is actually equally effective to control attained with nebulized administration. Currently, there is no inhaled glucocorticoid in the dry powder or metered dose inhaler formulation available in the United States that is approved for use in children less than four years of age. Understandably, it is rare that a dry powder formulation will be administered to a young child since this device requires the generation of a sufficient inspiratory flow rate to generate the necessary fine particle size for sufficient pulmonary deposition. In addition, it is likely that the current pressurized metered dose formulations with the chlorofluorocarbon propellants will be removed from the market once the alternative devices are fully accepted. It will therefore be important to evaluate the new hydrofluoroalkane-based metered dose inhalers along with spacer/face mask for their appropriate use in young children including dose definition and safety.

Following the publication of the updated asthma guidelines (3), a study was published that compared nebulized budesonide to inhaled cromolyn via nebulizer (8). This study by Leflein et al. (8) clearly demonstrated superiority in asthma control in the nebulized budesonide formulation group with all measures of symptom control and time for supplementary medication as compared to the cromolyn group. However, the number of hospitalizations and emergency department visits were similar in the two treatment groups.

For the treatment of moderate persistent asthma in young children, the asthma guidelines recommend either a medium dose of inhaled glucocorticoid or the addition of a long-acting β2-adrenergic agonist to low or medium dose inhaled glucocorticoid (3). These recommendations are clearly based on conclusions derived from adult studies in lieu of adequate controlled studies performed in children. However, there is currently no long-acting β2-adrenergic agonist formulation approved for use in children less than four years of age. Admittedly, there are no dosing guidelines that would assure safety. Therefore, it is important to develop and test a hydrofluoroalkane preparation or a nebulized form of a long-acting β2-adrenergic agonist. An alternative decision is to utilize the approved form of a leukotriene antagonist for supplementary therapy with the inhaled glucocorticoid. High dose inhaled glucocorticoids plus a long-acting β2-adrenergic agonist are recommended for more severe asthma. If needed, a systemic glucocorticoid may be added. The dose of the glucocorticoid should be adjusted to the lowest dose required to minimize symptoms and adverse effects.

The updated asthma guidelines also address criteria to consider for early intervention in young children, namely those who are at risk for persistent asthma (3). Recent studies by the Tucson Children's Respiratory Study following analysis of respiratory patterns in children for the first 15 years of life reported that children who wheeze during lower respiratory tract illnesses in the first three years of life and who still wheeze at age six ("persistent wheezers") have lower levels of pulmonary function than children who have not had wheezing illnesses before age six years (21). They reported that the lowest levels of lung function in early childhood are observed among children who wheeze before age three and were not current wheezers at age six. These patients are considered "transient wheezers" as compared to the "persistent wheezers" who have comparably normal pulmonary function in the first three years of life but lower pulmonary function thereafter (14,21). This raises the question whether the observed decline in pulmonary function in "persistent wheezers" can be prevented with early utilization of either environmental control or anti-inflammatory therapy.

This natural history study was also useful in deriving risk factors for the development of persistent asthma. An Asthma Predictive Index, introduced by Castro-Rodriguez et al. (22), documents that frequent wheezing during the first three years of life associated with either one major risk factor (parental history of asthma or eczema in the child), or two of three minor risk factors (eosinophilia >4%, wheezing without colds, and allergic rhinitis), significantly increases the risk of developing asthma by age six years.

It has also been suggested that a loss of pulmonary function over time is associated with airway remodeling (23). This loss of pulmonary function is comparable to the pattern observed in chronic obstructive pulmonary disease in adults and cystic fibrosis in children except that asthma retains a reversible component. It thus appears that patients differ considerably in both clinical presentation and susceptibility to impairment in lung growth. It remains to be seen whether early intervention with anti-inflammatory therapy, such as an inhaled glucocorticoid, can alter the natural history of asthma, especially the component of progressive loss in pulmonary function. Nevertheless, it is already clear that intervention with inhaled glucocorticoids improves asthma control based on well-controlled studies in both young and older children including adolescents (8,12). The NHLBI Childhood Asthma Research and Education Network is now conducting an early intervention study with inhaled glucocorticoid therapy in young children at risk for childhood asthma applying the Asthma Predictive Index (22) as an entry criteria. The results of this study should be available within the next year. This study is designed to answer a number of questions relating to the effect of early intervention with anti-inflammatory therapy on altering clinical and pulmonary function features associated with the development of asthma.

IV. When Should Long-Term Asthma Controller Therapy Be Initiated in Children?

The revised NAEPP asthma guidelines now recommend intervention at several points (3). First, bronchodilators should be administered for symptoms and systemic glucocorticoids for significant exacerbations regardless of the patient's age. Second, intervention with long-term control therapy has been recommended for children with symptoms that occur more than twice per week, nocturnal symptoms that occur more than two times per month, and with pulmonary function that is less than 80% predicted or within day variability in PEF that exceeds 20% (Tables 2 and 3).

Table 2 Guidelines—Classification of Asthma Severity

	Symptoms	Night-time symptoms	Lung function
Step 4 Severe persistent	Continual symptoms Limited physical activity Frequent exacerbations	Frequent	$FEV_1/PEF \leq 60\%$ predicted PEF variability $>30\%$
Step 3 Moderate persistent	Daily symptoms Daily use of inhaled short-acting β2-agonist Exacerbations affect activity Exacerbations ≥ 2 times a week; may last days	>1 time a week	$FEV_1/PEF \leq 60\%$ - $<80\%$ predicted PEF variability $>30\%$
Step 2 Mild persistent	Symptoms >2 times a week, but <1 time a day Exacerbations may affect activity	≥ 2 times a month	$FEV_1/PEF \geq 80\%$ predicted PEF variability >20–30%
Mild intermittent	Symptoms ≤ 2 times a week Asymptomatic and normal PEF between exacerbations Exacerbations brief (from a few hours to a few days), intensity may vary	≤ 2 times a month	$FEV_1/PEF \geq 80\%$ predicted PEF variability $<20\%$

Source: NIH Guidelines for the Diagnosis and Treatment of Asthma, 1997

Table 3 Stepwise Approach for Managing Asthma in Adults and Children Older than 5 Years of Age

	Clinical features before treatment or adequate control			Daily medications required to maintain long-term control[a]
	Daytime symptoms	Nighttime symptoms	PEF (% of personal best) or FEV_1 (% of predicted)	PEF variability (%)	
Step 4 Severe persistent	Continual	Frequent	<60	≥30	*Preferred treatment:* High-dose inhaled corticosteroids and long-acting inhaled β2-agonists *Additional treatment (if needed):* Corticosteroid tablets or syrup, long term (2 mg/kg/day, generally without exceeding 60 mg per day)[b]
Step 3 Moderate persistent	Daily	>1 night per week	>60–<80	>30	*Preferred treatment* Low- to medium-dose inhaled corticosteroids and long-acting inhaled β2-agonists *Alternate treatment:* Increased inhaled corticosteroids within medium-dose range, or low- to medium-dose inhaled corticosteroids and either leukotriene modifier or theophylline

	Days	Nights			Treatment
					If needed, particularly in patients with recurring severe exacerbations:
					Preferred treatment: Increased inhaled corticosteroids within medium-dose range, and add long-acting inhaled β2-agonists
					Alternate treatment: Increased inhaled corticosteroids in medium-dose range, and add either leukotriene modifier or theophylline
Step 2 Mild persistent	>2/week but < 1x/day	>2 nights/ month	≥80	20–30	*Preferred treatment:* Low-dose inhaled corticosteroids
					Alternate treatment: Cromolyn, leukotriene modifier, nedocromil, or sustained-release theophylline to serum concentration of 5–15 mcg/mL
Step 1 Mild intermittent	≤2 days/week	≤2 nights/ month	>80	<20	No daily medication needed. Severe exacerbations may occur, separated by long periods of normal lung function and no symptoms. A course of systemic corticosteroids is recommended.

(Continued)

Table 3 Stepwise Approach for Managing Asthma in Adults and Children Older than 5 Years of Age (*Continued*)

Step down	Goals of asthma management
Review treatment every 1–6 months; a gradual stepwise reduction in treatment may be possible	Minimal or no chronic symptoms day or night
	Minimal or no exacerbations
	No limitations on activities; no school/work missed
	PEF >80% of personal best
	Minimal use of inhaled short-acting β2-agonists (<1x per day)
	Minimal or no adverse effects from medications

The stepwise approach is meant to assist, not replace, the clinical decision-making required to meet individual patient needs. Classify severity by assigning the patient to the most severe step in which any feature occurs (PEF is percent of personal best; FEV$_1$ is % predicted). Gain control as quickly as possible (consider a short course of systemic corticosteroids) then step down to the least medication necessary to maintain control. Provide education on self-management and controlling environmental factors that make asthma worse (e.g., allergens and irritants). Refer to an asthma specialist if there are difficulties controlling asthma or if step 4 care is required. Referral may be considered if step 3 care is required.

[a]For all patients: (1) Short-acting bronchodilator (2–4 puffs short-acting inhaled β2-agonists as needed for symptoms). (2) Intensity of treatment will depend on severity of exacerbation; up to three treatments at 20-minute intervals or a single nebulizer treatment, as needed. Course of systemic corticosteroids may be needed. (3) Use of short-acting inhaled β2-agonists on a daily basis or increasing their use indicates the need to initiate or increase long-term control therapy.

[b]Make repeat attempts to reduce systemic corticosteroids and maintain control with high-dose inhaled corticosteroids.

In addition, the guidelines suggest that intervention with long-term controller therapy should be considered in young children when they have significant acute exacerbations that recur within six weeks. The updated guidelines also suggest a consideration for intervention with long-term therapy in the young child who is at risk for persistent asthma based on frequent episodes of wheezing and major or minor risk factors that comprise the Asthma Predictive Index as described previously (22).

V. Evolution of Asthma Therapy and Potential for Future Developments

The treatment of asthma, less than 50 years ago, was originally focused on alleviating episodes of bronchospasm using short acting bronchodilators that included epinephrine, isoproterenol, and metaproterenol. Less than 20 years ago theophylline, a long acting bronchodilator, was the preferred maintenance therapy for asthma. Alteration of the oral release characteristics resulted in the development of products that facilitated twice-and even once-daily administration and also offered benefits in reducing the number of nighttime asthma episodes. Subsequently, it was recognized that inhaled cromolyn administered prior to an allergen challenge in a sensitized patient offered advantages in attenuating the early and late pulmonary response to an allergen challenge and also blocking the development of airways hyperresponsiveness. These observations helped introduce the concept of preventative therapy.

Although the benefits of inhaled glucocorticoid therapy dosing were recognized in the late 1970s, they were not considered preferred therapy until the clear documentation of efficacy in the long-term management of asthma for both adults and children. Several new classes of medications were introduced in the last ten years including the long-acting $\beta2$-adrenergic agonists and the leukotriene modifiers. The long acting $\beta2$-adrenergic agonists, specifically salmeterol and formoterol, have a 12-hour duration of bronchodilator action, and are now approved for use in children four years of age and older. The oral leukotriene antagonist, montelukast, has emerged as the most popular first-line long-term control therapy in children with asthma due to the availability of product information regarding dosage and the demonstration of safety in children as young as one year of age.

To limit the adverse effects of short-acting $\beta2$-agonists, the stereoisomer of albuterol, levalbuterol was developed and introduced (24). Levalbuterol, the active bronchodilator component of albuterol, has less adverse effect with comparable doses of albuterol especially for cardiac stimulation. This is an advantage for continuous administration schedules. Also, renewed interest has developed for the combination of medications in one formulation, such as an inhaled steroid and a long-acting $\beta2$-adrenergic agonist, based on evidence of additive effects, convenience for the patient, and the potential to further reduce the risk for significant exacerbation (18). This combination has the benefits of the unique effects of each medication including bronchodilator, bronchoprotective, and anti-inflammatory effects. Combination therapy is now approved for use in children as young as four years old. Physicians now have the opportunity to individualize the patient's treatment plan with this selection of potent medications that can address concerns of cost, taste, and ease of administration.

The research discoveries based on information from bronchoscopy, bronchoalveolar lavage, biopsy, molecular biology, along with non-invasive measures of airway inflammation, stimulate new considerations for the use of approved medications, and also a base for developing new entities. For example, the observation that certain mediators are present in airway inflammation, such as IL-4, IL-5, IL-13, and interferon gamma, has generated the development and clinical trial evaluation of drugs that block or enhance these mediators (25), [also see chapter by Dr. Barnes in this book]. Another concept being evaluated is a DNA vaccine therapy with antisense oligonucleotides to block the inflammatory response (26). Currently, the immunomodulator that is now approved is anti-IgE. Several reports have indicated that anti-IgE has the potential to reduce the frequency of acute exacerbations and improve asthma control (27–29). Phosphodiesterase 4 inhibitors are also undergoing early clinical trials.

VI. Variable Response to Treatment and Relevance of the Asthma Phenotype

The National Heart, Lung, and Blood Institute Asthma Clinical Research Network (ACRN) identified significant variability in response associated with inhaled glucocorticoid therapy in adults with compromised pulmonary function and persistent asthma (30). The effect of increasing doses of inhaled glucocorticoids on improvement in pulmonary function and reduction in airways hyperresponsiveness was evaluated in 30 adult participants with persistent asthma and FEV_1 percent predicted between 55% and 85%.

Several key observations were reported in this study related to measures of response. It was noted that near maximal FEV_1 and methacholine PC_{20} change was obtained with low to medium dose for both inhaled glucocorticoids evaluated, fluticasone propionate and beclomethasone dipropionate, administered with a metered dose inhaler and a spacer device. The highest dose of each inhaled glucocorticoid did not result in a further increase in efficacy for either outcome measure, but did show an increased systemic effect as determined by overnight plasma cortisol concentrations. Of interest, there was significant variability in response among the participants with both inhaled glucocorticoids. The investigators cautioned that it is possible that higher doses of inhaled glucocorticoids may be necessary to manage more severe patients or to prevent significant asthma exacerbations.

About one-third of the subjects had a good pulmonary response as determined by greater than 15% improvement in FEV_1, while another third had a marginal response, between 5% and 15% increase in FEV_1, and another third failed to respond showing less than 5% increase in FEV_1. A similar pattern was observed with the reduction in methacholine PC_{20}. The FEV_1 improvement did not correlate to the PC_{20} improvement and therefore, patients can improve with one measure of response without showing an effect with the other response measure. Thus, the type of response and the magnitude of effect can vary among patients. Certain biomarkers, specifically exhaled nitric oxide and sputum eosinophils, along with asthma characteristics including duration of asthma and their bronchodilator response, could be associated with these two response parameters (30). The ACRN is currently conducting studies to define the mechanisms of poor response to inhaled glucocorticoid therapy.

In addition, the NHLBI Childhood Asthma Research and Education (CARE) Network is completing a study to determine if poor response to inhaled glucocorticoid therapy can occur in children and whether the biomarkers that predict response in adults are similar in children. A unique feature of this study will be to determine whether the response to an inhaled glucocorticoid is proportional to the response to a leukotriene antagonist. An assessment of asthma-associated phenotypic characteristics similar to that conducted by the ACRN in adults as well as genotypic analysis will be evaluated in these children to further identify predictors of response to the two medications.

There are a number of factors that can lead to disease variability within patients over time including environmental exposure and sensitivity to allergens, tobacco smoke exposure, environmental irritants, medication adherence, etc. However, there are also a number of variables that can effect the response to medications among a group of patients and these factors include, medication pharmacokinetics, genetic variability in receptor response, severity of disease including features of airway remodeling or irreversible changes in lung function, and perception of symptoms, to name a few.

A review by Payne and Balfour-Lynn (31) provides an approach to the management of severe, persistent asthma in children. They proposed that tools to measure airway inflammation such as exhaled nitric oxide, induced sputum, bronchoalveolar lavage and biopsy could be used to assist with decisions regarding alternative anti-inflammatory therapy or bronchodilator therapy. Other measures of airway inflammation, such as interleukin-4 and interferon gamma, can be measured in exhaled breath condensates (32). The field of biomarker measurement is rapidly progressing with the recent ability to measure carbon monoxide, pH and even leukotrienes in exhaled condensates (33–36). Biomarkers can also be measured in induced sputum. For example, levels of matrix metalloproteinase (MMP)-9 and the tissue inhibitor of matrix metalloproteinase (TIMP) -1 can be measured in induced sputum (37). The balance of MMP-9 and TIMP has been associated with the airway remodeling process. Thus, there are growing opportunities to incorporate biomarkers in the assessment of disease control, potential prediction of medication response, as well as indicators of treatment effect on inflammation control and long-term sequelae of uncontrolled inflammation. These measures could also be applied to investigate the mechanisms associated with treatment failure.

However, there is little evidence in children that these markers or indicators of airway inflammation can be reliably applied to clinical management. In an innovative study conducted by Sont et al. (38), it was observed that a treatment plan based on measures of methacholine PC_{20} along with the guidelines approach could lead to better asthma control as compared to the guidelines approach alone. They also observed a greater reduction in subepithelial fibrosis in the airway hyperresponsiveness-based group suggesting a potential reversal in airway remodeling. The studies from the ACRN (30) provide a note of caution in applying this approach since patients may not be able to reduce airway hyperresponsiveness or improve pulmonary function with inhaled glucocorticoid doses beyond the medium dose range. This raises the question whether those patients who fail to respond have persistent inflammation as previously recognized or perhaps structural airway changes that are unresponsive to any form of available anti-inflammatory therapy. It is possible that new medications or approaches need to be developed to treat these refractory patients.

A similar study conducted by Green et al. (39) utilized sputum eosinophil counts as a guide for making adjustments in asthma therapy as compared to a conventional guidelines approach. Of interest, the investigators reported a sixfold reduction in asthma exacerbations with the treatment strategy that was directed at normalization of the induced sputum eosinophils. Curiously, it did not result in a greater need for additional anti-inflammatory therapy on average as compared to the guidelines-based approach. Therefore, the biomarker-based approach stimulates interest in treatment strategies directed at reducing markers of inflammation resulting in an overall improvement in asthma management.

Chan et al. (40) reported that patients classified as severe "steroid resistant" asthma have at least two different patterns of pulmonary function in the presence of optimal therapy. One group of patients with low pulmonary function had a fixed pattern of pulmonary function despite high dose systemic glucocorticoid therapy, while another group had apattern of variable pulmonary function. Of interest is the observation that African Americans had a greater prevalence of steroid resistant asthma, as defined by failure to improve FEV_1, as compared to Caucasians. It will therefore be important to obtain further information on the mechanisms for these two patterns of apparent steroid resistance along with the reason for the higher prevalence of steroid resistance in the African American population.

The area of pharmacogenetics could provide additional information on the relationships of genetics to medication response (41–43). Advances in this area could be useful in defining asthma phenotypes and genotypes for associations with good or poor response to medications and assist the clinician in selecting treatment approaches that are tailored for the individual patient. The response to medications could be related to specific genetic polymorphisms that alter the drug response at the receptor or cellular level, influence drug metabolism pathways (43), or modify asthma-associated disease features, such as increased IgE production, that could influence the level of response to available asthma medications (44–53). This information could provide unique opportunities to understand variability in drug response as well as new methods to select medications to optimize response. The following section will summarize available information in several categories of genetics and the potential impact on medication response.

VII. Genetic and Pharmacogenetic Advances in Asthma Research

Traditionally, pharmacogenetics is associated with understanding variability in drug metabolizing enzymes (DMEs) that alter the pharmacokinetic profile of a medication, ultimately resulting in alteration in the pharmacologic response. Knowledge of relevant polymorphisms has been useful in dosing medications with narrow margins of safety, such as succinylcholine. This section will not address DMEs with asthma medications, but will focus on drug targets, such as receptors, enzymes and enzyme systems. A pharmacodynamic approach will be emphasized, for example β2 adrenergic receptor genotypes (Fig. 2) are examples of changes in a drug target, illustrating the lack of pharmacokinetic involvement. (54). Pharmacogenetics of asthma medications also includes genetic polymorphisms related to the disease process since medications used in asthma either augment or inhibit the body's endogenous cellular messengers, including epinephrine, cortisol, and leukotrienes. Table 4 provides a list of candidate genes that may influence response to asthma medications.

In the study of pharmacogenetics, the Hardy–Weinberg equilibrium is utilized to determine if the population in question is an appropriate population. The Hardy–Weinberg equation is defined as $p^2 + 2pq + q^2 = 1$; where p is the wild type allele, and q is the mutant. It is important to describe the population being evaluated since genetic variation may differ due to severity of disease, ethnicity, and population geography.

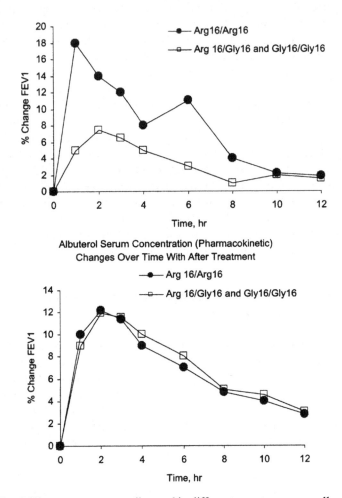

Figure 2 Different response to albuterol in different genotypes, regardless of serum concentrations. This demonstrates how the pharmacogenetics of asthma medications is driven by response (pharmacodynamics), but not serum concentrations (pharmacokinetics). *Source*: From Ref. 54.

A. β2-Adrenergic Receptor (β2AR)

One of the most carefully examined and also the most controversial area of asthma pharmacogenetics is related to the polymorphisms of the β2AR. The β2AR is coded on the intronless ADRB2 gene located on chromosome 5q31–5q33. In this gene, several Single Nucleotide Polymorphisms (SNPs–a

Table 4 List of Candidate Genes That May Affect Response to Asthma Medications

Gene	Gene locus	Protein
B2AR	5q31–33	β2-Adrenergic receptor
ADCY9	16pl3.3	Adenylate cyclase type 9
ALOX5	10	5-Lipoxygenase
LTA4H	12q22	LTA_4 Hydrolase
LTC4S	5q35	LTC_4 Synthase
ABCC1	16pl3.1	Multi-drug resistant protein 1
GGT1	22q11.1–11.2	Gamma glutamyl transferase
GCR	5q31	Glucocorticoid receptor
NOS1	12q24.2–24.31	Nitric oxide synthase 1
NOS2	17cent-q11.2	Nitric oxide synthase 2
NOS3	7q35–36	Nitric oxide synthase 3
TNFα	6p21.3	Tumor necrosis factor α
TNFRSF1A	12pl3.2	Tumor necrosis factor α receptor I
TNFRSF1B	lp36.3–36.2	Tumor necrosis factor α receptor II
NFKB1,NFKB2	4q23–24, 10q24	NF-κB
IKBKG	Xq28	NF-κB essential modulator (NEMO)

SNP is a single change in the nucleic acid sequence of a gene, that may or may not have resultant changes in the amino acid sequence of the translated protein) have been described. At amino acid position 16 and 27, these changes contribute to tachyphylaxis. At amino acid position 164, this change alters receptor binding to agonists. However, because the frequency of this SNP is low, it is not usually addressed in pharmacogenetic studies of the β2AR (Table 5). There are also at least eight SNPs upstream relative to the initiation site in the nucleic acid sequence. A part of the upstream region codes for a 19 amino acid peptide cistron leader to the β2AR, is of interest due to a SNP at nucleic acid position -47 that codes for a change in the amino acid sequence altering β2AR expression (Table 5).

Table 5 β$_2$-adrenergic receptor SNPs and Their Corresponding Amino Acid Changes

Nucleotide change	Amino acid change	Function of amino acid change
1. $A_{46}G$	$Arg_{16}Gly$ ($R_{16}G$)	These two changes may influence the ability of the receptor to
2. $C_{79}G$	$Gln_{27}Glu$ ($Q_{27}E$)	Insert into the cell's membrane (148)
3. $C_{491}T$	$Thr_{164}Ile$ ($T_{164}I$)	Proximal to β$_2$-adrenergic agonist binding site; alters binding affinity (149)
4. $T_{-47}C$	$Cys_{-19}Arg$ ($C_{-19}R$)	Affects transcription of β$_2$AR (150)

Glycine (Gly) at position 16 has been associated with an increase in nocturnal asthma (55) and steroid dependent asthma. Glutamine (Gln) at position 27 has reported associations with childhood asthma (56), increased bronchial hyperresponsiveness (57), and increased IgE (58). These SNPs are also associated with changes in β2AR function. Lima et al. (54) observed response to oral albuterol (8 mg) in moderate asthmatics. They reported a more rapid increase and greater response (change in FEV_1% predicted) to albuterol in patients homozygous for Arg16 when compared to patients homozygous for Gly16 and heterozygous for both. There were no differences in albuterol peak concentrations or AUC between the two groups (Fig. 3).

Green et al. (59) examined β-agonist function characteristics associated with the 16 and 27 amino acid positions. Through receptor expression studies in Chinese hamster fibroblasts, they reported that Glu27 was not associated with down-regulation; whereas Gly16 was associated with significant down-regulation (41%). The Gly16 with Glu27 was associated with 39% down-regulation (wildtype was 26% down-regulation). It was concluded that Gly16 has the greatest influence on down-regulation (59). They also evaluated individual polymorphisms on the expression of β2ARby observing surface density on human airway smooth muscle after prolonged (24 hours) exposure to isoproterenol. The homozygote for Arg16 had approximately 78% down-regulation, while homozygotes for Gly16 demonstrated 96% down-regulation, and homozygotes for Glu27 had 30% down-regulation. There were no homozygotes for Gln27 and Glu27 showed less desensitization compared to the other two genotypes (59).

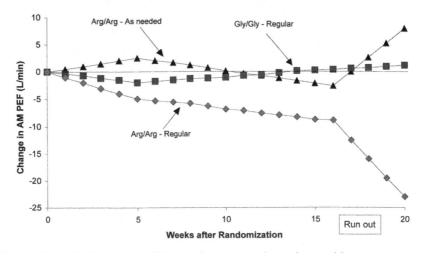

Figure 3   This shows the difference in response in patients with same genotype (Arg16/Arg16), based on as needed albuterol (1.25 puffs/day) compared to scheduled albuterol (7.2 puffs/day). *Source*: From Ref. 60.

Israel et al. (60) observed different features of response. This group reported that in asthma subjects receiving regular albuterol use versus as needed use (7.2 vs. 1.25 puffs/day), participants who were homozygotes for Arg16 had significantly greater deterioration in morning peak expiratory flow rate (PEFR)(-30.5 L/min ± 12.1) as compared to those who received as needed β2-agonists ($p = 0.012$). Participants who were homozygous for Gly16 demonstrated no changes in pulmonary function with regular use of β2-agonists (Fig. 3). There were no significant changes at the 27 position (60). It was postulated that this variable effect following β-agonist administration in patients with different genotypes may be due to the possibility that the β2AR exists in a dynamic state. The β2AR may produce seemingly paradoxical results when patients adminsiter β2-agonists on a scheduled regimen versus intermittent use (61). McGraw et al. (62) examined function related to alterations in the 5′ cistron leader peptide at position -19. Through receptor density studies, they reported that patients who were homozygous for Cys had a greater receptor density when compared to patients who were homozygous for Arg at the -19 position.

Haplotypes have also been investigated for their disease modifying properties as well as their association with response to β2-agonists. Haplotypes are multiple alleles that are in linkage disequilibrium with one another. Linkage disequilibrium is described as the occurrence of

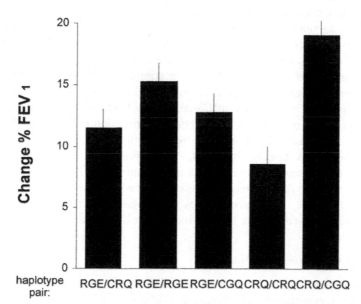

Figure 4 Heterogeneity in response with different haplotype pairs. Unfortunately there were no CGQ haplotype pairs in this population to offer comparison. *Source*: From Ref. 64.

multiple SNPs (or polymorphisms) with one another at a greater frequency than would be predicted by random observation. Ulbrecht et al. (63) observed linkage disequilibrium in the combinations of Arg16Gln27, Gly16Gln27, and Gly16Glu27. Those with the Gly16Gln27 haplotype had greater bronchial hyperresponsiveness to methacholine. The haplotype Arg16Glu27 was not observed (62). They observed linkage disequilibrium between the three alleles (positions −19, 16, and 27). The haplotypes of Arg-19, Gly16, and Glu27 (with single letter designations of RGE) were seen in combination with one another. Cys-19, Arg16, and Gln27 (CRQ) were also seen in combination with one another (62).

Drysdale et al. (64) examined 13 SNPs across four ethnic groups. Twelve haplotypes were observed (out of the possible 8192 combinations). In these 12 haplotypes, three of the most common were investigated, containing three of the previously described alleles. The haplotypes were Arg-19Gly16Glu27 (RGE), Cys-19Arg16Gln27 (CRQ), and Cys-19Gly16Gln27 (CGQ). The three most common haplotype pairs were then observed in relationship to their percent change in FEV_1 (Fig. 4). After examination of this figure, it is difficult to make intuitive remarks on the haplotype pairs, especially with the lack of a CRQ homozygote. These unexpected results emphasize the importance of examining haplotypes of the gene rather than a single genotype for linking a response to the β2-agonist (64).

Adenylate cyclase is an important second messenger enzyme associated with the activation of the β2AR. Recently a polymorphism has been reported in the coding region of the gene ($A_{2316}G$) that translates to a change in the amino acid sequence ($Ile_{772}Met$) of adenylate cyclase isoform 9 (AC9) (65). In vitro studies demonstrated that this change in amino acid sequence results in a loss of catalytic activity of AC9 after stimulation of the β2AR by isoproterenol, both at baseline and at maximal stimulation. The allele frequency for the mutant $_{2316}G$ was similar in Caucasian and Asian populations (0.3 and 0.37), but lower in the African American population (0.19) (65). Although there was no linkage disequilibrium between the SNP in AC9 and SNPs in β2AR, the observation is significant. Needless to say more work is needed to define the relevance of the various β2AR polymorphisms to predict functional response to β2-adrenergic agonists. This will be necessary for the application of β2AR pharmacogenetics to decisions around initiating or discontinuing β2-adrenergic agonist therapy in individual patients.

B. Leukotriene Synthesis

The leukotriene synthesis pathway has multiple target proteins for pharmacologic intervention through either synthesis inhibitors or leukotriene receptor antagonists (Fig. 5). These protein enzymes or receptors contain polymorphisms that contribute to the variation in response to the pharmacologic interventions. In the initial steps of leukotriene synthesis, nuclear

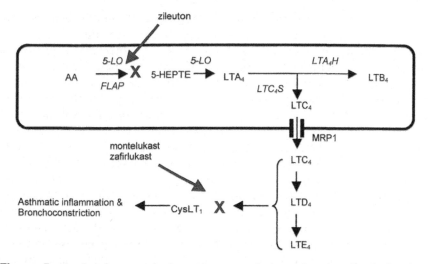

Figure 5 Leukotriene synthesis pathway, and sites of action for leukotriene modifiers.

membrane-bound phospholipase A_2 (PLA2) liberates arachadonic acid (AA) from phosphatidyl choline in the nuclear membrane of the cell. AA is then presented to 5-lipoxygenase (5-LO coded by the ALOX5 gene) by 5-LO activating protein (FLAP, coded by the ALOX5AP gene). The genes that code for these two enzymes contain polymorphisms that alter response to 5-LO inhibitors (zileuton), and also have an association with the incidence of asthma. Koshino et al. (66) demonstrated an association between Japanese asthmatics and increased amounts of 5-LO and FLAP enzymes in their peripheral blood leukocytes. In the FLAP enzyme, two types of polymorphisms have been reported, both in the promoter region of the enzyme. When polymorphisms occur in the promoter region, they may alter the transcription of DNA, rather than modifying the function of the final protein. In the promoter region of FLAP, they investigated triple adenine repeats, that are recognized as 18A and 21A repeats. They reported that patients with the 21A repeat had a greater incidence of asthma when compared to healthy controls (71 patients in each group, 73.2% vs. 54.9%, $p = 0.035$); the functional significance of this polymorphism is unknown (66), Sayers et al. evaluated this polymorphism as well as a SNP in the promoter region of FLAP ($G_{-336}A$) in 341 Caucasian families. Contrary to the report of Koshino et al. (66) they did not find an association with asthma for any of the polymorphisms in the promoter region with asthma (67).

In the coding region of 5-LO, there are three SNPs: $C_{21}T$, $G_{270}A$, and $A_{1738}G$ (68). These changes are considered to be synonymous, as they do not produce a change in the amino acid sequence. Within the gene promoter region, the SNPs $G_{-1708}A$, and $G_{-1761}A$, are present but are not associated with altered function (68). A family of polymorphisms is located in the promoter region of 5-LO that are 212–88 base pairs upstream from the transcription initiation site, composed of glycine and cytosine (G,C) rich repeats. This area is recognized as binding motifs for the zinc finger transcription factors Spl and Egr-1. The binding area for Spl and Egr-I are GGGCGG and GCGGGGGCG, respectively; and these binding motifs overlap (Fig. 6). The three polymorphisms in this region are considered to be the deletion of one, two, or addition of one six base pair binding motif. In assays that measure activity and binding affinity, these polymorphisms may bind to Sp 1 and Egr-1, but all with lower activity. It may be speculated that these polymorphisms contribute to less 5-LO expression, and thus lower overall production of leukotrienes. Evidence for the association of these polymorphisms in the ALOX5AP and ALOX5 genes is somewhat conflicting. However, it should be noted that although these genes are not associated with a causing for asthma, but they may modify the disease severity (68).

To examine the relation of these polymorphisms to drug response, Drazen et al. (69) utilized a second generation 5-LO inhibitor, ABT-761. Participants ($n = 114$) were genotyped for the 5-LO wild type and mutant alleles; the mutant alleles of the one or two deletion, or one addition of the six-base pair binding motifs were combined as the mutant allele. The wild type had the greatest allele frequency (0.772) and homozygote frequency (0.602). Carriers of the wild type allele (homozygote plus heterozygotes) made up 95% of the study population; 5% were homozygotes for the

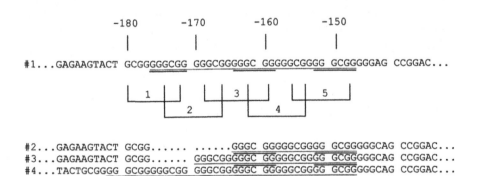

Figure 6 The 5-LO promoter region containing deletion and addition polymorphisms. The GGGCGG polymorphism (consecutively underlined and double underlined) denotes the SP1 binding motif, and the (G)GCGGGGGCG polymorphism (overlapping) denotes the Egr-1 binding motif (68). *Source:* Modified from In KH, et al. J Clin Invest 1997;99(5):1 130–1137.

mutant allele. Utilizing FEV_1 as the indicator of response, participants homozygous or heterozygous for the wild type allele had significantly greater response to treatment than the homozygotes for the mutant allele ($p < 0.0001$, and $p = 0.0006$, respectively). None of the participants who were homozygotes for the mutant allele had an FEV_1 response greater than 12%. There were no significant differences noted between the wild type or mutant alleles when other outcome indicators were examined, such as peak expiratory flow rates (PEFRs) and β2 agonist rescue therapy (69). These observations support an alteration in response that is derived from the promoter region.

The LTA_4 is a product of 5-LO and FLAP that is quickly converted to either LTB_4 (by LTA_4 hydrolase, LTA4H) or by conjugation with reduced glutathione, to the cysteinyl leukotriene, LTC_4 (by LTC_4 synthase, LTC4S) (Fig. 5). Two SNPs have been identified in the promoter region of the gene that code for the LTC4S enzyme. The first SNP is 444 basepairs upstream from the site of transcription initiation which changes from adenine to cytosine ($A_{-444}C$). Aspirin intolerance is observed in 10–20% of adult asthmatics. This polymorphism occurs with increased frequency in aspirin intolerant asthmatics (AIA) when compared to aspirin tolerant asthmatics (ATA) and normal controls (70–72). For the $_{-444}C$ allele, Sanak et al. (73) observed an allele frequency of 39% in ATA, 27% in ATA and 27% in normal controls ($p = 0.01$, and 0.025, respectively). There was a significant increase in urinary LTE_4 in carriers of the C allele compared to homozygotes for the A allele ($p < 0.006$), but no significant changes in PD_{20} for methacholine challenges. The proposed function of the $_{-444}C$

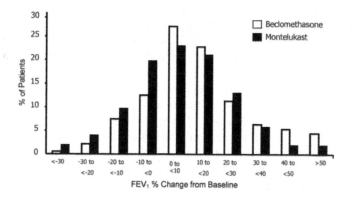

Figure 7 This figure exemplifies the gradient-like response that is observed with asthma medications in a population. Full knowledge polymorphisms in the asthma pharmacogenetic candidate genes discussed may be superimposable to this chart. In this figure from Malmstrom et al. striped bars represent montelukast 10 mg once daily and white bars represent beclomethasone 200 µg inhaled twice daily. *Source*: Adapted from Ref. 147.

polymorphism is that it provides an additional binding site for histone H4 transcription factor and thus facilitates increased synthesis of the enzyme.

The $_{-444}$C polymorphism has been associated with increased pulmonary function following leukotriene modifier administration; however, the available data are not conclusive. Sampson et al. (74) demonstrated a non-significant trend in the $_{-444}$C carrier, as an increased response to zafirlukast when given 20 mg twice daily for two weeks in addition to regular treatment in severe asthmatics with a 9% and 15% improvement in FEV_1 and FVC, compared to controls who had a –12% and –18% change, respectively ($p = 0.1$). In a study conducted on patients with asthma in Japan, a better response to a leukotriene modifier (pranlukast, 225 mg twice daily for four weeks) was observed if they were carriers of the $_{-444}$C allele. Heterozygotes for the mutant C allele showed a 14.3% $\pm$ 5.3% improvement in FEV_1 when compared to homozygotes for the A allele (3.1% $\pm$ 2.4%, $p < 0.01$). However, there was no significant difference in urinary LTE_4 concentrations between the groups (75). Whelan et al. (76) reported that children who were carriers of the C allele responded more favorably to montelukast when compared to children who were carriers of the A allele as indicated by reduction in exhaled NO ($p < 0.05$). Thus, selection of patients for treatment with a leukotriene antagonist based on the presence of this polymorphism could provide a useful technique for optimizing response. The SNP $G_{-1072}A$ in the promoter region of LTC4S has also been evaluated in asthmatics. Although it is associated with increase LTC4S transcription in vitro, it has not associated with any functional activity in lung function (77,78).

Once LTC_4 is synthesized, it is then transported out of the cell to be further transformed into the more active form, LTD_4. Multidrug resistance protein (MRP1) is the transport protein for LTC_4. There are multiple SNPs encoded in this gene ($G_{816}A$, $T_{825}C$, $T_{1684}C$, and $G_{4002}A$) that are candidate sites for an association with asthma as well as response to leukotriene modifying drugs (79). Currently, there are no identified polymorphisms in the genes that code for cysteinyl leukotriene receptor-1 (Cys-LTl) and associated with altered expression or function of the protein receptor that binds leukotriene receptor antagonists. However, IL-4 and IL-13 can up-regulate expression of Cys-LTl. These two cytokines have several polymorphisms that could potentially alter response to leukotriene modifiers (80–83).

The LTA4H is also of interest since elevated concentrations of LTB_4 have been reported in asthmatic children (84). The gene encoding LTA4H has several sites of interest. When these sites are altered by mutagenesis they influence expression of LTA4H (85–87). There may be a dynamic interplay between LTA4H and LTC4S that modulates the severity of asthma. Phospholipase A_2 (PLA_2) is an early enzyme in the pathway of LT synthesis; Clara Cell secretory protein (CC16) is an endogenous protein that may exhibit anti-inflammatory properties via blockage (at least one mechanism) of PLA_2 (88,89). A SNP has been identified ($A_{38}G$) that results in increased amounts of CC16 in the respiratory tract, suggesting that homozygotes for the A allele are at greater risk for asthma (90,91). Although investigation in the area of leukotriene synthesis genetics has been extensive, a practical clinical model has not been established. Perhaps, the techniques used or the number of patients studied has not been adequate.

C. Glucocorticoid Receptor (GR)

Another area of interest in asthma pharmacogenetics relates to the gluco-corticoid receptor (GR) and other proteins associated with response to glucocorticosteroids (GCs). The pathway through which GCs control inflammation is complex with numerous cytosolic and nuclear proteins. Briefly, the lipid soluble GC enters the cell's cytoplasm through the cellular membrane via passive diffusion. The GC then interacts with the complexed GR. The GR is complexed with two heat shock proteins (HSP90), p23 protein, and an immunophillin related protein, all of which contribute to the stabilization of the GR for GC binding. The complex fragments and the new GR-GC complex is translocated into the nucleus, initiating numerous interactions with activator and co-activator proteins, transcription factors (TFs), and other basal transcriptional components. The result is alteration of transcriptional activity by repression of inflammatory proteins (IL-1 through 6, 11, 13, 16, TNFα, NOS2, NF-KB, MMP9, and RANTES, etc.,) and induction of anti-inflammatory proteins (lipocortin-l, IL-1 receptor decoy, and proteinase inhibitor, etc.) (92).

Currently, inhaled glucocorticoids are the cornerstone of asthma therapy; however, there is great variability in response to these medications for efficacy and systemic adverse effects (Fig. 7). This variability in response may be due to genetic polymorphisms in the GR, as well as other proteins involved in this pathway. Generally, the GR exists in two isoforms: α and β. The GRα isoform binds ligand, whereas the GRβ does not. GRα and β are identical through amino acid 727, at which point GRα has an additional 50 amino acids and GRβ has an additional 15 amino acids. The additional amino acid sequences are not synonymous between the isoforms. Because the GRβ isoform does not bind ligand, it has been associated with glucocorticoid resistance as well as fatal asthma (93–95). There are five known SNPs in the GR gene that lead to the amino acid changes $Arg_{23}Lys$, $Asn_{363}Ser$, $Ile_{559}Asn$, $Asp_{641}Val$, and $Val_{729}Ile$. The mutation of $A_{2054}T$ leads to the $Asp_{641}Val$ change that, in vitro, leads to a threefold reduction in binding affinity (Kd) when compared to the wild type (96). The $A_{2317}G$ mutation leads to the $Val_{729}Ile$ change, also resulting in an increased Kd in vitro (twofold) (97). These mutations, as well as the $Asn_{336}Ser$ have been linked to familial glucocorticoid resistance in a small subset of patients (96–98).

De Lange et al. (99) evaluated the effects of these mutations. Five mutations, as well as the GRα/β isoforms, were compared to the wild type GR in vitro with the addition of 10^{-7} M dexamethasone. Several markers of GC-GR activity were investigated. With transcription activation, Val641 and ILe729 had markedly lower activity, whereas Asn559 and GRβ demonstrated no activity. In glucocorticoid responsive element repression of transcription, Val641 and ILe729 showed similar activity to the wild-type, whereas Asn559 and GRB demonstrated no activity. In NF-KB transcription repression the rank order was Val641>wild-type=Lys23>IIe729>> Asn559=GRβ. With transcription factor AP-1 repression the rank order was wild-type=Val641=Lys23=ILe729=Ser363>Asn559=GRβ. There was variability in the results but overall the $ILe_{559}Asn$ mutation and the GRβ isoform did not demonstrate any viable GR activity (99).

Huizenga et al. (100) observed in a group of 219 elderly individuals that 13 were carriers of the SNP of the $A_{1220}G$ allele, resulting in heterozygous $Asn_{336}Ser$. This change gives an allele frequency of 0.03 for the mutant (q) G allele, compared to 0.97 for the wild-type (p) A allele. With the dexamethasone suppression test, carriers of the mutant allele had a more sensitive response in cortisol reduction, when comparing 1 mg to 0.25 mg of dexamethasone. With 1 mg of dexamethasone, no differences in response were observed between controls (wild-type homozygote) and the mutant carriers of the G allele with a change in cortisol -488.1 and -506.3 nmol/L, respectively ($p = 0.5$). However, with 0.25 mg of dexamethasone, there was a significant difference in decreased cortisol with -280.5 and -373.9 nmol/L for the controls compared to the mutants, respectively ($p < 0.05$ when adjusted for body mass index). Dexamethasone concentrations did not vary between the two groups ($p=0.48$). There was also a significant increase in insulin concentrations for the mutant group at both doses of dexamethasone when compared to the control group ($p < 0.01$, and $p < 0.03$, respectively) (100). These observations are consistent with those of De Lange et al. (99) reporting increased insulin sensitivity in vitro with this mutant form of the allele.

In another example, the $Arg_{23}Lys$ exists as part of a two-linked SNP as GAGAGG → GAAAAG. The first part of this sequence is considered a synonymous change, and the latter is non-synonymous; expressed as Glu22-Glu and Arg23Lys, or GluArg GluLys. The allele frequency for the mutant allele was 0.045, and as a result out of 202 individuals, only heterozygotes (carriers) were observed. After a 1 mg dexamethasone test, the GluLys carriers demonstrated significantly greater cortisol concentrations compared to the wild-types (54.8 vs. 26.4 nmol/L, respectively, $p < 0.0001$). This suggests that the mutant allele results in a degree of GC insensitivity (101). However, the investigators concluded there was no association of these polymorphisms witii glucocorticoid resistance. Therefore, additional investigation with larger sample size and functional tests are needed to resolve specific genetic mechanisms for steroid resistance.

D. Nitric Oxide Synthase (NOS)

Nitric oxide (NO) has different roles in various disease states. For asthma, NO plays both a positive and negative feature in the human airway, and is considered a potential surrogate marker of inflammation. Nitric oxide synthase (NOS) is an oxidizing enzyme with homology similar to that of the P450 drug metabolizing enzymes (103). The NO is produced by the interaction of arginine with NOS, NADPH, O_2, Ca^{2+}, and calmodulin, and other co-factors (103–105). This reaction yields citrulline and NO. There are three known isoforms of NOS; two are constitutive, calcium dependent enzymes, neuronal NOS (nNOS, or NOS1), and endothelial NOS (eNOS or NOS3). Both contribute to maintaining airway patency with a mild bronchodilator effect (determined by the method of NO induced muscle relaxation). The third, inducible NOS (iNOS or NOS2), is considered calcium independent since its activation only requires basal concentrations of cellular free calcium (106), Inducible NOS is thought to contribute to airway inflammation and tissue damage. The NO reacts with superoxide (O_2^-) in the lung to form the peroxynitrite ion $(OONO^-)$ and peroxynitrous acid (OONOH) (104), Both anions facilitate lipid peroxidation which results in lung tissue damage (107,108). Measurements of exhaled NO have been studied as noninvasive indicators of airway inflammation.

Inhaled corticosteroids clearly have a significant effect on reducing exhaled NO (109–115); whereas studies with leukotriene modifiers have shown a variable effect on reducing exhaled NO (116–123). Variability in response to medications, as well as heterogeneity within the asthma population, may be related to polymorphisms in the NOS genes.

The NOS2 isoform is upregulated in asthmatics, resulting in higher exhaled NO than a normal population (107). In the NOS2 gene, there are variable number tandem repeats (VNTR) of nucleotides, located in the promoter region, approximately 2.5 kilobases (kb) upstream from transcription initiation. The VNTR, CCTTT (8 through 21) occurs in humans, with 11, 12, and 13 being the highest in frequency. VNTR 14 is of particular interest, because it is associated with an increase in luciferase activity, suggesting greater NOS2 expression in those individuals with the VNTR polymorphism (124). Konno et al. (125) however, reported that carriers of this allele had an association with atopy ($p = 0.0063$), but not with asthma. Gao et al. (126) also examined a different VNTR (AAAT/AAAAT) polymorphism extending -756 to -716 base-pairs from transcription initiation. Similarly, no association was made to asthma or atopy with the VNTR studied (126,127). It is possible that NOS2 up-regulation for asthma-associated inflammation may be expected.

Three different locations in the NOS1 gene have been examined for associations with asthma and exhaled NO. A VNTR polymorphism comprised of AAT repeats at intron 20 has been associated with an increased incidence of asthma, as well as elevated exhaled NO concentrations. Wechsler et al. (128) observed a significantly greater amount of exhaled NO in mild asthmatics who were carriers of less than 12 AAT repeats, when compared to other asthmatics (10.8 ± 3.6 ppb $\geq$ (AAT)$_{12}$ and 16.6 ± 10.1 ppb $<$ (AAT)$_{12}$; $p = 0.00008$). This polymorphism has also been linked to atopy, but not to increased exhaled NO concentrations (129). Two different AC repeats in asthmatics ((AC)$_{17}$ (AC)$_{18}$) also demonstrate associations with asthma in exon 29 of the NOS1 gene (130). A group of moderate to severe Caucasian asthmatics had a higher frequency of the 17 repeat (0.828 vs. 0.763, $p = 0.0013$) and a lower frequency of the 18 repeat (0.061 vs. 0.119, $p = 0.00004$) when compared to a population of normal, healthy controls. Intron 2 contains VNTR of CA repeats (177–187 base-pairs). Gao et al. (126) observed a significantly greater number of asthmatics carried the 183 VNTR allele (OR $= 1.42$, $p = 0.034$), as well as homozygotes for the allele (OR$=2.08$, $p = 0.008$).

The NOS3 gene has two polymorphisms reportedly associated with asthma and increased exhaled NO (SNP of $G_{893}T$, and a VNTR) (131,132). Because of the growing interest and clinical application of exhaled NO as a marker of inflammation, these polymorphisms could be useful in understanding the response to anti-inflammatory medications, as well as disease heterogeneity.

E. TNFα and NF-κB

Because asthma is a complex disease involving many enzymatic pathways, the discovery of new pathways for asthma inflammation inherently allows for new drug targets and novel treatment modalities. TNFα, a TH1-type pro-inflammatory cytokine, is a component of allergic airway inflammation. TNFα is produced predominantly by inflammatory cells (macrophages, T lymphocytes, granulocytes and mast cells) (133). The TNFα gene is located in chromosome 6 near the major histocompatibility complex. TNFα binds to the TNFα receptor, TNF-R1, as a step in the inflammatory cascade.

TNFα is upregulated in asthma with elevated levels measured in BAL fluid of atopic asthmatics. TNFα can increase bronchial hyperresponsiveness, sputum neutrophilia, and cellular response, and it may be involved in tissue remodeling in asthma. Increased expression of TNFα has been observed in children with severe asthma and in wheezy infants (133–136).

A SNP is present at the -308 position in the promoter region of the gene that codes for TNFα. This SNP is observed as a change from guanine to adenine ($G_{-308}A$). The variant allele is associated with an increase in TNFα production, and has been associated with a higher frequency in asthmatics. Subsets of severe asthmatics with this SNP may respond more favorably to anti-TNFα agents such as etanercept, infliximab, and adalimumab (135–138).

There are other polymorphisms present in the TNFα gene, and there are known polymorphisms in the TNFα receptors (I and II), which may influence response to anti-TNFα agents (139–143). Nuclear Factor κB (NF-κB) is a pivotal transcription factor involved in inflammation pathways of asthma and a transcription factor for TNFα activation (as well as NOS2) (144,145). The NF-κB essential modulator NEMO (also known as IKK-γ) regulates the NF-κB pathway and also has polymorphisms (146). Considering the pathway of TNFα transcription activation, synthesis, and signalling—many steps involved contain genetic polymorphisms. Alteration in activity within these steps may influence the likelihood of response to anti-TNFα agent among patients with asthma.

VIII. Conclusions

The long-term CAMP clinical trial in childhood asthma has provided evidence-based support for the benefits of continuous long-term use of inhaled glucocorticoids on asthma control. Based on the limitations of effect identified in CAMP and other studies, clinical trials are now in progress to determine whether earlier intervention with inhaled glucocorticoids can influence the progression of asthma. Data are also being generated that help define the patient at risk for persistent asthma and thus identify the best candidates for early intervention. With the right medication and the correct patient profile, it is conceivable that remission could be induced. Unfortunately, patients with established severe asthma already have low pulmonary function that is difficult to reverse. Perhaps early intervention with effective therapy will also reduce the prevalence and morbidity of severe asthma.

Individual response to medications may be influenced by a person's genome. This may explain the variability in response to conventional asthma therapy (Fig. 7) (147). Current knowledge of the polymorphisms, SNPs, genotypes, and haplotypes is not sufficient to precisely predict clinical response, but rather provide assistance to the clinician of how a person *may* respond to a medication. Although this is a very exciting time for discovery, pharmacogenetics and pharmacogenomics are still in their infancy as disciplines. The development of new technologies such as pharmacoproteomics and pharmacophylogenomics could enhance the insight generated through pharmacogenomics. Insight into these areas may assist in the discovery of new treatment modalities.

Acknowledgment

We would to thank Gretchen Hugen for assistance in the manuscript preparation.

References

1. Mannino DM, Homa DM, Akinbami LJ, Moorman JE, Gwynn C, Redd SC. Surveillance for asthma—United States, 1980–1999. MMWR 2002; 51:1–13.
2. National Institutes of Health, National Heart, Lung, and Blood Institute. Global initiative for Asthma. Global strategy for asthma management and prevention, NHLBI/NIH workshop report. 2002.
3. National Asthma Education and Prevention Program Report. Guidelines for the diagnosis and management of asthma update on selected topics—2002. J Allergy Clin Immunol 2002; 110:S141–S219.
4. Busse WW, Lenfant C, Lemanske RF. Asthma guidelines: a changing paradigm to improve asthma care. J Allergy Clin Immunol 2002; 110:703–705.
5. Szefler SJ, Eigen H. Budesonide inhalation suspension: a nebulized corticosteroid for persistent asthma. J Allergy Clin Immunol 2002; 109:730–742.
6. Knorr B, Franchi LM, Bisgaard H, Vermeulen JH, LeSouef P, Santanello N, Michele TM, Reiss TF, Nguyen HH, Bratton DL. Montelukast, a leukotriene receptor antagonist, for the treatment of persistent asthma in children aged 2 to 5 years. Pediatrics 2001; 108(3):1–10.
7. Szefler SJ ed. Meeting the needs of the modernization act: challenges in developing pediatric therapies. J Allergy Clin Immunol 2000; 106(suppl 3):115–117.
8. Leflein JG, Szefler SJ, Murphy KR, Fitzpatrick S, Cruz-Rivera M, Miller CJ, Smith JA. Nebulized budesonide inhalation suspension compared with cromolyn sodium nebulizer solution for asthma in young children: Results of a randomized outcome trial. Pediatrics 2002; 109:866–872.
9. Naspitz C, Szefler SJ, Tinkelman D, Warner JO, eds. Textbook of Pediatric Asthma. London: Martin-Dunitz, 2001.
10. Spahn JD, Szefler SJ. Childhood asthma: new insights into management. J Allergy Clin Immunol 2002; 109:3–13.
11. Suissa S, Ernst P. Inhaled corticosteroids: impact on asthma morbidity and mortality. J Allergy Clin Immunol 2001; 107:937–944.
12. The Childhood Asthma Management Program Research Group. Long-term effects of budesonide or nedocromil in children with asthma. N Engl J Med 2000; 343:l054–1063.
13. Agertoft L, Pedersen S. Effects of long-term treatment with an inhaled corticosteroid on growth and pulmonary function in asthmatic children. Respir Med 1994; 88:373–381.
14. Covar RA, Spahn JD, Murphy JR, Szefler SJ. Childhood Asthma Management Program Research Group. Progression of asthma measured by lung function in the childhood asthma management program. Am J Respir Crit Care Med 2004; 170(3):234–241.
15. Martinez FD, Wright AL, Taussig LM, Holberg CJ, Halonen M, Morgan WJ, Associates TGHM. Asthma and wheezing in the first six years of life. N Engl J Med 1995; 332:133–138.
16. Phelan PD, Robertson CF, Olinsky A. The Melbourne asthma study: 1964–1999. J Allergy Clin Immunol 2002; 109:189–194.
17. Agertoft L, Pedersen S. Effect of long-term treatment with inhaled budesonide on adult height in children with asthma. N Engl J Med 2000; 343:1064–1069.

18. Matz J, Emmett A, Rickard K, Kalberg C. Addition of salmeterol to low-dose fluticasone versus higher-dose fluticasone: an analysis of asthma exacerbations. J Allergy Clin Immunol 2001; 107:783–789.

19. Soler M, Matz J, Townley R, Buhl R, O'Brien J, Fox H, Thirlwell J, Gupta N, Dellia Cioppa G. The anti-IgE antibody omalizumab reduces exacerbations and steroid requirement in allergic asthmatics. Eur Respir J 2001; 18:254–261.

20. Spahn JD, Covar RA, Gleason MC, Tinkelman DG, Szefler SJ. Pharmacologic management of asthma in infants and small children. In: Naspitz CK, Szefler SJ, Tinkelman D, Warner JO, eds. Textbook of Pediatric Asthma. London: Martin Dunitz Ltd., 2001:121–147.

21. Martinez FD. Development of wheezing disorders and asthma in preschool children. Pediatrics 2002; 109:362–367.

22. Castro-Rodriguez JA, Holberg CJ, Wright AL, Martinez FD. A clinical index to define risk of asthma in young children with recurrent wheezing. Am J Respir Crit Care Med 2000; 162:1403–1406.

23. Rasmussen F, Taylor DR, Flannery EM, Cowan JO, Greene JM, Herbison GP, Sears M. Risk factors for airway remodeling in asthma manifested by a low post-bronchodilator FEV_1/vital capacity ratio. Am J Respir Crit Care Med 2002; 165:1480–1488.

24. Milgrom H, Skoner DP, Bensch G, Kim KT, Claus R, Baumgartner RA for the Levalbuterol Pediatric Study Group. Low-dose levalbuterol in children with asthma: safety and efficacy in comparison with placebo and racemic albuterol. J Allergy Clin Immmunol 2001; 108:938–945.

25. Barnes P. New targets for future asthma therapy. In: Yeadon M, Diamont Z, eds. New and Exploratory Therapeutic Agents for Asthma, Lung Biology in Health and Disease. New York: Marcel Dekker, 2000:361–389.

26. Kline JN. DNA therapy for asthma. Curr Opin Allergy Immunol 2002; 2: 69–73.

27. Milgrom H, Fick RB, Su JQ, Reimann JD, Bush RK, Watrous ML, Metzger WJ. Treatment of allergic asthma with monoclonal anti-IgE antibody. N Engl J Med 1999; 341:1966–1973.

28. Holgate S, Bousquet J, Wenzel S, Fox H, Liu J, Castellsague J. Efficacy of omalizumab, an anti-immunoglobiln E antibody, in patients at high risk of serious asthma-related morbidity and mortality. Curr Med Res Opin 2001; 17:233–240.

29. Soler M, Matz J, Townley R, Buhl R, O'Brien J, Fox H, Thirlwell J, Gupta N, Dellia Cioppa G. The anti-IgE antibody omalizumab reduces exacerbations and steroid requirement in allergic asthmatics. Eur Respir J 2001; 18:254–261.

30. Szefler SJ, Martin RJ, King TS, Boushey HA, Cherniack RM, Chinchilli VM, Craig TJ, Dolovich M, Drazen JM, Fagan JK, et al. Significant variability in response to inhaled corticosteroids for persistent asthma. J Allergy Clin Immunol 2002; 109:410–418.

31. Payne DNR, Balfour-Lynn IM. Children with difficult asthma: a practical approach. J Asthma 2001; 38:189–203.

32. Shahid SK, Kharitinov SA, Wilson NM, Bush A, Barnes PJ. Increased interleukin-4 and decreased interferon-gamma in exhaled breath condensate of children with asthma. Am J Respir Crit Care Med 2002; 165:1290–1293.

33. Zanconato S, Scollo M, Zaramella C, Landi L, Zacchello F, Baraldi E. Exhaled carbon monoxide levels after a course of oral prednisone in children with asthma exacerbation. J Allergy Clin Immunol 2002; 109:440–445.

34. Terashima T, Amakawa K, Matsumaru A, Yamaguchi K. Correlation between cysteinyl leukotriene release from leukocytes and clinical response to a leukotriene inhibitor. Chest 2002; 122:1566–1570.

35. Csoma Z, Kharitonov SA, Baliant B, Bush A, Wilson NM, Barnes PJ. Increased leukotrienes in exhaled breath condensate in childhood asthma. Am J Respir Crit Care Med 2002; 166:1345–1349.

36. Antczak A, Montuschi P, Kharitonov S, Gorski P, Barnes PJ. Increased exhaled cysteinyl- leukotrienes and 8-isoprostane in aspirin-induced asthma. Am J Respir Crit Care Med 2002; 166:301–306.

37. Cataldo DD, Bettiol J, Noel A, Bartsch P, Foidart J-M, Louis R. Matrix metalloproteinase-9, but not tissue inhibitor of matrix metalloproteinase-1, increases in the sputum from allergic asthmatic patients after allergen challenge. Chest 2002; 122:1553–1559.

38. Sont JK, Willems LNA, Bel EH, van Krieken JHJM, Vendenbroucke JP, Sterk PJ and the AMPUL Study group. Clinical control and histopathologic outcome of asthma when using airway hyperresponsiveness as an additional guide to long-term treatment. Am J Respir Crit Care Med 1999; 159: 1043–1051.

39. Green RH, Brightling CE, McKenna S, Hargadon B, Parker D, Bradding P, Wardlaw AJ, Pavord I. Asthma exacerbations and sputum eosinophil counts: a randomized controlled trial. Lancet 2002; 360:1715–1721.

40. Chan MT, Leung DYM, Szefler SJ, Spahn JD. Difficult-to-control asthma: clinical characteristics of steroid- insensitive asthma. J Allergy Clin Immunol 1998; 101(5):594–601.

41. Ober C, Moffatt ME. Contributing factors to the pathobiology: the genetics of asthma. Clin Chest Med 2000; 21:245–261.

42. Fenech A, Hall EP. Pharmacogenetics of asthma. Br J Clin Pharmacol 2002; 53:2–15.

43. Palmer LJ, Silverman ES, Weiss ST, Drazen JM. Pharmacogenetics of asthma. Am J Respir Crit Care Med 2002; 165:861–866.

44. Marsh DG, Neely JD, Breazeale DR, Ghosh B, Freidhoff LR, Ehrlich-Kautzky E, Schou C, Krishnaswamy G, Beaty TH. Linkage analysis of IL4 and other chromosome 5q31.1 markers and total serum immunoglobulin E concentrations. Science 1994; 264:1152–1156.

45. Borish L, Mascali JJ, Klinnert M, Leppert M, Rosenwasser LJ. SSC polymorphisms in interleukin genes. Hum Mol Genet 1995; 4:974.

46. Rosenwasser LJ, Klemm DJ, Dresback JK, Inamura H, Mascali JJ, Klinnert M, Borish L. Promoter polymorphisms in the chromosome 5 gene cluster in asthma and atopy. Clin Exp Allergy 1995; 25(suppl 2):74–78; discussion 95–96.

47. Burchard EG, Silverman EK, Rosenwasser LJ, Borish L, Yandava C, Pillari A, Weiss ST, Hasday J, Lilly CM, Ford JG, Drazen JM. Association between a sequence variant in the IL-4 gene promoter and FEV(l) in asthma. Am J Respir Crit Care Med 1999; 160:919–922.

48. Hershey GK, Friedrich MF, Esswein LA, Thomas ML, Chatila TA. The association of atopy with a gain-of-function mutation in the alpha subunit of the interleukin-4 receptor. N Engl J Med 1997; 337:1720–1725.

49. Rosa-Rosa L, Zimmermann N, Bernstein JA, Rothenberg ME, Khurana Hershey GK. The R576 JJL-4 receptor alpha allele correlates with asthma severity. J Allergy Clin Immunol 1999; 104:1008–1014.

50. Martinez FD. Maturation of immune responses at the beginning of asthma. J Allergy Clin Immunol 1999; 103:355–361.

51. Spahn JD, Szefler SJ, Surs W, Doherty DE, Nimmagadda SR, Leung DYM. A novel action of IL-13: induction of diminished monocyte glucocorticoid receptor-binding affinity. J Immunol 1996; 157:2654–2659.

52. Kam JC, Szefler SJ, Surs W, Sher ER, Leung DYM. Combination IL-2 and IL-4 reduces glucocorticoid receptor binding affinity and T cell response to glucocorticoids. J Immunol 1993; 151:3460–3466.

53. Sher ER, Leung DYM, Surs W, Kam JC, Zieg, G, Kamada AK, Szefler SJ. Steroid resistant asthma: cellular mechanisms contributing to inadequate response to glucocorticoid therapy. J Clin Invest 1994; 93:33–39.

54. Lima JJ, Thomason DB, Mohamed MH, Eberle LV, Self TH, Johnson JA. Impact of genetic polymorphisms of the beta2-adrenergic receptor on albuterol bronchodilator pharmacodynamics. Clin Pharmacol Ther 1999; 65(5): 519–525.

55. Turki J, Pak J, Green SA, Martin RJ, Liggett SB. Genetic polymorphisms of the beta2-adrenergic receptor in nocturnal and nonnocturnal asthma. Evidence that Glyl6 correlates with the nocturnal phenotype. J Clin Invest 1995; 95(4):1635–1641.

56. Hopes E, McDougall C, Christie G, Dewar J, Wheatley A, Hall IP, Helms PJ. Association of glutamine 27 polymorphism of beta2 adrenoceptor with reported childhood asthma: population based study. BMJ 1998; 316(7132):664.

57. Hall IP, Wheatley A, Wilding P, Liggett SB. Association of Glu 27 beta2-adrenoceptor polymorphism with lower airway reactivity in asthmatic subjects. Lancet 1995; 345(8959):1213–1214.

58. Dewar JC, Wilkinson J, Wheatley A, Thomas NS, Doull I, Morton N, Lio P, Harvey JF, Liggett SB, Holgate ST, Hall IP. The glutamine 27 beta2-adrenoceptor polymorphism is associated with elevated IgE levels in asthmatic families. J Allergy Clin Immunol 1997; 100(2):261–265.

59. Green SA, Turki J, Bejarano P, Hall IP, Liggett SB. Influence of beta2-adrenergic receptor genotypes on signal transduction in human airway smooth muscle cells. Am J Respir Cell Mol Biol 1995; 13(1):25–33.

60. Israel E, Drazen JM, Liggett SB, Boushey HA, Cherniack RM, Chinchilli VM, Cooper DM, Fahy JV, Fish IE, Ford JG, et al. The effect of polymorphisms of the beta2-adrenergic receptor on the response to regular use of albuterol in asthma. Am J Respir Crit Care Med 2000; 162(1):75–80.

61. Liggett SB. Polymorphisms of the beta2-adrenergic receptor. N Engl J Med 2002; 346(7):536–538.

62. McGraw DW, Forbes SL, Kramer LA, Liggett SB. Polymorphisms of the 5' leader cistron of the human beta2-adrenergic receptor regulate receptor expression. J Clin Invest 1998; 102(11):1927–1932.

63. Ulbrecht M, Hergeth MT, Wjst M, Heinrich J, Bickeboller H, Wichmann HE, Weiss EH. Association of beta2-adrenoreceptor variants with bronchial hyperresponsiveness. Am J Respir Crit Care Med 2000; 161(2 Pt 1):469–474.

64. Drysdale CM, McGraw DW, Stack CB, Stephens JC, Judson RS, Nandabalan K, Arnold K, Ruano G, Liggett SB. Complex promoter and coding region beta2-adrenergic receptor haplotypes alter receptor expression and predict in vivo responsiveness. Proc Natl Acad Sci U.S.A. 2000; 97(19):10483–10488.

65. Small KM, Brown KM, Theiss CT, Seman CA, Weiss ST, Liggett SB. A ILe to Met polymorphism in the catalytic domain of adenylyl cyclase type 9 confers reduced beta2-adrenergic receptor stimulation. Pharmacogenetics 2003; 13(9): 535–541.

66. Koshino T, Takano S, Kitani S, Ohshima N, Sano Y, Takaishi T, Hirai K, Yamamoto K, Morita Y. Novel polymorphism of the 5-lipoxygenase activating protein (FLAP) promoter gene associated with asthma. Mol Cell Biol Res Commun 1999; 2(1):32–35.

67. Sayers I, Barton S, Rorke S, Sawyer J, Peng Q, Beghe B, Ye S, Keith T, Clough JB, Holloway JW, Sampson AP, Holgate ST. Promoter polymorphism in the 5-lipoxygenase (ALOX5) and 5-lipoxygenase-activating protein (ALOX5AP) genes and asthma susceptibility in a Caucasian population. Clin Exp Allergy 2003; 33(8):1103–1110.

68. In KH, Asano K, Beier D, Grobholz J, Finn PW, Silverman EK, Silverman ES, Collins T, Fischer AR, Keith TP, et al. Naturally occurring mutations in the human 5-lipoxygenase gene promoter that modify transcription factor binding and reporter gene transcription. J Clin Invest 1997; 99(5):1130–1137.

69. Drazen JM, Yandaval CN, Dubé L, Szczerback N, Hippensteel R, Pillari A, Israel E, Schork N, Silverman ES, Katz DA, Drajesk J. Pharmacogenetic association between ALOX5 promoter genotype and the response to anti-asthma treatment. Nat Genet 1999; 22:168–170.

70. Szczeklik A, Stevenson DD. Aspirin-induced asthma: advances in pathogenesis and management. J Allergy Clin Immunol 1999; 104(1):5–13.

71. Spector SL, Wangaard CH, Farr RS. Aspirin and concomitant idiosyncrasies in adult asthmatic patients. J Allergy Clin Immunol 1979; 64(6 Pt 1):500–506.

72. Bochenek G, Nizankowska E, Szczeklik A. The atopy trait in hypersensitivity to nonsteroidal anti-inflammatory drugs. Allergy 1996; 51(1):16–23.

73. Sanak M, Pierzchalska M, Bazan-Socha S, Szczeklik A. Enhanced expression of the leukotriene C(4) synthase due to overactive transcription of an allelic variant associated with aspirin-intolerant asthma. Am J Respir Cell Mol Biol 2000; 23(3):290–296.

74. Sampson AP, Siddiqui S, Buchanan D, Howarth PH, Holgate ST, Holloway JW, Sayers I. Variant LTC(4) synthase allele modifies cysteinyl leukotriene synthesis in eosinophils predicts clinical response to zafirlukast. Thorax 2000; 55(suppl 2):S28–S31.

75. Asano K, Shiomi T, Hasegawa N, Nakamura H, Kudo H, Matsuzaki T, Hakuno H, Fukunaga K, Suzuki Y, Kanazawa M, Yamaguchi K. Leukotriene C4 synthase gene A(-444)C polymorphism and clinical response to a CYS-LT(l) antagonist, pranlukast, in Japanese patients th moderate asthma. Pharmacogenetics 2002; 12(7):565–570.

76. Whelan GJ, Blake KV, Kissoon N, Duckworth LJ, Wang J, Sylvester IE, Lima JJ. Effect of montelukast on time-course as exhaled nitric oxide in asthma: influence of LTC$_4$ synthase A$_{444}$C polymorphism. Pediat Pulmonol 2003; 36:413–420.

77. Sayers I, Sampson AP, Ye S, Holgate ST. Promoter polymorphism influences the effect of dexamethasone on transcriptional activation of the LTC4 synthase gene. Eur J Hum Genet 2003; 11(8):619–622.

78. Sayers I, Barton S, Rorke S, Beghe B, Hayward B, Van Eerdewegh P, Keith T, Clough JB, Ye S, Holloway JW, Sampson AP, Holgate ST. Allelic association and functional studies of promoter polymorphism in the leukotriene C4 synthase gene (LTC4S) in asthma. Thorax 2003; 58(5):417–424.

79. Oselin K, Mrozikiewicz PM, Gaikovitch E, Pahkla R, Roots I. Frequency of MRP1 genetic polymorphisms and their functional significance in Caucasians: detection of a novel mutation G816A in the human MRP1 gene. Eur J Clin Pharmacol 2003; 59(4):347–350.

80. Kabesch M, Tzotcheva I, Carr D, Hofler C, Weiland SK, Fritzsch C, von Mutius E, Martinez FD. A complete screening of the IL4 gene: novel polymorphisms and their association with asthma and IgE in childhood. J Allergy Clin Immunol 2003; 112(5):893–898.

81. Heinzmann A, Mao XQ, Akaiwa M, Kreomer RT, Gao PS, Ohshima K, Umeshita R, Abe Y, Braun S, Yamashita T, et al. Genetic variants of IL-13 signalling and human asthma and atopy. Hum Mol Genet 2000; 9(4):549–559.

82. Heinzmann A, Jerkic SP, Ganter K, Kurz T, Blattmann S, Schuchmann L, Gerhold K, Berner R, Deichmann KA. Association study of the IL13 variant Arg110Gln in atopic diseases and juvenile idiopathic arthritis. J Allergy Clin Immunol 2003; 112(4):735–739.

83. He JQ, Connett JE, Anthonisen NR, Sandford AJ. Polymorphisms in the IL13, IL13RA1, and IL4RA genes and rate of decline in lung function in smokers. Am J Respir Cell Mol Biol 2003; 28(3):379–385.

84. Zaitsu M, Hamasaki Y, Matsuo M, Ichimaru T, Fujita I, Ishii E. Leukotriene synthesis is increased by transcriptional up-regulation of 5-lipoxygenase, leukotriene A4 hydrolase, and leukotriene C4 synthase in asthmatic children. J Asthma 2003; 40(2):147–154.

85. Mueller MJ, Andberg MB, Samuelsson B, Haeggstrom JZ. Leukotriene A4 hydrolase, mutation of tyrosine 378 allows conversion of leukotriene A4 into an isomer of leukotriene B4. J Biol Chem 1996; 271(40):24345–24348.

86. Wetterholm A, Medina JF, Radmark O, Shapiro R, Haeggstrom JZ, Vallee BL, Samuelsson B. Leukotriene A4 hydrolase: abrogation of the peptidase activity by mutation of glutamic acid-296. Proc Natl Acad Sci U.S.A. 1992; 89(19):9141–9145.

87. Andberg MB, Hamberg M, Haeggstrom JZ. Mutation of tyrosine 383 in leukotriene A4 hydrolase allows conversion of leukotriene A4 into 5S,6S-dihydroxy-7, 9-trans-11, 14-cis-eicosatetraenoic acid. Implications for the epoxide hydrolase mechanism. J Biol Chem 1997; 272(37):23057–23063.

88. Lesur O, Bernard A, Arsalane K, Lauwerys R, Begin R, Cantin A, Lane D. Clara cell protein (CC-16) induces a phospholipase A2-mediated inhibition of fibroblast migration in vitro. Am J Respir Crit Care Med 1995; 152(1): 290–297.

89. Miele L, Cordella-Miele E, Mukherjee AB. Uteroglobin: structure, molecular biology, and new perspectives on its function as a phospholipase A2 inhibitor. Endocr Rev 1987; 8(4):474–490.

90. Laing IA, Hermans C, Bernard A, Burton PR, Goldblatt J, Le Souef PN. Association between plasma CC16 levels, the A38G polymorphism, and asthma. Am J Respir Crit Care Med 2000; 161(1):124–127.

91. Laing IA, Goldblatt J, Eber E, Hayden CM, Rye PJ, Gibson NA, Palmer LJ, Burton PR, Le Souef PN. A polymorphism of the CC16 gene is associated with an increased risk of asthma. J Med Genet 1998; 35(6):463–467.

92. Leung DY, Bloom JW. Update on glucocorticoid action and resistance. J Allergy Clin Immunol 2003; 111(1):3–22.

93. Leung DY, Hamid Q, Vottero A, Szefler SJ, Surs W, Minshall E, Chrousos GP, Klemm DJ. Association of glucocorticoid insensitivity with increased expression of glucocorticoid receptor beta. J Exp Med 1997; 186(9):1567–1574.

94. Hamid QA, Wenzel SE, Hauk PJ, Tsicopoulos A, Wallaert B, Lafitte JJ, Chrousos GP, Szefler SJ, Leung DY. Increased glucocorticoid receptor beta in airway cells of glucocorticoid-insensitive asthma. Am J Respir Crit Care Med 1999; 159(5 Pt 1):1600–1604.

95. Christodoulopoulos P, Leung DY, Elliott MW, Hogg JC, Muro S, Toda M, Laberge S, Hamid QA. Increased number of glucocorticoid receptor-beta-expressing cells in the airways in fatal asthma. J Allergy Clin Immunol 2000; 106(3):479–484.

96. Hurley DM, Accili D, Stratakis CA, Karl M, Vamvakopoulos N, Rorer E, Constantine K, Taylor SI, Chrousos GP. Point mutation causing a single amino acid substitution in the hormone binding domain of the glucocorticoid receptor in familial glucocorticoid resistance. J Clin Invest 1991; 87(2): 680–686.

97. Malchoff DM, Brufsky A, Reardon G, McDermott P, Javier EC, Bergh CH, Rowe D, Malchoff CD. A mutation of the glucocorticoid receptor in primary cortisol resistance. J Clin Invest 1993; 91(5):1918–1925.

98. Karl M, Lamberts SW, Detera-Wadleigh SD, Encio IJ, Stratakis CA, Hurley DM, Accili D, Chrousos GP. Familial glucocorticoid resistance caused by a splice site deletion in the human glucocorticoid receptor gene. J Clin Endocrinol Metab 1993; 76(3):683–689.

99. de Lange P, Koper JW, Huizenga NA, Brinkmann AO, de Jong FH, Karl M, Chrousos GP, Lamberts SW. Differential hormone-dependent transcriptional activation and -repression by naturally occurring human glucocorticoid receptor variants. Mol Endocrinol 1997; 11(8):1156–1164.

100. Huizenga NA, Koper JW, De Lange P, Pols HA, Stolk RP, Burger H, Grobbee DE, Brinkmann AO, De Jong FH, Lamberts SW. A polymorphism in the glucocorticoid receptor gene may be associated with and increased sensitivity to glucocorticoids in vivo. J Clin Endocrinol Metab 1998; 83(1): 144–151.

101. van Rossum EF, Koper JW, Huizenga NA, Uitterlinden AG, Janssen JA, Brinkmann AO, Grobbee DE, de Jong FH, van Duyn CM, Pols HA, Lamberts SW. A polymorphism in the glucocorticoid receptor gene, which

decreases sensitivity to glucocorticoids in vivo, is associated with low insulin and cholesterol levels. Diabetes 2002; 51(10):3128–3134.

102. Koper JW, Stolk RP, de Lange P, Huizenga NA, Molijn GJ, Pols HA, Grobbee DE, Karl M, de Jong FH, Brinkmann AO, Lamberts SW. Lack of association between five polymorphisms in the human glucocorticoid receptor gene and glucocorticoid resistance. Hum Genet 1997; 99(5):663–668.

103. Bredt DS, Hwang PM, Glatt CE, Lowenstein C, Reed RR, Snyder SH. Cloned and expressed nitric oxide synthase structurally resembles cytochrome P-450 reductase. Nature 1991; 351(6329):714–718.

104. Gaston B, Drazen JM, Loscalzo J, Stamler JS. The biology of nitrogen oxides in the airways. Am J Respir Crit Care Med 1994; 149(2 Pt 1):538–551.

105. Xie QW, Cho H, Kashiwabara Y, Baum M, Weidner JR, Elliston K, Mumford R, Nathan C. Carboxyl terminus of inducible nitric oxide synthase. Contribution to NADPH binding and enzymatic activity. J Biol Chem 1994; 269(45):28500–28505.

106. Ruan J, Xie Q, Hutchinson N, Cho H, Wolfe GC, Nathan C. Inducible nitric oxide synthase requires both the canonical calmodulin-binding domain and additional sequences in order to bind calmodulin and produce nitric oxide in the absence of free Ca2+. J Biol Chem 1996; 271(37):22679–22686.

107. Saleh D, Ernst P, Lim S, Barnes PJ, Giaid A. Increased formation of the potent oxidant peroxynitrite in the airways of asthmatic patients is associated with induction of nitric oxide synthase: effect of inhaled glucocorticoid. FASEB J 1998; 12(11):929–937.

108. Beckman JS, Beckman TW, Chen J, Marshall PA, Freeman BA. Apparent hydroxyl radical production by peroxynitrite: implications for endothelial injury from nitric oxide and superoxide. Proc Natl Acad Sci 1990; 87(4):1620–1624.

109. Covar RA, Szefler SJ, Martin RJ, Sundstrom DA, Silkoff PE, Murphy J, Young DA, Spahn JD. Relations between exhaled nitric oxide and measures of disease activity among children with mild-to-moderate asthma. J Pediatr 2003; 142(5):469–475.

110. Beck-Ripp J, Griese M, Arenz S, Koring C, Pasqualoni B, Bufler P. Changes of exhaled nitric oxide during steroid treatment of childhood asthma. Eur Respir J 2002; 19(6):1015–1019.

111. Carra S, Gagliardi L, Zanconato S, Scollo M, Azzolin N, Zacchello F, Baraldi E. Budesonide but not nedocromil sodium reduces exhaled nitric oxide levels in asthmatic children. Respir Med 2001; 95(9):734–739.

112. Tsai YG, Lee MY, Yang KD, Chu DM, Yuh YS, Hung CH. A single dose of nebulized budesonide decreases exhaled nitric oxide in children with acute asthma. J Pediatr 2001; 139(3):433–437.

113. Visser MJ, Postma DS, Arends LR, de Vries TW, Duiverman EJ, Brand PL. One-year treatment with different dosing schedules of fluticasone propionate in childhood asthma. Effects on hyperresponsiveness, lung function, and height. Am J Respir Crit Care Med 2001; 164(11):2073–2077.

114. Lanz MJ, Eisenlohr C, Llabre MM, Toledo Y, Lanz MA. The effect of low-dose inhaled fluticasone propionate on exhaled nitric oxide in asthmatic patients and comparison with oral zafirlukast. Ann Allergy Asthma Immunol 2001; 87(4):283–238.

115. Jones SL, Herbison P, Cowan JO, Flannery EM, Hancox RJ, McLachlan CR, Taylor DR. Exhaled NO and assessment of anti-inflammatory effects of inhaled steroid: dose-response relationship. Eur Respir J 2002; 20(3):601–608.

116. Alessandra Sandrini, Ivone M. Ferreira, Carlos Gutierrez, Jose R. Jardim, Noe Zamel, and Kenneth R. Chapman Effect of montelukast on exhaled nitric oxide and nonvolatile markers of inflammation in mild asthma. Chest 2003; 124:1334–1340.

117. Bratton DL, Lanz MJ, Miyazawa N, White CW, Silkoff PE. Exhaled nitric oxide before and after montelukast sodium therapy in school-age children with chronic asthma: a preliminary study. Pediatr Pulmonol 1999; 28(6):402–407.

118. Bisgaard H, Loland L, Oj JA. NO in exhaled air of asthmatic children is reduced by the leukotriene receptor antagonist montelukast. Am J Respir Crit Care Med 1999; 160(4):1227–1231.

119. Dempsey OJ, Kennedy G, Lipworth BJ. Comparative efficacy and anti-inflammatory profile of once-daily therapy with leukotriene antagonist or low-dose inhaled corticosteroid in patients with mild persistent asthma. J Allergy Clin Immunol 2002; 109(1):68–74.

120. Wilson AM, Orr LC, Sims EJ, Dempsey OJ, Lipworth BJ. Antiasthmatic effects of mediator blockade versus topical corticosteroids in allergic rhinitis and asthma. Am J Respir Crit Care Med 2000; 162(4 Pt 1):1297–1301.

121. Wilson AM, Orr LC, Sims EJ, Lipworth BJ. Effects of monotherapy with intra-nasal corticosteroid or combined oral histamine and leukotriene receptor antagonists in seasonal allergic rhinitis. Clin Exp Allergy 2001; 31(1): 61–68.

122. Lipworth BJ, Dempsey OJ, Aziz I, Wilson AM. Effects of adding a leukotriene antagonist or a long-acting beta2-agonist in asthmatic patients with the glycine-16 beta2-adrenoceptor genotype. Am J Med 2000; 109(2):114–121.

123. Wilson AM, Dempsey OJ, Sims EJ, Lipworth BJ. Evaluation of salmeterol or montelukast as second-line therapy for asthma not controlled with inhaled corticosteroids. Chest 2001; 119(4):1021–1026.

124. Warpeha KM, Xu W, Liu L, Charles IG, Patterson CC, Ah-Fat F, Harding S, Hart PM, Chakravarthy U, Hughes AE. Genotyping and functional analysis of a polymorphic (CCTTT)(n) repeat of NOS2A in diabetic retinopathy. FASEB J 1999; 13(13):1825–1832.

125. Konno S, Hizawa N, Yamaguchi E, Jinushi E, Nishimura M. (CCTTT)n repeat polymorphism in the NOS2 gene promoter is associated with atopy. J Allergy Clin Immunol 2001; 108(5):810–814.

126. Gao PS, Kawada H, Kasamatsu T, Mao XQ, Roberts MH, Miyamoto Y, Yoshimura M, Saitoh Y, Yasue H, Nakao K, Adra CN, Kun JF, Moro-oka S, Inoko H, Ho LP, Shirakawa T, Hopkin JM. Variants of NOS1, NOS2, and NOS3 genes in asthmatics. Biochem Biophys Res Commun 2000; 267(3): 761–763.

127. Bellamy R, Hill AV. A bi-allelic tetranucleotide repeat in the promoter of the human inducible nitric oxide synthase gene. Clin Genet 1997; 52(3):192–193.

128. Wechsler ME, Grasemann H, Deykin A, Silverman EK, Yandava CN, Israel E, Wand M, Drazen JM. Exhaled nitric oxide in patients with asthma: association with NOS1 genotype. Am J Respir Crit Care Med 2000; 162(6):2043–2047.

129. Ali M, Khoo SK, Turner S, Stick S, Le Souef P, Franklin P. NOS1 polymorphism is associated with atopy but not exhaled nitric oxide levels in healthy children. Pediatr Allergy Immunol 2003; 14(4):261–265.

130. Grasemann H, Yandava CN, Storm van's Gravesande K, Deykin A, Pillari A, Ma J, Sonna LA, Lilly C, Stampfer MJ, Israel E, Silverman EK, Drazen JM. A neuronal NO synthase (NOS1) gene polymorphism is associated with asthma. Biochem Biophys Res Commun 2000; 272(2):391–394.

131. Lee YC, Cheon KT, Lee HB, Kim W, Rhee YK, Kim DS. Gene polymorphisms of endothelial nitric oxide synthase and angiotensin-converting enzyme in patients with asthma. Allergy 2000; 55(10):959–963.

132. van's Gravesande KS, Wechsler ME, Grasemann H, Silverman ES, Le L, Palmer LJ, Drazen JM. Association of a missense mutation in the NOS3 gene with exhaled nitric oxide levels. Am J Respir Crit Care Med 2003; 168(2): 228–231.

133. Shah A, Church MK, Holgate ST. Tumour necrosis factor alpha: a potential mediator of asthma. Clin Exp Allergy 1995; 25(11):1038–1044.

134. Thomas PS, Yates DH, Barnes PJ. Tumor necrosis factor-alpha increases airway responsiveness and sputum neutrophilia in normal human subjects. Am J Respir Crit Care Med 1995; 152:76–80.

135. Massoud MN, el-Nawawy AA, el-Nazar SY, Abdel-Rahman GM. Tumour necrosis factor-alpha concentration in severely asthmatic children. East Mediterr Health J 2000; 6(2–3):432–436.

136. Azevedo I, de Blic J, Dumarey CH, Scheinmann P, Vargaftig BB, Bachelet M. Increased spontaneous release of tumour necrosis factor-alpha by alveolar macrophages from wheezy infants. Eur Respir J 1997; 10(8):1767–1773.

137. Winchester EC, Millwood IY, Rand L, Penny MA, Kessling AM. Association of the TNF-alpha-308 (G→A) polymorphism with self-reported history of childhood asthma. Hum Genet 2000; 107(6):591–596.

138. Witte JS, Palmer LJ, O'Connor RD, Hopkins PJ, Hall JM. Relation between tumour necrosis factor polymorphism TNF-alpha-308 and risk of asthma. Eur J Hum Genet 2002; 10(1):82–85.

139. Kucukaycan M, Van Krugten M, Pennings HJ, Huizinga TW, Buurman WA, Dentener MA, Wouters EF. Tumor Necrosis Factor-alpha +489G/A gene polymorphism is associated with chronic obstructive pulmonary disease. Respir Res 2002; 3(1):29.

140. Bridges SL Jr, Jenq G, Moran M, Kuffner T, Whitworth WC, McNicholl J. Single-nucleotide polymorphisms in tumor necrosis factor receptor genes: definition of novel haplotypes and racial/ethnic differences. Arthritis Rheum 2002 46(8):2045–2050.

141. Sashio H, Tamura K, Ito R, Yamamoto Y, Bamba H, Kosaka T, Fukui S, Sawada K, Fukuda Y, Tamura K, Satomi M, Shimoyama T, Furuyama J. Polymorphisms of the TNF gene and the TNF receptor superfamily member 1B gene are associated with susceptibility to ulcerative colitis and Crohn's disease, respectively. Immunogenetics 2002; 53(12):1020–1027.

142. Nishimura M, Obayashi H, Mizuta I, Hara H, Adachi T, Ohta M, Tegoshi H, Fukui M, Hasegawa G, Shigeta H, Kitagawa Y, Nakano K, Kaji R, Nakamura N. TNF, TNF receptor type 1, and allograft inflammatory

factor-1 gene polymorphisms in Japanese patients with type 1 diabetes. Hum Immunol 2003; 64(2):302–309.

143. Ehling R, Gassner C, Lutterotti A, Strasser-Fuchs S, Kollegger H, Kristoferitsch W, Reindl M, Berger T. Genetic variants in the tumor necrosis factor receptor II gene in patients with multiple sclerosis. Tissue Antigens 2004; 63(1):28–33.

144. Hart LA, Krishnan VL, Adcock IM, Barnes PJ, Chung KF. Activation and localization of transcription factor, nuclear factor-kappaB, in asthma. Am J Respir Crit Care Med 1998; 158(5 Pt 1):1585–1592.

145. Barnes PJ, Karin M. Nuclear factor-kappaB: a pivotal transcription factor in chronic inflammatory diseases. N Engl J Med 1997; 336(15):1066–1071.

146. Aradhya S, Woffendin H, Jakins T, Bardaro T, Esposito T, Smahi A, Shaw C, Levy M, Munnich A, D'Urso M, Lewis RA, Kenwrick S, Nelson DL. A recurrent deletion in the ubiquitously expressed NEMO (IKK-gamma) gene accounts for the vast majority of incontinentia pigmenti mutations. Hum Mol Genet 2001; 10(19):2171–2179.

147. Malmstrom K, Rodriguez-Gomez G, Guerra J, Villaran C, Pineiro A, Wei LX, Seidenberg BC, Reiss TF. Oral montelukast, inhaled beclomethasone, and placebo for chronic asthma. A randomized, controlled trial. Montelukast/ Beclomethasone study group. Ann Intern Med 1999; 130(6):487–495.

148. Green SA, Turki J, Innis M, Liggett SB. Ammo-terminal polymorphisms of the human beta2-adrenergic receptor impart distinct agonist-promoted regulatory properties. Biochemistry 1994; 33(32):9414–9419.

149. Green SA, Cole G, Jacinto M, Innis M, Liggett SB. A polymorphism of the human beta2-adrenergic receptor within the fourth transmembrane domain alters ligand binding and functional properties of the receptor. J Biol Chem 1993; 268(31):23116–23121.

150. McGraw DW, Forbes SL, Kramer LA, Liggett SB. Polymorphisms of the 5' leader cistrom of the human beta2-adrenergic receptor regulate receptor expression. J Clin Invest 1998; 102(11):1927–1932.

18

Role of Allergen-Specific Immunotherapy in Childhood Asthma

ANDREW H. LIU

Department of Pediatrics, National Jewish Medical and Research Center, and University of Colorado Health Sciences Center Denver, Colorado, U.S.A.

HAROLD S. NELSON

Department of Medicine, National Jewish Medical and Research Center, and University of Colorado Health Sciences Center Denver, Colorado, U.S.A.

I. Introduction

Although allergen-specific immunotherapy by subcutaneous injections (SIT) is not standard therapy in the management of childhood asthma, a substantial body of evidence finds that SIT can achieve clinical and immune modulatory outcomes that can complement conventional pharmacotherapy for asthma. To provide a current basis for SIT in childhood asthma, this chapter will review the clinical rationale, mechanisms of action, and the key parameters for SIT administration in asthmatic children. Impediments to its widespread implementation include the complexity of optimal SIT administration and the risks of allergic reactions. Improvements in SIT that could lead to its widespread implementation for childhood asthma include: (a) safety; (b) ease and route of administration; (c) efficacy; and (d) costs. Recent and ongoing efforts to improve SIT in these ways will also be discussed.

II. Clinical Rationale for SIT in Childhood Asthma

A. Role of Allergy in Childhood Asthma

Childhood asthma is strongly linked to allergy. As an epidemiologic example, in the NIH-funded Childhood Asthma Management Program (CAMP) study of elementary school-age asthmatic children in the United States ($n = 1041$), 88% had at least one positive allergy prick skin test (PST) to a common panel of inhaled allergens (1). In a pediatric practice-based case-control study of childhood asthma risk factors ($n = 343$), allergen sensitization to mite, cat and/or alternaria, but not pollens, were the dominant correlates of recurrent wheezing (2). Asthma symptoms and severity have been correlated with allergen exposure in asthmatic children who are sensitized and exposed to higher levels of dust mite (3), cat (1), and cockroach (4) allergens. Thus, the combination of indoor allergen sensitization and exposure seems most problematic for asthmatic children.

Correspondingly, removal of allergen exposure in sensitized asthmatic children improves disease severity. In a study of 20 mite-sensitive asthmatic children, a controlled trial of extensive mite reduction measures in the patients' homes significantly reduced asthma symptoms and improved peak flows and bronchial hyperresponsiveness (BHR) (5). In a study of mite-sensitive asthmatic children who temporarily moved to a high-altitude locale in the Alps (i.e., without dust mites), total IgE, mite-specific IgE, and BHR to methacholine, exercise, and mite allergen all improved during their nine months in the Alps, and worsened upon returning to their mite allergen-containing homes (6). A three-month stay in the Alps was also associated with significant reductions in induced sputum eosinophil percentages and breath condensate concentrations of cysteinyl leukotrienes (LTC4/D4/E4), and nitrites and 8-isoprostane (i.e., markers of oxidant stress) (7,8).

In young children with recurrent wheezing, a number of well-performed, prospective natural history studies consistently reveal that the strongest risk factors for disease persistence into later childhood and adulthood include clinical allergy (e.g., atopic dermatitis and allergic rhinitis) and biological measures of atopy (e.g., inhalant allergen sensitization, food allergen sensitization, and elevated serum IgE levels) (9–15).

B. SIT Efficacy in Asthma

The clinical efficacy of SIT for asthma has been addressed in numerous randomized, double-blind, placebo-controlled studies over the past century. To critically evaluate this body of evidence, several meta-analyses have been recently published (16–18). A recent update to the Cochrane Database of Systematic Reviews for SIT efficacy for asthma (19) identified 75 randomized controlled SIT trials for asthma to June 2001. A total of 3188 participants with asthma were involved. There were 36 trials for house dust mite allergy, 20 for pollen allergy, 10 for animal dander allergy, two for cladosporium mold allergy, and six trials for multiple allergies. Overall, there was a significant improvement in asthma symptoms, asthma medication use, and BHR following SIT. Treating four patients with SIT would be necessary to avoid one with deterioration in asthma symptoms, and treating five patients with SIT would be necessary to avoid one increase in asthma medications.

Studies of the efficacy of SIT in children are relatively limited in number and scope. In the Cochrane Systematic Review described above, 13 studies were specifically of children with asthma, mostly older than seven years of age. Approximately one-half of all of the assessed randomized, controlled studies included some childhood participants. A separate or sub-analysis of the childhood participants has not been performed. In one study in which the efficacy of mite SIT in children vs. adults was compared, participants <20 years of age had significantly better clinical improvement to SIT (20).

C. Prevention of Neo-Sensitization and Asthma

SIT has recently been associated with substantial reductions in the development of new inhalant allergen sensitizations in asthmatic children. This prevention of new sensitization to inhalant allergens has persisted for several years after SIT discontinuation (21–23). As an example of these studies, in a group of mite-monosensitized asthmatic children treated with mite SIT or placebo for four years, re-evaluation of allergen sensitivities three years after SIT discontinuation revealed that 27% of treated vs. 77% of controls had developed hypersensitivity to new aeroallergens (i.e., in addition to mites) (22).

A classic study suggested that SIT can prevent the development of persistent asthma in children. Johnstone (24) randomized 200 children with perennial asthma into one of four SIT treatment groups for four years (parent-blinded to treatment group): (a) placebo; or all of the inhalant allergens to which they were positive on skin testing, but at maximum concentrations for each allergen of (b) 1:10,000,000 w/v (low dose); (c) 1:5000 w/v (medium dose); or (d) 1:250 w/v (high dose). The final determination of asthma status was reportedly made by a clerk who was blinded to treatment groups. Wheezing with exertion was reported by 54% in the placebo and low dose treatment groups, 31% receiving medium-dose SIT, and only 9% of those receiving high dose SIT. Similar differences were reported for wheezing with respiratory infections.

A randomized controlled trial (PAT-study) sought to determine if SIT in children with seasonal allergic rhinitis could prevent the development of asthma (25). A group of 208 children ages 6–14 years with grass and/or birch pollen allergy were randomized to SIT (weekly injections or rush schedule) in a controlled but open-label study, with maintenance injections every six weeks for three years. After three years of SIT, the proportion of the SIT versus placebo-treated groups with clinical asthma in the past year was 24% vs. 44%. This coincided with well-demonstrated improvement in BHR to methacholine in the SIT-treated group.

These studies provide compelling evidence for important beneficial outcomes beyond asthma control. However, neither the prevention of asthma development in children with allergic rhinitis nor prevention of persistent asthma into later childhood has been validated by randomized, double-blind, placebo-controlled studies.

D. Persistence of Clinical Improvement After Stopping SIT

Two studies have examined the persistence of clinical improvement after discontinuation of SIT with grass pollen extract for seasonal allergic rhinitis. In an uncontrolled study, grass SIT was discontinued after three to four years of treatment in 108 patients who had responded well to treatment (26). There was a progressive increase in the number of patients reporting a return of grass pollen symptoms, reaching 31% by the third year, but with no appreciable increase in the fourth and fifth years. A double-blind, placebo-controlled trial supported the findings of this open study (27). Thirty-two patients who had received grass SIT for three to four years were randomized to either continue to receive grass SIT or to receive placebo injections for the following three years. Untreated patients with grass-induced allergic rhini-tis constituted an additional control group. In annual evaluations, both those continuing to receive grass SIT or those receiving placebo SIT had significantly fewer symptoms and less need for medication than the untreated controls, and scores in the active and placebo groups were virtually identical. Three years after SIT discontinuation, both treated groups had similar suppression of conjunctival sensitivity as well as immediate and late cutaneous reactions to grass pollen extract. In addition, biopsies obtained from the grass pollen intradermal skin test sites revealed less CD3+ cells (i.e., T-lymphocytes) and less IL-4 mRNA + cells in both treated groups.

Persistence of clinical improvement has also been monitored after stopping mite SIT for asthma (28). In a group of 40 asthmatic patients who had received mite SIT for one to eight years and who no longer required medication to control their symptoms, SIT was discontinued. Over a three-year period following discontinuation, 55% had a relapse in asthma symptoms. A lower likelihood of relapse correlated with longer SIT duration. Furthermore, a correlation of asthma relapse with less suppression of immediate skin test reactivity to mite was even stronger.

E. Clinical Efficacy with Specific Allergens

A refined understanding of SIT efficacy in asthma can be obtained by considering the roles and efficacy of specific inhalant allergens. Aeroallergens can be generally categorized into those that are perennial or seasonal. In asthma, the perennial allergens (e.g., mite, cat, and cockroach) have received the most attention, perhaps because of their strong links to childhood asthma severity, and the commonly perennial nature of asthma.

House Dust Mites

"Mite" allergens (i.e., from *Dermatophagoides pteronyssinus* or *D. farinae*) are ubiquitous. Perennial mite exposure is common and occult, and mite sensitization in asthmatic children is common. For example, in the CAMP cohort of 1041 asthmatic children in the United States, 48% were PST-positive to mites (1). The degree of mite sensitization has also been associated with asthma severity. In a large population sample study of schoolchildren in Sydney, Australia, skin test wheal size to mite correlated with BHR and asthma morbidity (29). Accordingly, nearly one-half of the SIT studies for asthma that were entered into the meta-analysis studies were with mite extracts. In these analyses, there was a significantly greater probability for asthma symptom and medication use reduction with active treatment with mite SIT versus placebo.

Animal Danders

Like mites, the combination of animal dander sensitivity and exposure e.g., cat and dog is associated with increased asthma severity (1). Although animal dander exposure is potentially avoidable, many asthmatic children are pet owners, and good efforts to educate patients and families of the importance of eliminating pet allergen exposure in the home seems to be of low yield. For example, for asthmatic children in the CAMP study, 65% of participants had furred and/or feathered pets in their home, 49% were sensitized to cat, and 23% to dog. All CAMP participants received education to reduce pet allergen exposure through the five years of the study. At the end of the study, 68% of CAMP participants were pet owners. Of further relevance, significant cat allergen exposure occurs in schools for cat-sensitive asthmatic children. In a prospective Swedish study, children in classrooms with more cat owners had higher levels of airborne cat allergen exposure, and deterioration in their asthma in the first two months of the start of the school year (30). Cat dander allergens have also been measured in other public places (31) and homes without cats (32). For cat-sensitive asthmatic children, significant exposure to cat dander seems unavoidable.

Two studies have demonstrated that cat SIT in patients without cats in the home can reduce asthma symptom medication scores (33) and BHR to histamine (34). Although the efficacy of animal dander SIT while maintaining pets in the home have not been specifically studied, pet-owning participants have generally not been excluded from these SIT efficacy studies.

Molds

Airborne fungal spores have been recognized as causing epidemic outbreaks (35) and life threatening episodes (36) in asthmatic children. SIT to fungi continues to present additional challenges when compared with other inhalant allergens (37). There are estimated to be hundreds of thousands of different species of fungi. Accurate information on exposure patterns to most fungal species is lacking, in part because many fungi do not grow in artificial media. Expressed fungal proteins (i.e., allergens) are variable and change with different life stages. Given these difficulties in working with fungi, it is perhaps not surprising that the quality of fungal extracts has been highly variable (38).

Randomized, controlled trials with standardized extracts of two important outdoor seasonal fungi, *Cladosporium* and *Alternaria*, have demonstrated efficacy. Ten months of *Cladosporium* SIT in 30 asthmatic children significantly reduced medication use but not symptom scores (39). Six months of SIT in 22 adult asthmatics produced a significant reduction in symptom-medication scores compared to placebo (40). One year of SIT with a standardized *Alternaria* extract in 24 patients with rhinitis and/or asthma who were sensitive only to Alternaria significantly reduced symptom-medication scores, and skin and nasal reactivity to *Alternaria* (41).

Cockroach

Sensitivity and exposure to cockroach is now recognized as a major morbidity factor in inner city children with asthma (4). Significant exposure is probably also widespread in warmer climates. There is only one published study of SIT for cockroach; however, the small number of study participants in the control group that completed the study ($n = 2$ at 5 years) mitigates the statistical power of the study (42). Current limitations to performing a high-quality cockroach SIT clinical trial include the lack of a reference standard or standardized cockroach allergen extracts. A recent investigation of the quality of commercially available cockroach allergen extracts by U.S. Food and Drug Administration (FDA) investigators revealed that their allergen content was highly variable for major allergen content, differed from the FDA reference standard, and were generally low in potency (43).

Pollens

Seasonal allergic rhinitis due to grass in England (44,45), ragweed in the United States (46,47), and birch in Scandinavia (48,49) have long been the most popular human allergic conditions for investigating SIT efficacy and mechanisms of action. The combination of their predictable seasonality of allergen exposure, available methods of measuring airborne allergen levels, relative ease of obtaining high-quality allergens and stable extracts, and the corresponding ability to make an accurate diagnosis of pollen-induced rhinitis provide optimal circumstances for SIT investigations. In all of these studies, adequate doses of pollen extracts significantly reduced clinical symptoms of allergic rhinitis and, when present, asthma.

Multiple vs. Single Allergen SIT

The response of asthmatics to SIT with multiple allergens combined in a single mixed "vaccine" has also been investigated in several studies. Some of the original SIT studies suggested that treatment with multiple allergens was successful. In the studies of ragweed allergic rhinitis conducted by Lowell and Franklin, patients received vaccines containing multiple allergens. When only the ragweed was removed (46) or reduced (50) in the mixed SIT vaccine, ragweed pollen-induced symptoms increased. Similarly, the results in asthmatic children reported by Johnstone (24) suggested that a mixed vaccine containing multiple unrelated allergens can be effective in treating asthma, and that its effectiveness depended on the dose of each allergen administered.

In contrast, the response to SIT for grass pollen allergic rhinitis was compared in patients only allergic to grass pollen and patients with multiple sensitivities (51). Patients received maintenance doses of 2000 biologic units of only grass pollen extract, or same maintenance dose of a mixture of pollen extracts if they were also sensitive to these pollens. Despite similar grass-specific IgG responses, clinical improvement was limited to only those who were sensitive to and received only grass SIT. In a placebo-controlled trial of mixed allergen SIT for asthmatic children, a single mixture of different allergens was used based on each participant's specific allergen sensitivities (52). The SIT-treated group did not demonstrate significant improvement when compared with placebo. Some have interpreted these studies to mean that mixed allergens SIT is ineffective. Indeed, most of the studies that have demonstrated SIT efficacy have employed single allergens.

However, there are other possible explanations for the lack of SIT efficacy with mixed allergens. For example, in the SIT study of asthmatic children (52), mold allergen extracts were included that contain proteases capable of degrading all allergens except for mold and ragweed (53). In addition, although perennial allergens were reportedly prioritized in SIT (presumably to be consistent with the perennial nature of asthma in their subject population), their perennial allergens consisted of mites and some molds, but did not include cockroach, cat, dog, other indoor molds, mouse and/or rat—additional important perennial allergens.

Generally, SIT studies that have not demonstrated efficacy differ from those that have in the following ways:

a. *Inappropriate subject selection*: Patient history and examination were not consistent with inhalant allergen-mediated disease.
b. *Suboptimal allergen selection for SIT*: To identify true inhalant allergen offenders that are good targets for SIT, subjects' histories

of symptomatic asthma and/or rhinitis must be matched with their allergen sensitizations and exposures. When these are mismatched (e.g., seasonal allergen SIT given to perennial asthmatics), SIT is typically less effective or ineffective.

    c.   *Inadequate allergen dosing in SIT*: A therapeutic dose of each important allergen in the SIT extract must be reached and sustained. Protocols that combine allergens are vulnerable to allergen dilution such that therapeutic allergen concentrations are not reached.

    d.   *Allergen mixing can lead to degradation of the relevant allergens in SIT extract mixes*: such as the mold mixture problem described above.

III. Mechanisms of Action

SIT induces a broad range of immune modulatory effects. Most are allergen-specific, and some have correlated with clinical improvement and/or persisted for years after SIT discontinuation. This suggests antigen (i.e., allergen)-specific immune "re-education"—an optimal outcome of any immune modulatory therapy.

A. Reduction in Mucosal and Skin Reactivity to Allergen

For pollen-induced hay fever, SIT has long been shown to reduce conjunctival, nasal, and skin test responses to the specific allergen (54–57). A reduction in immediate and late-phase skin reactions within months of initiating SIT and within weeks of reaching maintenance doses has been repeatedly confirmed (55,56,58–60). In a grass SIT study, the nasal pollen challenge threshold and the endpoint of titrated PST after rush SIT correlated with symptoms during the grass pollen season (57).

B. Improvements in Bronchial Responses

Numerous SIT studies with differing allergens have demonstrated a reduction in nonspecific (i.e., histamine or methacholine) BHR, such that the efficacy of mite and cat SIT on BHR has been reported in a Cochrane Systematic Review (19). In asthmatic children, mite or grass SIT were shown to reduce the likelihood and severity of early- and late-phase allergen-induced airways responses to inhalation of mite or grass pollen (61).

C. Improvements in Inflammatory Responses: Reduced Eosinophils, Mast Cells, and Basophils

Eosinophils, basophils, and mast cells are principal effector cells of the allergic response. Increased levels of these cells have been seen during natural allergen exposure and reduced by allergen SIT. Most of these studies have been in adults with seasonal pollen-induced rhinitis. For example, in a dose–response SIT study using the major ragweed allergen *Amb aI* for seasonal rhinitis, the presence of eosinophils in nasal brushings during the peak of the ragweed pollen season was compared in four groups who received either (a) no treatment, (b) maintenance SIT with 2 μg *Amb aI* for one or (c) two years, or with (d) a maintenance SIT dose of 24 μg *Amb aI* for three years (62). Reduction in nasal eosinophils during the ragweed pollen season was present only in those receiving the high-dose 24 μg *Amb aI* injections. SIT was also associated with fewer nasal metachromatic cells (i.e., basophils and mast cells) with allergen challenge (63) and fewer dermal mast cells (64). Clinical improvement in hay fever was accompanied by a greater than 10-fold reduction in the immediate cutaneous response to grass pollen and a seven fold decrease in mast cell numbers in the skin. The number of mast cells after SIT correlated with the clinical response in terms of seasonal symptoms ($r = 0.61, p = 0.0001$) and rescue medication use ($r = 0.75, p = 0.0001$).

Analogous to seasonal rhinitis, birch pollen-sensitive asthmatics who had received high-dose SIT for the previous three years underwent bronchoalveolar lavage (BAL) prior to and during the peak of the birch pollen season (65). There was no seasonal increase in BAL eosinophils in SIT-treated versus untreated patients. There also was blocking of a seasonal rise in eosinophil and neutrophil chemotactic activity in the BAL fluid in the treated group. In another study, peripheral blood eosinophils were lower and comparable to normal levels in mite-sensitive asthmatic children treated with SIT versus nontreated controls (66). Serum eosinophil cationic protein values were significantly lower at the peak of the Parietaria pollen season in the group of Parietaria-sensitive patients receiving SIT than in untreated controls (67). SIT blocked the seasonal increase in both eosinophil and neutrophil chemotactic activity in serum (68) and BAL (65).

D. Reduced Histamine Release

After four months of SIT, spontaneous in vitro histamine release from peripheral blood was significantly reduced in 50% of the subjects (69). Peripheral blood mononuclear cells (PBMC) of grass-sensitive asthmatic patients, studied out of season, spontaneously released increased amounts of a histamine-releasing factor (HRF) that induced histamine release from leukocytes of a single donor (70). Histamine release was further increased by adding grass pollen extract to PBMC. During the first grass pollen season, patients treated with placebo developed typical symptoms and increased release of HRF. Both symptoms and histamine release were reduced in those receiving grass SIT, and the two strongly correlated in the SIT-treated group. Similarly, in untreated asthmatic children allergic to dust mites, increased levels of spontaneous and allergen-induced HRF were reduced in those who clinically responded to mite SIT (71). In children treated with ragweed SIT, decreased sensitivity of basophils to release histamine in vitro on exposure to ragweed was reported (72). Subsequently, decreased basophil histamine releasability was also shown to a non-cross-reacting antigen (73).

E. Effects on B Lymphocytes

Prior to the discovery of IgE in the 1960s, the skin-sensitizing antibody, or "reagin," was measured by passive transfer of serial dilutions of serum. Using this method, Sherman demonstrated that the amount of skin-sensitizing antibody increased during the first few months of SIT and subsequently decreased (56). He also reported on 27 patients who had received SIT for 10–23 years with outstanding clinical improvement (74). Sera from seven patients could no longer be shown to contain skin-sensitizing antibodies; 18 others did, but only at very low titers.

Allergen-Specific IgE

SIT produces initially an increase in allergen-specific IgE antibodies; however, the normal seasonal rise in specific IgE is blunted, while the post-seasonal decline is unaffected (75). This was followed by a progressive decline in ragweed-specific IgE in the SIT-treated group when compared with the levels in an untreated group.

Allergen-Specific IgG1, IgG4, and Blocking Antibody

In 1935, Cooke reported that ragweed SIT resulted in the generation of an antibody which, when mixed with serum from a ragweed allergic donor, would inhibit the immediate reaction to ragweed at a passive transfer site (76). He suggested the term "blocking antibody" for this activity, although blocking antibody activity or allergen-specific IgG has not correlated with clinical improvement (20,57,77).

It has since been shown that SIT typically induces a prompt rise in allergen-specific IgG1 and IgG4 antibodies, but not the IgG2 or IgG3 subclasses (78). Initially, IgG1 antibodies predominated, but by the second year of SIT, the IgG4 response was more pronounced. No correlation was found between preseasonal levels of allergen-specific IgG1 or IgG4 and symptoms scores during the season. However, a good clinical outcome has been correlated with the rate of rise of allergen-specific IgG4 antibodies (79). In a rush SIT study with cat allergen, serum cat-specific IgG4 was increased one week after maintenance dosing was reached and in a dose-dependent manner (60). An effect of rush SIT on cat-specific IgE levels was not observed.

Perhaps the most compelling evidence to date of a role for blocking IgG antibodies in the clinical response to SIT was a recent demonstration that serum from grass SIT-treated people with rhinitis inhibited in vitro allergen-specific IgE binding to B cells, and subsequent allergen presentation to T cells (80). This activity was eliminated by depleting serum of IgG; IgG-containing fractions exhibited this blocking activity. The allergen specificity of this effect was demonstrated using serum from grass- and birch-sensitive patients who had received only grass SIT. Although grass allergen-IgE binding was inhibited by their serum, birch allergen-IgE binding was not. A possible explanation is SIT induces high-affinity IgG antibodies capable of out-competing allergen-specific IgE for allergen binding.

Other B Lymphocyte Effects

Expression of the low-affinity IgE receptor (FceRII/CD23) is regulated by the Th-2 cytokine IL-4. Two groups of mite-sensitive asthmatic versus non-asthmatic children were shown to have increased percentages of $CD23^+$ B lymphocytes (81,82). Mite SIT resulted in a significant reduction in the percentage of $CD23^+$ B lymphocytes in both studies; however, no significant correlation was found between changes in $CD23^+$ B-lymphocytes and clinical improvement (82). In another study, grass SIT reduced CD23 expression on B lymphocytes (83). Reduction in the severity of allergic symptoms and medication requirement during the following grass pollen season correlated closely with the SIT-induced reduction in the proportion of $CD23^+$ B lymphocytes. In another study, grass SIT also blocked the seasonal increase in several B cell activation antigens—CD23, CD40, and HLA-DR—which was observed during the pollen season in placebo-treated subjects (84).

F. Effects on T Lymphocytes

$CD4^+$ T Lymphocytes: Type 2 (Th-2), Type 1 (Th-1), and Regulatory (Treg)

The paradigm of two types of $CD4^+$ helper T-lymphocytes has emerged, with those from patients with allergic diseases (Th-2) secreting preferentially IL-4 and those from non-allergic subjects (Th-1) preferentially secreting interferon-gamma (IFN-γ) in response to allergen stimulation (85,86). Using a number of different approaches to investigate SIT effects on these T lymphocyte types, SIT appears to reduce Th-2 and increase Th-1 cell numbers, and cytokine expression and release.

In patients who had received mite or grass SIT for a mean duration of five years versus controls, in vitro cultures of $CD4^+$ T-lymphocytes with specific allergen resulted in increased IL-4 secretion by cells from untreated subjects, but lower, normal levels from the cells of those who had received

SIT (85). No differences in IL-2 or IFN-γ secretion between the treated and untreated patients were observed. A prospective, controlled study was conducted of patients with perennial allergic rhinitis treated with mite SIT for nine years (87). Serum IL-4 levels were markedly elevated prior to treatment, but declined from 13.3 to 4.3 pg/mL with SIT. This decline correlated with the degree of reduction in allergen-specific IgE. In a study from Scandinavia, allergen-induced IL-4 and IL-13 from PBMC were increased during the birch pollen season in placebo-treated subjects, but did not occur in SIT-treated subjects (88).

Patients who underwent rush SIT to mites had an increase in peripheral blood CD4$^+$ lymphocytes producing IFN-γ, which correlated with the decrease in sensitivity to mite PST (59). One year of mite SIT progressively increased the IFN-γ/IL-4 ratio in CD4 T-lymphocytes, but not in CD8$^+$ T-lymphocytes (89). Secretion of IL-5 by allergen-stimulated PBMC has also been reported to be increased in allergic patients (90,91). This was reduced by SIT in one study (91), but not in another (90). Using flow cytometry to assess PBMC responses to high-dose rush SIT to cat, CD4$^+$/IL-4$^+$ PBMC were decreased one week after high-dose maintenance SIT was reached; no SIT-induced differences were seen with CD4$^+$/IL-5$^+$ or CD4$^+$/IFN-γ^+ PBMC (60).

Complementary observations have been made in mucosal tissues and skin. Following one year of grass SIT, treated patients had a decrease in the size of the late-phase skin response to injection of grass pollen extract (86). Biopsies of the skin test site 24 hr following injection of the allergen revealed a reduction in the number of infiltrating CD4$^+$ T-lymphocytes, increased expression of the T lymphocyte activation markers, IL-2 receptor and HLA-DR, and, in one-half of the treated patients, IL-2 and IFN-γ mRNA. In the same study, patients underwent nasal challenge with grass pollen extract, followed by nasal biopsy 24 hours later—the results were similar (92). Subjects treated with SIT had significantly fewer infiltrating CD4$^+$ T-lymphocytes and fewer total and activated eosinophils. There were more IFN-γ mRNA-expressing cells in the treated patients, and the number of IFN-γ^+ cells was inversely correlated with patients' pollen seasonal symptoms-medication scores. In a follow-up study after four years of SIT, skin biopsies obtained 24 hours after intradermal allergen injection revealed increased IL-12 mRNA-expressing cells (93). The number of IL-12$^+$ cells correlated positively with the number of IFN-γ^+ cells and negatively with IL-4$^+$ cells. Since IL-12 promotes Th-1 and suppresses Th-2 lymphocyte proliferation, these findings favor the induction of allergen-specific Th-1 response after SIT.

There is evolving evidence for the induction of suppressor or regulatory T-lymphocytes by SIT. Ragweed SIT has been shown to reduce the allergen-specific proliferative response of PBMC (94). Recently, SIT has been shown to induce a CD4$^+$ subset of "regulatory" T-lymphocytes (i.e., CD4$^+$ CD25$^+$ IL-10$^+$ cells). Using grass pollen PBMC in vitro stimulation studies, grass

SIT patients versus controls had higher levels of allergen-induced IL-10 release, higher numbers of $CD4^+$ $CD25^+$ cells, and $IL-10^+$ cells that were almost exclusively $CD4^+$ $CD25^+$ cells (95). In another study of mite-allergic asthmatics who received mite SIT in a cluster protocol, in vitro Der p 1-stimulated PBMC from SIT patients released more IL-10 and TGF-β, primarily from $CD4^+$ $CD25^+$ cells (i.e., regulatory T-lymphocytes) (96). Antigen-specific suppressor activity by these cells was also demonstrated, and was IL-10 and TGF-β-dependent. Regulatory T-lymphocytes may suppress T-lymphocyte proliferation by inhibiting IL-2 receptor expression. SIT has been demonstrated to reduce the release of soluble IL-2 receptors (sIL-2R) (97). Serum levels of sIL-2R have also been reported to be lower in children receiving mite SIT compared to untreated asthmatic children (66).

$CD8^+$ T Lymphocytes

Similar observations to those described with $CD4^+$ helper T-lymphocytes have been made with $CD8^+$ T-lymphocytes. $CD8^+$ lymphocytes were increased in the peripheral blood following rush mite SIT (59). In mite-stimulated PBMC from children who received house dust SIT vs. controls, $CD8^+$ $CD25^+$ T-cells were increased only in those children with a good SIT response (98). The number of these cells also correlated with the cumulative dose of house dust SIT that they had received. Similarly, following two years of sublingual/swallow immunotherapy (SLIT) with a standardized mite extract, percentage of $CD8^+$ T-lymphocytes in the treated group increased, with a concomitant reduction in the $CD4^+/CD8^+$ ratio (99).

Interestingly, the allergen-specific suppressive effects of SIT (94) were originally attributed to $CD8^+$ cells. SIT was shown to induce allergen-specific cells that would suppress allergen-induced lymphocyte proliferative responses (100,101). Anti-CD8 antibody plus complement (which would lyse $CD8^+$ cells) abrogated this suppressive effect (101). Ragweed SIT also induced mononuclear cells that suppressed the in vitro production of anti-ragweed IgE (102). This suppressor activity was again reversed by treating the cells with the anti-CD8 antibody plus complement.

G. Other Cytokines Influenced by SIT

Peripheral blood monocytes manifest reductions in pro-inflammatory cytokine release following SIT. The previously described suppression of allergen-induced lymphocyte proliferation by ragweed SIT was accompanied by a marked reduction in ragweed-induced release of mitogenic and macrophage inhibitory factors from PBMC (94). In allergic asthmatic children, adherent peripheral blood monocytes released significantly more IL-1 and TNF-α on stimulation with house dust mite allergen (103). After one year of mite SIT, stimulated release of both cytokines was reduced, but the difference was significant only for TNF-α. Plasma platelet activating factor (PAF) production was also reduced in SIT responders (104). Both spontaneous and mite-induced PAF secretion was increased in asthmatic children who had not received SIT, and was reduced to normal levels in good but not poor SIT responders. Calcium ionophore-stimulated secretion of PAF increased in all patient groups and was not affected by SIT.

IV. Key Parameters for Effective SIT

In both clinical studies and patient care, optimally effective SIT depends on optimizing patient selection and a number of features of allergen extracts administered in SIT: quality, dose, selection, mixing, and storage. Inadequate optimization of any of these parameters can markedly reduce or lose SIT efficacy. A variety of SIT schedules seem to be equally effective in inducing clinical and immunologic responses. To optimize the safety of SIT, adverse reactions risk factors, monitoring during SIT administration, preparation for allergic reactions, and pharmacotherapeutic pretreatment(s) can reduce the occurrence of allergic reactions to SIT and the severity of allergic reactions that occur.

A. Optimizing Patient Selection

National and international asthma guidelines and allergy societies have addressed the role of SIT for asthma, with differing recommendations. For example, the Expert Panel of the National Asthma Education and Prevention Program (NAEPP), sponsored by the National Heart, Lung, & Blood Institute (NHLBI) of the U.S. National Institutes of Health, stated that SIT may be considered for asthma patients when: (a) there is clear evidence of a relationship between symptoms and exposure to an unavoidable allergen to which the patient is sensitive; (b) symptoms occur all year or during a major portion of the year; and (c) there is difficulty controlling symptoms with pharmacologic management because the medication is ineffective, multiple medications are required, or the patient is not accepting of medications (105). Other groups, also convened by the NHLBI, endorsed this recommendation while listing certain considerations that should be weighed in making the decision (106,107): (a) asthma severity; (b) efficacy of the available immunotherapy; and (c) the cost, risk and duration of pharmacologic therapy versus SIT. Among the specific factors to consider were the potentially greater SIT efficacy in children and young adults (20) the greater likelihood of success in patients with a single sensitivity (51), and the increased risk of SIT administration in asthmatic patients who are symptomatic and/or have a spirometric FEV1 of less than 70% of predicted (108).

*Matching Symptom Patterns with Allergen Exposure and
Sensitization (Table 1)*

Although authorities differ in whom they consider to be suitable SIT candidates with asthma, current evidence suggests that asthma patients must meet three essential conditions to have a high likelihood of benefiting from SIT:

    a. significant allergen *exposure,*
    b. a significant level of *hypersensitivity* to the allergen,
    c. the patterns of *asthma symptoms conform to the exposure patterns* with sensitized allergens.

Significant exposure may be difficult to define, however, there are some general rules. For potential perennial allergens, an understanding of common regional perennial allergens and some questions about household environments for asthmatic patients can provide major clues for perennial allergen exposures. Dust mites are generally ubiquitous indoor allergens unless patients live in dry climates, such as at high altitudes (32), or are taking extensive household measures to substantially reduce dust mites (109). Water damage, visible mold, basement pooling of water, and/or evidence of home dampness are clues that homes may have high levels of molds. Both pets (e.g., cats and dogs) and pests (e.g., cockroaches and rats) generate high levels of allergens that can increase asthma severity and morbidity. Asking about pets and pests in the home often provides enlightening exposure information. However, this is not

Table 1 Worksheet for Identifying Allergen Candidates for SIT

Allergens	History	Exposure	Allergen-specific IgE
Seasonal			
Trees			
Grasses			
Weeds			
Molds			
Perennial			
Animals			
Mites			
Pests			
Molds			
Other			

Allergens with the highest likelihood of worsening asthma are those to which the patient has (i) significant exposure, (ii) a pattern of symptoms that conforms with the exposure patterns, and (iii) objective evidence of hypersensitivity to the allergens (e.g., allergy prick skin test wheal ≥3 mm in diameter). Optimal allergens for SIT meet all three criteria.

always the case. For example, inner city asthmatic children were provided with video camcorders to make video diary movies about their lives with asthma (110). This was compared with information that providers obtained in the clinic through conventional medical history interviews. The video vignettes revealed that 95% of the asthmatic children were exposed to high levels of asthma irritants in their daily living environment despite reporting little to no exposures during clinic-based interviews (molds 91%, ETS 63%, furry pets 43%, and noxious fumes 25%). Home visits with environmental surveys can help to clarify significant allergen exposures. House dust samples can be analyzed for quantitative major allergen content for mites (Der p 1 and Der f 1), cat (Fel d 1), dog (Can f 1), cockroach (Bla g 1 and Bla g 2), rat (Rat n 1), and mouse (Mus m 1) with commercially available tests. With cat allergen, asthmatic children can experience significant occult exposure outside of their homes. A study of cat-sensitive asthmatic schoolchildren in Sweden demonstrated that those who were assigned to classrooms with more cat owners were exposed to higher levels of respirable cat allergen in the classroom, and subsequently experienced greater asthma severity on their return to school (30).

Seasonal locale-specific pollen and mold exposures can be determined from quantitative pollen sampling data. Local allergists often collect this information and cultivate an understanding of the relevant aerobiology. Nationally, the American Academy of Allergy, Asthma & Immunology has an Aeroallergen Network including 77 pollen-counting stations in North America. Seasonal regional and local pollen counts are available through this "National Allergy Bureau" at http://www.aaaai.org.

Most of the studies that demonstrated SIT efficacy have selected patients on the basis of positive allergy PSTs and have often required positive in vitro tests for allergen sensitivity as well (20,45,111–114). With potent grass pollen (53) and cat dander (115) extracts, the sensitivity detectable by intradermal testing in patients with negative PSTs does not appear to be clinically relevant (116); therefore, the use of positive intradermal skin tests following negative PST with these extracts and others of similar potency does not form a strong basis for selecting patients and allergens for SIT. On the other hand, with allergen extracts of poor quality, it may not be feasible to administer an effective subcutaneous dose.

Finally, the pattern of allergen exposure and sensitivity should be consistent with the patient's pattern of symptoms. For example, in patients with perennial asthma, the allergens of primary concern would be those causing year-round exposure and with PST sensitization. Historical evidence of asthma worsening with high levels of exposure (e.g., asthma worsening when visiting homes with cats) and/or asthma improvement with allergen exposure reduction (e.g., asthma improvement) when on vacation in dry, mountain climates with negligible mite allergen is further evidence of a pattern of asthma symptoms that matches changes in exposure levels. In contrast,

SIT to a few pollen extracts is unlikely to benefit patients with perennial asthma symptoms without seasonal variation.

SIT Adverse Reactions and Contraindications

The main complication and concern of SIT is the potential occurrence of systemic allergic and/or asthmatic reactions (SAR). Two studies prospectively monitored ~15,000 patients who received ~850,000 injections during SIT for SARs (116,117). The SIT SAR rate over one year was 2.1% of patients (117) and, over a 13-year period, was 2.9% of patients (116). In both studies, the majority of SARs occurred during the build-up phase of SIT. In one study, 90% of SARs occurred between 100–1000 PNU/mL SIT vaccine concentrations (full range of SIT concentrations was 10–2000 PNU/mL) (116). In this same study, the highest incidence of SARs occurred in patients ages 10–39 years, and 95% occurred with SIT to pollens.

Two retrospective surveys of fatal reactions to allergen injections from skin testing or SIT were performed by the Committee on Allergen Standardization of the American Academy of Allergy, Asthma & Immunology (118,119). Through a collective effort of the American Academy of Allergy, Asthma & Immunology and the American College of Allergy, Asthma & Immunology, from 1945 to 1989, 63 fatalities associated with allergen injections were identified, mostly due to SIT. The estimated SIT fatality rate per injection was one fatality per two million injections (119). The mean age of SIT fatalities was 35 years (range 7–77 years), in slightly more women than men. Nineteen of 31 cases occurred during the increasing-dose phase of SIT. A risk factor assessment of the available case histories revealed that administration errors may have occurred in six cases, and five cases occurred with the first injection of a newly prepared allergen vaccine. Seventy-three percent occurred during the build-up phase of SIT, 77% occurred in patients with asthma, and 36% had a prior history of SARs. Out of 13 identified asthma patients, four had asthma symptoms at the time of SIT injection, of whom two were also taking β-adrenergic blocker medication (119). Two did not wait for observation after injections, and one died at home after home SIT.

Patients with asthma versus allergic rhinitis alone have a greater risk of having a fatal reaction to SIT (118,119). This is particularly true if the asthma is labile or symptomatic at the time of the injection, requires oral corticosteroid treatment, has resulted in hospitalization or emergency room visits, or if the patient has a complicating cardiovascular condition (119). In patients with asthma receiving mite SIT with a rapid build-up schedule (i.e., "rush"), an asthma episode was the most common form of systemic allergic reaction (108). Patients whose initial FEV1 was less than 80% of their predicted were more prone to developing bronchospasm. Some studies and guidelines have recommended that SIT be withheld in asthmatic patients with FEV1 less that 70% of predicted (106,107,120). Other suggestions include having asthma patients perform peak expiratory flow measurements prior to an SIT injection and again before leaving the clinic, and optimizing asthma management prior to an SIT course with conventional controller pharmacotherapy, environmental control measures, and management of co-morbid conditions.

The interval between allergen extract injection and development of a systemic reaction is of considerable importance, because it dictates the period of time that patients should remain in the physician's office after receiving treatment for close monitoring. Severe reactions tend to occur quickly; one study reported that all severe reactions occurred within 30 minutes (121). In the retrospective surveys of SIT-associated case fatalities described above, the onset of systemic reactions generally occurred within minutes of allergen injection, with 29 of 32 cases occurring within 30 minutes (118,119). After reviewing the fatalities associated with SIT, a suggested recommendation for the duration of observation after SIT injections was 20 minutes for "usual" cases, and 30 minutes for "high-risk" patients, with acknowledgement that asthmatics may deserve special considerations (119).

Large local skin reactions at the SIT injection site, and SIT build-up injections during the pollen season (i.e., time of greatest exposure) are often believed to increase the likelihood of a systemic reaction. The occurrence of large local skin reactions was not found to be predictive of the occurrence of a systemic reaction (122). In a prospective study, local reactions were found to be an insensitive predictor of systemic reactions with the next SIT injection (123). It was concluded that local reactions do not require dose adjustments. Studies of large numbers of patients receiving SIT have not demonstrated an increased risk of systemic allergic reactions due to SIT during the pollen seasons (116,117). However, one study observed an increased occurrence of systemic reactions during August–October, coincident with the peak of outdoor mold spores (117).

Premedication to reduce systemic reactions to SIT have been tested in patients receiving rush (120,124,125) or cluster (126) SIT, both of which may be associated with a higher incidence of systemic reactions than conventional dosing because of the relatively rapid build-up. Prior to rush SIT (i.e., eight build-up injections given over three consecutive days), pretreatment for SIT injections with oral corticosteroids (methylprednisolone 0.5 mg/kg), ketotifen (1 mg, with additional 1 mg post-AIT), and long-acting theophylline (5 mg/kg, with additional 5 mg/kg post-AIT) (120,124), or with oral corticosteroids and the combination of H1 and H2 antagonists (125) reduced systemic reactions during rush SIT to less than one-half of expected. A similar reduction in both the number and severity of systemic reactions during cluster SIT was reported with pretreatment with the antihistamine loratadine each day, given two hours before beginning injections (126). In two studies, the addition of a step to withhold SIT advancement for large local reactions (i.e., >10 cm) or FEV1 <70% of predicted further reduced the rate of SIT SAR during the build-up phase by an additional ~50% (120,124). In these studies, further spreading out of the SIT injections over 5–6 days reduced SIT SARs by an additional ~50%.

Non-IgE Mediated Adverse Reactions

Injection of foreign proteins to which patients will develop IgG antibodies can theoretically cause the formation of antigen-antibody complexes and induce immune complex-mediated disease. In one report, six of 20 consecutive patients with polyarteritis nodosa were receiving SIT at the time of onset of their vasculitic symptoms (127). It was pointed out, however, that no anti-allergen precipitating antibodies were detected in these patients. In three other studies, a total of 151 SIT patients revealed no evidence of autoimmune or immune complex disorders (128–130). When relevant blood tests were compared in SIT versus controls (144 control participants in these three studies), the SIT group had no significantly increased incidence of circulating immune complexes, C1q binding complexes, cryoglobulinemia, ANA, rheumatoid factor, or complement depletion. Additionally, several recently published SIT trials in children have not reported any autoimmune disease complications from SIT (25,52,131).

B. Optimizing Allergen Vaccines

In addition to optimal patient selection, SIT efficacy is strongly dependent on a number of features of the allergen-containing vaccine that is administered. Key among them is the *dosage* of the relevant allergen(s) administered per maintenance injection. Allergen extracts of variable, poor and/or deteriorating quality pose a two-headed problem. Not only are potent allergen extracts essential for achieving effective SIT, varying potency of allergen extracts can increase the risks of SIT administration. For example, if an allergen vaccine does not maintain its potency over time, then the patient is becoming tolerant of a lower-than-expected dose of allergen. When the deteriorating allergen vaccine runs out, the new vaccine can be substantially more potent, leading to an increased risk of a systemic allergic reaction. As a precaution, some allergists, when starting a new maintenance vial of allergen vaccine, will reduce the dosage to one-half to one-quarter of the most recent maintenance dosage and build up to maintenance again.

Aspects of allergen vaccines that are essential to attain and maintain allergen vaccines of adequate potency for SIT include:

a. commercial availability of potent and consistent (e.g., standardized) allergen extracts,
b. allergen cross-reactivity,

c. some allergens contain proteases that, when combined with other allergens, will degrade them,

d. sub-optimal buffers, diluents and storage conditions can lead to degradation of allergen extract potency.

Dosage

SIT consists of a "build-up" phase of gradually increasing allergen dosage, in order to safely reach effective "maintenance" doses. Clinically effective maintenance doses have been determined for mites, cat, grass, and ragweed, defined in terms of their major allergen content (132) Collectively, these studies suggest that an effective maintenance allergen dose for SIT is about 10 μg (range 6–20 μg) of major allergen per injection.

The methods of allergen extract standardization employed in the United States are not based on major allergen content determination by weight (i.e., microgram (mcg)), and vary for different allergens. For cat dander and short ragweed extracts, the U.S. FDA standardizes by major allergen content, expressed in FDA units. For mite and grass extracts, the FDA uses the "ID$_{50}$EAL" method to quantify "Bioequivalent Allergy Units" (BAU) in lots of allergen extracts based on titrated intradermal skin testing in allergic subjects in comparison with a reference standard. Because FDA-standardized extracts are compared to a single national potency standard, patients and physicians can switch from one manufacturer's product to another with knowledge of their comparative potency. There are other methods of allergen standardization; however, these methods use in-house reference standards without comparison to an external (e.g., national) standard.

There are currently 19 allergen extracts that meet the U.S. FDA criteria for allergen standardization. Representative lots of FDA-standardized extracts have been assessed for their major allergen content (Table 2) (132). Although this information allows an approximation of proven doses, the range of major allergen content for extracts labeled with the same standardized potency is quite broad.

In the United States, hundreds of unstandardized allergen extracts still meet a number of consistency and safety criteria for use in humans. The U.S. FDA Center for Biologics Evaluation and Research (CBER) enforces "current good manufacturing practice" standards for allergen extracts, including manufacturing standards, consistent allergen sources, consistent methods of allergen extract preparation, and sterility and preservative requirements and testing. Although unstandardized allergen extracts usually provide a unitage measure that denotes a consistent extraction approach, such as weight per volume ("w:v") or protein concentration in Protein Nitrogen Units (PNU/ml), these measures generally do not correlate well with allergen content.

In many cases, allergen extract manufacturers can provide major allergen potency for a particular lot of their extract. Unstandardized extracts can only

Table 2 Major Allergen Content of U.S. Standardized Aeroallergen Extracts

Allergen extract (No. of extracts tested)	Expressed potency	Major allergen	Mean content of major allergen (μg/mL)	Minimum content of major allergen (μg/mL)	Maximum content of major allergen (μg/mL)
Orchard (n=14)	100,000 BAU/mL	Dac g 5	918	294	2414
Fescue (n=12)	100,000 BAU/mL	Fes p 5	152	75	204
Rye (n=14)	100,000 BAU/mL	Lol p 5	337	157	526
Kentucky Blue (n=15)	100,000 BAU/mL	Poa p 5	262	118	338
Timothy (n=12)	100,000 BAU/mL	Phl p 5	743	354	1336
Short Ragweed (n=13)	1:10 w/v	Amb a 1	268	87	458
Mixed Ragweed (n=10)	1:10 w/v	Amb a 1	174	56	402
D. pteronyssinus (n=28)	10,000 AU/mL	Der p 1	172	68	385
D. Farinae (n=18)	10,000 AU/mL	Der f 1	44	30	72
Cat hair (n=12)	10,000 BAU/mL	Fel d 1	40	26	52
Dog hair (n=4)	1:10 w/v	Can f 1	5.4	2.7	7.2

Abbreviations: BAU, bioequivalent allergy units; mL, milliliters; μg, micrograms; w/v, weight/volume (extraction ratio); AU, arbitrary units (FDA equivalent to BAU).
Source: From Ref. 132.

be dosed based on analogy to standardized extracts or by what is known or suspected to be their potency (43,133). Unstandardized pollen extracts can be assumed to approximate standardized grass and ragweed extracts in potency. The potency of the currently available cockroach extracts is widely variable, and significantly different and generally less potent than an FDA reference standard (43). There is no data by which to extrapolate the potency of fungal extracts.

Cross-Reactive Allergens

If each allergen group should be present in the treatment extract in therapeutic amounts, then botanical cross-reactivity must be considered when selecting the extracts to be included in the skin test panel and in formulating the treatment extract. Some of the common allergens are highly cross-reactive. The general patterns of botanical cross-allergenicity are listed (Table 3).

Allergen Extract Proteases

Some allergen extracts contain proteases that can degrade the allergens in other extracts when they are mixed. Proteases have been reported in fungal and whole body insect extracts, and many of the major allergens of dust mites (e.g., Der p1 and Der f1), cockroach (e.g., Bla g2), and molds (e.g., penicillium, aspergillus, cladosporium, and alternaria) have protease activity (134,135). Commonly used fungal and cockroach allergen extracts have been shown in mixture to cause loss of allergenic potency of many pollen and cat extracts (53). Mite extract, when in a 25% glycerin diluent, does not appear to cause degradation of these pollen extracts, perhaps because glycerin inhibits protease activity. Perhaps the best general rule is to not mix cockroach or fungal extracts with pollen or mite extracts (except ragweed).

Storing and Handling Allergen Extracts

Once an allergen vaccine has been prepared for administration, its components are vulnerable to loss of potency, particularly when in more dilute concentrations (136). Degradation of allergen extract potency is accelerated at higher temperatures, including room temperature; therefore, allergen extracts should be kept at refrigerator temperature at all times except when in use (136). Loss of potency can be retarded by the addition of protein stabilizers such as 0.03% human serum albumin or 10–50% glycerin (136). Although 50% glycerin is probably the best preservative of allergen potency, its use is limited by the discomfort that accompanies its injection. In a study of painful reactions from SIT of glycerin at differing concentrations (10–30%), "annoying" or "intolerable pain" was unusual when the total dose of injected glycerin (i.e., volume × %glycerin) was less than 0.05 mL (e.g., 0.5 mL of 10% glycerin) (137). Increasing amounts of glycerin correlated well with an

Table 3 Allergen Cross-Reactivities

Trees
Cuppressaceae
  Juniper
  Cedar
  Cypress
Betulaceae
  Birch
  Alder
  Hazel
  Hornbeam
  Hophornbeam
Fagaceae
  Beech
  Oak
  Chestnut
Oleaceae
  Ash
  European olive
  Privet
Populus
  Aspen
  Poplar
  Cottonwood
Grasses
Gramineae
  Meadow fescue
  Timothy
  Rye
  Kentucky Blue
  Orchard
  Red top
Weeds
  Compositae
Ambrosia
  Short ragweed
  Giant ragweed
  False ragweed
  Western ragweed
Artemisia
  Sages
  Mugworts
  Wormwood
Chenopodiaceae
  Salsola
  Russian thistle

(Continued)

Table 3   Allergen Cross-Reactivities (*Continued*)

Chenopodium
Lambs quarter
Kochia
Burning bush
Atriplex
Wingscale
Salt bush
Amaranthaceae
Pigweed
Red root pigweed
Palmer's Amaranth
Dust mites
D. pteronyssinus
D. farinae
Cockroach
German cockroach
American cockroach

The *allergen groups* of tribes, genera, or species (underlined and italicized) show strong cross-reactivity within each group.
Source: Adapted from the Standardized Skin Test and Immunotherapy Forms, American Academy of Allergy, Asthma and Immunology, 2003 (www.aaaai.org).

increasing frequency of painful reactions. Individual variation in perceived discomfort was substantial.

C.   Prescribing and Administering SIT

To summarize, important considerations when writing an individualized allergen vaccine prescription for SIT include:

    a.   which allergen extracts to include,
    b.   potency of available allergen extracts,
    c.   patterns of allergenic cross-reactivity,
    d.   mixing effects,
    e.   effective maintenance dose for each allergen,
    f.   safe starting dose.

    When multiple major allergens are identified for SIT, combining allergens into one or two mixed allergen "vaccine(s)" can reduce the number of injections needed and thereby improve the convenience, ease, and comfort of the process. However, these benefits must be balanced with the potential deleterious effects of protease-containing allergens (e.g., molds and cockroaches) on the potency of others. Because some allergen extracts may be more irritating to the subcutaneous tissue due to such elements as endotoxins, mycotoxins, proteases, glycerin, or even the allergens in them, combined allergen extracts may slow or limit the achievable dosage of all allergens in the mix due to the adverse local reactions to one or a few allergens. In addition, mixing allergen extracts of low potency may lead to sub-therapeutic maintenance dosing.

D. Prescriptions and Injection Schedules

A comprehensive approach to prescribing, administering and managing SIT has an important role in optimizing SIT efficacy and safety. An excellent example of such an SIT program is sponsored by the AAAAI, and is available on its website (www.aaaai.org). This set of template forms provides detailed outlines for formulating and prescribing SIT vaccines, delivering and tracking SIT injections, and documenting adverse reactions. An SIT prescription generally includes an SIT vaccine for maintenance injections, with dilutions of this maintenance vaccine such that SIT injections begin at a safe dose of low potency, and can be safely advanced to reach maintenance.

SIT Injection Schedules

The initial build-up to maintenance is conventionally achieved by twice-weekly to weekly injections of SIT vaccine (138). An example of a conventional SIT schedule of a stock or maintenance allergen vaccine (i.e., Vial #1) with dilutions of the stock to be used as build-up injections to achieve an effective maintenance dose (Vials #2–5), is presented (Table 4).

To hasten SIT's build-up process to reach therapeutic maintenance doses sooner, alternative build-up schedules such as cluster (139), daily (140), or rush (20,125,141) have been studied and utilized. A daily SIT schedule revealed no increase in the incidence of systemic reactions over the conventional weekly schedule (140). A cluster SIT schedule [e.g., multiple injections of increasing amount given once weekly (139) or twice weekly (60)] was found to have a similar rate of adverse reactions and similar efficacy to weekly injections, although in some studies, a higher rate of systemic reactions was reported (126,142). Even more rapid rush SIT schedules have been studied (108,125). Such protocols have reduced the number of build-up injections to reach maintenance to eight over a period of three days (108), and even to eight injections in a single day (143). Both protocols have resulted in a significant increase in systemic adverse reactions in asthma patients. Systemic reactions were reduced from 73% to 27% with premedication with a combination of medications that included antihistamines and oral corticosteroids (125), from 36% to 7% with a similar premedication regimen plus not treating patients with reduced pulmonary function (FEV1 < 70% predicted) or very large injection site reactions (> 10 cm) (120). With both rush protocols, patients tolerated weekly maintenance injections after completion of the rush build-up without a high incidence of systemic reactions.

Once patients reach maintenance doses of their SIT vaccine, it is customary to give the maintenance injections at less frequent intervals, typically

Table 4 Example of SIT Treatment Schedule

Vial #5 (1:10,000 dilution of stock) (mL)	Vial #4 (1:1000 dilution of stock) (mL)	Vial #3 (1:100 dilution of stock) (mL)	Vial #2 (1:10 dilution of stock) (mL)	Vial #1 (stock allergen vaccine) (mL)
0.05	0.05	0.05	0.05	0.05
0.10	0.10	0.10	0.07	0.07
0.20	0.20	0.20	0.10	0.10
0.40	0.40	0.40	0.15	0.15
			0.25	0.20
			0.35	0.30
			0.50	0.40
				0.50[a]

This example begins with a concentrated "stock allergen vaccine" such that the final "maintenance" dose provides the target dose of allergen(s) for SIT. The stock allergen vaccine can then be diluted to make much lower dilutions to begin with, and then "build-up" tolerance to reach the target maintenance dose. SIT typically begins with the smallest dose of Vial #4 (0.05 mL of 1:1000 dilution of stock). Initial doubling-dose increases are subsequently reduced to 50% increases, then ultimately 25% increases in dose, as tolerated. The frequency of build-up injections has varied widely (e.g., weekly, twice weekly, daily, "cluster," and "rush").
[a]Maintenance dose.
Source: Adapted from Ref. 157.

increasing over a period of time to once monthly injections. Optimally safe spacing of SIT injections after maintenance is reached has not been specifically studied.

A few studies have addressed the question of SIT duration to optimize its efficacy. Benefit can be demonstrated after only a single series of preseasonal injections (47). Clinical benefits may increase with continuation of the same dose over several consecutive seasons (111). Furthermore, the benefit from a brief course of SIT may be rapidly lost, while that from a longer course may persist after injections are discontinued (28). Several studies have demonstrated the persistence of clinical benefits after SIT discontinuation when the SIT course was for three to four years (26,27). On this basis, general guidelines are that the SIT course, if successful and well tolerated, should be continued until the patient has been symptom-free or markedly improved for at least two years, and in most cases for three to five years (144).

SIT Considerations Unique to Children

Although, in the treating of asthma with SIT, children may experience greater benefit and optimal outcomes (e.g., reduce neo-sensitization and asthma persistence into adulthood), there are some additional considerations for children. There is relatively little information on the safety of SIT in children with asthma. Although the incidence of SIT SARs is less in children < 10 years of age (116), SARs and SIT fatalities in children < 10 years of age have been consistently reported (116,117,119). For allergic rhinitis, a recent study of 225 children using a cluster schedule and rapidly advancing dosages for pollen SIT reported an adverse reaction rate of 16% (injection site pruritis, site edema, rhinitis, asthma, and/or eczema), with no serious SARs (145). Children may indeed be more physiologically able to weather systemic adverse reactions to SIT. However, children are presumed to be less able to perceive or report the severity of their asthma or the onset of subtle systemic allergic symptoms. Younger children (i.e., less than seven years of age) may not provide valid spirometry or peak flow results for assessing lung function. Furthermore, spirometric criteria for assessing asthma severity that were developed in adults may not apply to children (146). Obtaining informed assent for SIT in children is an additional consideration.

V. Alternative Routes of Administration for SIT

In efforts to improve the safety, expense, appeal, and efficacy of SIT, administration of allergen by the oral, intranasal, or inhaled/intra-bronchial routes have been studied.

A. Sublingual/Swallow (SLIT) and Oral Immunotherapy

SLIT has been of particular interest as a form of allergen immunotherapy for children, because of its relative safety and subsequent potential for home administration. SLIT and oral immunotherapy are similar to SIT in providing a build-up of allergen dose to give daily oral maintenance doses that cumulatively exceed what is considered therapeutic by the subcutaneous route. SLIT differs from oral immunotherapy in that SLIT has a brief period ([i.e.], 1–2 minutes) of retaining each oral allergen dose under the tongue before being swallowed. Both SLIT and oral immunotherapy have demonstrated clinical efficacy for allergic rhinitis and supportive immune biological effects in randomized, controlled studies. SLIT has recently undergone a renaissance of interest for the treatment of allergic rhinitis. A recent Cochrane Systematic Review on this subject identified 22 randomized controlled trials (seven for perennial allergens mites or cat; 14 for seasonal allergens) for meta-analysis (147). SLIT significantly reduced rhinitis symptoms and relevant medication use. A broad variation in response to SLIT could be attributed to variations in allergens used, age of participants, and dose, schedule and duration of treatment, as well as differences in study designs. Two studies comparing the efficacy of SLIT to subcutaneous SIT (mite and grass) reported similar improvements in symptoms and medication requirements for these two routs of administration (148,149).

The efficacy of SLIT in pediatric patients was also recently reviewed, and seven studies of pediatric patients were identified with evidence for clinical efficacy of SLIT (150). In children with allergic rhinitis, a 3-year double-blind, placebo-controlled study of oral mite immunotherapy employed cumulative doses of five times those employed for injection SIT (151). In the second and third years of treatment, symptoms and conjunctival sensitivity were significantly decreased, allergen-specific IgG1 and IgG4 increased, and IgE declined.

Three studies of mite-sensitive asthmatic children with mite SLIT revealed significant reductions in asthma episodes and medication use (152–154), as well as improvement in allergen-specific and non-specific BHR and increased peripheral blood allergen-specific IgG and CD8+ cells (99,152). In an intriguing, prospective (open) study of mite-sensitive asthmatic children who had received a four to five year course of SLIT and were re-evaluated for the persistence of asthma four to five years later, ~10% of SLIT-treated asthmatic children had persistent asthma at the end of SLIT and four to five years after SLIT discontinuation vs. 96% in the untreated control group had persistent asthma (155).

Although it appears that allergen-specific immune responses, symptom improvement, and BHR reduction can result from SLIT, this route of treatment requires cumulative allergen doses that exceed injection SIT as well as a prolonged period of administration, suggesting that the oral route is relatively ineffective. Other fundamental limitations in our current understanding of optimal SLIT and oral immunotherapy include the lack of a consensus or evidence-based "maintenance" allergen dose (5–300 times SIT maintenance have been given). Accordingly, dose-response effect with SLIT has not yet been demonstrated.

Although serious adverse reactions have not been reported form SLIT, some local (oral itching) side effects and rare allergic (urticaria, rhinoconjunctivitis, and asthma) and gastrointestinal (nausea, vomiting, and cramping) effects have been reported in children receiving SLIT (150). In a postmarketing surveillance study of adverse reactions to SLIT in children, the incidence of systemic side effects was reported to be 3% of patients and 1/12,000 doses (156). Since SLIT protocols are generally designed for home administration on a daily basis, the safety concerns of such an approach to allergen immunotherapy, especially in children with asthma, deserves careful consideration.

B. Intranasal and Intrabronchial Immunotherapy

Topical allergen immunotherapy of the airways has been investigated primarily for allergic rhinitis. Its use is complicated by the respiratory symptoms induced by allergen inhalation in sensitized patients. A number of studies have demonstrated that inhalation allergen immunotherapy can improve respiratory symptoms and induce supportive changes in immune responses and inflammation that are primarily localized to the airways (reviewed in Ref. 157). Topical cromolyn pretreatment can markedly reduce or eliminate symptoms due to either intranasal or intrabronchial allergen administration. Two small studies of mite inhalation immunotherapy in asthmatic children decreased asthma symptoms, improved peak flows, and reduced airway sensitivity to inhaled mite (158,159). For a complete review of this topic, please see Ref. 157.

VI. Modified Allergen Extracts

Attempts to improve the efficacy, safety, and ease of SIT administration have also led to numerous alterations of allergens in extracts to achieve these aims (reviewed in Ref. 157). These allergen extract modifications have included: (a) attempts to retard allergen extract absorption after injection by emulsifying in mineral oil or precipitating with alum; (b) reducing allergenicity without reducing immunogenicity, with formaldehyde or glutaraldehyde treatment, or binding to alginate; and (c) recombinant allergen production. Many of these alterations have demonstrated improvements in efficacy and safety of allergen extracts in human studies, such as reductions in systemic adverse reactions, fewer injections during the build-up phase, and prolonged shelf life, while retaining the same clinical and immunologic results as with conventional aqueous allergen extracts.

A. Purified and Recombinant Allergens

The concept of major allergenic proteins driving most of the allergic response to complex allergenic sources has led to attempts to improve SIT by focusing on these major allergens. Purified major pollen allergens have been compared with conventional allergen extracts for SIT. The immune response to injections of the major ragweed allergen Antigen E (Amb a I) were considered to be equivalent to those obtained with the whole unmodified extract of ragweed (160). However, SIT with the two major allergens of timothy grass was not as effective as those with a partially purified whole timothy grass pollen extract in a three-year, blinded study (161).

The identification, cloning and sequencing of many of the major allergens have led to the production of some of these major allergens using recombinant expression systems, as whole allergens or their immunodominant peptides (i.e., T lymphocyte epitopes). Using major allergen peptides for SIT had the further appeal of essentially eliminating their IgE epitopes and the subsequent likelihood of triggering IgE-mediated adverse reactions with SIT. This approach was employed to develop peptide vaccines for ragweed pollen, containing epitopes from Amb A I, and from cat dander, containing epitopes from Fel d I. Clinical trials of these vaccines demonstrated some reduction in symptoms in comparison to placebo treatment (162). However, administration of the higher doses of the peptides caused late-phase respiratory symptoms several hours following injection (162,163). Although these became less with repeated dosing, a number of patients developed peptide-specific IgE, which resulted in some patients developing systemic allergic reactions with succeeding injections.

B. Enhancing Immune Modulatory Effects of Allergen Extracts

Several strategies have been pursued to improve the therapeutic immune response to allergen extracts used in SIT. In order to target allergen uptake by antigen-presenting cells, allergen has been combined with an excess of autologous allergen-specific IgG antibody to generate allergen: IgG complexes, and injected intradermally to treat asthma, rhinitis, and atopic dermatitis (164). Although the amount of allergen injected in this form of therapy is 500–1000 times less than used in conventional SIT, the effort required to generate this product has been a limitation to broader investigation.

Bacterial DNA: Allergen Conjugates

Recently, microbial (e.g., bacterial and viral) DNA has been found to be a Toll-like receptor (TLR9) ligand that stimulates innate immune responses and induces Th-1-type immunity (165,166). The specific TLR9 ligand, unmethylated CG motifs in microbial DNA sequence, is currently being exploited as conjugates to allergen to potentially improve the efficacy of allergen extracts used in SIT. At this early stage of development in human studies, "Immunostimulatory DNA" containing CG motifs has been conjugated to Amb a 1 and studied in ragweed allergic rhinitis patients. DNA conjugation to allergen markedly reduced the allergen-induced basophil histamine release, suggesting reduced IgE-mediated allergenicity (167). In a randomized controlled trial for ragweed-induced rhinitis, DNA: Amb a 1 conjugate was administered as SIT in only six build-up injections (168). After the first post-SIT ragweed season, nasal biopsies obtained after allergen challenge revealed less eosinophils, less IL-4 + mRNA cells, and more IFN-γ^+mRNA cells. Although clinical improvement was not observed in the SIT-treated group during the first post-treatment season, significantly less chest symptoms were reported during the second ragweed season.

VII. Conclusion

Effective SIT can be achieved in the majority of those who receive it. Optimal requirements include careful patient and allergen selection, composing individualized SIT vaccines to achieve effective maintenance dosing, and using administration schedules with close monitoring and rapid responses to rare systemic allergic and asthmatic reactions. Despite an extensive body of work on SIT, clear indications for its use in asthmatic children have not been established. Broad-based immune modulation, persistent efficacy for years after SIT discontinuation, reduction in neo-sensitization to inhalant allergens, and the possible prevention of disease progression are unique outcomes of any currently available asthma therapy. In this regard, SIT is a prototypical immune modulatory therapy for asthma, with the potential in children to achieve optimal outcomes beyond asthma control. Improvements in SIT safety and ease of administration continue to be sought, and such improvements could lead to SIT's widespread use.

Acknowledgment

We appreciate Ms. Jan Manzanares' help with the preparation of this chapter.

Abbreviations

SIT	Allergen-specific immunotherapy (by subcutaneous injections)
PST	Allergy prick skin test
BHR	Bronchial hyperresponsiveness
CAMP	Childhood Asthma Management Program
FDA	Food and Drug Administration
BAL	Bronchoalveolar lavage
PBMC	Peripheral blood mononuclear cells
Th-2	$CD4^+$ helper T-lymphocyte, type 2
Th-1	$CD4^+$ helper T-lymphocyte, type 1
Treg	$CD4^+$ Regulatory T-lymphocyte
IFN-γ	Interferon-gamma
sIL-2R	Soluble IL-2 receptor
mite	House dust mite
SAR	Systemic adverse reaction to SIT (allergic, asthmatic, and/or anaphylactic)
SLIT	Sublingual/swallow allergen-specific immunotherapy
CD23	Low-affinity IgE receptor (FCϵRII)
NHLBI	National Heart, Lung, & Blood Institute, U.S. National Institutes of Health
mcg	Microgram

References

1. Nelson HS, Szefler SJ, Jacobs J, Huss K, Shapiro G, Sternberg AL. The relationships among environmental allergen sensitization, allergen exposure, pulmonary function, and bronchial hyperresponsiveness in the Childhood Asthma Management Program. J Allergy Clin Immunol 1999; 104(4 Pt 1): 775–785.
2. Henderson FW, Henry MM, Ivins SS, Morris R, Neebe EC, Leu SY, Stewart PW. Correlates of recurrent wheezing in school-age children. The Physicians of Raleigh Pediatric Associates. Am J Respir Crit Care Med 1995; 151(6): 1786–1793.
3. Zock JP, Brunekreef B, Hazebroek-Kampschreur AA, Roosjen CW. House dust mite allergen in bedroom floor dust and respiratory health of children with asthmatic symptoms. Eur Respir J 1994; 7:1254–1259.
4. Rosenstreich DL, Eggleston P, Kattan M, Baker D, Slavin RG, Gergen P, Mitchell H, McNiff-Mortimer K, Lynn H, Ownby D, Malveaux F. The role of cockroach allergy and exposure to cockroach allergen in causing morbidity among inner-city children with asthma. N Engl J Med 1997; 336(19):1356– 1363.
5. Murray AB, Ferguson AC. Dust-free bedrooms in the treatment of asthmatic children with house dust or house dust mite allergy: a controlled trial. Pediatrics 1983; 71:418–422.
6. Peroni DG, Boner AL, Vallone G, Antolini I, Warner JO. Effective allergen avoidance at high altitude reduces allergen-induced bronchial hyperrespon-siveness. Am J Respir Crit Care Med 1994; 149:1442–1446.
7. Bodini A, Peroni D, Vicentini L, Loiacono A, Baraldi E, Ghiro L, Corradi M, Alinovi A, Boner AL, Piacentini GL. Exhaled breath condensate eicosanoids and sputum eosinophils in asthmatic children: a pilot study. Pediatr Allergy Immunol 2004; 15:26.
8. Straub DA, Ehmann R, Hall GL, Moeller A, Hamacher J, Frey U, Sennhauser FH, Wildhaber JH. Correlation of nitrites in breath condensates and lung function in asthmatic children. Pediatr Allergy Immunol 2004; 15(1):20–25.
9. Kulig M, Bergmann R, Tacke U, Wahn U, Guggenmoos-Holzmann I. Long-lasting sensitization to food during the first two years precedes allergic airway disease. The MAS Study Group, Germany. Pediatr Allergy Immunol 1998; 9(2):61–67.
10. Illi S, von Mutius E, Lau S, Nickel R, Niggemann B, Sommerfeld C, Wahn U. The pattern of atopic sensitization is associated with the development of asthma in childhood. J Allergy Clin Immunol 2001; 108:709–714.
11. Zeiger RS, Heller S. The development and prediction of atopy in high-risk children: follow-up at age seven years in a prospective randomized study of combined maternal and infant food allergen avoidance. J Allergy Clin Immunol 1995; 95:1179–1190.
12. Oswald H, Phelan PD, Lanigan A, Hibbert M, Bowes G, Olinsky A. Outcome of childhood asthma in mid-adult life. BMJ 1994; 309:95–96.
13. Jenkins MA, Hopper JL, Bowes G, Carlin JB, Flander LB, Giles GG. Factors in childhood as predictors of asthma in adult life. BMJ 1994; 309:90–93.

14. Strachan DP, Butland BK, Anderson HR. Incidence and prognosis of asthma and wheezing illness from early childhood to age 33 in a national British cohort. BMJ 1996; 312:1195–1199.

15. Sears MR, Greene JM, Willan AR, Wiecek EM, Taylor DR, Flannery EM, Cowan JO, Herbison GP, Silva PA, Poulton R. A longitudinal, population-based, cohort study of childhood asthma followed to adulthood. N Engl J Med 2003; 349(15):1414–1422.

16. Ross RN, Nelson HS, Finegold I. Effectiveness of specific immunotherapy in the treatment of asthma: a meta-analysis of prospective, randomized, double-blind, placebo-controlled studies. Clin Ther 2000; 22(3):329–341.

17. Abramson MJ, Puy RM, Weiner JM. Is allergen immunotherapy effective in asthma? A meta-analysis of randomized controlled trials. Am J Respir Crit Care Med 1995; 151(4):969–974.

18. Abramson M, Puy R, Weiner J. Allergen immunotherapy for asthma. Cochrane Database Syst Rev 2000; 2:CD001186.

19. Abramson M, Puy R, Weiner J. Allergen immunotherapy for asthma. Cochrane Database Syst Rev 2003; 4:CD001186.

20. Bousquet J, Hejjaoui A, Clauzel AM, Guerin B, Dhivert H, Skassa-Brociek W, Michel FB. Specific immunotherapy with a standardized Dermatophagoides pteronyssinus extract. II. Prediction of efficacy of immunotherapy. J Allergy Clin Immunol 1988; 82:971–977.

21. Des Roches A, Paradis L, Menardo JL, Bouges S, Daures JP, Bousquet J. Immunotherapy with a standardized Dermatophagoides pteronyssinus extract. VI. Specific immunotherapy prevents the onset of new sensitizations in children. J Allergy Clin Immunol 1997; 99:450–453.

22. Purello-D' Ambrosio F, Gangemi S, Merendino RA, Isola S, Puccinelli P, Parmiani S, Ricciardi L. Prevention of new sensitizations in monosensitized subjects submitted to specific immunotherapy or not. A retrospective study. Clin Exp Allergy 2001; 31(8):1295–1302.

23. Pajno GB, Barberio G, De Luca F, Morabito L, Parmiani S. Prevention of new sensitizations in asthmatic children monosensitized to house dust mite by specific immunotherapy. A six-year follow-up study. Clin Exp Allergy 2001; 31(9):1392–1397.

24. Johnstone DE, Crump L. Value of hyposensitization therapy for perennial bronchial asthma in children. Pediatrics 1961; 27:39–44.

25. Moller C, Dreborg S, Ferdousi HA, Halken S, Host A, Jacobsen L, Koivikko A, Koller DY, Niggemann B, Norberg LA, Urbanek R, Valovirta E, Wahn U. Pollen immunotherapy reduces the development of asthma in children with seasonal rhinoconjunctivitis (the PAT-study). J Allergy Clin Immunol 2002; 109(2):251–256.

26. Ebner C, Kraft D, Ebner H. Booster immunotherapy (BIT). Allergy 1994; 49:38–42.

27. Durham SR, Walker SM, Varga EM, Jacobson MR, O'Brien F, Noble W, Till SJ, Hamid QA, Nouri-Aria KT. Long-term clinical efficacy of grass-pollen immunotherapy. N Engl J Med 1999; 341:468–475.

28. Des Roches A, Paradis L, Knani J, Hejjaoui A, Dhivert H, Chanez P, Bousquet J. Immunotherapy with a standardized Dermatophagoides ptero-

nyssinus extract. V. Duration of the efficacy of immunotherapy after its cessation. Allergy 1996; 51(6):430–433.

29. Peat JK, Tovey E, Gray EJ, Mellis CM, Woolcock AJ. Asthma severity and morbidity in a population sample of Sydney schoolchildren: Part II—Importance of house dust mite allergens. Aust N Z J Med 1994; 24(3):270–276.

30. Almqvist C, Wickman M, Perfetti L, Berglind N, Renstrom A, Hedren M, Larsson K, Hedlin G, Malmberg P. Worsening of asthma in children allergic to cats, after indirect exposure to cat at school. Am J Respir Crit Care Med 2001; 163:694–698.

31. Custovic A, Taggart SCO, Woodcock A. House dust mite and cat allergen in different indoor environments. Clin Exp Allergy 1994; 24:1164–8.

32. Ingram JM, Sporik R, Rose G, Honsinger R, Chapman MD, Platts-Mills TA. Quantitative assessment of exposure to dog (Can f 1) and cat (Fel d 1) allergens: relation to sensitization and asthma among children living in Los Alamos, New Mexico. J Allergy Clin Immunol 1995; 96:449–456.

33. Alvarez-Cuesta E, Cuesta-Herranz J, Puyana-Ruiz J, Cuesta-Herranz C, Blanco-Quiros A. Monoclonal antibody-standardized cat extract immunotherapy: risk benefit effects from a double-blind placebo study. J Allergy Clin Immunol 1994; 93:556–566.

34. Hedlin G, Graff-Lonnevig V, Heilborn H, Lilja G, Norrlind K, Pegelow K, Sundin B, Lowenstein H. Immunotherapy with cat- and dog-dander extracts. V. Effects of 3 years of treatment. J Allergy Clin Immunol 1991; 87:955–964.

35. Salvaggio J, Aukrust L. Mold-induced asthma. J Allergy Clin Immunol 1981; 68:327–346.

36. O'Hollaren MT, Yunginger JW, Offord KP, Somers MJ, O'Connell EJ, Ballard DJ, Sachs MI. Exposure to an aeroallergen as a possible precipitating factor in respiratory arrest in young patients with asthma. N Engl J Med 1991; 324:359–363.

37. Salvaggio JE, Burge HA, Chapman JA. Emerging concepts in mold allergy: what is the role of immunotherapy. J Allergy Clin Immunol 1993; 92(2): 217–222.

38. Yunginger JW, Jones RT, Gleich GJ. Studies on alternaria allergens. II. Measurement of the relative potency of commercial alternaria extracts by the direct RAST and by RAST inhibition. J Allergy Clin Immunol 1976; 58:405–413.

39. Dreborg S, Argell B, Foucard T, Kjellman NI, Koivikko A, Nilsson S. A double-blind, multicenter immunotherapy trial in children using a purified and standardized Cladosporium herbarum preparation. Allergy 1986; 41:131–140.

40. Malling HJ, Dreborg S, Weeke B. Diagnosis and immunotherapy of mould allergy. V. Clinical efficacy and side effects of immunotherapy with Cladosporium herbarum. Allergy 1986; 41d:507–519.

41. Horst M, Hejjaoui A, Horst V, Michel FB, Bousquet J. Double-blind, placebo-controlled rush immunotherapy with a standardized Alternaria extract. J Allergy Clin Immunol 1990; 85:460–472.

42. Kang BC, Johnson J, Morgan C, Chang JL. The role of immunotherapy in cockroach asthma. J Asthma 1988; 25:206–218.

43. Patterson ML, Slater JE. Characterization and comparison of commercially available German and American cockroach allergen extracts. Clin Exp Allergy 2002; 32(5):721–727.
44. Frankland AW, Augustin R. Prophylzsis of summer hay-fever and asthma: a controlled trial comparing crude grass-pollen extracts with the isolated main protein component. Lancet 1954; i:1055–1057.
45. Varney VA, Gaga M, Frew AJ, Aber VR, Kay AB, Durham SR. Usefulness of immunotherapy in patients with severe summer hay fever uncontrolled by antiallergic drugs. BMJ 1991; 302:265–269.
46. Lowell FC, Franklin W. A double-blind study of the effectiveness and specificity of injection therapy in ragweed hay fever. N Engl J Med 1965; 273: 675–679.
47. Norman PS, Winkenwerder WL, Lichtenstein LM. Immunotherapy of hay fever with ragweed antigen E: comparisons with whole pollen extract and placebos. J Allergy 1968; 42:93–108.
48. Bodtger U, Poulsen LK, Jacobi HH, Malling HJ. The safety and efficacy of subcutaneous birch pollen immunotherapy—a one-year, randomized, double-blind, placebo-controlled study. Allergy 2002; 57(4):297–305.
49. Hedlin G, Wille S, Browaldh L, Hildebrand H, Holmgren D, Lindfors A, Nordvall SL, Lowenstein H. Immunotherapy in children with allergic asthma: effect on bronchial hyperreactivity and pharmacotherapy. J Allergy Clin Immunol 1999; 103(4):609–614.
50. Franklin W, Lowell FC. Comparison of two dosages of ragweed extract in the treatment of pollenosis. JAMA 1967; 201(12):915–917.
51. Bousquet J, Becker WM, Hejjaoui A, Chanal I, Lebel B, Dhivert H, Michel FB. Differences in clinical and immunologic reactivity of patients allergic to grass pollens and to multiple-pollen species. II. Efficacy of a double-blind, placebo-controlled, specific immunotherapy with standardized extracts. J Allergy Clin Immunol 1991; 88:43–53.
52. Adkinson NFJ, Eggleston PA, Eney D, Goldstein EO, Schuberth KC, Bacon JR, Hamilton RG, Weiss ME, Arshad H, Meinert CL, Tonascia J, Wheeler B. A controlled trial of immunotherapy for asthma in allergic children. N Engl J Med 1997; 336(5):324–331.
53. Nelson HS, Ikle D, Buchmeier A. Studies of allergen extract stability: the effects of dilution and mixing. J Allergy Clin Immunol 1996; 98:382–388.
54. Noon L. Prophylactic inoculation against hay fever. Lancet 1911; i:1572–1573.
55. Colmes A, Rackemann FM. Further observations on the changes in skin tests following specific pollen therapy. J Allergy 1932; 3(4):473–480.
56. Sherman WB. Changes in serological reactions and tissue sensitivity in hay fever patients during the early months of treatment. J Immunol 1941; 40: 289–309.
57. Bousquet J, Maasch H, Martinot B, Hejjaoui A, Wahl R, Michel FB. Double-blind, placebo-controlled immunotherapy with mixed grass-pollen allergoids. II. Comparison between parameters assessing the efficacy of immunotherapy. J Allergy Clin Immunol 1988; 82(3 Pt 1):439–446.

58. Nish WA, Charlesworth EN, Davis TL, Whisman BA, Valtier S, Charlesworth MG, Leiferman KM. The effect of immunotherapy on the cutaneous late phase response to antigen. J Allergy Clin Immunol 1994; 93:484–493.

59. Lack G, Nelson HS, Amran D, Oshiba A, Jung T, Bradley KL, Giclas PC, Gelfand EW. Rush immunotherapy results in allergen-specific alterations in lymphocyte function and interferon-γ production in CD4+ T cells. J Allergy Clin Immunol 1997; 99:530–538.

60. Ewbank PA, Murray J, Sanders K, Curran-Everett D, Dreskin S, Nelson HS. A double-blind, placebo-controlled immunotherapy does-response study with standardized cat extract. J Allergy Clin Immunol 2003; 111(1):155–161.

61. Van Bever HP, Bosmans J, De Clerck LS, Stevens WJ. Modification of the late asthmatic reaction by hyposensitization in asthmatic children allergic to house dust mite (Dermatophagoides pteronyssinus) or grass pollen. Allergy 1988; 43:378–385.

62. Furin MJ, Norman PS, Creticos PS, Proud D, Kagey-Sobotka A, Lichenstein LM, Naclerio RM. Immunotherapy decreases antigen-induced eosinophil cell migration into the nasal cavity. J Allergy Clin Immunol 1991; 88(1):27–32.

63. Otsuka H, Mezawa A, Ohnishi M, Okubo K, Seki H, Okuda M. Changes in nasal metachromatic cells during allergen immunotherapy. Clin Exp Allergy 1991; 21:115–119.

64. Durham SR, Varney VA, Gaga M, Jacobson MR, Varga EM, Frew AJ, Kay AB. Grass pollen immunotherapy decreases the number of mast cells in the skin. Clin Exp Allergy 1999; 29:1490–1496.

65. Rak S, Bjornson A, Hakanson L, Sorenson S, Venge P. The effect of immunotherapy on eosinophil accumulation and production of eosinophil chemotactic activity in the lung of subjects with asthma during natural pollen exposure. J Allergy Clin Immunol 1991; 88(6):878–888.

66. Moens MM, Van Bever HP, Stevens WJ, Mertens AV, Bridts CH, De Clerck LS. Influence of hyposensitization on soluble interleukin-2 receptor, eosinophil cationic protein, in vitro lymphocyte proliferation, in vitro lymphocyte adhesion, and lymphocyte membrane markers in childhood asthma. Allergy 1994; 49:653–658.

67. D'Amato G, Liccardi G, Russo M, Saggese M, D'Amato M. Measurement of serum levels of eosinophil cationic protein to monitor patients with seasonal respiratory allergy induced by Parietaria pollen (treated and untreated with specific immunotherapy). Allergy 1996; 51:245–250.

68. Rak S, Hakanson L, Venge P. Immunotherapy abrogates he generation of eosinophil and neutrophil chemotactic activity during pollen season. J Allergy Clin Immunol 1990; 86:706–713.

69. Wantke F, Gotz M, Janisch R. Spontaneous histamine release in whole blood in patients before and after 4 months of specific immunotherapy. Clin Exp Allergy 1993; 23:992–995.

70. Kuna P, Alam R, Kuzminska B, Rozniecki J. The effect of preseasonal immunotherapy on the production of histamine-releasing factor (HRF) by mononuclear cells from patients with seasonal asthma: results of a double-blind, placebo-controlled, randomized study. J Allergy Clin Immunol 1989; 83: 816–824.

71. Liao TN, Hsieh KH. Altered production of histamine-releasing factor (HRF) activity and responsiveness to HRF after immunotherapy in children with asthma. J Allergy Clin Immunol 1990; 86:894–901.
72. Sadan N, Rhyne MB, Mellits ED, Goldstein EO, Levy DA, Lichtenstein LM. Immunotherapy of pollinosis in children: investigation of the immunologic basis of clinical improvement. N Engl J Med 1969; 280:623–627.
73. Lichtenstein LM, Levy DA. Is desensitization for ragweed hay fever immunologically specific? Int Arch Allergy 1972; 42:615–626.
74. Sherman WB. Serologic changes in hay fever cases treated over a period of years. J Allergy 1940; 11:225–244.
75. Norman PS, Lichtenstein LM, Marsh DG. Studies on allergoids from naturally occurring allergens. IV. Efficacy and safety of long-term allergoid treatment of ragweed hay fever. J Allergy Clin Immunol 1981; 68:460–470.
76. Cooke RA, Barnard JH, Hebald S, Stull A. Serological evidence of immunity with coexisting sensitization in a type of human allergy (hay fever). J Exp Med 1935; 62:733–750.
77. Alexander HL, Johnson Mc, Bukantz SC. Studies on correlation between symptoms of ragweed, hay fever and titer of thermostable antibody. J Allergy 1948; 19:1–8.
78. Djurup R, Osterballe O. IgG subclass antibody response in grass pollen-allergic patients undergoing specific immunotherapy. Prognostic value of serum IgG subclass antibody levels early in immunotherapy. Allergy 1984; 39:433–441.
79. Nakagawa T, Kozeki H, Katagiri J, Fujita Y, Yamashita N, Miyamoto T, Skvaril F. Changes of house dust mite-specific IgE, IgG and IgG subclass antibodies during immunotherapy in patients with perennial rhinitis. Int Arch Allergy Appl Immunol 1987; 82:95–99.
80. Wachholz PA, Soni NK, Till SJ, Durham SR. Inhibition of allergen-IgE binding to B cells by IgG antibodies after grass pollen immunotherapy. J Allergy Clin Immunol 2003; 112(5):915–922.
81. Gagro A, Rabatic S, Trescec A, Dekaris D, Medar-Lasic M. Expression of lymphocytes Fc epsilon RII/CD23 in allergic children undergoing hyposensitization. Int Arch Allergy Immunol 1993; 101:203–208.
82. Kljaic-Turkalj M, Cvoriscec B, Tudoric N, Stipic-Markovic A, Rabatic S, Trescec A, Gagro A, Dekaris D. Decrease in CD23+ B lymphocytes and clinical outcome in asthmatic patients receiving specific rush immunotherapy. Int Arch Allergy Immunol 1996; 111:188–194.
83. Jung CM, Prinz JC, Rieber EP, Ring J. A reduction in allergen-induced FceR2/CD23 expression on peripheral B cells correlates with successful hyposensitization in grass pollinosis. J Allergy Clin Immunol 1995; 95:77–87.
84. Hakansson L, Heinrich C, Rak S, Venge P. Activation of B-lymphocytes during pollen season. Effect of immunotherapy. Clin Exp Allergy 1998; 28: 791–798.
85. Secrist H, Chelen CJ, Wen Y, Marshall JD, Umetsu DT. Allergen immunotherapy decreases interleukin 4 production in CD4+ T cells from allergic individuals. J Exp Med 1993; 178:2123–2130.
86. Varney VA, Hamid QA, Gaga M, Ying S, Jacobson M, Frew AJ, Kay AB, Durham SR. Influence of grass pollen immunotherapy on cellular infiltration

cytokine mRNA expression during allergen-induced late-phase cutaneous responses. J Clin Invest 1993; 92:644–651.

87. Ohashi Y, Nakai Y, Okamoto H, Ohno Y, Sakamoto H, Sugiura Y, Kakinoki Y, Tanaka A, Kishimoto K, Washio Y, Hayashi M. Serum level of interleukin-4 in patients with perennial allergic rhinitis during allergen-specific immunotherapy. Scand J Immunol 1996; 43:680–686.

88. Gabrielsson S, Soderlund A, Paulie S, van der Pouw Kraan TC, Troye-Blomberg M, Rak S. Specific immunotherapy prevents increased levels of allergen-specific IL-4 and IL-13-producing cells during pollen season. Allergy 2001; 56:293–300.

89. Majori M, Caminati A, Corradi M, Brianti E, Scarpa S, Pesci A. T-cell cytokine pattern at three times points during specific immunotherapy for mite-sensitive asthma. Clin Exp Allergy 2000; 30:341–347.

90. Till S, Walker S, Dickason R, Huston D, O'Brien F, Lamb J, Kay AB, Corrigan C, Durham S. IL-5 production by allergen stimulated T cells following grass pollen immunotherapy for seasonal allergic rhinitis. Clin Exp Immunol 1997; 110:114–121.

91. Meissner N, Kochs S, Coutelle J, Kussebi F, Baumgarten C, Lowenstein H, Kunkel G, Renz H. Modified T-cell activation pattern during specific immunotherapy (SIT) in cat-allergic patients. Clin Exp Allergy 1999; 29:618–625.

92. Durham SR, Ying S, Varney VA, Jacobson MR, Sudderick RM, Mackay IS, Kay AB, Hamid QA. Grass pollen immunotherapy inhibits allergen-induced infiltration of CD4+ T-lymphocytes and eosinophils in the nasal mucosa and increases the number of cells expressing messenger RNA for interferon-gamma. J Allergy Clin Immunol 1996; 97:1356–1365.

93. Hamid Q, Schotman E, Jacobson MR, Walker SM, Durham SR. Increases in IL-12 messenger RNA+ cells accompany inhibition of allergen-induced late skin responses after successful grass pollen immunotherapy. J Allergy Clin Immunol 1997; 99:254–260.

94. Evans R, Pence H, Kaplan H, Rocklin RE. The effect of immunotherapy on humoral and cellular responses in ragweed hayfever. J Clin Invest 1976; 57:1378–1385.

95. Francis JN, Till SJ, Durham SR. Induction of IL-10+CD4+CD25+ T-cells by grass pollen immunotherapy. J Allergy Clin Immunol 2003; 111(6):1255–1261.

96. Jutel M, Akdis M, Budak F, Abebischer-Casaulta C, Wrzyszcz M, Blaser K, Akdis CA. IL-10 and TGF-beta cooperate in the regulatory T cell response to mucosal allergens in normal immunity and specific immunotherapy. Eur J Immunol 2003; 33(5):1205–1214.

97. Hsieh KH. Decreased production of interleukin-2 receptors after immunotherapy to house dust. J Clin Immunol 1988; 8:171–177.

98. Bonno M, Fujisawa T, Iguchi K, Uchida Y, Kamiya H, Komada Y, Sakurai M. Mite-specific induction of interleukin-2 receptor on T-lymphocytes from children with mite-sensitive asthma: modified immune response with immunotherapy. J Allergy Clin Immunol 1996; 97(2):680–688.

99. Tari MG, Mancino M, Madonna F, Buzzoni L, Parmiani S. Immunologic evaluation of 24-month course of sublingual immunotherapy. Allergol Immunopathol 1994; 22(5):209–216.

100. Rocklin RE, Sheffer AL, Greineder DK, Melmon KL. Generation of antigen-specific suppressor cells during allergy densensitization. N Engl J Med 1980; 302:1214–1219.

101. Nagaya H. Induction of antigen-specific suppressor cells in patients with hay fever receiving immunotherapy. J Allergy Clin Immunol 1985; 75:388–394.

102. Tamir R, Castracane JM, Rocklin RE. Generation of suppressor cells in atopic patients during immunotherapy that modulate IgE synthesis. J Allergy Clin Immunol 1987; 79:591–598.

103. Wang J-Y, Lei H-Y, Hsieh K-H. The effect of immunotherapy on interleukin-1 and tumor necrosis factor production of monocytes in asthmatic children. J Asthma 1992; 29:193–201.

104. Hsieh K-H, Ng C-K. Increased plasma platelet activating factor in children with acute asthmatic attacks and decreased in vivo and in vitro production of platelet activating factor after immunotherapy. J Allergy Clin Immunol 1993; 91:60–67.

105. NAEPP Expert Panel Report II. Guidelines for the diagnosis and management of asthma/National Asthma Education and Prevention Program. NIH/NHLBI. NIH publication No 97–4051A page 29, 1997.

106. NHLBI. International consensus report on diagnosis and management of asthma. U.S. Department of Health and Human Services. Public Health Service. National Institutes of Health. Publication No. 92–3091, 1992.

107. NHLBI. Global initiative for asthma: Global strategy for asthma management and prevention. NIH/HLBI, Bethsada, MD. Publication No 95–3659, 1995.

108. Bousquet J, Hejjaoui A, Dhivert H, Clauzel AM, Michel FB. Immunotherapy with a standardized Dermatophagoides pteronyssinus extract. Systemic reactions during the rush protocol in patients suffering from asthma. J Allergy Clin Immunol 1989; 83:797–802.

109. Arlian LG, Neal JS, Morgan MS, Vyszenski-Moher DL, Rapp CM, Alexander AK. Reducing relative humidity is a practical way to control dust mites and their allergens in homes in temperate climates. J Allergy Clin Immunol 2001; 107(1):99–104.

110. ich M, Lamola S, Amory C, Schneider L. Asthma in life context: video intervention/prevention assessment (VIA). Pediatrics 2000; 105:469–477.

111. Dolz I, Martinez-Cocera C, Bartolome JM, Cimarra M. A double-blind, placebo-controlled study of immunotherapy with grass-pollen extract Alutard SQ during a 3-year period with initial rush immunotherapy. Allergy 1996; 51: 489–500.

112. Walker SM, Pajno GB, Lima MT, Wilson DR, Durham SR. Grass pollen immunotherapy for seasonal rhinitis and asthma: a randomized, controlled trial. J Allergy Clin Immunol 2001; 107:87–93.

113. Varney VA, Edwards J, Tabbah K, Brewster H, Mavroleon G, Frew AJ. Clinical efficacy of specific immunotherapy to cat dander: a double-blind placebo-controlled trial. Clin Exp Allergy 1997; 27(8):860–867.

114. Olsen OT, Larsen KR, Jacobsan L, Svendsen UG. A 1-year, placebo-controlled, double-blind house-dust-mite immunotherapy study in asthmatic adults. Allergy 1997; 52(8):853–859.

115. Wood RA, Phipatanakul W, Hamilton RG, Eggleston PA. A comparison of skin prick tests, intradermal skin tests, and RAST's in the diagnosis of cat allergy. J Allergy Clin Immunol 1999; 103(5 Pt 1):773–779.

116. Lin MS, Tanner E, Lynn J, Friday GAJ. Nonfatal systemic allergic reactions induced by skin testing and immunotherapy. Ann Allergy 1993; 71: 557–562.

117. Tinkelman DG, Cole WQI, Tunno J. Immunotherapy: a one-year prospective study to evaluate risk factors of systemic reactions. J Allergy Clin Immunol 1995; 95:8–14.

118. Lockey RF, Benedict IM, Turkeltaub PC, Bukantz SC. Fatalities from immunotherapy (IT) and skin testing (ST). J Allergy Clin Immunol 1987; 79: 660–677.

119. Reid MJ, Lockey RF, Turkeltaub PC, Platts-Mills TAE. Survey of fatalities from skin testing and immunotherapy 1985–1989. J Allergy Clin Immunol 1993; 92:6–15.

120. Hejjaoui A, Dhivert H, Michel FB, Bousquet J. Immunotherapy with a standardized Dermatophagoides pteronyssinus extract. IV. Systemic reactions according to the immunotherapy schedule. J Allergy Clin Immunol 1990; 85: 473–479.

121. Bousquet J, Hejjaoui A, Michel FB. Specific immunotherapy in asthma. J Allergy Clin Immunol 1990; 86:292–305.

122. Nelson BL, Dupont LA, Reid MJ. Prospective survey of local and systemic reactions to immunotherapy with pollen extracts. Ann Allergy 1986; 56: 331–334.

123. Tankersley MS, Butler KK, Butler WK, Goetz DW. Local reactions during allergen immunotherapy do not require dose adjustment. J Allergy Clin Immunol 2000; 106:840–843.

124. Hejjaoui A, Ferrando R, Dhivert H, Michel FB, Bousquet J. Systemic reactions occurring during immunotherapy with standardized pollen extracts. J Allergy Clin Immunol 1992; 89:925–933.

125. Portnoy J, Bagstad K, Kanarek H, Pacheco F, Hall B, Barnes C. Premedication reduces the incidence of systemic reactions during inhalant rush immunotherapy with mixtures of allergenic extracts. Ann Allergy 1994; 73:409–418.

126. Nielsen L, Johnsen CR, Mosbech H, Poulsen LK, Malling HJ. Antihistamine premedication in specific cluster immunotherapy: a double-blind, placebo-controlled study. J Allergy Clin Immunol 1996; 97:1207–1213.

127. Phanuphak P, Kohler PF. Onset of polyarteritis nodosa during allergic hyposensitization treatment. Am J Med 1980; 68(4):479–485.

128. Negrini AC, Troise C, Voltollini S, Siccardi M, Grassia L. Long-term hyposensitization and adverse immunologic responses. A laboratory evaluation. Ann Allergy 1985; 54(6):534–537.

129. Levinson AI, Summers RJ, Lawley TJ, Evans Rr, Frank MM. Evaluation of the adverse effects of long-term hyposensitization. J Allergy Clin Immunol 1978; 62(2):109–114.

130. Stein MR, Brown GL, Lima JE, Nelson HS, Carr RI. A laboratory evaluation of immune complexes in patients on inhalant immunotherapy. J Allergy Clin Immunol 1978; 62(4):211–216.

131. Tabar AI, Muro MD, Garcia BE, Alvarez MJ, Acero S, Rico P, Olaguibel JM. Dermatophagoides pteronyssinus cluster immunotherapy. A controlled trial of safety and clinical efficacy. J Invest Allergol Clin Immunol 1999; 9(3): 155–164.

132. Nelson HS. The use of standardized extracts in allergen immunotherapy. J Allergy Clin Immunol 2000; 106:41–45.

133. Meiser JB, Nelson HS. Comparing conventional and acetone-precipitated dog allergen extract skin testing. J Allergy Clin Immunol 2001; 107(4): 744–745.

134. Aalberse RC. Structural biology of allergens. J Allergy Clin Immunol 2000; 106:228–238.

135. Kauffman HF, Tomee JF, van de Riet MA, Timmerman AJ, Borger P. Protease-dependent activation of epithelial cells by fungal allergens leads to morphologic changes and cytokine production. J Allergy Clin Immunol 2000; 105(6 Pt 1): 1185–1193.

136. Nelson HS. Effect of preservatives and conditions of storage on the potency of allergy extracts. J Allergy Clin Immunol 1981; 67:64–69.

137. Van Metre TE Jr, Rosenberg GL, Vaswani SK, Ziegler SR, Adkinson NF. Pain and dermal reaction caused by injected glycerin in immunotherapy solutions. J Allergy Clin Immunol 1996; 97:1033–1039.

138. Malling H-J, Weeke B. Position paper: immunotherapy. Allergy 1993; 48(suppl 14):9–35.

139. Van Metre TE Jr, Adkinson NF, Amodio FJ, Kagey-Sobotka A, Lichtenstein LM, Mardiney MR Jr, Norman PS, Rosenberg GL. A comparison of immunotherapy schedules for injection treatment of ragweed pollen hay fever. J Allergy Clin Immunol 1982; 69(2):181–193.

140. Tipton WR, Nelson HS. Experience with daily immunotherapy in 59 adult allergic patients. J Allergy Clin Immunol 1982; 69:194–199.

141. Freeman J. "Rush" inoculation with special reference to hay-fever treatment. Lancet 1930; i:744–747.

142. Mellerup MT, Hahn GW, Poulsen LK, Malling H. Safety of allergen-specific immunotherapy. Relation between dosage regimen, allergen extract, disease and systemic side-effects during induction treatment. Clin Exp Allergy 2000; 30(10):1423–1429.

143. Sharkey P, Portnoy J. Rush immunotherapy: experience with a one-day schedule. Ann Allergy Asthma Immunol 1996; 76(2):175–180.

144. WHO/IUIS Working Group Report. Current status of allergen immunotherapy. Lancet 1989; I:259–256.

145. Kuehr J, Brauburger J, Zielen S, Schauer U, Wolfgang K, Von Berg A, Leupold W, Bergmann K-C, Rolinck-Weminghaus C, Grave M, Hultsch T, Wahn U. Efficacy of combination treatment with anti-IgE plus specific immunotherapy in polysensitized children and adolescents with seasonal allergic rhinitis. J Allergy Clin Immunol 2002; 109:274–280.

146. Spahn JD, Cherniack R, Paull K, Gelfand EW. Is forced expiratory volume in one second the best measure of severity in childhood asthma? Am J Respir Crit Care Med 2004; 169(7):784–786.

147. Wilson DR, Torres LI, Durham SR. Sublingual immunotherapy for allergic rhinitis. Cochrane Database Syst Rev 2003; 2:CD002893.
148. Mungan D, Misirligil Z, Gurbuz L. Comparison of the efficacy of subcutaneous and sublingual immunotherapy in mite-sensitive patients with rhinitis and asthma—a placebo controlled study. Ann Allergy Asthma Immunol 1999; 82(5):485–490.
149. Quirino T, Iemoli E, Siciliani E, Parmiani S, Milazzo F. Sublingual Vs. injective immunotherapy in grass pollen allergic patients: a double blind (double dummy) study. Clin Exp Allergy 1996; 26(11):1253–1261.
150. Passalacqua G, Baena-Cagnani CE, Beradi M, Canonica GW. Oral and sublingual immunotherapy in paediatric patients. Curr Opin Allergy Clin Immunol 2003; 3:139–145.
151. Giovane AL, Bardare M, Passalacqua G, Ruffoni S, Scordamaglia A, Ghezzi E, Canonica GW. A three-year double-blind, placebo-controlled study with specific oral immunotherapy to Dermatophagoides: evidence of safety and efficacy in paediatric patients. Clin Exp Allergy 1994; 24:53–59.
152. Tari MG, Mancino M, Monti G. Efficacy of sublingual immunotherapy in patients with rhinitis and asthma due to house dust mite. A double-blind study. Allergo et Immunopathol 1990; 18:277–284.
153. Pajno GB, Morabito L, Barberio G, Parmiani S. Clinical and immunologic effects of long-term sublingual immunotherapy in asthmatic children sensitized to mites: a double-blind, placebo-controlled study. Allergy 2000; 55(9): 842–849.
154. Bahceciler NN, Isik U, Barlan IB, Basaran MM. Efficacy of sublingual immunotherapy in children with asthma and rhinitis: a double-blind, placebo-controlled study. Pediatr Pulmonol 2001; 32(1):49–55.
155. Di Rienzo V, Marcucci F, Puccinelli P, Parmiani S, Frati F, Sensi L, Canonica GW, Passalacqua G. Long-lasting effect of sublingual immunotherapy in children with asthma due to house dust mite: a 10-year prospective study. Clin Exp Allergy 2003; 33:206–210.
156. Di Rienzo V, Pagani A, Parmiani S, Passalacqua G, Canonica GW. Postmarketing surveillance study on the safety of sublingual immunotherapy in pediatric patients. Allergy 1999; 54(10):1110–1113.
157. Nelson HS. Immunotherapy for Inhalant Allergens. In: Adkinson NF, Yunginger JW, Busse WW, Bochner BS, Holgate ST, Simon FER. Middleton's Allergy: Principles and Practice:Mosby Inc., 2003:1455–1473.
158. Moscato G, Rossi GA, Dellabianca A, Pisati A, Vinci G, Biale C. Local immunotherapy by inhalation of a powder extract in asthma due to house dust mite Dermatophagoides pteronyssinus. A double-blind comparison with parenteral immunotherapy. J Invest Allergo Clin Immunol 1991; 1:383–394.
159. Tari MG, Mancino M, Monti G. Immunotherapy by inhalation of allergen in powder in house dust allergic asthma. A double-blind study. J Invest Allergo Clin Immunol 1992; 2:59–67.
160. Norman PS. A rational approach to desensitization. J Allergy 1969; 44: 129–145.
161. Osterballe O. Immunotherapy with grass pollen major allergens. Clinical results from a prospective 3-year double blind study. Allergy 1982; 37:379–388.

162. Norman PS, Ohman JLJ, Long AA, Creticos PS, Gefter MA, Shaked Z, Wood RA, Eggleston PA, Hafner KB, Rao P, Lichtenstein LM, Jones NH, Nicodemus CF. Treatment of cat allergy with T-cell reactive peptides. Am J Respir Crit Care Med 1996; 154:1623–1628.

163. Maguire P, Nicodemus C, Robinson D, Aaronson D, Umetsu DT. The safety and efficacy of ALLERVAX CAT in cat allergic patients. Clin Immunol 1999; 93:222–231.

164. Saint-Remy JMR, Machiels JJ. Allergen-antibody complexes in the treatment of Dermatophagoides pteronyssinus hypersensitivity diseases. Clin Exp Allergy 1994; 24:1091–1093.

165. Hemmi H, Takeuchi O, Kawai T, Kaisho T, Sato S, Sanjo H, Matsumotoi M, Hoshino K, Wagner H, Takeda K, Akira S. A Toll-like receptor recognizes bacterial DNA. Nature 2000; 408:740–745.

166. Krieg AM. CpG motifs in bacterial DNA and their immune effects. Annu Rev Immunol 2002; 20:709–760.

167. Tighe H, Takabayashi K, Schwartz D, van Nest G, Tuck S, Eiden JJ, Kagey-Sobotka A, Creticos PS, Lichtenstein LM, Spiegelberg H, Raz E. Conjugation of immunostimulatory DNA to the short ragweed allergen amb a 1 enhances its immunogenicity and reduces its allergenicity. J Allergy Clin Immunol 2000; 106:124–134.

168. Tulic MK, Fiset PO, Christodoulopoulos P, Vaillancourt P, Desrosiers M, Lavigne F, Eiden J, Hamid Q. Amb a 1-immunostimulatory oligodeoxynucleotide conjugate immunotherapy decreases the nasal inflammatory response. J Allergy Clin Immunol 2004; 113(2):235–241.

19

Inner-City Asthma

MEYER KATTAN

Department of Pediatrics, Mount Sinai School of Medicine
New York, New York, U.S.A.

I. Introduction

Over the last two decades asthma prevalence, morbidity, and mortality have increased (1). The self-reported 12-month prevalence of asthma increased 73.9% from 1980 to 1996 in the United States (1). There are differences in prevalence among ethnic groups. Hispanics reported wide discrepancies in prevalence: Mexican American children reported low rates and Puerto Rican children predominantly living in the northeast United States reported some of the highest rates (2). Small-area analyses have demonstrated asthma period prevalence rate in poor urban communities in the United States to be twice the national prevalence rate (3). Although most of the regional analyses with high prevalence rates have been carried out in highly populated urban areas, less populated areas have also been reported to have high prevalence rates (4).

There has been a disproportionate increase in morbidity and mortality in urban areas that parallels the rise in prevalence (5). Hospitalization rates and emergency department (ED) visits are highest in poor urban areas (6,7). The rate of hospitalization in black children has increased over the last 30 years and is 3.5 times that of whites (1,8). The ED visit rates for blacks were greater than three times the rates for whites, and the youngest children consistently had the highest rates (1).

As a result of these disparities, these so-called "inner cities" have become the focus of studies to determine the characteristics of these locations and their populations that contribute to high prevalence and morbidity. The populations in the inner cities are predominantly racial and ethnic minorities that are socioeconomically disadvantaged.

The relationship of race/ethnicity, environment, and social class to prevalence and morbidity is complex (9). Studies show that racial differences in asthma prevalence could be explained by adjustment for social and environmental factors and living in an urban setting (10,11). A study in Philadelphia found that diagnosis of asthma was more common in African American children than among white children, but no difference in persistent wheeze, indicating that a racial difference exists in the acquisition of a diagnosis of asthma (12). Some studies in the United States have reported that diagnosed asthma, but not prevalence of wheezing, is associated with social class or family income (3,13). In contrast, no excess of wheezing or diagnosed asthma among lower social classes was found in Great Britain and Canada (14,15). African American children are at increased risk of hospitalization for asthma, but some of this increase is related to poverty rather than to race (16).

The interaction of genetic and environmental factors could potentially contribute to asthma morbidity. The frequency of alleles in the gene encoding the β2-adrenergic receptor varies among ethnic groups (17). The variability in the distribution of genetic polymorphisms may modify responses to pharmacologic agents or environmental factors. This area requires further study.

Other factors may contribute to the higher morbidity among urban children (Fig. 1). These fall into categories that relate predominantly to access to medical care, patterns of medical care, adherence issues, environmental exposures, and exposure to psychosocial problems within the family and community.

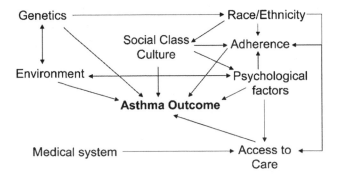

Figure 1   The interaction of factors affecting asthma outcome.

II. Access to and Patterns of Care

Families with lower socioeconomic status have patterns of health care utilization that differ from other groups. Poor children with asthma have fewer doctor visits despite more hospitalizations (18). Most children have a usual source of care, but when sick with asthma have difficulty finding care outside EDs (19,20). They are four times more likely to report an ED as a source of acute care (6). Use of the ED for asthma leads to more fragmented care. Thus, a major goal of ED intervention is to establish a link between the patient and the provider of ongoing asthma care, where complete education can be achieved and reinforced over time (21). There is room for improvement in inner-city EDs to achieve this goal. Leickly et al. reported that 31% of caregivers were neither told to make nor given a follow-up appointment after an ED visit (22). If they were given an appointment, 69% kept the appointment. In comparison, only 25% of children had a follow-up appointment after an ED visit if they were not told to make an appointment.

Inner-city children are undertreated despite guidelines recommending the use of anti-inflammatory medications in children with persistent asthma. Children use reliever medications more frequently than anti-inflammatory medications (23,24). Butz et al. found that 33% of children ages 5–12 years with persistent asthma used a nebulizer but only 15% reported inhaled steroid use (23,25). In children with persistent asthma, only 42% of their physicians reported prescribing a controller (25).

A growing number of children living in inner cities are uninsured. Diagnosis of asthma and treatment are related to health care coverage (26). Lack or type of insurance may limit children's access to quality care. Insurance, however, is not the only limiting factor affecting health care. In the National Cooperative Inner-City Asthma Study (NCICAS), 91% of children with current symptoms had insurance, but only 28% were receiving anti-inflammatory medications (19). Medicaid is a major insurer of inner-city children in the United States. Medicaid and non-Medicaid children within a health maintenance organization were equally likely to have controller medications prescribed, but Medicaid children were less likely to have them dispensed (27). This suggests that Medicaid members were somewhat less likely to fill or refill prescriptions for controller medications.

III. Adherence

Adherence to a medical regimen is a major challenge to the effective management of most chronic diseases, including asthma. Overall estimates for adherence to medications in both the pediatric and adult asthma populations are about 50% (28–30). When prescribed, more than one-third of caretakers reported not having a controller prescription (25). Factors associated with adherence include complexity of the treatment regimen, caretaker/patient beliefs regarding efficacy, adequacy of patient-provider communication, and psychological factors (22,25,30,31).

Adherence can be measured by self-report or by objective measures such as electronic counters, but these methods have shortcomings. Bauman et al. developed two measures of adherence for inner-city families with asthma: "admitted non-adherence" and "risk of non-adherence." "admitted non-adherence" is a summary score of the number of times that caregivers admitted non-compliance. "risk of non-adherence" is a summary score of characteristics of the child's regimen and characteristics of the child or caregiver that previous research had demonstrated to be associated with non-adherence. Children of caregivers who were less adherent assessed with either measure had more symptoms, more school days missed, and unscheduled doctor visits, but the "risk for non-adherence" was more strongly related to morbidity than "admitted non-adherence" (32). Given the difficulties of measuring adherence in research studies, this approach may be useful in asthma studies in inner-city children.

Many asthma interventions target the child's or caretaker's lack of knowledge. Interestingly, the NCICAS study found that asthma knowledge assessed by a multiple-choice test was reasonably good with an average of 85% correct responses (33). However, when caretakers were asked to respond to hypothetical vignettes, they had difficulty providing even one helpful response per situation and gave solutions that were considered medically undesirable. This indicates that knowledge does not necessarily translate into effective asthma management behaviors. Furthermore, children of caregivers with ineffective problem-solving strategies had more days of wheeze (33).

In focus groups involving caretakers of asthmatic children, asthma knowledge was perceived as a barrier in 20% of the comments (34). Therefore, the caretaker's perceptions and health beliefs may contribute to lack of adherence to medical regimens. In addition to asthma education, interventions need to focus on problem solving and address health beliefs in order to have a positive impact on outcome.

The level of responsibility for asthma management increases with the age of the child (35). A Baltimore/Washington survey of medication use by children with asthma found that 17% of 5- and 6-year-old children and more than 50% of 9-year-old children assumed responsibility for supervising their own medications (36). A complicating factor was the discordance between the caretaker and the child regarding responsibility for the management of the child's asthma, with up to 16% of children reporting less responsibility for self-care than was indicated by the caregiver (35).

Another underemphasized factor relating to adherence is the role of other caretakers such as grandparents, babysitters, and older siblings. Additional caretakers may provide much needed social support, but there is a risk that medical instructions may not be accurately transmitted from one caretaker to another. Over one-third of children in the NCICAS study reported having two or more caregivers in addition to the primary caregiver (35). Identifying those persons responsible for care could enhance education efforts for asthma management.

IV. Psychosocial Factors

Behavioral and psychosocial factors can affect asthma morbidity and asthma morbidity can precipitate psychological distress. Lower socioeconomic status and stressful life events are predictive of less optimal psychological adjustment (37). In the large NCICAS study, 77% of the caretakers were women who were single, separated, divorced, or widowed. An assessment of caretaker mental health using the brief symptom inventory (BSI) revealed that 50% of the caretakers met criteria indicating clinically important psychological symptoms. The child behavior checklist (CBCL), an instrument to assess child adjustment, indicated that 35% of children had clinically significant mental health problems. Children of caretakers who exceeded the clinical cutoff on the BSI were almost twice as likely to be hospitalized for asthma (38). Bartlett et al. reported that mothers of inner-city children with asthma with high depressive symptoms reported more problems with their child using inhalers improperly and forgetting doses (39).

Families living in disadvantaged neighborhoods have a high prevalence of exposure to crime and violence (40). Increased exposure to violence predicted a higher number of symptom days in a graded fashion. Over one-third of caretakers in the Inner-City Asthma Study (ICAS) reported keeping their child indoors owing to fear of violence (40). More time spent, indoors could potentially increase exposure to aeroallergens and irritants, but the effect on morbidity needs to be elucidated.

V. Outdoor Environmental Exposures

Higher levels of ambient air pollutants are associated with increased symptoms in children with asthma (41,42). Particulate pollution in outdoor air has been associated with a number of adverse health effects (43). Fine particles, those with an aerodynamic diameter $< 2.5\mu m$ ($PM_{2.5}$), may produce most of these harmful effects, although coarse particles (those with diameters $2.5-10\,\mu m$) have also been implicated in some studies of childhood asthma (44,45).

Despite this evidence, increasing asthma morbidity has been observed during a period of declining air pollution in American cities (46). This should not be interpreted as a lesser role for air pollution in asthma. Although ambient air quality has generally improved, these improvements have not reached minority communities in equal proportions. Those who live in underserved communities may be particularly at risk because environmental pollution has been found to be disproportionately distributed among communities (47).

Few air pollution studies have focused on the health of inner-city asthmatic children. In a time-series study of 846 asthmatic children living in eight urban areas in the Northeast and Midwest United States, Mortimer and coworkers observed that the morning peak expiratory flow rate (PEFR) was reduced in association with increased ozone (O_3) concentration and that asthma symptoms were increased in association with increases in O_3, sulfur dioxide (SO_2), and nitrogen dioxide (NO_2) concentrations (48). In a time-series study of 71 asthmatic children in Mexico City, both PEFR and respiratory symptoms were associated with outdoor ambient levels of PM_{10} and O_3 (41). Among 22 Hispanic children with asthma living in Los Angeles, the concentrations of O_3, NO_2, SO_2, and PM_{10} were associated with symptoms but not with reductions in PEFR (49).

VI. Indoor Environmental Exposures

Indoor air quality is of concern because children in urban areas spend over 70% of their time indoors, where they are exposed to irritants and allergens (50). Exposure to environmental tobacco smoke (ETS) in asthmatic children living in inner cities is high. Studies report that 32% to 39% of primary caretakers of children with asthma are smokers and 48% to 59% have one or more smokers in the household (19,51,52). Elevated levels of urinary cotinine (>30 ng/g creatinine) were found in 38% to 48% of asthmatic children, confirming the high level of personal exposures to ETS in this population (19,51). African Americans are more likely to be exposed than Latino children (51).

ETS exposure doubles the risk of having asthma and is associated with wheezing in younger children (51). An association of smoking with morbidity in older children is less clear. Ehrlich et al. did not find differences in cotinine levels between asthmatic children seen in the ED and children with stable asthma and those without a history of asthma followed in an inner-city clinic (51).

Indoor concentrations of particulate matter are related to the sources of combustion products, as well as to variation in ventilation and air filtration (53,54). The high prevalence of parental smoking, poor ventilation, and other environmental factors found in many inner-city homes may expose asthmatic children in this setting to relatively high levels of particles (19,52).

The Inner-City Air Pollution Study (ICAP) measured fine particles ($PM_{2.5}$) in 294 homes drawn from seven U.S. cities (55). The most important particle source in these homes was smoking. The mean indoor value in the 101 smoking homes was 46.5 µg/m³, compared with 17.8 µg/m³ in the 193 non-smoking homes. A second less powerful source was cooking, particularly frying/sautéing, or a smoky cooking event. Mean indoor values were 31 µg/m³ in homes with cooking and 23.5 µg/m³ in homes without cooking. Use of incense also led to significant increases in particle concentrations. Infiltration of outdoor air added about half of the outdoor air concentration to the concentrations produced by the indoor sources. The health effects of these exposures to indoor particulates have not yet been reported.

Nitrogen dioxide, a by-product of combustion sources, is an air pollutant that is found indoors. Household appliances fueled by gas, such as gas stoves and space heaters, are the major indoor sources of NO_2 (56). In the seven cities participating in NCICAS, 89% of families had gas stoves. Venting results in a significant reduction in indoor NO_2, but the majority of stoves in those households were not vented (57). Levels of 40 ppb or greater were found in 24% of households. There are no indoor air standards, but the U.S. Environmental Protection Agency environmental outdoor standard for NO_2 is an annual average level of 50 ppb or greater. NO_2 increases the risk of asthmatic exacerbations following respiratory infections, even at relatively low levels of exposure (58). The contribution to asthma morbidity of higher levels of exposures found in inner cities needs further study.

Exposure and sensitization to allergens increase asthma morbidity. Information on exposures in the home can be obtained from caretaker reports, inspection, and measurement of allergens in dust samples. Comparison of caretaker reports with home inspection reveals that caretaker reports are reliable for furry pets, but underestimate cockroach and rodent exposure and dampness or water leaks (52). Caretaker reports in ICAS reveal that 45% of homes had water leaks, 58% had cockroach problems, 40% had rodents, and 28% currently had a furry pet. Allergen concentrations in bedroom dust samples of asthmatic children living in inner cities confirms the high exposure with 50% to 70% of homes having high exposures to cockroach (>8 U/g) and 10% to 80% to house dust mite (>2 U/g) (59,60).

There are racial/ethnic disparities in rates of sensitization to allergens. Black and Puerto Rican children are more likely to be sensitized to cockroach and dust mite (61,62). The NCICAS study, which included asthmatics living in impoverished urban areas with a wide range of severity, reported that 77% of children had at least one positive skin test to a panel of 14 indoor and outdoor allergens and 47% had three or more positive tests (19). In the ICAS cohort of more severe asthmatic children, 94% had a positive skin test to indoor allergens and more than 50% had three or more positive tests (52). The skin test results from the two studies are shown in Table 1.

Table 1 Allergy Skin Test Results in NCICAS[a] ($n = 1286$) and ICAS[b] ($n = 937$)

Allergen sensitivities	NCICAS	ICAS
Dust mites		
D. farinae	24	47
D. pteronyssinus	31	57
Cockroach mix	36	69
Rodent		
Rat epithelia	19	19
Mouse epithelia	15	28
Molds		
Alteneria tenuis	38	36
Penicillium notatum	20	13
Furry pets		
cat	24	44
dog	16	21

[a]National Cooperative Inner-City Asthma Study (eight U.S. sites) (19)
[b]Inner-City Asthma Study (seven U.S. sites) (52)

Exposure and sensitization to cockroach allergen increases morbidity. Rosenstreich et al. showed that children exposed and sensitized to cockroach had more days of wheeze, unscheduled doctor visits, and hospitalizations compared to those children who were only exposed, only sensitized, or neither exposed nor sensitized (59). These authors did not demonstrate an association between sensitization and exposure to dust mite or cat allergen and asthma morbidity, but the sample size limited the power of the study to test this association.

VII. Overcoming the Barriers to Improve Morbidity

Issues related to access and patterns of care need interventions that change both provider and patient behavior. One challenge is to direct patients from episodic and fragmented care into an outpatient setting where prevention, education, and monitoring are more easily done. Interventions aimed at providers working in the inner city need to be developed and evaluated.

Successful approaches need to set realistic goals that account for limitations imposed by the inner-city setting. For example, only 38% of homes in NCICAS had functioning vacuum cleaners (63). Therefore, asthma education involving vacuuming to reduce allergens would not be effective without supplying the appropriate resources. Telephone-based interventions would not be successful in inner-city areas where there are a substantial number of families without telephone service. There are diverse cultural beliefs and complementary and alternative medicine approaches in urban communities that need to be considered in developing and implementing interventions (64).

Partnering with the community increases the probability of success in implementation of interventions and in conducting research. Involvement of advisory boards, asthma coalitions, and community health care workers in programs and research can be helpful in developing a trusting relationship between health care institutions and urban communities.

VIII. Interventions

The multiple factors associated with increased morbidity in children with asthma living in inner cities present a major challenge in disease management. Inner-city populations are heterogeneous and interventions need to be tailored to the problems both at the community level and individual level. This would increase the chance of success and also be more efficient and cost-effective. Numerous interventions have been developed and implemented in a variety of settings, including EDs, clinics, schools, and homes. The approaches include educational interventions aimed either at patients and their families or heath care providers, counseling, and environmental control strategies. Interventions that have been most successful are those that target asthmatic children with greater morbidity and address multiple risk factors. Limitations of many asthma intervention studies are that few are aimed at inner-city children, are culturally sensitive, or provide an economic evaluation. The study sample sizes have been small and few of these have been subjected to randomized, controlled clinical trials. The importance of this study design is underscored by the fact that there is a significant improvement in outcome in children with asthma enrolled in control arms of these trials (65).

To assist in the identification of effective interventions, the National Center for Environmental Health (NCEH) of the Centers for Disease Control and Prevention (CDC) has identified on its Web site potentially effective interventions and described and documented research-based asthma-control interventions that are being implemented in communities. Database searches focused on pertinent articles published from January 1980 through October 2002. Of the interventions identified in the 202 articles reviewed, 42 interventions met their criteria and were included in the group of potentially effective approaches (1). Randomized, controlled clinical trials in inner-city children are summarized in Table 2.

Several studies have investigated the effect of nurse-led education on admissions to the hospital. Inpatient asthma education programs led by nurse educators for inner-city adults with asthma have been successful in achieving

Table 2 Randomized, Controlled Clinical Trials of Asthma Interventions in Inner-City Children

Program	No. intervention/ control	Follow-up	Outcome	Economic analysis	Comment
Inner-city pediatric home intervention ™ (72)	35/35/34*	12 months	Decreased acute visits	No	No difference between active and placebo group; both different from control
Health Buddy ™ (72)	66/68	12 weeks	Less limitation of activity	No	Short follow-up
Pediatric asthma center program (85)	60/69	24 months	Fewer ED visits/month	No	43% completed year 1 25% completed year 2
Wee wheezers (71)	49/46	12 months	Decreased asthma symptoms	No	30% refusal rate for participation; 29% dropout
Hospital discharge program (69)	80/80	6 months	Lower readmission rate	No	Brief education during hospital stay
Asthma education program (86)	38/40	12 months	Decreased ED visits Decreased hospitalization	Yes	Intervention group received specialty care as well as education
Asthma outreach program (87)	28/29	12–24 months	Decreased ED visits Decreased hospitalization	Yes	Education plus nurse case manager

NCICAS asthma counselor (77,88)	515/518	24 months	Decreased symptom days	Yes	Multicenter; social worker trained as asthma counselor
Open airways (89)	310/290	12 months	No decrease in hospitalization/ED visits	Yes	Decrease in hospitalization in those with prior hospitalization
ICAS environmental intervention (82)	469/468	24 months	Decreased symptom days	No	Multicenter; reduction in home allergen correlated with decreased symptoms
Home management (68)	96/105	14 months	Lower readmission rate	No	Nurse-led program; free access to medical care
Family coordinator asthma education program (90)	50/50	3 months	Decreased symptoms and activity restriction	No	Labor-intensive; participation rate—28%
Patient education (HMO) (91)	127/126	12 months	No decrease in ED visits or hospital days	No	Health maintenance organization intervention

higher follow-up rates with outpatient appointments and reductions in hospitalizations and ED visits (66,67). A nurse-led education program in Glasgow, Scotland, for children hospitalized for asthma who were predominantly of lower social class implemented home management training that incorporated written and verbal information and was reinforced with outpatient follow-up appointments and telephone advice (68). This study demonstrated a significant reduction in hospital readmissions during a 12-month follow-up period from 25% in the control group to 8% in the intervention group. A brief, individual, and simple educational program in Leicester, England, which provided a specific, written management plan together with instructions on the use of inhalers and peak flow devices for hospitalized children, reduced the likelihood of readmission to the hospital during a six-month follow-up period, but the social status of this urban population was not reported (69). A similar intervention in hospitalized preschool children (age 18 months to 5 years) did not reduce morbidity over the subsequent 12 months (70).

Home-based interventions for inner-city children have been studied. A home-based education intervention adapted from the Wee Wheezers program for young low-income children, 1–6 years of age, and their families was assessed (71). This program consisted of eight 90-minute educational sessions. There was a reduction in morbidity for children aged 1–3 years, but not children aged 4–6 years. There was no effect on asthma management behaviors. The refusal rate for participation in the study was 30% and dropout rate after randomization to the treatment group was 29%. A home-based intervention reported by Carter et al. demonstrated a reduction in acute visits in both the intervention and placebo groups (72). The effect in both was significantly better than that of a placebo group who received no home visits, indicating that home visits by themselves have a beneficial effect.

Interactive computer education programs have been developed but have had little effect on asthma outcome (73). An interactive home-based communication device, Health Buddy℠, has been developed and evaluated in inner-city children (74). This device enabled children to assess and monitor symptoms and to transmit this information to a nurse coordinator. Compared with a control group using an asthma diary, the Health Buddy group had significantly less limitation of activity over the 12-week follow-up period. There was no difference between the groups in coughing or wheezing, ED visits, or hospitalizations. The daily compliance rate with the device and the diaries declined over the study period. Decreased compliance with daily monitoring has been observed in studies of inner-city children using peak flow meters (75). The short duration of follow-up and the small sample size limit interpretation of the results.

Care by asthma specialists improves outcome compared to generalists (76). In inner cities there is limited access to specialty care, and extensive changes to the preexisting medical services are not practical in the short term. The asthma counselor intervention program developed by NCICAS took a different approach to empower the family to increase asthma self-management and to improve their interaction with the primary care provider (77). This was a one-year multifaceted intervention that was tailored to the patient's risk factors for asthma. Social workers were trained as asthma counselors and met with patients and caretakers initially in two group asthma education sessions. After the group sessions, the asthma counselor met patients in person every two months and spoke on the telephone on the alternate months. Content of the meetings was determined by an initial assessment of risk using an asthma risk assesssment tool (ARAT). The topics included environmental control, improving communication with providers, adherence, and assistance with psychological and social issues. The intervention reduced symptom days overall by about half a month compared to controls and by more than one and a half months for children with the most severe symptoms. The beneficial effects of the intervention continued in the second year, at which time they did not have access to an asthma counselor.

Exposure of asthma patients to irritants or allergens to which they are sensitive increases asthma symptoms. Recent asthma management guidelines have stressed environmental control measures as an integral part of treatment. Shapiro et al. attempted dust mite mitigation in a low-income urban population (78). Dust mite levels and bronchial reactivity to methacholine were reduced, but symptoms and quality of life did not differ between intervention and control groups. Attempts to reduce cockroach allergens in the home have had varied success (79). Integrated pest management, which consists of filling holes with copper mesh, vacuuming and cleaning, and low-toxicity pesticides and traps, can control cockroach infestation. Reduction of cockroach allergen levels to less than 8 U/g in bedrooms is feasible and can be maintained in some, but not all, multifamily dwellings in the inner city (80,81).

Most studies have focused on a single allergen or ETS rather than on the multiple exposures encountered by many urban asthmatic children. ICAS developed an intervention tailored to each child's sensitization and environmental risk profile (52). The goal of the intervention was to provide the child's caretaker with the knowledge, skills, motivation, equipment, and supplies necessary to perform comprehensive environmental remediation. The intervention was organized into six modules, including remediation of exposure to dust mites, passive smoking, cockroaches, pets, rodents, and mold. Intervention activities were tailored to each child's skin test sensitization profile and environmental exposures. Reducing exposure to indoor allergens, including cockroach and dust mite, and ETS resulted in 34 fewer days with reported wheeze over the two years of study for children in the intervention group compared to the control group (82).

There are few interventions aimed at providers in inner cities. Evans et al. found that in New York City, clinics receiving intensive staff educational training in current guidelines for asthma care, coupled with administrative support for change in practice behavior, increased the number of patients with asthma receiving continuing care and improved the quality of care they received compared to control clinics (83). The research design did not allow for a determination of the relative contributions of the training to the study outcomes and the strong organizational commitment by the health department leadership to improve asthma care. The effect on patient outcome was not reported. Easy Breathing was a management program instituted in primary care clinics in Hartford, Connecticut (84). There was a positive effect on clinicians' knowledge and adherence to asthma guidelines, but the program was not subjected to a controlled clinical trial. The ICAS is currently evaluating an intervention aimed at primary care providers, but the results are not available.

IX. Conclusions

The management of asthma in inner cities presents a formidable challenge. The multiple factors contributing to morbidity are interdependent. Targeting one aspect of the problem may result in some improvement, but may not have a major impact on the large number of asthmatic children living in inner cities. Research on interventions will require large clinical trials to assess effects on outcome. Data are needed on the success of translation of potentially effective programs into the community. The barriers to implementation of these programs in the inner city need to be documented.

References

1. Mannino DM, Homa DM, Akinbami LJ, Moorman JE, Gwynn C, Redd SC. Surveillance for asthma—United States, 1980–1999. MMWR Surveill Summ 2002; 51:1–13 (http://www.cdc.gov/asthma/interventions/interventions.htm).
2. Carter-Pokras OD, Gergen PJ. Reported asthma among Puerto Rican, Mexican-American, and Cuban children, 1982 through 1984. Am J Public Health 1993; 83:580–582.
3. Crain EF, Weiss KB, Bijur PE, Hersh M, Westbrook L, Stein RE. An estimate of the prevalence of asthma and wheezing among inner-city children. Pediatrics 1994; 94:356–362.
4. Sporik R, Ingram JM, Price W, Sussman JH, Honsinger RW, Platts-Mills TA. Association of asthma with serum IgE and skin test reactivity to allergens among children living at high altitude. Tickling the dragon's breath. Am J Respir Crit Care Med 1995; 151:1388–1392.
5. Carr W, Zeitel L, Weiss K. Variations in asthma hospitalizations and deaths in New York City. Am J Public Health 1992; 82:59–65.

6. Halfon N, Newacheck PW. Childhood asthma and poverty: differential impacts and utilization of health services. Pediatrics 1993; 91:56–61.
7. Gottlieb DJ, Beiser AS, O'Connor GT. Poverty, race, and medication use are correlates of asthma hospitalization rates. A small area analysis in Boston. Chest 1995; 108:28–35.
8. Crater DD, Heise S, Perzanowski M, Herbert R, Morse CG, Hulsey TC, Platts-Mills T. Asthma hospitalization trends in Charleston, South Carolina, 1956 to 1997: twenty-fold increase among black children during a 30-year period. Pediatrics 2001; 108:E97.
9. Gergen P. Social class and asthma—distinguishing between the disease and the diagnosis. Am J Public Health 1996; 86:1361–1362.
10. Weitzman M, Gortmaker S, Sobol A. Racial, social, and environmental risks for childhood asthma. Am J Dis Child 1990; 144:1189–1194.
11. Aligne CA, Auinger P, Byrd RS, Weitzman M. Risk factors for pediatric asthma. Contributions of poverty, race, and urban residence. Am J Respir Crit Care Med 2000; 162:873–877.
12. Cunningham J, Dockery DW, Speizer FE. Race, asthma, and persistent wheeze in Philadelphia schoolchildren. Am J Public Health 1996; 86:1406–1409.
13. Schwartz J, Gold D, Dockery DW, Weiss ST, Speizer FE. Predictors of asthma and persistent wheeze in a national sample of children in the United States. Association with social class, perinatal events, and race. Am Rev Respir Dis 1990; 142:555–562.
14. Strachan DP, Anderson HR, Limb ES, O'Neill A, Wells N. A national survey of asthma prevalence, severity, and treatment in Great Britain. Arch Dis Child 1994; 70:174–178.
15. Ernst P, Demissie K, Joseph L, Locher U, Becklake MR. Socioeconomic status and indicators of asthma in children. Am J Respir Crit Care Med 1995; 152: 570–575.
16. Wissow LS, Gittelsohn AM, Szklo M, Starfield B, Mussman M. Poverty, race, and hospitalization for childhood asthma. Am J Public Health 1988; 78:777–782.
17. Weir TD, Mallek N, Sandford AJ, Bai TR, Wadh NA, Fitzgerald JM, Cockcroft D, James A, Liggett SB, Paré PD. β2-Adrenergic receptor haplotypes in mild, moderate and fatal/near fatal asthma. Am J Respir Crit Care Med 1998; 158:787–791.
18. Halfon N, Newacheck PW, Wood DL, St Peter RF. Routine emergency department use for sick care by children in the United States. Pediatrics 1996; 98:28–34.
19. Kattan M, Mitchell H, Eggleston P, Gergen P, Crain E, Redline S, Weiss K, Evans III R, Kercsmar C, Leickly F, Malveaux F, Wedner HJ. Characteristics of inner-city children with asthma: the National Cooperative Inner-City Asthma Study. Pediatr Pulmonol 1997; 24:253–262.
20. Crain EF, Kercsmar C, Weiss KB, Mitchell H, Lynn H. Reported difficulties in access to quality care for children with asthma in the inner city. Arch Pediatr Adolesc Med 1998; 152:333–339.
21. Petersen DL, Murphy DE, Jaffe DM, Richardson MS, Fisher EB, Shannon W, Sussman L, Strunk RC. A tool to organize instructions at discharge after treat-

ment of asthmatic children in an emergency department. J Asthma 1999;
36:597–603.

22. Leickly FE, Wade SL, Crain E, Kruszon-Moran D, Wright EC, Evans R, 3rd.
    Self-reported adherence, management behavior, and barriers to care after an
    emergency department visit by inner city children with asthma. Pediatrics
    1998; 101:E8.

23. Butz AM, Eggleston P, Huss K, Kolodner K, Rand C. Nebulizer use in inner-
    city children with asthma: morbidity, medication use, and asthma management
    practices. Arch Pediatr Adolesc Med 2000; 154:984–990.

24. Warman KL, Silver EJ, Stein RE. Asthma symptoms, morbidity, and antiin-
    flammatory use in inner-city children. Pediatrics 2001; 108:277–282.

25. Riekert KA, Butz AM, Eggleston PA, Huss K, Winkelstein M, Rand CS. Care-
    giver-physician medication concordance and undertreatment of asthma among
    inner-city children. Pediatrics 2003; 111:e214–e220.

26. Freeman NC, Schneider D, McGarvey P. The relationship of health insurance
    to the diagnosis and management of asthma and respiratory problems in chil-
    dren in a predominantly Hispanic urban community. Am J Public Health 2003;
    93:1316–1320.

27. Finkelstein JA, Barton MB, Donahue JG, Algatt-Bergstrom P, Markson LE,
    Platt R. Comparing asthma care for Medicaid and non-Medicaid children in
    a health maintenance organization. Arch Pediatr Adolesc Med 2000; 154:
    563–568.

28. Celano M, Geller RJ, Phillips KM, Ziman R. Treatment adherence among low-
    income children with asthma. J Pediatr Psychol 1998; 23:345–349.

29. Bender B, Wamboldt FS, O'Connor SL, Rand C, Szefler S, Milgrom H, Wam-
    boldt MZ. Measurement of children's asthma medication adherence by self
    report, mother report, canister weight, and Doser CT. Ann Allergy Asthma
    Immunol 2000; 85:416–421.

30. Apter AJ, Reisine ST, Affleck G, Barrows E, ZuWallack RL. Adherence with
    twice-daily dosing of inhaled steroids. Socioeconomic and health-belief differ-
    ences. Am J Respir Crit Care Med 1998; 157:1810–1817.

31. Yoos HL, Kitzman H, McMullen A. Barriers to anti-inflammatory medication
    use in childhood asthma. Ambul Pediatr 2003; 3:181–190.

32. Bauman LJ, Wright E, Leickly FE, Crain E, Kruszon-Moran D, Wade SL, Vis-
    ness CM. Relationship of adherence to pediatric asthma morbidity among
    inner-city children. Pediatrics 2002; 110:e6.

33. Wade S, Weil C, Holden G, Mitchell H, Evans III R, Kruszon-Moran D, Bau-
    man L, Crain E, Eggleston P, Kattan M, Kercsmar C, Leickly F, Malveaux F,
    Wedner HJ. Psychosocial characteristics of inner-city children with asthma: a
    description of the NCICAS psychosocial protocol. National Cooperative
    Inner-City Asthma Study. Pediatr Pulmonol 1997; 24:263–276.

34. Mansour ME, Lanphear BP, DeWitt TG. Barriers to asthma care in urban
    children: parent perspectives. Pediatrics 2000; 106:512–519.

35. Wade SL, Islam S, Holden G, Kruszon-Moran D, Mitchell H. Division of
    responsibility for asthma management tasks between caregivers and children
    in the inner city. J Dev Behav Pediatr 1999; 20:93–98.

36. Eggleston PA, Malveaux FJ, Butz AM, Huss K, Thompson L, Kolodner K, Rand CS. Medications used by children with asthma living in the inner city. Pediatrics 1998; 101:349–354.
37. MacLean WE, Jr, Perrin JM, Gortmaker S, Pierre CB. Psychological adjustment of children with asthma: effects of illness severity and recent stressful life events. J Pediatr Psychol 1992; 17:159–171.
38. Weil CM, Wade SL, Bauman LJ, Lynn H, Mitchell H, Lavigne J. The relationship between psychosocial factors and asthma morbidity in inner-city children with asthma. Pediatrics 1999; 104:1274–1280.
39. Bartlett SJ, Kolodner K, Butz AM, Eggleston P, Malveaux FJ, Rand CS. Maternal depressive symptoms and emergency department use among inner-city children with asthma. Arch Pediatr Adolesc Med 2001; 155:347–353.
40. Wright RJ, Mitchell H, Visness CM, Cohen S, Stout J, Evans R, Gold DR. Community violence and asthma morbidity: the inner-city asthma study. Am J Public Health 2004; 94:625–632.
41. Romieu I, Meneses F, Ruiz S, Sienra JJ, Huerta J, White MC, Etzel RA. Effects of air pollution on the respiratory health of asthmatic children living in Mexico City. Am J Respir Crit Care Med 1996; 154:300–307.
42. Slaughter JC, Lumley T, Sheppard L, Koenig JQ, Shapiro GG. Effects of ambient air pollution on symptom severity and medication use in children with asthma. Ann Allergy Asthma Immunol 2003; 91:346–353.
43. Lippmann M, Frampton M, Schwartz J, Dockery D, Schlesinger R, Koutrakis P, Froines J, Nel A, Finkelstein J, Godleski J, Kaufman J, Koenig J, Larson T, Luchtel D, Liu LJS, Oberdörster G, Peters A, Sarnat J, Sioutas C, Suh H, Sullivan J, Utell M, Wichmann E, Zelikoff J. The U.S. Environmental Protection Agency Particulate Matter Health Effects Research Centers Program: a midcourse report of status, progress, and plans. Environ Health Perspect 2003; 111:1074–1092.
44. Schwartz J, Neas LM. Fine particles are more strongly associated than coarse particles with acute respiratory health effects in schoolchildren. Epidemiology 2000; 11:6–10.
45. Lin M, Chen Y, Burnett RT, Villeneuve PJ, Krewski D. The influence of ambient coarse particulate matter on asthma hospitalization in children: case-crossover and time-series analyses. Environ Health Perspect 2002; 110:575–581.
46. Lang DM, Polansky M. Patterns of asthma mortality in Philadelphia from 1969 to 1991. N Engl J Med 1994; 331:1542–1546.
47. Claudio L, Torres T, Sanjurjo E, Sherman LR, Landrigan PJ. Environmental health sciences education–a tool for achieving environmental equity and protecting children. Environ Health Perspect 1998; 106(suppl 3):849–855.
48. Mortimer KM, Neas LM, Dockery DW, Redline S, Tager IB. The effect of air pollution on inner-city children with asthma. Eur Respir J 2002; 19:699–705.
49. Delfino RJ, Gong H, Jr, Linn WS, Pellizzari ED, Hu Y. Asthma symptoms in Hispanic children and daily ambient exposures to toxic and criteria air pollutants. Environ Health Perspect 2003; 111:647–656.
50. Kleipes N, Tsang A, Behar J. Analysis of the national human activity pattern (NHAPS) Respondents From A standpoint of Exposure Assessment. Final Report. Las Vegas, NV: Environmental Protection Agency, 1995.

51. Ehrlich R, Kattan M, Godbold J, Saltzberg DS, Grimm KT, Landrigan PJ, Lilienfeld DE. Childhood asthma and passive smoking. Urinary cotinine as a biomarker of exposure. Am Rev Respir Dis 1992; 145:594–599.

52. Crain EF, Walter M, O'Connor GT, Mitchell H, Gruchalla RS, Kattan M, Malindzak GS, Enright P, Evans R, Morgan M, Stout J. Home and allergic characteristics of children with asthma in seven u.s. Urban communities and design of an environmental intervention: the inner-city asthma study. Environ Health Perspect 2002; 110:939–945.

53. Sarnat JA, Koutrakis P, Suh HH. Assessing the relationship between personal particulate and gaseous exposures of senior citizens living in Baltimore, MD. J Air Waste Manag Assoc 2000; 50:1184–1198.

54. Wallace LA, Emmerich SJ, Howard-Reed C. Continuous measurements of air change rates in an occupied house for 1 year: the effect of temperature, wind, fans, and windows. J Expo Anal Environ Epidemiol 2002; 12:296–306.

55. Wallace LA, Mitchell H, O'Connor GT, Neas L, Lippmann M, Kattan M, Koenig J, Stout JW, Vaughn BJ, Wallace D, Walter M, Adams K, Liu L-JS. Particle concentrations in inner-city homes of children with asthma: the effect of smoking, cooking, and outdoor pollution. Environ Health Perspect 2003; 111:1265–1272.

56. Neas LM, Dockery DW, Ware JH, Spengler JD, Speizer FE, Ferris BG, Jr. Association of indoor nitrogen dioxide with respiratory symptoms and pulmonary function in children. Am J Epidemiol 1991; 134:204–219.

57. Farrow A, Greenwood R, Preece S, Golding J. Nitrogen dioxide, the oxides of nitrogen, and infants' health symptoms. ALSPAC Study Team. Avon Longitudinal Study of Pregnancy and Childhood. Arch Environ Health 1997; 52: 189–194.

58. Chauhan AJ, Inskip HM, Linaker CH, Smith S, Schreiber J, Johnston SL, Holgate ST. Personal exposure to nitrogen dioxide (NO2) and the severity of virus-induced asthma in children. Lancet 2003; 361:1939–1944.

59. Rosenstreich DL, Eggleston P, Kattan M, Baker D, Slavin RG, Gergen P, Mitchell H, McNiff-Mortimer, Lynn H, Ownby D, Malveaux F. The role of cockroach allergy and exposure to cockroach allergen in causing morbidity among inner-city children with asthma. N Engl J Med 1997; 336:1356–1363.

60. Call RS, Smith TF, Morris E, Chapman MD, Platts-Mills TA. Risk factors for asthma in inner city children. J Pediatr 1992; 121:862–866.

61. Stevenson LA, Gergen PJ, Hoover DR, Rosenstreich D, Mannino DM, Matte TD. Sociodemographic correlates of indoor allergen sensitivity among United States children. J Allergy Clin Immunol 2001; 108:747–752.

62. Celedon JC, Sredl D, Weiss ST, Pisarski M, Wakefield D, Cloutier M. Ethnicity and skin test reactivity to aeroallergens among asthmatic children in Connecticut. Chest 2004; 125:85–92.

63. Eggleston PA. Environmental causes of asthma in inner city children. The National Cooperative Inner City Asthma Study. Clin Rev Allergy Immunol 2000; 18:311–324.

64. Pachter LM, Weller SC, Baer RD, de Alba Garcia JE, Trotter RT, Glazer M, Klein R. Variation in asthma beliefs and practices among mainland Puerto

Ricans, Mexican-Americans, Mexicans, and Guatemalans. J Asthma 2002; 39:119–134.

65. Greineder DK, Loane KC, Parks P. Outcomes for control patients referred to a pediatric asthma outreach program: an example of the Hawthorne effect. Am J Manag Care 1998; 4:196–202.

66. George MR, O'Dowd LC, Martin I, Lindell KO, Whitney F, Jones M, Ramondo T, Walsh 1, Grinsinger J, Hansen-Flaschen, Panettieri RA. A comprehensive educational program improves clinical outcome measures in inner-city patients with asthma. Arch Intern Med 1999; 159:1710–1716.

67. Castro M, Zimmermann NA, Crocker S, Bradley J, Leven C, Schechtman KB. Asthma intervention program prevents readmissions in high healthcare users. Am J Respir Crit Care Med 2003; 168:1095–1099.

68. Madge P, McColl J, Paton J. Impact of a nurse-led home management training programme in children admitted to hospital with acute asthma: a randomised controlled study. Thorax 1997; 52:223–228.

69. Wesseldine LJ, McCarthy P, Silverman M. Structured discharge procedure for children admitted to hospital with acute asthma: a randomised controlled trial of nursing practice. Arch Dis Child 1999; 80:110–114.

70. Stevens CA, Wesseldine LJ, Couriel JM, Dyer AJ, Osman LM, Silverman M. Parental education and guided self-management of asthma and wheezing in the pre-school child: a randomised controlled trial. Thorax 2002; 57:39–44.

71. Brown JV, Bakeman R, Celano MP, Demi AS, Kobrynski L, Wilson SR. Home-based asthma education of young low-income children and their families. J Pediatr Psychol 2002; 27:677–688.

72. Carter MC, Perzanowski MS, Raymond A, Platts-Mills TA. Home intervention in the treatment of asthma among inner-city children. J Allergy Clin Immunol 2001; 108:732–737.

73. Homer C, Susskind O, Alpert HR, Owusu C, Schneider L, Rappaport LA, Rubin DH. An evaluation of an innovative multimedia educational software program for asthma management: report of a randomized, controlled trial. Pediatrics 2000; 106:210–215.

74. Guendelman S, Meade K, Benson M, Chen YQ, Samuels S. Improving asthma outcomes and self-management behaviors of inner-city children: a randomized trial of the Health Buddy interactive device and an asthma diary. Arch Pediatr Adolesc Med 2002; 156:114–120.

75. Redline S, Wright EC, Kattan M, Kercsmar C, Weiss K. Short-term compliance with peak flow monitoring: results from a study of inner city children with asthma. Pediatr Pulmonol 1996; 21:203–210.

76. Zeiger RS, Heller S, Mellon MH, Wald J, Falkoff R, Schatz M. Facilitated referral to asthma specialist reduces relapses in asthma emergency room visits. J Allergy Clin Immunol 1991; 87:1160–1168.

77. Evans R, III, Gergen PJ, Mitchell H, Kattan M, Kercsmar C, Crain E, Anderson J, Eggleston P, Malveaux F, Wedner J. A randomized clinical trial to reduce asthma morbidity among inner-city children: results of the National Cooperative Inner-city Asthma Study. J Pediatr 1999; 135:332–338.

78. Shapiro GG, Wighton TG, Chinn T, Zuckrman J, Eliassen AH, Picciano JF, Platts-Mills TAE. House dust mite avoidance for children with asthma in homes of low-income families. J Allergy Clin Immunol 1999; 103:1069–1074.

79. Eggleston PA. Cockroach allergen abatement: the good, the bad, and the ugly. J Allergy Clin Immunol 2003; 112:265–267.

80. Arbes SJ Jr, Sever M, Archer J, Long EH, Gore JC, Schal C, Walter M, Nuebler B, Vaughn B, Mitchell H, Liu E, Collette N, Adler P, Sandel M, Zeldin DC. Abatement of cockroach allergen (Bla g 1) in low-income, urban housing: a randomized controlled trial. J Allergy Clin Immunol 2003; 112:339–345.

81. Arbes SJ Jr, Sever M, Mehta J, Gore JC, Schal C, Vaughn B, Mitchell H, Zeldin DC. Abatement of cockroach allergens (Bla g 1 and Bla g 2) in low-income, urban housing: month 12 continuation results. J Allergy Clin Immunol 2004; 113:109–114.

82. Morgan WJ, Crain E, Gruchalla RS, O'Connor GT, Kattan M, Evans RE, Stout J, Malindzak G, Smartt E, Plaut M, Walter M, Vaughn B, Mitchell H. The Inner-City Asthma Study: A home based environmental intervention. New Engl J Med 2004; 351:1068–1080.

83. Evans D, Mellins R, Lobach K, Ramos-Bonoan C, Pinkett-Heller M, Wiesemann S, Klein I, Donahue C, Burke D, Levison M, Levin B, Zimmerman B, Clark N. Improving care for minority children with asthma: professional education in public health clinics. Pediatrics 1997; 99:157–164.

84. Cloutier MM, Wakefield DB, Carlisle PS, Bailit HL, Hall CB. The effect of Easy Breathing on asthma management and knowledge. Arch Pediatr Adolesc Med 2002; 156:1045–1051.

85. Harish Z, Bregante AC, Morgan C, Fann CS, Callaghan CM, Witt MA, Levison KA, Caspe WD. A comprehensive inner-city asthma program reduces hospital and emergency room utilization. Ann Allergy Asthma Immunol 2001; 86:185–189.

86. Kelly CS, Morrow AL, Shults J, Nakas N, Strope GL, Adelman RD. Outcomes evaluation of a comprehensive intervention program for asthmatic children enrolled in medicaid. Pediatrics 2000; 105:1029–1035.

87. Greineder DK, Loane KC, Parks P. A randomized controlled trial of a pediatric asthma outreach program. J Allergy Clin Immunol 1999; 103:436–440.

88. Sullivan SD, Weiss KB, Lynn H, Mitchell H, Kattan M, Gergen PJ, Evans R. The cost-effectiveness of an inner-city asthma intervention for children. J Allergy Clin Immunol 2002; 110:576–581.

89. Clark NM, Feldman CH, Evans D, Levison MJ, Wasilewski Y, Mellins RB. The impact of health education on frequency and cost of health care use by low income children with asthma. J Allergy Clin Immunol 1986; 78:108–115.

90. Bonner S, Zimmerman BJ, Evans D, Irigoyen M, Resnick D, Mellins RB. An individualized intervention to improve asthma management among urban Latino and African-American families. J Asthma 2002; 39:167–179.

91. Shields MC, Griffin KW, McNabb WL. The effect of a patient education program on emergency room use for inner-city children with asthma. Am J Public Health 1990; 80:36–38.

20

Asthma in Adolescence

**ROBERT C. STRUNK, LEONARD B. BACHARIER, and
GORDON R. BLOOMBERG**

Department of Pediatrics, Washington University School of Medicine, and the Division
  of Allergy and Pulmonary Medicine, St. Louis Children's Hospital
St. Louis, Missouri, U.S.A.

Perhaps the title of this edition of *Lung Biology in Health and Disease*, *Childhood Asthma*, is most appropriate for this chapter on adolescence. In caring for the adolescent with asthma, a clinician must break the barriers of adolescent disinterest in caring for a chronic illness to attain the confidence of the adolescent patient in developing a functioning partnership. The task of developing a partnership with the adolescent must be done while helping the family in their process of allowing their adolescent to become independent and take over care for the asthma.

Adolescence is defined by *Webster's College Dictionary* as "the transitional period between puberty and adulthood in human development, terminating legally when the age of majority is reached" or "the process of growing to maturity." Whatever the actual ages of adolescence, it is a period of dramatic developmental maturation that can impact asthma management and outcomes. Adolescents present challenging variations in mood and capabilities to society, their families, and their health care providers. Further complicating care, adolescence is the time of high variability in the course of asthma, with asthma appearing to improve or even be "outgrown" in many, but it is also the time when the prevalence of mortality from asthma has increased greater than any other age group over the past decades. The clinician must recognize that adolescents with asthma have the same issues dealing with peers and family that all adolescents undergo. The drive to conform, to take risks, to be normal, to not be different, to worry about body image are all very real and can have a tremendous impact on asthma care and outcomes. To effectively treat asthma in an adolescent, a physician must understand development and its impact on asthma self-care expectations. No longer can a clinician talk just to the parent and expect that instructions will be followed. The adolescent becomes the real patient and the real subject of interaction.

Adolescence is characterized by moving through the developmental stages of industry versus inferiority (approximately 11–12 years of age), when a child begins to have the ability to think abstractly an0d enjoys challenges, on to identity versus role confusion in later adolescence, when work on becoming psychologically independent from the family occurs. These changes are accompanied by both an increase in decision-making capability and the capacity to become responsible for day-to-day care. The change across the developmental continuum is not smooth and rates vary widely among individuals. The health care provider must recognize the variability in the attainment of developmental stages and assist in the process of the adolescent gaining independence appropriate for the actual development level, hile helping the parent relinquish control. The adolescents must be the subject of questioning at the time of visits and the person who agrees to the plan. Many adolescent patients are best seen by themselves, with a review with the parents at the end of the visit.

Physicians and parents have long assumed that children will outgrow asthma in adolescence. Health care utilization for asthma decreases throughout childhood, but overall asthma prevalence actually increases (1). Roorda et al. followed 8- to 12-year-old children into young adulthood (2). Only 19% of the young adults were still under a physician's supervision, in contrast to the 76% who continued to have respiratory symptoms. Further emphasizing the under-treatment of symptoms by adolescents and young adults, only 32% used maintenance medication with most using the medications only intermittently. Even among children in whom symptoms improve and even resolve completely, pulmonary function abnormalities remain. Taken together, these issues leave the adolescent at risk for asthma symptoms that are often minimized and can result in severe episodes of morbidity and even mortality. Rather than decreasing visits as desired by these patients, adolescence is an age group that requires increased attention and ongoing regular visits to assess asthma objectively and review the approach to increased symptoms.

I. The Myth of "Outgrowing Asthma": Natural History of Asthma from Childhood to Adolescence

Long-term studies of outcome of childhood asthma have been published from as early as 1945 (3–29). While these studies have widely different

Table 1 Factors Associated with Persistence and Relapse of Asthma

Persistence: atopy (positive skin tests, eczema early in life and its persistence, allergic rhinitis, elevated level of IgE, peripheral blood eosinophilia, and family history of asthma or an allergic disease) (158–169), both passive and active smoking (111,167,170), airway hyper responsiveness (161,171,172), and more severe asthma in childhood (173).

Relapse history of any wheeze, chronic productive cough, personal smoking, persistent airway hyper responsiveness, and atopy (18,174). Further emphasizing the importance of hyper responsiveness in outcome, Grol et al. found airway hyper responsiveness present at ages 5–14 years to be an independent risk factor for a low level of FEV$_1$ in early adulthood (175).

methodologies, it is possible to make some estimates of percentages of children who improve and those who remain with symptoms as they grow into adulthood. By early adulthood, 37% (range: 14–65%) of school-age children with doctor-diagnosed asthma were in remission (generally defined as no asthma symptoms in three years) and another 32% were improved (generally defined as symptoms within 1–3 years, but not within 12 months, or significantly less severe symptoms than at the time of the last survey). However, significant disease persisted in approximately 36% of patients. An outcome of equal importance to persistence of asthma is relapse of wheeze/asthma symptoms after a period of wellness. Relapse occurs in 20% to 36% of the populations studied in early adulthood (3,5,14,15,17,18,20–22,27). Factors that may promote persistence and relapse of asthma are presented in Table 1.

It is well known that children with asthma who become asymptomatic during adolescence continue to have spirometric abnormalities and airway responsiveness to methacholine or cold air challenge (30–36). A significant proportion of children who are free of symptoms and have normal forced expiratory volume in 1 second (FEV$_1$), and even normal FEV$_1$/FVC ratios, continue to have bronchial lability (37). Adolescents in clinical remission have been shown to have significant airway inflammation and airway remodeling on biopsy (38), have eosinophils in bronchoalveolar lavage fluid (39), and have eosinophils and eosinophil cationic protein in induced sputum (36). Children who have continuous respiratory symptoms are most likely to have lower levels of lung function and a worse prognosis (21,40,41). Finally, the duration of disease is associated with the degree of abnormality in pulmonary function (42,43). (see Chapter 10).

II. The Paradox of Asthma Mortality in the Period of Wellness That Occurs in Adolescence

Most deaths due to asthma occur in adults, particularly in those over 65 years of age. Deaths due to asthma in children are uncommon, but approximately

200 occur in the United States each year. In 2000 there were 223 children aged 0 to 17 years who died (44). Concern about deaths in children is heightened because most deaths are thought to be preventable, and asthma death rates increased by an average of 3.4% per year from 1980 to 1998 (1). Increases in asthma mortality have been greatest in 11- to 17-year-old children among all age groups, except those greater than 65 years old (1,45,46). Among children, black non-Hispanics have the highest asthma death rates and the greatest increase over time (1,45).

Early work suggested that the most common course leading to death was gradual deterioration and late arrival for medical care (47–49). Subsequently there have been case reports providing evidence of wellness until shortly before a rapid deterioration and then death (50–54). These patterns were termed types 1 (slow-onset, late arrival) and 2 (sudden onset) (55). The latter pattern is of uncertain frequency. Recently, Jorgensen et al. examined all deaths in the Danish child population from 1993 to 1994 (56). They found that issues in all age groups were gradual deterioration during the last month and delay in seeking medical help during the final attack, consistent with the type 1 pattern.

Risk factors for asthma mortality are presented in Table 2. Most patients who die have severe disease. Severe disease can be manifest in the short term, such as by recent hospitalization, or chronically by lability of course and pulmonary function and repeated need for oral steroids (54). With the many examples of severe disease collected (54), there seems to be no unifying theme beyond the clear risk of the most severe forms of asthma: respiratory failure requiring ventilation or hypoxic seizure.

Atopy seems to be a feature that occurs in many patients who have died, but it is clearly not sufficient alone to produce asthma mortality. However, two types of allergen sensitivity appear to be related more closely to adverse outcomes. Alternaria sensitivity was associated with near-fatal and fatal events occurring in Rochester, Minnesota (57). Roberts et al. found food allergy to be a risk factor for near-fatal asthma independent of gender, age, and ethnicity (58).

Psychological factors have been shown to be present more frequently in patients with near-fatal and fatal outcomes than controls (47,49,59–61).

Table 2 Risk Factors for Death Due to Asthma

Severe disease (although patients with mild disease can have a severe sudden attack and die)

Atopy, particularly to alternaria and food (peanut most notable)

Psychological factors, especially depression

Difficulties in delivery of medical care

Low socioeconomic status

Adolescence, probably related to poor adherence and late arrival for care

---

The specific factors found vary with the methodology, but are distinguished between those who died and the case controls in each study when examined. Particularly concerning is depression, as it can lead to discouragement with having asthma and having to take asthma medications, and result in abruptly discontinuing medications and then not seeking help when symptoms start.

Difficulties in delivery of medical care are commonly identified in case–control studies and in individual reports. Both doctor issues (quality of care, in particular with inadequate frequency of follow-up visits and planning for exacerbations) and patient issues (poor response to increased symptoms) have been identified. Related to quality of care is prescription and use of inhaled corticosteroids, as use of these drugs even intermittently clearly decreases the risk of death (e.g., see Ref. 62).

Low socioeconomic status shows up as a factor in many published surveys of asthma deaths (63–66). The issue of low socioeconomic status may just be another example of psychological issues and/or medical care barriers leading to late arrival for care (66).

The role of adolescence in poor asthma outcomes is as difficult to determine as it is to address in individual patients. There are multiple issues of adolescence that could result in poor outcomes. There is a clear association between adverse outcomes from asthma and difficulties in self care (47), and adolescents are subject to poor self care as they seek independence from their families. The general tendency to-ward wave decreased doctor visits in adolescence would result in decreased identification of severe disease by objective measures of pulmonary function, as well as absence of planning for acute attacks. Risk-taking behavior that becomes more prominent in adolescents can have serious outcomes if there is an underlying medical problem. This has been highlighted by peanut ingestion by children known to be peanut allergic in situations where there is no care available (67). Aside from the psychological issues so obvious in these patients, adolescents are also undergoing rapid changes in maturation, which may prompt changes in physiologic responses that may play a role in the adverse outcomes. The combination of observations on adolescence being the largest age group for deaths among children and the prominence of sleep-associated severe events prompted an evaluation of circadian variation of airway reactivity and hypoxic ventilatory drive in adolescents with severe asthma (68). No systematic variation in these measures was found in adolescents, and there was no association of the variations observed by maturation stage (68). The idea that sexual maturation plays a role in outcomes is intriguing and requires further exploration.

Efforts should be made to identify patients at risk for death. While there have been significant efforts toward understanding reasons that fatal and near-fatal asthma episodes occur, the identification of patients at risk for dying remains an art with no single set of criteria able to identify all patients who will die. History of a prior severe event, especially respiratory failure requiring intubation, is an obvious risk factor. However, while as many as 25% of patients with a history of respiratory failure were found to have died in a three- to five-year follow-up, most patients who die have not had respiratory failure (54). Most studies indicate that a high proportion of patients who have died have had severe asthma, but the number of patients with severe disease is large and only 1% to 3% will die over an extended follow-up period. Death in patients with otherwise mild disease has been documented (69). The importance of psychological factors in poor outcomes from asthma (47) indicates that patient and family factors resulting in psychological dysfunction need to be identified and referral made for treatment. There are certain time intervals when risk is increased. For example, patients may need extra care and communication in periods following hospitalization, as bronchial hyperresponsiveness persists after hospitalization much longer than abnormalities in spirometry, and oral steroids are being weaned, further increasing risk.

Clinician judgment is required to identify patients at risk. Such judgments will continue to have low specificity, with over identification, and may even have low sensitivity, as even patients with mild disease can die suddenly and unexpectedly.

III. Changing Gender Relationships of Asthma from Preteen Years to Adult

A. Incidence and Prevalence

Differences in prevalence of asthma in males and females have been of interest for many years. During childhood, boys have a greater prevalence than girls, with the maximum difference occurring before puberty. In adult years, asthma is more common in females. The shift from male to female predominance has been documented in several studies (70–72). For example, in the Teumseh study, the prevalence of both "probably" and "suggestive" asthma was higher in males than females through age 24, with mean rates from birth to 24 years 4.8% for "probably" asthma in males and 3.0 for females, compared to rates of 3.6% and 5.2%, respectively, in the 25 to 34 age group (70). Detailed analysis of asthma-related symptoms in Swiss children follows the same pattern (73,74). For example, night cough had a male predominance at age 7, equal male/female prevalence at age 12, and a female predominance at age 15.

Differences in male and female prevalence rates over increasing age can be explained by changes in incidence rates. In the Tucson epidemiologic study, males had an incidence of 1.4% per year between birth and four years, 1% per year between five and nine years, and were stable at 0.2% over the rest of the age range (72). Females had a slightly lower incidence of 0.9% between birth and four years, 0.7% between five and nine-years, and then fluctuating from

0.4% to 0.8% per year over the rest of the age range (72). A study of incidence rates in Rochester, Minnesota, found similar changes occurring with increasing age (71). The incidence rates for "definite" and "probably" asthma cases were higher for males than for females from infancy through nine years of age, but the reverse was true for the age group of 15 thorough 49 years of age (71). Recently a large survey in Europe estimated the age- and gender-specific incidence of asthma from birth to age 44 in men and women, and documented the same pattern of changes in incidence noted in Tecumseh, Tucson, and Rochester across the decades of life in all 16 countries studied (75).

The only study to demonstrate continued male predominance in incidence rates through adolescence was the National Child Development Study in the United Kingdom, following all children born in one week of 1958 and then through age 16 years (17). Anderson and colleagues found that boys were more likely to have both higher rates of current prevalence and development of new asthma through age 16 years (17). These investigators defined asthma as a positive response to questions of whether the child had had "attacks of asthma" or "attacks of bronchitis with wheezing" ever and then the number of attacks over the past 12 months. This study raises the issue of the impact of how asthma is defined on prevalence of asthma and gender differences in prevalence. Hendriksen and coworkers suggest that asthma may be under-diagnosed in adolescent girls (76). Most studies examining prevalence and incidence use a doctor diagnosis of asthma. In their study of children with current wheeze, more boys than girls with symptoms reported doctor diagnosis of asthma (44% vs. 32%, $p<0.02$) (76). In addition, patterns of asthma-related symptoms may differ in boys and girls, with boys having wheeze and night cough and girls having night cough alone (74). These different patterns may secondarily influence asthma diagnosis (73,74,77). While the weight of evidence on the effect of gender on asthma occurrence indicates an early male predominance followed by a switch to female predominance, careful attention to the details of asthma ascertainment must be considered in examining the details in individual studies.

B. Health Care Utilization

Much of the attention to gender differences has come from data related to health care utilization, indicating a much higher rate of hospital admission for asthma among prepubertal males than females (males were admitted nearly twice as often as females from birth through 10 years of age), a small but statistically significant female predominance during the ages of 11 to 20, with the continuing trend resulting in a female to male ratio of three to one between the ages of 20 and 50 (78–87). These patterns have been observed in an evaluation of hospital admissions in 67 hospitals in five counties of southeastern Pennsylvania for the period of 1986 through 1989 (78), in Canada for both admissions and readmissions from 1994 to 1997 (79), and in both admissions and readmissions over a 10-year period (1990–1999) in the St. Louis metropolitan area (85). Horwood compared rates of admission and readmission for asthma between boys and girls in three age groups, 0 to 4, 5 to 9 and 10 to 13 (81). Rates of admission were highest among preschoolers and lowest for 10 to 13-year-old. The male to female admission rates over the period of the survey were significantly greater for the 0 to 9 age groups with almost unity for the 10 to 13-year-old. Studies from the United States, Canada, England, New Zealand, the European community, and Finland all confirm this gender difference in hospitalization for asthma among children, with adolescent females being hospitalized more often than their male counterparts. Health care utilization for outpatient and emergency department visits also follow a similar pattern. In patients 2 to 13 years of age, utilization and medication variables within a health maintenance organization were significantly greater for male children, but females had more outpatient and emergency department visits and used more oral corticosteroids than males over the age range of 14 to 22 years. This difference was even greater for asthma utilization and severity during the adult years (88).

The reversal in asthma prevalence by gender during adolescence is not completely understood, but may relate to several factors, including hormonal and anatomical relationships. There is considerable evidence that estrogen and progesterone modify airway responsiveness (89). Female susceptibility to asthma in adulthood is at least partly explained by gender differences in the rate of lung growth and in airway size, with young males having smaller airways relative to lung size than girls, with equalization of airways caliber in adolescence (75,90,91). Gender differences in asthma with increasing age may relate to differences in hormonal status, potentially influencing airway inflammation and smooth muscle and vascular functions, although the specific effects have not been thoroughly defined (90). With increasing age, allergy rather than mechanical factors appear to become a predominant factor (77). Recently the increase in weight among preteen girls seems to be a factor influencing the tendency for more girls to have asthma in adolescence (92). A complete review of the evidence concerning gender (the sociocultural effect of being female or male) and sex concerning their complex interactions with the development of asthma and severity is discussed by Fuhlbrigge et al. (93).

C. Differential Diagnosis of Asthma

Given that symptoms of cough and wheeze can occur in many diseases, clinicians must be prepared to consider causes other than asthma when a patient presents with lower respiratory tract symptoms. Diseases that result in cough and wheeze other than asthma are particularly important to consider and should prompt the appropriate investigations to diagnose them

Table 3 Differential Diagnosis

Primarily cough
Rhinitis/sinusitis/post-nasal drip
Lower respiratory tract infection
 Mycoplasma pneumoniae
 Chlamydia pneumoniae
 Bordetella pertussis and *Bordetella parapertussis*
 Adenovirus pneumonia/bronchiolitis obliterans
 Cystic fibrosis (even presenting at a later age)
 Bronchiectasis (idiopathic or associated with immune deficiency)
Habit (psychogenic) cough
Drug-induced (ACE inhibitors)
 Cough associated with wheeze
Asthma
VCD, or primary vocal cord pathology
GER, with or without aspiration
Extrinsic airway compression
 Mediastinal mass producing narrowing of the airway (e.g., Hodgkin's disease, lymphoma, teratoma, other tumors)
 Granulomatous disease (e.g., histoplasmosis) causing mediastinal lymphadenopathy
 Other anatomic abnormalities, such as vascular ring, less likely to present in adolescence
Mass intrinsic to the airway (tumor such as bronchial adenoma)
Foreign body aspiration
Cardiac disease

---

in the setting of new onset symptoms or a sudden change in the severity of the clinical course. This is particularly important in the adolescent. While asthma may develop at any age, asthma symptoms begin prior to the age of five years in 80% of cases (71), and thus the development of symptoms in an adolescent without a prior history of asthma-like symptoms should prompt careful investigation. Table 3 gives some diseases that can cause symptoms similar to asthma.

Asthma is under-diagnosed in the adolescent age group. A study of 12- to 15-year old in Denmark without previously diagnosed asthma identified asthma in 29% of subjects (94). Undiagnosed asthma was associated with low physical activity, high body mass index (BMI), serious family problems, passive smoke exposure, and the absence of rhinitis. The authors note that two-thirds of those with undiagnosed asthma did not report their symptoms to a doctor, emphasizing the importance of routine screening for asthma during all physician contacts and the need for public education aimed at raising the awareness of asthma in the adolescent population.

Table 4 Factors That Increase Asthma Severity in Adolescence

Risk-taking behaviors
Cigarette smoking
Obesity
Exposure to violence
Stress and depression
Non-adherence

D. Vocal Cord Dysfunction (VCD)

VCD, a functional respiratory tract disorder resulting from paradoxical adduction of the vocal cords during inspiration, complicates the diagnosis and management of asthma (95). The recognition of VCD in a patient with atypical or difficult-to-control asthma is critical in minimizing symptoms and potential side effects associated with treatment of severe asthma.

VCD commonly presents during the period of adolescence (96,97). The true prevalence of VCD is unknown, but reports from tertiary care referral centers estimate that up to 40% of adult patients hospitalized for refractory asthma had VCD either independent (10%) or coexistent (30%) with asthma (98). Similar data are not available for children. The largest report of childhood VCD, consisting of 37 patients with laryngoscopy-confirmed VCD found VCD more commonly among females (68% of the 37 patients) and Caucasians (81%) (99). Twenty-nine of these children had coexisting asthma of apparently sufficient severity to have led to frequent acute care visits and a prior hospitalization in one-half of the patients. The majority of patients were academic achievers (84%) and/or athletes (61%). One-third of patients had prior psychiatric illness and 70% were identified as having a component of family dysfunction. Twenty-seven percent had either confirmed or strongly suspected prior sexual abuse.

IV. Factors That Increase Asthma Severity in Adolescence

A. Risk Behaviors

Overall risk for asthma severity, morbidity, and mortality must be considered in the context of risk factors that account for poor health outcomes in this age group in general. In the United States, approximately three-fourths of all deaths among persons aged 10 to 24 result from four causes: motor vehicle accidents, other unintentional injuries, homicide, and suicide (100). This survey demonstrates that numerous high school students engage in behaviors that increase their likelihood of death from these four causes. Additional other risk factors affecting health, which may relate to asthma, are noted. Nationwide, 63.9% of students had tried cigarette smoking.

Smoking cigarettes is particularly problematic given the effect on FEV_1 (discussed in the next section). Obesity has become a significant problem, with 10.5% of adolescents being overweight and 13.6% being at risk for obesity nationwide (100) (the relationship between obesity and asthma is discussed below). A related risk factor is the lack of exercise for adolescents. In the survey noted above 67.8% did not attend physical education class on a daily basis. On a national basis, 38.3% watched television three or more hours per day on an average school day (100). Exposure to violence is a contributor to unintentional injuries, and is a risk factor for asthma morbidity (101,102). Nationwide, 6.6% of students had missed one day of school or more during the preceding 30 days because they felt unsafe at school or on their way to school. Hispanic and African American students were significantly more likely to have missed school than white students because they felt unsafe. Six percent of students carried a weapon on school property and 9% had been threatened or injured with a weapon on school property one or more times during the previous 12 months (100). One can imagine the stress and anxiety a school child experiences under such circumstances, easily leading to a lowered priority for asthma management and possibly exaggerated bronchial lability.

B. Cigarette Smoking

Active cigarette smoking among children is for before the ages of 9 to 10, but the U.S. national statistics from the Centers for Disease Control suggest that experimentation with cigarettes (i.e., smoking less than one cigarette per day on a regular basis) occurs in as many as 15% in 9- to 11-year olds (103–105). By the time children attend high school, the prevalence of smoking as much as one cigarette per day is as high as 25% (103–105).

Several risk factors for smoking initiation in adolescence have been identified. Females are more likely to begin smoking than males, and smoking initiation among females has been associated with low self-esteem, desire to improve negative mood, control of weight, and rebelliousness (106). There appears to be a racial difference in smoking in adolescence, as it is highest among Caucasians (31.9%) and lowest among African Americans (14.7%) (106). Other risk factors include exposure to parents who smoke, lower levels of physical activity (107), and the presence of symptoms of depression (108).

The rate of smoking among asthmatic adolescents is comparable to that of non-asthmatics, and the risk factors for smoking initiation are similar between asthmatics and non-asthmatics (109). However, among 15- to 20-year-old students in Denmark, there were more daily smokers with asthma than without asthma (109), and those smokers with asthma smoked more than non-asthmatic smokers. However, if an asthmatic was taking asthma medications, they were less likely to smoke than those asthmatics not using asthma medications.

Active cigarette smoking by asthmatics in adolescence and early adulthood is associated with increased numbers of hospitalizations and emergency department visits, increased respiratory symptoms, lower levels of lung function, and increased levels of airways responsiveness (110–112).

The effects of cigarette smoking on pulmonary function can be divided into environmental tobacco smoke exposure and active smoking. In normal subjects, environmental tobacco smoke exposure is associated with 2.5% to 5% decrement in maximally attained level of FEV_1 by age 16 to 18 (112). It is currently thought that most of this effect in normal subjects occurs as a result of in utero exposure (111). However, childhood asthmatics exposed to environmental tobacco smoke have increased hospitalizations and emergency department visits, decreased levels of lung function, and increased airways responsiveness (111).

Unfortunately, the timing of cigarette smoking with regard to lung function and growth is critical in determining an effect. Children who smoke one cigarette per day between the ages of 10 and 16 can reduce their maximally attained level of FEV_1 by 10% (110–112). Comparable figures for childhood asthmatics are not available, but would be expected to be at least the effect seen in non-asthmatics. The extent to which the combination of asthma and smoking can lead to early and premature decline in FEV_1 and, hence, the development of chronic airflow obstruction, is currently unknown.

C. Obesity

The increasing prevalence of obesity in childhood represents one of the most urgent public health concerns today. The proportion of adolescents in the United States at or above the gender- and age-specific 95th percentile for BMI from 1963 to 1965 has increased markedly over the past three decades. Specifically, the proportion of overweight children so defined more than doubled from 1988 to 1994 to 11% among children aged 6 to 11 years (113). The prevalence of asthma has increased significantly during the last decades in a manner that appears parallel to that of obesity (114), suggesting to some that these trends may be related (115).

Large longitudinal studies have shown an association between incidence of asthma and BMI in female children (115,116). In females, becoming overweight or obese between 6 and 11 years of age increases the risk of developing new asthma symptoms and increased bronchial responsiveness during the early adolescent period (116).

The mechanisms that underlie the association between obesity and asthma are not well understood. It does not appear that the presence of asthma results in a restricted lifestyle with less physical activity, which could increase the risk of becoming overweight, as weight gain precedes the development of new asthma symptoms (117). A linear association has been reported between bronchial responsiveness to methacholine and BMI in adults (118), suggesting that the association is not due to either over-reporting or increased perception of asthma symptoms by overweight subjects. Bronchial hyperresponsiveness predisposes are to exercise-induced airway narrowing and symptoms, potentially leading obese asthmatics to restrict their lifestyle in an effort to prevent symptoms. Altered breathing patterns in overweight children may modify actin/myosin latching, thereby altering airway smooth muscle responsiveness (114). The effect of obesity on allergic sensitization has been inconsistent, with some studies suggesting either an increase (119) or lack of association between obesity and allergen sensitization (116,118). Overweight status has been shown to upregulate the production of leptin, a hormone that modifies responsiveness at both the β2-adrenergic and corticosteroid receptors (120,121). Finally, obesity is associated with an increased likelihood of gastroesophageal reflux (GER) (122), which may worsen asthma (123), although the role of GER as a determinant of increased asthma symptoms in overweight children has not been established.

If the association between overweight status and asthma is causal, weight reduction in overweight children with asthma should be associated with significant reduction in asthma symptoms. This has not been studied in the pediatric age group, but two studies in adults suggest that weight reduction in obese adult asthmatics improves peak flow variability (124) and lung function (124,125) and decreases rescue medication use (125).

D. Psychologic Factors: Stress and Depression

Stress is associated with worse asthma outcomes. Among children with moderate to severe asthma, experiencing an acute negative life event increased children's risk for an asthma attack four to six weeks after the event (126). Moreover, of children with ongoing chronic stress, those experiencing an acute life event had greater risk for an asthma attack within two weeks of the acute event (126). Life stressors have been associated with lower same-day peak expiratory flow and greater self-report of asthma symptoms (127). Additionally, the number of asthma exacerbations induced by colds was higher in adults with asthma who had high numbers of negative life events and low social support (128). Finally, perceived stress has been linked to the development of asthma-related symptoms. Reports of parental stress have been prospectively associated with risk of wheezing among children during the first two years of life (129).

In addition to stress, children with asthma are at increased risk for psychological distress and adjustment problems compared to healthy children (130). Furthermore, children with asthma appear to be at greater risk for depression than children with other chronic illnesses such as cystic fibrosis and cancer (131). The presence of depression impacts substantially upon asthma care and control through poor medication compliance (132). Alternatively, asthma may predispose individuals to emotional distress and depression as patients suffer through issues of self-image related to the fear of side effects (real and perceived) of asthma medications (133), and/or develop a sense of learned helplessness as they experience the unpredictability of asthma episodes (134).

The effects of stress and depression are most prominent in patients of lower socioeconomic status who experience greater exposure to stressful life events. In a study comparing adolescents with persistent asthma from high socioeconomic status to those from low socioeconomic status, we found that low socioeconomic status adolescents with asthma had higher levels of chronic stress, lower beliefs of control over their health, were more likely to report a severe acute life event during the previous six months, and were more likely to interpret an ambiguous life situation in a threatening manner (80). The low socioeconomic status children differed immunologically from the high socioeconomic status children, as reflected by elevated IL-5 and IFN-γ stimulated cytokine levels. These findings indicate that socioeconomic status affects multiple dimensions of stress in adolescents, including both stress exposure (more ongoing burdens, events of greater severity) and stress appraisals (perceiving the same event in a more threatening fashion).

V. Issues of Adherence and Self Care

A. Asthma in the Context of Adolescence

It should be as apparent to the asthma specialist as it is to the primary care physician that asthma in the adolescent represents not only the problem of the chronic illness, but of the unique issues concerning adolescence generally. This is especially of concern when it comes to adherence to prescribed medication, as well as avoiding those behaviors and activities that could lead to asthma exacerbations.

B. Chronic Illness and Adolescence

The problems that adolescents have in dealing with their asthma are no different than the problems they have in dealing with chronic disease in general. The thinking of the adolescent is widely different from doctors who prescribe therapies. While doctors think of future consequences and potential risks and benefits, adolescents are oriented in the present time (135). Even in as serious a situation as continuing immunosuppressive medication in post-transplant cases, non-adherence is a leading cause of morbidity. A postrenal transplant adolescent will risk transplant rejection by discontinuing immunosuppressive medications because of side effects of the medications, especially those that affect their appearance (136). Recently, a report of medication adherence among pediatric and adolescent liver transplant recipients noted that the transition of responsibility for medication taking occurred approximately at 12 years of age. Forgetfulness was cited as the most common reason for non-adherence by patients and caregivers (137). Psychological factors such as the personal meaning of illness and its treatment, attitude, and emotional well-being all exert a great influence on the adolescent's adherence, but family, peer, and health provider support are also essential to good outcomes. Adolescent-s needs attention as an individual and consideration of lifestyle (138). Adolescents and doctors often emphasize different aspects of the illness. Adolescents may feel stigmatized by having asthma and attempt to conceal their disease and its medications (139). The patient may focus on the difficulties in the social domain and the impact of their illness on their lives, while the physician sees the illness primarily as a pathophysiologic problem that affects the patient's physical body or may focus on the task of intervening rather than relating to the patient (140).

Non-adherence with chronic illness regimens is high among school aged children and adolescents with rates ranging from 17% to 64%. Non-adherence rates are higher among adolescents than adults (141) and school children (140,141). In diabetes mellitus, parents often withdrew from the insulin adjustment process as their adolescent became older, with parental participation virtually eliminated by the time the child reached 15 years of age (142). Parental withdrawal, though, was not always balanced by the adolescent's assumption of responsibility for insulin adjustments. Adolescents who are less cognitively mature than expected by their age may be given responsibility for self-managerial behaviors for which they are not capable. This situation in respect to asthma is exemplified by the study of Walders and colleagues (143). They examined the allocation of family responsibility for asthma management tasks in African American adolescents. Caretakers overestimated the capability of their older adolescents to assume responsibility and overlooked evidence of declining responsibility for asthma management with older adolescents. These patterns resulted in increased non-adherence and functional morbidity. Primary maternal factors may also be a factor in non-adherence to prescribed asthma medications. A study of elementary school children showed that maternal high depressive symptoms were related to children not using their inhalers properly and forgetting doses (144).

C. Adherence to Asthma Treatment

In children with asthma the average medication adherence rate is 48% (145). Adolescents are repeatedly reported to have less adherence to treatment than younger children or adults (141,145–147). This issue is exacerbated among those families living in the inner-city environment (143,148–150).

In general, children with asthma take only 40% to 70% of prescribed medication when estimated by canister weight (145,151,152). Adherence measured by electronic devices is even lower (145). There is individual variation in adherence and resulting morbidity because of non-adherence. Children who had frequent exacerbations requiring oral corticosteroid bursts had a median adherence of 13.7% compared to a median adherence of 68.2% in those who were well controlled (153).

There is little concurrence about the best intervention to correct the problem of poor adherence to treatment regimens (154). In the review by Bender, Milgrom, and Apter, one-half of the studies reviewed found that the experimental intervention did not change adherence; behavior change reported by patients was often not accompanied by changes in treatment success; and a variety of methods were used among the studies resulting in contradictory findings and varying quality (154). Physicians must also take some responsibility for adherence by their adolescent patients. Following the National Asthma Education and Prevention Program Guidelines for the Diagnosis and Management of Asthma (155) reflects good care, but there are still deficits in physician understanding and implementation of these guidelines (156). Adherence must be addressed during visits using approaches that give permission for more honest answers rather than prompting the adolescent to say what is expected to please the physician. Questions such as, "What happens when you miss your medicine?" or, "Are you having any difficulty remembering to take your medicine?" may be useful. The ability of the physician to practice the art of care may influence the patient's perception of the doctor more than the doctor's technical quality of care. In the absence of artful care the patient may then perceive the technical quality as being less than adequate and lose confidence, leading to non-adherence (140). Non-adherence in the adolescent is best identified early by these non-judgmental questions about current or previous regimen behavior. An appreciation of the relevant psychological and social issues can suggest to the clinician which adolescents are at high risk for non-adherence. Even if there are no proven intervention techniques, the personal characteristics of the physician may determine whether the physician can work productively with the non-adherent adolescent (157).

VI. Conclusion

The approach to the adolescent presenting with recurrent cough and wheeze presents complex diagnostic and management challenges to the clinician. While adolescents can be frustrating, caring for a chronic disease in partnership with them can be very rewarding. Essential to the development of these rewards is establishing a good relationship with the adolescent. A clinician must respect the adolescent and the capacity of the adolescent to deal with the illness in cooperation with the medical team. The clinician must look the adolescent in the eye, shake hands, and conduct the interview and negotiations about care with the adolescent, seeking support from the parents, but dealing with the patient directly and not through the parents. Even more than in other age groups, the major barrier to improving outcomes is adherence to medical regimens and lifestyles known to be beneficial. Medications have improved both in effectiveness and ease of use, but understanding of behavior and development of techniques to promote the use of effective medications remain elusive. Only good patient–physician relationships can improve adherence and outcomes.

References

1. Akinbami LJ, Schoendorf KC. Trends in childhood asthma: prevalence, health care utilization, and mortality. Pediatrics 2002; 110:315–322.
2. Roorda RJ, Gerritsen J, Van Aalderen WM, Schouten JP, Veltman JC, Weiss ST, Knol K. Risk factors for the persistence of respiratory symptoms in childhood asthma. Am Rev Respir Dis 1993; 148:1490–1495.
3. Flensborg E. The prognosis for bronchial asthma arisen in infancy, after the nonspecific treatment hitherto applied. Acta Paediatr (Uppsala) 1945; 33: 4–24.
4. Rackemann F, Edwards M. Asthma in children—a follow-up study of 688 patients after an interval of twenty years. N Engl J Med 1952; 246:815–823, 858–863.
5. Ryssing E. Continued follow-up investigation concerning the fate of 298 asthmatic children. Acta Paediatr 1959; 48:255–260.
6. Ogilvie A. Asthma: a study in prognosis of 1000 patients. Thorax 1962; 17: 183–189.
7. Aas K. Prognosis for Asthmatic Children. Acta Paediatr Scand 1963; 52: 87–88.
8. Kraepelien S. Prognosis of asthma in childhood with special reference to pulmonary function and the value of specific hyposensitization. Acta Paediatr (Uppsala) 1963; 140:92–93.
9. McNicol K, Williams H. Spectrum of asthma in children—I, clinical and physiological components. Br Med J 1973; 4:7–11.
10. Ryssing E, Flensborg E. Prognosis after puberty for 442 asthmatic children examined and treated on specific allergologic principles. Acta Paediatr 1963; 52:97–105.
11. Barr L, Logan G. Prognosis of children having asthma. Pediatrics 1964; 34: 856–860.
12. Buffum W, Settipane G. Prognosis of asthma in childhood. Am J Dis Child 1966; 112:214–217.
13. Johnstone D. A study of the natural history of bronchial asthma in children. Am J Dis Child 1968; 115:213–216.
14. Blair H. Natural history of childhood asthma. Arch Dis Child 1977; 52: 613–619.

15. Martin A, McLennan L, Landau L, Phelan P. The natural history of childhood asthma to adult life. Br Med J 1980; 281:1397–1400.

16. Martin A, Landau L, Phelan P. Asthma from childhood at age 21: the patient and his disease. Br Med J 1982; 284:380–382.

17. Anderson H, Bland J, Patel S, Peckham C. The natural history of asthma in childhood. J Epidemiol Community Health 1986; 40:121–129.

18. Bronnimann S, Burrows B. A prospective study of the natural history of asthma. Chest 1986; 90:480–484.

19. Burrows B. The natural history of asthma. J All Clin Immunol 1987; 80: 373–377.

20. Jonsson J, Boe J, Berlin E. The long-term prognosis of childhood asthma in a predominantly rural Swedish county. Acta Paediatr Scand 1987; 76:950–954.

21. Kelly W, Hudson I, Phelan P, Pain M, Olinsky A. Childhood asthma in adult life: a further study at 28 years of age. Br Med J 1987; 294:1059–1062.

22. Cserhati E, Mezei G, Kelemen J. Late prognosis of bronchial asthma in children. Respiration 1984; 46:160–165.

23. Gerritsen J, Koeter G, Postma D, Schouten J, Knol K. Prognosis of asthma from childhood to adulthood. Am Rev Respir Dis 1989; 140:1325–1330.

24. Lebowitz M, Holberg C, Martinez F. A longitudinal study of risk factors in asthma and chronic bronchitis in childhood. Eur J Epidemiol 1990; 6: 341–347.

25. Godden D, Ross S, Abdalla M, McMurray D, Douglas A, Oldman D, Friend JAR, Legge JS, Douglas JG. Outcome of wheeze in childhood: symptoms and pulmonary function 25 years later. Am J Respir Crit Care Med 1994; 149:106– 112.

26. Jenkins M, Hopper J, Bowes G, Carlin J, Flander L, Giles G. Factors in childhood as predictors of asthma in adult life. Br Med J 1994; 309:90–93.

27. Ulrik C, Backer V, Dirksen A, Pedersen M, Koch C. Extrinsic and intrinsic asthma from childhood to adult age: a 10-year follow-up. Respir Med 1995; 89:547–554.

28. Strachan DP, Butland BK, Anderson HR. Incidence and prognosis of asthma and wheezing illness from early childhood to age 33 in a national British cohort. BMJ 1996; 312:1195–1199.

29. Panhuysen C, Vonk J, Koeter G, Schouten JP, van Altena R, Bleecker ER, Postma DS. Adult patients may outgrow their asthma: a 25-year follow-up study. Am J Respir Crit Care Med 1997; 155:1267–1272.

30. Gold D, Wypij D, Wang X, Speizer FE, Pugh M, Ware JH, Ferris BG, Dockery DW. Gender- and race-specific effects of asthma and wheeze on level and growth of lung function in children in sex U.S. cities. Am J Respir Crit Care Med 1994; 149:1198–1208.

31. Kerrebijn K, Fioole A, van Bentveld R. Lung function in asthmatic children after year or more without symptoms or treatment. Br Med J 1978; 1: 886–888.

32. Gruber W, Eber E, Steinbrugger B, Modl M, Weinhandl E, Zach MS. Atopy, lung function and bronchial responsiveness in symptom-free paediatric asthma patients. Eur Respir J 1997; 10:1041–1045.

33. Canny G, Levison H. Pulmonary function abnormalities during apparent clinical remission in childhood asthma. J All Clin Immunol 1988; 82:1–3.
34. Cooper D, Cutz E, Levison H. Occult pulmonary abnormalities in asymptomatic asthmatic children. Chest 1977; 71:361–365.
35. Cade J, Pain M. Pulmonary function during clinical remission of asthma: How reversible is asthma? Aust N Z J Med 1973; 3:545–551.
36. Obase Y, Shimoda T, Kawano T, Saeki S, Tomari S, Izaki K, Fukushima C, Matsuse H, Kohno S. Bronchial hyperresponsiveness and airway inflammation in adolescents with asymptomatic childhood asthma. Allergy 2002; 58:213–220.
37. Blackhall MI. Ventilatory function in subjects with childhood asthma who have become symptom free. Arch Dis Child 1970; 45:363–366.
38. van den Toorn LM, Overbeek SE, de Jongste JC, Leman K, Hoogsteden HC, Prins JB. Airway inflammation is present during clinical remission of atopic asthma. Am J Respir Crit Care Med 2001; 164:2107–2113.
39. Warke T, Fitch P, Brown V, Taylor R, Lyons JD, Ennis M, Shields MD. Outgrown asthma does not mean no airways inflammation. Eur Respir J 2002; 19:284–287.
40. Kelly W, Hudson I, Raven J, Phelan P, Pain M, Olinsky A. Childhood asthma and adult lung function. Am Rev Respir Dis 1988; 138:26–30.
41. Martin D, Landau K, Phelan P. Lung function in young adults who had asthma in childhood. Am Rev Respir Dis 1980; 122:609–616.
42. Zeiger R, Dawson C, Weiss S. Relationships between duration of asthma and asthma severity among children in the Childhood Asthma Management Program (CAMP). J All Clin Immunol 1999; 103:376–387.
43. Weiss ST, Van Natta ML, Zeiger RS. Relationship between increased airway responsiveness and asthma severity in the childhood asthma management program. Am J Respir Crit Care Med 2000; 162:50–56.
44. National Center for Health Statistics. Asthma prevalence, health care use and mortality, 2000–2001. Hyattsville, MD: U.S. Department of Health and Human Services, Centers for Disease Control and Prevention, National Center for Health Statistics, 2003.
45. Mannino D, Homa D, Pertowski C, Ashizawa A, Nixon LL, Johnson CA, Ball LB, Jack E, Kang DS. Surveillance for Asthma—United States, 1960–1995. CDC Surveillance Summaries, April 24, 1998. MMWR. Vol. 47 (No. SS-1), 1998.
46. Moorman JE, Mannino DM. Increasing U.S. asthma mortality rates: who is really dying? J Asthma 2001; 38:65–71.
47. Strunk R, Mrazek D, Fuhrmann G, LaBrecque J. Physiologic and psychological characteristics associated with deaths due to asthma in childhood. A case-controlled study. JAMA 1985; 254:1193–1198.
48. Strunk R. Deaths from asthma in childhood: patterns before and after professional intervention. Pediatr Asthma All Immunol 1987; 1:5–13.
49. Rea H, Scragg R, Jackson R, Beaglehole R, Fenwick J, Sutherland D. A case-control study of deaths of asthma. Thorax 1986; 41:833–839.
50. Bateman JRM, Clarke SW. Sudden death in asthma. Thorax 1979; 34:40–44.

51. Wasserfallen J-B, Schaller M-D, Feihl F, Perret C. Sudden asphyxic asthma: a distinct entity? Am Rev Respir Dis 1990; 142:108–111.

52. Sur S, Crotty T, Kephart G, Hyma BA, Colby TV, Reed CE, Hunt LW, Gleich GJ. Sudden-onset fatal asthma. A distinct entity with few eosinophils and relatively more neutrophils in the airway submucosa? Am Rev Respir Dis 1993; 148:713–719

53. Saetta M, Thiene G, Crescioli S, Fabbri L. Fatal asthma in a young patient with severe bronchial hyperresponsiveness but stable peak flow records. Eur Respir J 1989; 2:1008–1012.

54. Strunk R, Nicklas R, Milgrom H, Davis M, Ikle D. Risk factors for fatal asthma. In: Sheffer AL, ed. Fatal Asthma. Vol. 115. New York: Marcel Dekker Inc., 1998:31–44.

55. Strunk R. Death due to asthma. New insights into sudden unexpected deaths, but the focus remains on prevention. Am Rev Respir Dis 1993; 148:550–552.

56. Jorgensen IM, Jensen VB, Bulow S, Dahm TL, Prahl P, Juel K. Asthma mortality in the Danish child population: risk factors and causes of asthma death. Pediatr Pulmonol 2003; 36:142–147.

57. O'Hallaren M, Yuninger J, Offord K, Somers MJ, O'Connell EJ, Ballard DJ, Sachs MI. Exposure to an aeroallergen as a possible precipitating factor in respiratory arrest in young patients with asthma. N Engl J Med 1991; 324:359–363.

58. Roberts G, Patel N, Levi-Schaffer F, Habibi P, Lack G. Food allergy as a risk factor for life-threatening asthma in childhood: a case-controlled study. J All Clin Immunol 2003; 112:168–174.

59. Miller B, Strunk R. Circumstances surrounding the deaths of children due to asthma. Am J Dis Child 1989; 143:1294–1299.

60. Boulet LP, Deschesnes F, Turcotte H, Gignac F. Near-fatal asthma: clinical and physiologic features, perception of bronchoconstriction, and psychologic profile. J All Clin Immunol 1991; 88:838–846.

61. Sturdy PM, Victor CR, Anderson HR, Bland JM, Butland BK, Harrison BD, Peckitt C, Taylor JC. Psychological, social and health behaviour risk factors for deaths certified as asthma: a national case-control study. Thorax 2002; 57:1034–1039.

62. Goldman M, Rachmiel M, Gendler L, Katz Y. Decrease in asthma mortality rate in Israel from 1991–1995: is it related to increased use of inhaled corticosteroids? J All Clin Immunol 2000; 105:71–74.

63. Targonski P, Persky V, Orris P, Addington W. Trends in asthma mortality among African Americans and whites in Chicago, 1968–1991. Am J Public Health 1994; 84:1830–1833.

64. Lang D, Polansky M. Patterns of asthma mortality in Philadelphia from 1969–1991. N Engl J Med 1994; 331:1542–1546.

65. Marder D, Targonski P, Orris P, Persky V, Addington W. Effect of racial and socioeconomic factors on asthma mortality in Chicago. Chest 1992; 101: 426s–429s.

66. Grant E, Weiss K. Socioeconomic risk factors for asthma mortality. In: Sheffer A, ed. Fatal Asthma. Vol. 115. New York: Marcel Dekker Inc., 1998:237–255.

67. Bock S, Munoz-Furlong A, Sampson H. Fatalities due to anaphylactic reactions to foods. J All Clin Immunol 2001; 107.

68. Porter FL, White D, Attaway N, Miller JP, Strunk RC. Absence of diurnal variability of airway reactivity and hypoxic ventilatory drive in adolescents with stable asthma. J All Clin Immunol 1999; 103:804–809.

69. Robertson C, Rubinfeld A, Bowes G. Pediatric asthma deaths in Victoria: The mild are at risk. Ped Pulm 1992; 13:95–100.

70. Broder I, Higgins M, Matthew K, Keller J. Epidemiology of asthma and allergic rhinitis in a total community: Tecumseh, Michigan: III second survey of the community. J All 1974; 53:127–138.

71. Yunginger J, Reed C, O'Connell E, Melton LI, O'Fallon W, Silverstein M. A community-based study of the epidemiology of asthma. Am Rev Respir Dis 1992; 146:888–894.

72. Dodge R, Burrows B. The prevalence and incidence of asthma-like symptoms in a general population sample. Am Rev Respir Dis 1980; 122:567–575.

73. Sennhauser FH, Kuhni C. Prevalence of respiratory symptoms in swiss children: Is bronchial asthma really more prevalent in boys? Pediatr Pulmonol 1995; 19:161–166.

74. Kuhni C, Sennhauser FH. The yentl syndrome in childhood asthma: risk factors for undertreatment in swiss children. Pediatr Pulmonol 1995; 19: 156–160.

75. de Marco R, Locatello F, Sunyer J, Burney PG, Group ECRHSS. Differences in incidence of reported asthma related to age in men and women, a retrospective analysis of the data of the European Respiratory Health Survey. Am J Respir Crit Care Med 2000; 162:68–74.

76. Hendriksen A, Holmen T, Bjermer L. Gender differences in asthma prevalence may depend on how asthma is defined. Respir Med 2003; 97:491–497.

77. Weiss S, Gold DR. Gender differences in asthma: guest editorial. Pediatr Pulmonol 1995; 19:153–155.

78. Skobeloff EM, Spivey WH, St Clair SS, Schoffstall JM. The influence of age and sex on asthma admissions. JAMA 1992; 268:3437–3440.

79. Chen Y, Stewart P, Johansen H, McRae L, Taylor G. Sex difference in hospitalization due to asthma in relation of age. J Clin Epidemiol 2003; 56: 180–187.

80. Chen E, Fisher EB, Bacharier LB, Strunk RC. Socioeconomic status, stress, and immune markers in adolescents with asthma. Psychosom Med 2003; 65: 984–992.

81. Horwood LJ, Dawson KP, Mogridge N. Admission patterns for childhood acute asthma: Christchurch 1974–1989. N Z Med J 1991; 104:277–279.

82. Wilkins K, Mao Y. Trends in rates of admission to hospital and death from asthma among children and young adults in Canada during the 1980's. Can Med Assoc J 1993; 148:185–190.

83. Mitchell EA, Borman B. Demographic characteristics of asthma admissions to hospitals. N Z Med J 1986; 99:576–579.

84. Korhonen K, Reifonen T, Malmstrom K, Klaukka T, Remes K, Korppi M. Hospitalization trends for paediatric asthma in eastern Finland: a 10 year survey. Eur Respir J 2002; 19:1035–1039.

85. Bloomberg GR, Trinkaus KM, Fisher EB Jr, Musick JR, Strunk RC. Hospital readmissions for childhood asthma: a 10-year metropolitan study. Am J Respir Crit Care Med 2003; 167:1068–1076.
86. Morrison DS, McLoone P. Changing patterns of hospital admission for asthma, 1981–1997. Thorax 2001; 56:687–690.
87. Gergen P, Weiss K. Changing patterns of asthma hospitalization among children: 1979–1987. AJDC 1990; 144:1189–1194.
88. Schatz M, Camargo CA Jr. The relationship of sex to asthma prevalence, health care utilization, and medications in a large managed care organization. Ann All Asthma Immunol 2003; 91:553–558.
89. Haggerty CL, Ness RB, Kelsey S, Waterer G. The impact of estrogen and progesterone on asthma. Ann All Asthma Immunol 2003; 90:284–291.
90. Redline S, Gold DR. Challenges in interpreting gender differences in asthma. Am J Respir Crit Care Med 1994; 150:1219–1221.
91. Kanner R, Connett J, Altose M, Buist AS, Lee WW, Tashkin DP, Wise RA. Lung Health Study Research Group. Gender Difference in Airway Hyperresponsiveness in Smokers with Mild COPD. Am J Respir Crit Care Med 1994; 150:956–961.
92. Castro-Rodriguez JA, Holberg CJ, Morgan WJ, Wright AL, Martinez FD. Increased incidence of asthmalike symptoms in girls who become overweight or obese during the school years. Am J Respir Crit Care Med 2001; 163: 1344–1349.
93. Fuhlbrigge AL, Jackson B, Wright R. Gender and asthma. Immunol All Clin North Am 2002; 22:753–789.
94. Siersted HC, Boldsen J, Hansen HS, Mostgaard G, Hyldebrandt N. Population based study of risk factors for underdiagnosis of asthma in adolescence: odense schoolchild study. Br Med J 1998; 316:651–655.
95. Bacharier LB, Strunk RC. Vocal cord dysfunction: a practical approach. J Respir Dis 2001; 3:42–48.
96. Landwehr LP, Wood RP II, Blager FB, Milgrom H. Vocal cord dysfunction mimicking exercise-induced bronchospasm in adolescents. Pediatrics 1996; 98: 971–974.
97. Powell DM, Karanfilov BI, Beechler KB, Treole K, Trudeau MD, Forrest LA. Paradoxical vocal cord dysfunction in juveniles. Arch Otolaryngol Head Neck Surg 2000; 126:29–34.
98. Newman K, Dubester S. Vocal cord dysfunction: masquerader of asthma. Sem Respir Crit Care Med 1994; 15:161–167.
99. Brugman S, Howell J, Rosenberg D, Blager F, Lack G. The spectrum of pediatric vocal cord dysfunction. Am J Respir Crit Care Med 1994; 149:A353.
100. Grunbaum J, Kann L, Kinchen S, Williams B, Ross JG, Lowry R, Kolbe L. Youth Risk Behavior Surveillance-United States, 2001. Surveillance Summaries. MMWR 2002; 51:1–64.
101. Wright RJ, Steinbach SF. Violence: an unrecognized environmental exposure that may contribute to greater asthma morbidity in high risk inner-city populations. Environ Health Perspect 2001; 109:1085–108.

102. Wright R, Mitchell H, Visness C, Cohen S, Stout JW, Evans R, Gold DR. Community violence and athma morbidity: the inner-city asthma study. Am J Public Health 2004; 94:625–632.

103. MacDorman M, Minino A, Strobino D, Guyer B. Annual summary of vital statistics—2001. Pediatrics 2002; 110:1037–1052.

104. Kann L, Kinchen S, Williams B, Ross JG, Lowry R, Grunbaum JA, Kolb LL. Youth risk behavior surveillance—United States, 1999. MMWR CDC Surveill Summ 2000; 49:1–32.

105. Martin J, Peruga A. The global youth tobacco survey: results in the Americas. Epidemiol Bull 2002; 23:6–9.

106. Vickers KS, Thomas JL, Patten CA, Mrazek DA. Prevention of tobacco use in adolescents: review of current findings and implications for healthcare providers. Curr Opin Pediatr 2002; 14:708–712.

107. DuRant RH, Smith JA. Adolescent tobacco use and cessation. Prim Care 1999; 26:553–575.

108. Tercyak KP. Psychosocial risk factors for tobacco use among adolescents with asthma. J Pediatr Psychol 2003; 28:495–504.

109. Precht DH, Keiding L, Madsen M. Smoking patterns among adolescents with asthma attending upper secondary schools: a community-based study. Pediatrics 2003; 111:e562–e568.

110. Tager I. Smoking and childhook asthma-where do we stand? Am J Respir Crit Care Med 1998; 158:349–351.

111. Tager I, Weiss S, Munoz A, Rosner B, Speizer F. Longitudinal study of the effects of maternal smoking on pulmonary function in children. N Engl J Med 1983; 309:699–703.

112. Tager I, Segal M, Speizer F, Weiss S. The natural history of forced expiratory volumes. Effect of cigarcttc smoking and respiratory symptoms. Am Rev Resir Dis 1988; 138:837–849.

113. Troiano RP, Flegal KM. Overweight children and adolescents: description, epidemiology, and demographics. Pediatrics 1998; 101:497–504.

114. Tantisira KG, Weiss ST. Complex interactions in complex traits: obesity and asthma. Thorax 2001; 56(suppl 2):ii64–ii73.

115. Chinn S. Obesity and asthma: evidence for and against a causal relation. J Asthma 2003; 40:1–16.

116. Castro-Rodriquez J, Holberg C, Morgan W, Wright AL, Martinez FD. Increased incidence of asthma-like symptoms in girls who become overweight or obese during the school years. Am J Respir Crit Care Med 2001; 163: 1344–1399.

117. Chinn S, Rona RJ. Can the increase in body mass index explain the rising trend in asthma in children? Thorax 2001; 56:845–850.

118. Jarvis D, Chinn S, Potts J, Burney P. Association of body mass index with respiratory symptoms and atopy: results from the European Community Respiratory Health Survey. Clin Exp All 2002; 32:831–837.

119. Huang SL, Shiao G, Chou P. Association between body mass index and allergy in teenage girls in Taiwan. Clin Exp All 1999; 29:323–329.

120. Ogard CG, Bratholm P, Kristensen LO, Almdal T, Christensen NJ. Lymphocyte glucocorticoid receptor mRNA correlates negatively to serum leptin in normal weight subjects. Int J Obes Relat Metab Disord 2000; 24:915–919.
121. Eikelis N, Schlaich M, Aggarwal A, Kaye D, Esler M. Interactions between leptin and the human sympathetic nervous system. Hypertension 2003; 41: 1072–1079.
122. Locke GR III, Talley NJ, Fett SL, Zinsmeister AR, Melton LJ III. Risk factors associated with symptoms of gastroesophageal reflux. Am J Med 1999; 106:642–649.
123. Gislason T, Janson C, Vermeire P, Plaschke P, Bjornsson E, Gislason D, Boman G. Respiratory symptoms and nocturnal gastroesophageal reflux: a population-based study of young adults in three European countries. Chest 2002; 121:158–163.
124. Hakala K, Stenius-Aarniala B, Sovijarvi A. Effects of weight loss on peak flow variability, airways obstruction, and lung volumes in obese patients with asthma. Chest 2000; 118:1315–1321.
125. Stenius-Aarniala B, Poussa T, Kvarnstrom J, Gronlund EL, Ylikahri M, Mustajoki P. Immediate and long term effects of weight reduction in obese people with asthma: randomised controlled study. Br Med J 2000; 320:827–832.
126. Sandberg S, Paton JY, Ahola S, McCann DC, McGuinness D, Hillary CR, Oja H. The role of acute and chronic stress in asthma attacks in children. Lancet 2000; 356:982–987.
127. Smyth J, Spoefer M, Hurewitz A, Kliment A, Stone A. Daily psychosocial factors predict levels and diurnal cycles of asthma symptomatology and peak flow. J Behavioral Med 1999; 22:1999.
128. Smith A, Nicholson K. Psychosocial factors, respiratory viruses and exacerbation of asthma. Psychoneuroendocrinology 2001; 26:411–420.
129. Wright RJ, Cohen S, Carey V, Weiss ST, Gold DR. Parental stress as a predictor of wheezing in infancy: a prospective birth-cohort study. Am J Respir Crit Care Med 2002; 165:358–365.
130. Gillaspy SR, Hoff AL, Mullins LL, Van Pelt JC, Chaney JM. Psychological distress in high-risk youth with asthma. J Pediatr Psychol 2002; 27:363–371.
131. Bennett DS. Depression among children with chronic medical problems: a meta-analysis. J Pediatr Psychol 1994; 19:149–169.
132. Galil N. Depression and asthma in children. Curr Opin Pediatr 2000; 12: 331–335.
133. Gizynski M, Shapiro V. Depression and childhood illness. Child Adolesc Social Work 1990; 7:179–197.
134. Chaney JM, Mullins LL, Uretsky DL, Pace TM, Werden D, Hartman VL. An experimental examination of learned helplessness in older adolescents and young adults with long-standing asthma. J Pediatr Psychol 1999; 24:259–270.
135. Blum R. Compliance in the adolescent with chronic illness. Semin Adolesc Med 1987; 3:157–162.
136. Korsch B, Fine R, Negrette V. Non-compliance in children with renal transplants. Pediatrics 1976; 61:872–876.
137. Shemesh E, Shneider BL, Savitzky JK, Arnott, Lindsay, Gondolesi, Gabriel E, Krieger, Nancy R, Kerkar, Nanda, Magid, Margret S , Stuber, Margaret L,

Schmeidler, James, Yehuda, Rachel, Emre, Sukru. Medication adherence in pediatric and adolescent liver transplant recipients. Pediatrics 2004; 113:825–832.

138. Kyngas H, Kroll T, Duffy M. Compliance in adolescents with chronic diseases: a review. J Adolesc Health 2000; 26:379–386.

139. George MR, Apter A. Improving adherence to asthma medications. Clin Pulmonary Med 2001; 8:257–264.

140. Liptac G. Enhancing patient compliance in pediatrics. Pediatr Rev 1996; 17: 128–134.

141. Pidgeon V. Compliance with chronic illness regimens: school aged children and adolescents. J Pediatric Nursing 1989; 4:36–47.

142. Ingersoll G, Orr D, Herrold A, Golden M. Cognitive maturity and self-management among adolescents with insulin-dependent diabetes mellitus. J Pediatr 1986; 108:620–623.

143. Walders N, Drotar D, Kercsmar C. The allocation of family responisibility for asthma management tasks in African-American adolescents. J Asthma 2000; 37:89–99.

144. Bartlett SJ, Krishnan JA, Riekert KA, Butz A, Malveaux F, Rand C. Maternal depressive symptoms and adherence in inner-city children with asthma. Pediatrics 2004; 113:229–237.

145. Bender B, Wamboldt FS, O'Connor SL, Rand C, Szefler SJ, Milgrom H. Measurement of children's asthma medication adherence by self report, mother report, canister weight, and Doser CT. Ann All Asthma Immunol 2000; 85:416–421.

146. Fotheringham M, Sawyer M. Adherence to recommended medical regimens in childhood and adolescence. J Paediatr Child Health 1995; 31:72–78.

147. McQuaid EL, Kopel S, Klein R, Fritz GK. Medication adherence in pediatric asthma: Reasoning, responsibility, and behavior. J Pediatr Psychol 2003; 28: 323–333.

148. Redline S, Wright E, Kattan M, Kercsmar C, Weiss K. Short-term compliance with peak flow monitoring: results from a study of inner-city children with asthma. Pediatr Pulmonol 1996; 21:203–210.

149. Eggleston P, Malveaux F, Butz A, Huss K, Thompson L, Kolodner K, Rand CS. Medications used by children with asthma living in the inner city. Pediatrics 1998; 101:349–354.

150. Winkelstein ML, Huss K, Butz AM, Eggleston P, Vargas P, Rand CS. Factors associated with medication self-administration in children with asthma. Clin Pediatr 2000; 39:337–345.

151. Burkhart P, Dunbar-Jacob J, Rohav J. Accuracy of children's self-reported adherence to treatment. J Nurs Scholarsh 2001; 33:27–32.

152. Celano M, Geller R, Phillips K, Ziman R. Treatment adherence among low-income children with asthma. J Pediatr Psychol 1998; 23:345–349.

153. Milgrom H, Bender B, Ackerson L, Bowry P, Smith B, Rand C. Noncompliance and treatment failure in children with asthma. J All Clin Immunol 1996; 98:1051–1057.

154. Bender B, Milgrom H, Apter A. Adherence intervention research: What have we learned and what do we do next? J All Clin Immunol 2003; 112:489–494.

155. Expert Panel Report 2: National Heart, Lung, and Blood Institute, National Institutes of Health. Guidelines for the Diagnosis and Management of Asthma: NIH Publication No. 97–4053, 1997.

156. Doerschug K, Peterson M, Dayton C, Kline J. Asthma guidelines, An assessment of physician understanding and practice. Am J Respir Crit Care Med 1999; 159:1735–1741.

157. Friedman I, Litt I. Promoting adolescent's compliance with therapeutic regimens. Pediatr Clinics N Am 1986; 33:955–973.

158. Martin A, Landau L, Phelan P. Natural history of allergy in asthmatic children followed to adult life. Med J Aust 1981; 2:470–474.

159. Roorda R, Gerritsen J, van Aaderen W, Knol K. Skin reactivity and eosinophil count in relation to the outcome of childhood asthma. Eur Respir J 1993; 6:509–516.

160. Kelly W, Hudson I, Phelan P, Pain M, Olinsky A. Atopy in subjects with asthma followed to age of 28 years. J All Clin Immunol 1990; 85:548–557.

161. O'Connor G, Sparrow D, Weiss S. The role of allergy and nonspecific airway hyperresponsiveness in the pathogenesis of chronic obstructive pulmoanry disease. Am Rev Resir Dis 1989; 140:225–252.

162. Platts-Mills T, Sporik R, Wheatley L, Heymann P. Is there a dose-response relationship between exposure to indoor allergens and symptoms of asthma? Editorial. J All Clin Immunol 1995; 96:435–440.

163. Popp W, Bock A, Herkner K, Wagner C, Zwick H, Sertl K. Factors contributing to the occurrence and predictability of bronchial hyperresponsiveness to methacholine in children. J All Clin Immunol 1994; 93:735–742.

164. Platts-Mills T, Carter M. Asthma and indoor exposure to allergens. N Engl J Med 1997; 336:1382–1384.

165. Sherrill D, Lebowitz M, Halonen M, Barbee R, Burrows B. Longitudinal evaluation of the association between pulmonary function and total serum IgE. Am J Respir Crit Care Med 1995; 152:98–102.

166. Mensinga T, Schouten J, Weiss S, van der Lende R. Relationship of skin test reactivity and eosinphilia to level of pulmonary function in a community-based population study. Am Rev Respir Dis 1992; 146:638–643.

167. Henderson F, Henry M, Ivins S, Morris R, Neebe ED, Leu S-Y, Stewart PW. Correlates of recurrent wheezing in school-age children. Am J Respir Crit Care Med 1995; 151:1786–1793.

168. Rijcken B, Schouten JP, Weiss ST, Rosner B, de Vries K, van der Lende R. Long-term variability of bronchial responsiveness to histamine in a random population sample of adults. Am Rev Respir Dis 1993; 148:944–949.

169. Rijcken B, Xu X, Schouten JP, Rosner B, Weiss ST. Airway hyperresponsiveness to histamine associated with accelerated decline in FEV1. Am J Respir Crit Care Med 1995; 151:1377–1382.

170. Lebowitz M, Holberg C, Knudson R, Burrows B. Longitudinal study of pulmonary function development in childhood, adolescence, and early adulthood. Am Rev Respir Dis 1987; 136:69–75.

171. Gerritsen J, Koeter G, Postma D, Schouten J, van Aalderen W, Knol K. Airway responsiveness in childhood as a predictor of the outcome of asthma in adulthood. Am Rev Respir Dis 1991; 143:1468–1469.

172. Carey V, Weiss S, Tager I, Leeder S, Speizer F. Airways responsiveness, wheeze onset, and recurrent asthma episodes in young adolescents. The East Boston Childhood Respiratory Disease Cohort. Am J Respir Crit Care Med 1996; 153:356–361.
173. Martin A, Landau L, Phelan P. Predicting the course of asthma in children. Aust Paediatr J 1982; 18:84–87.
174. Phelan P. Hyperresponsiveness as a determinant of the outcome in childhood asthma. Am Rev Respir Dis 1991; 143:1463–1467.
175. Grol MH, Gerritsen J, Vonk JM, Schouten JP, Koeter GH, Rijcken B, Postma DS. Risk factors for growth and decline of lung function in asthmatic individuals up to age 42 years. A 30-year follow-up study. Am J Respir Crit Care Med 1999; 160:1830–1837.

21

Exercise-Induced Asthma in the Competitive Athlete

HENRY MILGROM

Department of Pediatrics and Medicine, National Jewish Medical and Research
Center, and Department of Pediatrics, University of Colorado
Health Sciences Center
Denver, Colorado, U.S.A.

...if from running, gymnastic exercises, or any other work, the breathing
becomes difficult, it is called *Asthma* ... The symptoms of its approach are
heaviness of the chest; sluggishness to one's accustomed work, and to every
other exertion; difficulty of breathing in running or on steep road; they are
hoarse and troubled with cough.... But, during the remissions, though they
may walk about erect, they bear the traces of the affection (1).

Aretaeus, the Cappadocian, Second Century

The terms exercise-induced bronchospasm, exercise-induced bronchoconstriction, and exercise-induced asthma (EIA) all stand for transient airflow obstruction associated with physical exertion. EIA is a problem in all
age groups, but it is most frequently observed in children and young adults
because of their enthusiasm for vigorous activities. It occurs during or more
frequently after exercise in 10–50% of elite athletes with the highest prevalence among competitors in winter sports. Clinical presentation and timing
of EIA may point to the diagnosis, but the association of airway obstruction
and exercise alone is not sufficient for confirmation, and the use of objective
measures of lung function is well advised. Although most exacerbations are

self-limited or subside readily with medication, mortality comparable to that of trauma and cardiac disease, generally regarded as the main cause of unexpected death in young, highly trained athletes, has been reported (2,3). It is important to anticipate EIA in all patients with asthma. Prompt and accurate diagnosis together with sound treatment should keep the athletes with EIA safe, allow them to enjoy the benefits of an active lifestyle, and help them fulfill their competitive potential (4).

I. Diagnosis and Screening

The EIA should be considered in all athletes with established or suspected asthma as well as relatively healthy individuals with a history of wheezing, cough, shortness of breath, chest pain, or tightness associated with exertion. All athletes thought to have EIA should be questioned about personal and family history of allergies and asthma as well as how much exercise they perform, their exercise tolerance, and symptoms following physical effort. The same inquiries should be addressed to children with chronic cough or allergic rhinitis, and those at risk for developing asthma such as youngsters with atopic dermatitis and first-degree relatives of asthma patients. It is important to establish that children who avoid vigorous activity are not so constrained by disagreeable experiences deriving from EIA. This also applies to elite athletes, who should be questioned about activities that cause respiratory symptoms or prolonged shortness of breath and about avoidance of events that cause them undue distress.

There are no established guidelines for the diagnosis of EIA in elite athletes. Some authorities recommend thermal and others hyperpneic or osmotic challenges (5,6). Recently, measurement of exhaled nitric oxide has been proposed as a less demanding alternative to the challenge protocols (7). The pathogenesis of EIA in elite athletes may be distinct from that of asthma, and neither the pre-exercise forced expiratory volume in 1 sec (FEV_1) nor the methacholine challenge predicts the severity of response or the presence of EIA (8,9). Athletes with a history suggestive of EIA should undergo a diagnostic evaluation comprising baseline spirometry, followed by a challenge and repeat spirometry after the provocation. The International Olympic Committee required documentation by eucapnic voluntary hyperpnea (hyperventilation challenge with dry air) or field exercise challenge prior to allowing the use of inhaled $\beta2$-agonists by competitors at the Salt Lake City Olympic Winter Games in 2002 (10–12). In the future it is likely that such documentation will be required of athletes who take medication while they participate at lower levels of competition (13,14) (Table 1).

After strenuous physical exercise subjects may report dyspnea, but even in patients with EIA, it is only loosely correlated to the decrease in FEV_1 (15). Children's symptom perception correlates weakly to change

Table 1 IAAF β2-Agonists Exemption Procedure

The IAAF will now require applicants to provide an accompanying letter to their exemption applications, signed by a respiratory specialist or a National Federation Team Physician, including the following documentation:

1. *Detailed medical records*
Medical records should include:
- A precise diagnosis of the individual's condition requiring the use of β2-agonists.
- All relevant information concerning the individual concerned and his condition:
  - Age of onset.
  - Symptoms suggesting airway obstruction following exercise, upper respiratory infection at rest and at night and/or during the pollen season.
  - Identified triggering factors.
  - Past history of atopic disorders and/or childhood asthma.
  - Past physical examinations.
  - Results of skin prick tests or RAST to document the presence of allergic hypersensitivity.
- Any specific information concerning the individual's coughing during or postexercise, dyspnea, shortness of breath, wheezing, chest tightness, or excess sputum.
- Details of all consultations with physicians qualified in the treatment of asthma and details of any attendance in hospital emergency departments for treatment or admission to hospital for treatment of acute exacerbation of asthma.
- Details of the individual's currently prescribed medication and any other medication prescribed in the last 6 months. Details of medication in the 3 months prior to provocation tests (see below) must also be notified.

2. *Resting spirometry test results*
Athletes must present the results of a spirometry test (resting) together with the following data: FEV_1, FVC, FEV_1/FVC presented both as an actual and percent predicted value. Graphic evidence (spirometry of flow volume tracings) must also be submitted.

3. *Provocation test results*
Athletes must also present a positive test result from one of the following recognized provocation tests:
(a) Bronchodilator test:
A positive test result shall be defined as:
- A 15% or greater increase in FEV_1 calculated as a percentage of the baseline FEV_1 OR
- A 12% or greater increase in FEV_1 on predicted FEV_1 in either case, after the administration of an inhaled permitted β2-agonist. Graphic evidence (spirometry of flow volume tracings) must be submitted in support of the result.
(b) Bronchial provocation test:
A bronchial provocation test will take the form of an exercise test in the laboratory or in the field or a EVH test. A positive test result will be obtained if AHR is confirmed with a fall of 10% or more in FEV_1 in the post-test period. Graphic evidence (spirometry of flow volume tracings) must be submitted in support of the result.

(Continued)

Table 1 IAAF β2-Agonists Exemption Procedure (*Continued*)

(c) Bronchial provocation test with inhaled methacholine:
A positive test result will be obtained if AHR is confirmed with:
 • A PC20 FEV$_1$ ≤ 2 mg/mL; OR
 • A PD20 FEV$_1$ equal to or less than a cumulative dose of 1 μmol or 200 μg or 20 breath units in steroid-naïve subjects.
In the case of individuals on daily inhaled corticosteroid treatment of more than 3-month duration, a positive test result will be obtained if AHR is confirmed with:
 • A PC20 FEV$_1$ equal to or less than 13.2 mg/mL; OR
 • A PD20 FEV$_1$ equal to or less than a cumulative dose of 6.6 μmol, or equal to or less than 1320 μg or 130 breath units.
(d) Broncho constrictor test:
A positive test result for a bronchoconstriction test is defined as a fall of 15% or more in FEV$_1$ after the subject inhaling a hypertonic aerosol (4.5% saline commonly used).

Under IAAF rules, the administration of the β2-agonists albuterol, formoterol, salmeterol, or terbutaline may be permitted by inhalation where prescribed for therapeutic purposes by properly qualified medical personnel and prior clearance has been given for such administration.
The PEFR measurements will not be accepted.
Abbreviations: IAAF, International Association of Athletics Federations; RAST, radioactive allergosorbent test; FEV, forced expiratory volume; EVH, eucapneic voluntary hyperpnea; AHR, airway hyper-responsiveness. http://www.iaaf.org/downloads/antidoping/index.html

in FEV$_1$, and parents' reports bear no relationship to physiologic measures (16). Physical examinations and screening questionnaires do not detect EIA with sufficient accuracy. Hallstrand and colleagues obtained a screening history from 256 adolescent athletes suggesting that 39.5% of them had EIA, but the diagnosis was established by exercise challenge and spirometry in only 9.4%, even as persons who screened negative accounted for 45.8% of the confirmed cases (17). The usefulness of questionnaires is undermined by their failure to address varying perceptions of symptoms. In studies of asthma the use of self-reported respiratory symptoms produces unacceptable rates of both false-negative and false-positive diagnoses (18). Even exercise challenges are often misleading when they rely on self-report, as shown recently by only 25% of athletes with physician-diagnosed asthma reporting symptoms following exercise (19). Rundell and colleagues compared self-reported symptoms of EIA to postexercise pulmonary function test results in elite athletes. Twenty-six percent of the study population demonstrated >10% postexercise drop in FEV$_1$ and 29% reported two or more symptoms. The proportions of PFT-positive and PFT-normal athletes reporting two or more symptoms were not different (39% vs. 41%). The authors' sensitivity/ specificity analysis demonstrated a lack of effectiveness of self-reported symptoms to identify athletes with positive findings on pulmonary function tests or to exclude those with normal results (18).

Rundell recommends standard pulmonary function testing before and after a high-intensity exercise challenge conducted while the subject is breathing dry air. He considers a 10% postchallenge fall in FEV_1 diagnostic. Godfrey and colleagues carried out comparisons of the sensitivity and specificity of the challenges and determined that the optimal cutoff point for the fall in FEV_1 after exercise is 13%, with a sensitivity (power) of 63% and specificity of 94% (20). Others prefer to base the diagnosis on a reduction in peak expiratory flow rate (PEFR) or FEV_1 that exceeds 15% because the postexercise fall in PEFR of normal children may be as great as 15% (21,22). Another approach to gain greater diagnostic accuracy might be to base the judgment on more than one maximum expiratory flow–volume measure (23).

In the course of exercise challenge bronchospasm typically follows a brief period of bronchodilation. Strenuous physical activity lasting more than 2 minutes is necessary to initiate bronchospasm. Most often bronchospasm develops within 10–15 minutes of the start of exercise or at its conclusion; it peaks 8–15 minutes later and resolves spontaneously over about 30–40 minutes (24). The existence of a much weaker delayed response 4–12 hours after exercise is a subject of some controversy (25). Six minutes of continuous exercise at an intensity sufficient to raise the heart rate to 80% of the maximum predicted value usually yields satisfactory results. However, in severe asthmatics even minimal exertion may be sufficient to produce symptoms. Patients with normal lung function at rest may have severe air flow limitation induced by exercise (26). As many as 50% of asthmatics who appear to be well controlled with inhaled corticosteroids still exhibit EIA (27), one of the last signs of asthma to disappear during treatment (28). Protocols based on duration of work or the achievement of specific heart rate may not incorporate all the relevant variables, and a standard challenge may be inadequate to elicit symptoms in highly trained athletes (29). In such cases the best course is to replicate the activity and the ambient conditions that incited the original complaint or to conduct a field test. Still, an athlete's response to exercise may change from day to day.

It depends on the nature of the exercise, the ambient conditions, and airway responsiveness that may be affected by viral infections, exposure to allergens, and the use of medications. When the underlying asthma is unstable, only minimal physical effort is required to produce symptoms. As the patient's disease improves, greater stimulation is necessary to produce the same airway narrowing. Even so, a challenge of sufficient magnitude will likely provoke EIA in all patients with asthma (30).

II. Differential Diagnosis

Airflow obstruction caused by strenuous activity may not develop until airway rewarming. For this reason it is important to obtain expiratory flow measurements after exercise has been completed. Preexisting airflow limitation or upper airway obstruction in all probability causes symptoms that develop immediately upon the initiation of exercise. Failure to reduce the symptoms with appropriate medications should direct diagnostic considerations away from EIA. Patients with exercise-induced respiratory symptoms that are refractory to treatment may not be using their prophylactic treatment appropriately or may be suffering from another condition (31,32).

Although disorders affecting other organ systems enter into the differential diagnosis (Table 2), vocal cord dysfunction (VCD), an abnormal adduction of the vocal cords, is the most common in the author's experience and perhaps the most underdiagnosed. The situation is confounded by the fact that VCD frequently coexists with asthma, and establishing one diagnosis does not rule out the other. The signs and symptoms of VCD—throat tightness, change in voice quality and airflow obstruction sufficient to cause wheezing, chest tightness, shortness of breath, and cough—are commonly precipitated by exercise. The presence of inspiratory wheezing most prominent over the neck or sternum points toward the diagnosis of VCD. This diagnosis is best established by observing the vocal cords of a symptomatic patient through a fiberoptic rhinolaryngoscope. In normal individuals the cords abduct during inspiration and adduct only slightly, if at all, during expiration; forced inspiratory or expiratory maneuvers may cause the cords to hyper-abduct briefly. In patients with typical VCD the anterior two-thirds of the cords adduct during inspiration, forming a small diamond-shaped or triangular aperture posteriorly (Fig. 1). It is possible to provoke VCD in asymptomatic patients prior to rhinolaryngoscopy. A positive study is diagnostic, but a negative one does not rule out this condition. Without rhinolaryngoscopy the diagnosis of VCD is strongly supported by the presence of truncated inspiratory loops and the absence of bronchospasm in patients experiencing symptoms of airway obstruction following exercise or methacholine challenge (32–34) (Fig. 2). In our experience, the most successful treatment of VCD is derived from breathing exercises used for hyperfunctional voice disorders to decrease the laryngeal muscle tone (35).

Table 2 Differential Diagnosis of EIA

Deconditioning
Vocal cord dysfunction
Cardiac disease
Central airway obstruction
Pulmonary disorders
Muscle disorders

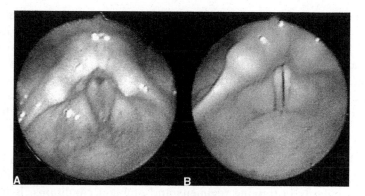

Figure 1 (**A**) Vocal cords of patient with VCD; note the diamond-shaped posterior chink. (**B**) Normal vocal cords in adducted position.

III. Prevalence

Against expectation the prevalence of asthma and EIA in athletes is higher than in the general population (19,36–38). The prevalence of EIA in the general population is between 6% and 13%; among athletes estimates reach 50%; it occurs in up to 90% of asthmatics and 40% of patients with allergic rhinitis (37,39). Approximately 90% of individuals with EIA have a history of asthma or allergy (40). EIA frequently goes undiagnosed. Fifty percent of children with asthma who gave a negative history for

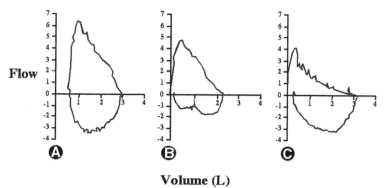

Volume (L)

Figure 2 (**A**) Normal flow–volume curve of a patient with VCD during an asymptomatic period. (**B**) Flow–volume curve of a patient with VCD following exercise while the patient was experiencing dyspnea and chest tightness. Note the truncated inspiratory portion of the loop. (**C**) The characteristic findings pictured here followed an 8-minute exercise challenge in a patient with EIA. Note the prolonged expiratory phase and concave expiratory portion of the loop, common to patients with asthma.

EIA had a positive response to exercise challenge (22). The prevalence is highest in winter sports among athletes who train and compete in cold, dry air or polluted indoor ice arenas (39). Airway hyperresponsiveness is found among athletes more frequently than symptomatic asthma, with prevalence ranging from 13% to 60% (19,41–44). The discrepancy in the prevalence of asthma and airway hyperresponsiveness may be due to a lack of recognition or underreporting of exercise-induced respiratory symptoms by athletes, and the possibility that training at the elite level raises the threshold for respiratory nociceptive sensations (19).

The differences in reported prevalence rates may result from the use of inconsistent criteria for diagnosis, inter- and intra-individual variability, and dissimilarity in training regimens and ambient conditions. Before the 1984 summer Olympic games, of the 597 members of the U.S. team, 67 (11%) were found to have EIA. Remarkably, only 26 of these competitors who trained under close medical supervision had been previously identified, emphasizing the importance of screening for EIA even among well-conditioned individuals who appear to be in excellent health (45). Athletes competing in seven sports (biathlon, cross-country skiing, figure skating, ice hockey, Nordic combined, long-track speedskating, and short-track speedskating) on the 1998 U.S. winter Olympic team were evaluated for EIA. The overall prevalence was 23%. It was highest among cross-country skiers, where 50% of the athletes (57% of the women and 43% of the men) were diagnosed with EIA (37).

There are many high school–age athletes with undiagnosed asthma or EIA. In one study, 12% of subjects not considered to be at risk by history or baseline spirometry tested positive (46). In another, 801 athletes were screened for asthma as part of their sports physicals. Forty-six had been previously diagnosed with asthma or EIA. Of the remaining 755 athletes, 49 were newly diagnosed with asthma by a simple protocol consisting of a brief questionnaire, PEFR measurements, and a free-run exercise challenge (47). Although the prevalence of EIA is greater in individuals with more severe asthma, the magnitude of the response to exercise is not consistently related to the intensity of the disease, and even individuals with severe persistent asthma may test negative (8).

IV. Pathophysiology of EIA

The acute EIA response is characterized by airway smooth muscle contraction, membrane swelling, and/or mucous plug formation. Its severity is related to the level of ventilation. Hyperventilation results in bronchoconstriction even in the absence of exercise. Reduction of the temperature and water content of inspired air enhances bronchoconstriction caused by isocapneic hyperventilation (48). Two possibly reconcilable hypotheses have been advanced to account for the mechanism of airway narrowing provoked by exercise. One holds that an increase in osmolarity, resulting from evaporative water loss, triggers the release of mediators from resident inflammatory cells leading to bronchoconstriction and airway edema (49,50). The rate and amount of water loss have been proposed as the main determinants of the scale of airway response (51). Kotaru and colleagues cast some doubt on this concept by collecting airway surface fluid of normal subjects breathing dry, frigid air and then showing that hyperpnea has no influence on the amount of fluid recovered or its osmolarity (52). The other hypothesis proposes that EIA is set off by the thermal effects of exercise—initial airway cooling and subsequent rapid rewarming as the rate of ventilation drops. These thermal effects are proposed to cause a reactive hyperemia of the bronchial microvasculature and edema of the airway wall. The narrowing of the airways in this scenario is a direct consequence of the vascular events (5,53,54). Its severity depends predominantly on the rate of airway rewarming after the challenge (55,56). To give emphasis to these associations McFadden and colleagues have proposed the term "thermally induced asthma."

The EIA is commonly associated with positive skin tests and raised IgE levels (28). An increase in CD23-positive B cells and CD25-positive T cells has been documented in patients with mild asthma after development of EIA symptoms (57). But the most important inflammatory cells in EIA are the mast cell and the eosinophil. Mast cells are capable of inducing immediate bronchospasm following allergen exposure, but their degranulation has also been demonstrated following non-IgE-mediated stimuli such as cold, dry air (58,59). They also readily degranulate in response to a change in osmolarity, constituting a link between the loss of water from hyperventilation during exercise and subsequent mediator release (60). The mediators released by these cells include histamine, leukotrienes, and prostaglandins. Mast cells, eosinophils, and alveolar macrophages, all resident in the airways, have the capacity to synthesize leukotrienes. Concentrations of leukotrienes in the nasal lavage rise fourfold after cold, dry air exposure in subjects with rhinitis (58). Isocapneic hyperpnea is associated with increased concentrations of leukotrienes B4, C4, D4, and E4 in the bronchoalveolar lavage fluid (61), and of leukotriene E4 in the urine of children with EIA after exercise challenge (62).

The severity of bronchoconstriction evoked by exercise is more closely related to eosinophilic airway inflammation than to airway hyperresponsiveness to methacholine (63), and an acute increase in the proportion of eosinophils in the sputum after exercise has been demonstrated in asthma patients with EIA, but not in those without EIA (64). On the other hand, increased bronchial responsiveness to exercise in asymptomatic children and adolescents was not a strong predictor for subsequent development of symptomatic asthma (65), and exercise-induced bronchoconstriction did not cause eosinophilic airway inflammation in subjects with asthma who developed airway inflammation with the same degree of allergen-induced bronchoconstriction (66).

One group of investigators devised an animal model for athletic competition in the cold. They demonstrated hyperosmolarity of the surface lining fluid in canine airways after peripheral airway exposure to cool, dry air (67). They subsequently studied inflammation in racing sled dogs 24 to 48 hours after completion of an 1100-mile endurance race (68). Of the 59 canine elite athletes examined, 81% had abnormal accumulation of debris on bronchoscopy, and 46% had moderate to severe accumulation of exudate. Bronchoalveolar lavage revealed statistically significant increases in macrophages, lymphocytes, and eosinophils. Bonsignore et al. found large increases in airway eosinophils and lymphocytes but no evidence of inflammatory cell activation in elite swimmers and skiers (69). Helenius and colleagues carried out a five-year prospective study to compare the effects of continuation as opposed to retirement from elite swimming competition on bronchial hyperresponsiveness, asthma symptoms, and airway inflammation. Sixteen (38%) of the swimmers continued their competitive careers (active swimmers), while 26 (62%) stopped competing (past swimmers) more than three months prior to the follow-up examination. Bronchial responsiveness was increased in seven (44%) of the active swimmers at baseline and in eight (50%) at follow-up; it was increased in eight (31%) of past swimmers at baseline but only in three (12%) at follow-up (McNemar test, $p = 0.025$). Current asthma (defined as bronchial hyperresponsiveness and EIA) was observed in five (31%) of the active swimmers at baseline and in seven (44%) at follow up; among past swimmers, it occurred in six (23%) at baseline and in one (4%) at follow-up (McNemar test, $p = 0.025$). Eosinophils and lymphocytes in the sputum increased significantly during the follow-up period in the active swimmers but tended to decrease in the past swimmers (70). Thus, airway inflammation may subside in athletes after they give up competition. These changes may represent chronic adaptive responses to hyperventilation associated with exercise. They do not prove that long-lasting strenuous exercise is detrimental to respiratory health (69).

V. Pharmacologic Therapy

It is important that not only the athletes but also their parents, coaches, team physicians, and trainers be informed of the athletes' diagnosis, condition, and therapeutic plan. With appropriate therapy, 90% of athletes with EIA can control their symptoms and should be able to participate in vigorous activities (71). Exercise, unlike exposure to allergens, does not produce a long-term increase in airway reactivity. Accordingly, patients whose symptoms occur only after strenuous activity may be treated prophylactically and do not require continuous therapy (72). Most asthma and antihistamine medications, and diverse others such as heparin, furosemide, and calcium channel blockers, given before exercise, reduce EIA (73). McFadden accounts for the effectiveness of these disparate classes of drugs by their effect on the bronchial vasculature that modulates the cooling and/or rewarming of the airways (5).

Since 1997 the Expert Panel, convened by the National Heart, Lung, and Blood Institute, has issued guidelines for the treatment of asthma that include recommendations for EIA. These guidelines put forward a stepwise approach to treat patients with asthma of varying severity. The Panel endorsed the use of short-acting β2-agonists and salmeterol, nedocromil, and cromolyn for the prevention of EIA (74). At present formoterol is approved as well. Short-acting inhaled β2-agonists used shortly before exercise last 2–3 hours while long-acting β2-agonists (LABA) may prevent EIA for 9–12 hours. Short-acting β2-agonists provide protection in 80% to 95% of affected individuals and have been regarded for many years as first-line therapy (75). Cromolyn sodium is also effective in 70% to 87% of those diagnosed with EIA and has minimal side effects (75). Nedocromil sodium provides protection equal to that of cromolyn in children (76). It is important to note that the effectiveness of cromolyn and nedocromil against EIA is limited to pre-exercise administration and that continuous treatment does not offer satisfactory protection. One-week's treatment with salmeterol 50 μg bid in asthmatic children and adolescents provided better protection against EIA than cromolyn taken four times daily (77).

Zafirlukast, a D4 leukotriene receptor blocker, attenuates exercise-induced bronchoconstriction in children for four hours after dosing (78). Both zafirlukast and zileuton, a 5-lipoxygenase inhibitor, suppress EIA by about 50% (60). The inability of these agents to inhibit EIA fully suggests that other mediators are also involved in this process (61). Once-a-day treatment with montelukast attenuates the immediate-phase response and abolishes the late-phase response to exercise challenge in asthmatic children (79). On the other hand, it provides no benefit in the treatment of asthma-like symptoms, increased bronchial hyperresponsiveness, and a mixed type of eosinophilic and neutrophilic airway inflammation in highly trained ice hockey players (80). A single dose of the antihistamine, terfenadine 180 mg, inhibits EIA by approximately 35% (81). It increases the intensity of exercise required to provoke bronchospasm to the same extent as cromolyn. When the dose is raised beyond 180 mg, protection against the challenge does not increase further.

Spooner and colleagues performed a quantitative comparison of the effects of either nedocromil or cromolyn to a single dose of a short-acting β2-agonist or an anti-cholinergic agent in patients over six years old with reproducible EIA. They analyzed 24 trials with 518 participants conducted in 13 countries between 1976 and 1998 to conclude that in a population of stable asthmatics, short-acting β2-agonists suppress EIA more effectively than chromones, while the latter are more effective than anti-cholinergic agents, and that combining short-acting β2-agonists and chromones may be appropriate in selected cases (82).

The LABA used intermittently in the absence of daily treatment with short-acting β2-agonists offer the most effective protection against EIA (83). Inhaled short-acting β2-agonists are effective as bronchodilators for up to four hours, but they act as prophylactic agents for EIA for less than three (84). The training sessions of many competitive athletes last longer than three hours. Children commonly engage in unplanned physical activity, and when exercise is scheduled, it frequently takes place on school grounds where they may be unable or unwilling to take medicine. Thus, a LABA regimen given at home is likely to be more effective than short-acting drugs that must be administered in a timely manner. The nine hour duration of action for single-dose administration reported for salmeterol should be sufficient in most cases (85–87).

Henriksen and Dahl were the first to demonstrate the importance of inflammation and the value of inhaled corticosteroids in the treatment of EIA (88,89). The severity of EIA was markedly reduced by one to four weeks of treatment with 400 µg of budesonide (88,89), and after 12 weeks' treatment with one of three budesonide regimens (100 or 200 µg once daily in the morning, or 100 µg twice daily) (90). The fall in FEV_1 after exercise was 7.2% to 7.8% compared to 16.7% for placebo (90). In a study of 19 children with severe EIA who demonstrated a 55% fall in FEV_1 after exercise, Pedersen and colleagues showed that the low dose of 100 µg budesonide daily for four weeks stabilized symptoms and peak flow variability. Although budesonide did completely control EIA, the severity of the EIA diminished with increasing doses. Thus, the mean percentage fall in FEV_1 was 55.4% after placebo, 25.7% after 100 µg/day, 20.1% after 200 µg/day, and 9.9% after 400 µg/day (91). After three weeks of treatment with fluticasone the geometric mean percentage fall in FEV_1 was reduced from 34.1% to 9.9% for 100 µg bid, and from 35.9% to 7.6% for 250 µg bid ($p < 0.05$) (92,28,83). Anderson points out that when potent inhaled corticosteroids were introduced into the care of children with asthma, the need for high doses of β2-agonists dropped precipitously. But children with good control of symptoms and normal spirometry at rest may still have EIA. Anderson gives warning that EIA may be one of the last problems to disappear during treatment with steroids, a sign of ongoing inflammation, and an indication for continued treatment with these medications (28,83).

A single 50 µg dose of salmeterol has been found to protect against EIA, but the time of protection appears to wane from 12 to 9 hours in the course of daily therapy (85–87). Hancox and colleagues published similar findings relating to patients who used a short-acting β2-agonist for EIA on a regular basis (93). These workers carried out a double-blind crossover trial in eight subjects randomized to albuterol (200 µg four times daily) or placebo for one week. After withholding therapy for eight hours, the subjects performed an exercise challenge known to produce a 15% fall in FEV_1. After exercise, there was a significantly greater fall in FEV_1 in the albuterol arm at one, three, and five minutes ($P < 0.001$); at five minutes the fall was 90% greater in the albuterol arm. The FEV_1 remained significantly lower in the albuterol arm throughout the dose-response curve ($p < 0.001$) (Fig. 3).

Anderson sounds another cautionary note. When β2-agonists are used on a regular basis the duration of the protective effect may be reduced, multiple doses of rescue medication may be required, and the time of recovery to pre-exercise lung function may be prolonged. Further, there are likely to be individuals at risk for severe attacks that may be difficult to reverse. She questions whether we compromise the prevention and recovery from an attack of asthma provoked by exercise by using β2-agonists daily in high doses. She argues that consideration should be given to treatment with twice-daily low-dose inhaled steroids as this may be all that is required to prevent the problem in the majority of children (83). Gibson and colleagues showed that the activity of childhood asthma, assessed by the frequency of symptoms over the preceding 12 months, is related to sputum eosinophilia,

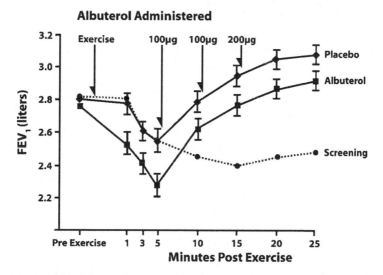

Figure 3 Double-blind crossover trial in eight subjects randomized to albutuol (20 µg four times daily) or placebo for one week. An exercise challange was carried out eight hours after witholding therapy. The figure shows FEV_1 before and after exercise and doing a dose–response study of albutuol. FEV_1 measurements from the prerandomization screening challenge are shown to illustrate the effect of one week of daily administration of albuterol or placebo. Error bars represent 95% confidence intervals.

sputum ECP, and desquamation of bronchial epithelial cells (94). The potency of the required asthma treatment was related to sputum eosinophilia. They proposed using the frequency of wheezing episodes over the past 12 months rather than current symptoms to determine the requirement for anti-inflammatory treatment and an examination of the induced sputum for eosinophils in patients not controlled by initial treatment. Perhaps the presence of eosinophils in the sputum of patients with EIA should serve as an indication for treating with inhaled corticosteroids.

VI. Non-pharmacologic Therapy

There is evidence that dietary fish oil supplementation provides significant protection against EIA. Elite athletes with EIA who received fish oil capsules containing 3.2 g eicosapentaenoic acid and 2.2 g docohexaenoic acid improved their post-exercise pulmonary function. At 15 minutes post-exercise FEV_1 decreased by $3 \pm 2\%$ in athletes on the fish oil diet, $14.5 \pm 5\%$ in those on placebo diet, and $17.3 \pm 6\%$ on the normal diet. Leukotriene E4, 9α, 11β-prostaglandin F2, leukotriene B4, tumor necrosis factor-α, and interleukin-1β all significantly decreased in those on the fish oil diet rich in polyunsaturated fatty acids (95).

At rest, inspired air is warmed and humidified primarily in the nose and trachea. As the rate of ventilation increases, the air is conditioned predominantly in the intrathoracic airways. Breathing through the nose rather than the mouth, or through a mask that reduces the loss of heat and moisture during physical exertion, has been shown to minimize EIA (96,97).

About 40% to 50% of patients with EIA experience a refractory period following an earlier exercise stimulus. This protection has a half-life of about 45 minutes and dissipates over two to three hours (98). For this reason, a prolonged warm-up that includes brief periods of intense activity is beneficial for athletes with EIA, and for some may even preclude the need for medication (71). A gradual cooling off, rather than sudden cessation of activity, reduces the rate of rewarming of airways and may also protect against bronchospasm (5). And finally, deep inhalation promotes bronchodilation during episodes of EIA (99).

Athletes whose asthma is well managed and who do not have significant fixed airflow obstruction tolerate aerobic training regimens (100). Specific training of individuals with mild to moderate asthma enhances both aerobic and anaerobic exercise fitness (101). Improved physical fitness raises exercise tolerance and capacity resulting in increased oxygen uptake (VO_2) and a reduction in ventilatory requirement, cardiac frequency, and lactic acid production at any given workload (100). Although there is no consistent evidence that physical training decreases the incidence of EIA or improves pulmonary function, it allows athletes to increase their exercise load before reaching the threshold for EIA (100,102). They develop improved ventilatory capacity and decreased hyperpnea of exercise, but their pulmonary function remains unchanged (103).

VII. Conclusion

Exercise is a powerful trigger for asthma symptoms. The EIA is a common problem, not limited to patients with asthma, and one that occurs even in individuals with normal spirometry at rest. It affects many athletes who compete successfully in aerobic events. EIA is a manifestation of airway hyperresponsiveness and a marker of airway inflammation. It endangers athletes and limits their ability to compete. It is likely that individuals with EIA have a threshold ventilatory rate, modulated by inspired air conditions, that triggers bronchoconstriction. When athletes reach or exceed this threshold, bronchoconstriction is likely to occur regardless of the level of their fitness. Although improved physical condition of patients with asthma is highly desirable, we must emphatically discourage the view that they can overcome their disease by being fit. Happily, appropriate therapy limits exacerbations and allows most athletes with EIA to train and compete for the most part free of respiratory symptoms.

References

1. Adams F. The Extant Works of Aretaeus the Cappadocian. London: The Syndenham Society, 1856.
2. Rossini A, Crocetti J, Rogers J, Quedenfeld T, D'Alonzo G. Asthma deaths associated with sporting activities (abstract). Am J Respir Crit Care Med 2000; 161:623.
3. Maron BJ. Sudden death in young athletes. N Engl J Med 2003; 349: 1064–1075.
4. Milgrom H, Taussig LM. Keeping children with exercise-induced asthma active. Pediatrics 1999; 104:e38.
5. McFadden ER Jr. Respiratory heat exchange. In: McFadden ER Jr, ed. Exercise-Induced Asthma. Vol. 130. New York: Marcel Dekker Inc., 1999:47–76.
6. Anderson SD, Argyros GJ, Magnussen H, Holzer K. Provocation by eucapnic voluntary hyperpnoea to identify exercise induced bronchoconstriction. Br J Sports Med 2001; 35:344–347.
7. ElHalawani SM, Ly NT, Mahon RT, Amundson DE. Exhaled nitric oxide as a predictor of exercise-induced bronchoconstriction. Chest 2003; 124: 639–643.
8. Cabral AL, Conceicao GM, Fonseca-Guedes CH, Martins MA. Exercise-induced bronchospasm in children: effects of asthma severity. Am J Respir Crit Care Med 1999; 159:1819–1823.

9. Holzer K, Anderson SD, Douglass J. Exercise in elite summer athletes: challenges for diagnosis. J Allergy Clin Immunol 2002; 110:374–380.

10. Capao-Filipe M, Moreira A, Delgado L, Rodrigues J, Vaz M. Exercise-induced bronchoconstriction and respiratory symptoms in elite athletes. Allergy 2003; 58:1196.

11. Holzer K, Anderson SD, Chan HK, Douglass J. Mannitol as a challenge test to identify exercise-induced bronchoconstriction in elite athletes. Am J Respir Crit Care Med 2003; 167:534–537.

12. Weiler JM. Why must Olympic athletes prove that they have asthma to be permitted to take inhaled beta2-agonists? J Allergy Clin Immunol 2003; 111: 36–37.

13. IAAF Beta-2-Agonists Exemption Procedure, 2004. http://www.iaaf.org/downloads/antidoping/index.html.

14. Anderson SD, Fitch K, Perry CP, Sue-Chu M, Crapo R, McKenzie D, Magnussen H. Responses to bronchial challenge submitted for approval to use inhaled beta2-agonists before an event at the 2002 Winter Olympics. J Allergy Clin Immunol 2003; 111:45–50.

15. Melani AS, Ciarleglio G, Pirrelli M, Sestini P. Perception of dyspnea during exercise-induced bronchoconstriction. Respir Med 2003; 97:221–227.

16. Panditi S, Silverman M. Perception of exercise induced asthma by children and their parents. Arch Dis Child 2003; 88:807–811.

17. Hallstrand TS, Curtis JR, Koepsell TD, Martin DP, Schoene RB, Sullivan SD, Yorioka GN, Aitken ML. Effectiveness of screening examinations to detect unrecognized exercise-induced bronchoconstriction. J Pediatr 2002; 141:343–348.

18. Rundell KW, Im J, Mayers LB, Wilber RL, Szmedra L, Schmitz HR. Self-reported symptoms and exercise-induced asthma in the elite athlete. Med Sci Sports Exerc 2001; 33:208–213.

19. Turcotte H, Langdeau JB, Thibault G, Boulet LP. Prevalence of respiratory symptoms in an athlete population. Respir Med 2003; 97:955–963.

20. Godfrey S, Springer C, Bar-Yishay E, Avital A. Cut-off points defining normal and asthmatic bronchial reactivity to exercise and inhalation challenges in children and young adults. Eur Respir J 1999; 14:659–668.

21. Weiler JM. Exercise-induced asthma: a practical guide to definitions, diagnosis, prevalence, and treatment. Allergy Asthma Proc 1996; 17:315–325.

22. Kattan M, Keens TG, Mellis CM, Levison H. The response to exercise in normal and asthmatic children. J Pediatr 1978; 92:718–721.

23. Fonseca-Guedes CH, Cabral AL, Martins MA. Exercise-induced bronchospasm in children: comparison of FEV1 and FEF25–75% responses. Pediatr Pulmonol 2003; 36:49–54.

24. Tan RA, Spector SL. Exercise-induced asthma. Sports Med 1998; 25:1–6.

25. Zawadski DK, Lenner KA, McFadden ER Jr. Re-examination of the late asthmatic response to exercise. Am Rev Respir Dis 1988; 137:837–841.

26. Anderson SD. Exercise-induced asthma. In: Middleton E, Reed C, Ellis E, Adkinson NF Jr, Yunginger JW, Busse WW, eds. Allergy: Principles and Practice. Vol. II. St. Louis: Mosby, 1993:1343–1368.

27. Waalkens HJ, van Essen-Zandvliet EE, Gerritsen J, Duiverman EJ, Kerrebijn KF, Knol K. The effect of an inhaled corticosteroid (budesonide) on exercise-induced asthma in children. Dutch CNSLD Study Group. Eur Respir J 1993; 6:652–656.
28. Anderson SD. Exercise-induced asthma in children: a marker of airway inflammation. Med J Aust 2002; 177(suppl):S61–S63.
29. McFadden ER Jr. Historical review. In: McFadden ER Jr, ed. Exercise-Induced Asthma. Vol. 130. New York: Marcel Dekker Inc., 1999:1–10.
30. McFadden ER Jr. Exercise-induced asthma. Assessment of current etiologic concepts. Chest 1987; 91:151S–157S.
31. Milgrom H, Bender B, Ackerson L, Bowry P, Smith B, Rand C. Noncompliance and treatment failure in children with asthma. J Allergy Clin Immunol 1996; 98:1051–1057.
32. Landwehr LP, Wood RP II, Blager FB, Milgrom H. Vocal cord dysfunction mimicking exercise-induced bronchospasm in adolescents. Pediatrics 1996; 98:971–974.
33. Wood RP II, Milgrom H. Vocal cord dysfunction. J Allergy Clin Immunol 1996; 98:481–485.
34. Milgrom H, Wood RI, Ingram D. Respiratory conditions that mimic asthma. Immunol Allergy Clin N Am 1998; 18:113–132.
35. Blager FB, Gay ML, Wood RP. Voice therapy techniques adapted to treatment of habit cough: a pilot study. J Commun Disord 1988; 21:393–400.
36. Weiler JM, Layton T, Hunt M. Asthma in United States Olympic athletes who participated in the 1996 Summer Games. J Allergy Clin Immunol 1998; 102: 722–726.
37. Wilber RL, Rundell KW, Szmedra L, Jenkinson DM, Im J, Drake SD. Incidence of exercise-induced bronchospasm in Olympic winter sport athletes. Med Sci Sports Exerc 2000; 32:732–737.
38. Langdeau JB, Boulet LP. Prevalence and mechanisms of development of asthma and airway hyperresponsiveness in athletes. Sports Med 2001; 31: 601–616.
39. Rundell KW, Jenkinson DM. Exercise-induced bronchospasm in the elite athlete. Sports Med 2002; 32:583–600.
40. Mehta H, Busse WW. Prevalence of exercise-induced asthma in the athlete. In: Weiler JM, ed. Allergic and Respiratory Disease in Sports Medicine. New York: Marcel Dekker Inc., 1997:81–86.
41. Leuppi JD, Kuhn M, Comminot C, Reinhart WH. High prevalence of bronchial hyperresponsiveness and asthma in ice hockey players. Eur Respir J 1998; 12:13–16.
42. Helenius IJ, Tikkanen HO, Sarna S, Haahtela T. Asthma and increased bronchial responsiveness in elite athletes: atopy and sport event as risk factors. J Allergy Clin Immunol 1998; 101:646–652.
43. Potts J. Factors associated with respiratory problems in swimmers. Sports Med 1996; 21:256–261.
44. Langdeau JB, Turcotte H, Bowie DM, Jobin J, Desgagne P, Boulet LP. Airway hyperresponsiveness in elite athletes. Am J Respir Crit Care Med 2000; 161:1479–1484.

45. Voy RO. The U.S. Olympic Committee experience with exercise-induced bronchospasm. Med Sci Sports Exerc 1984; 18:328–330.
46. Rupp NT, Brudno DS, Guill MF. The value of screening for risk of exercise-induced asthma in high school athletes. Ann Allergy 1993; 70:339–342.
47. Hammerman SI, Becker JM, Rogers J, Quedenfeld TC, D'Alonzo GE Jr. Asthma screening of high school athletes: identifying the undiagnosed and poorly controlled. Ann Allergy Asthma Immunol 2002; 88:380–384.
48. Deal EC Jr, McFadden ER Jr, Ingram RH Jr, Strauss RH, Jaeger JJ. Role of respiratory heat exchange in production of exercise-induced asthma. J Appl Physiol 1979; 46:467–475.
49. Anderson SD, Daviskas E. The airway microvasculature and exercise induced asthma. Thorax 1992; 47:748–752.
50. Anderson S, Daviskas E. Airway drying and exercise induced asthma. In: McFadden E, ed. Exercise Induced Asthma—Lung Biology in Health and Disease. New York: Marcel Dekker, 1999:77–113.
51. Hahn A, Anderson SD, Morton AR, Black JL, Fitch KD. A reinterpretation of the effect of temperature and water content of the inspired air in exercise-induced asthma. Am Rev Respir Dis 1984; 130:575–579.
52. Kotaru C, Hejal RB, Finigan JH, Coreno AJ, Skowronski ME, Brianas LJ, McFadden ER Jr, Influence of hyperpnea on airway surface fluid volume and osmolarity in normal humans. J Appl Physiol 2002; 93:154–160.
53. McFadden ER Jr. Hypothesis: exercise-induced asthma as a vascular phenomenon. Lancet 1990; 335:880–883.
54. McFadden ER Jr, Nelson JA, Skowronski ME, Lenner KA. Thermally induced asthma and airway drying. Am J Respir Crit Care Med 1999; 160:221–226.
55. McFadden ER Jr, Lenner KA, Strohl KP. Postexertional airway rewarming and thermally induced asthma. New insights into pathophysiology and possible pathogenesis. J Clin Invest 1986; 78:18–25.
56. McFadden ER Jr, Gilbert IA. Exercise-induced asthma. N Engl J Med 1994; 330:1362–1367.
57. Hallstrand TS, Ault KA, Bates PW, Mitchell J, Schoene RB. Peripheral blood manifestations of T(H)2 lymphocyte activation in stable atopic asthma and during exercise-induced bronchospasm. Ann Allergy Asthma Immunol 1998; 80:424–432.
58. Togias AG, Naclerio RM, Peters SP, et al. Local generation of sulfidopeptide leukotrienes upon nasal provocation with cold, dry air. Am Rev Respir Dis 1986; 133:1133–1137.
59. Varner AE, Busse WW. Inflammatory mediators in exercise-induced asthma. In: McFadden ER Jr, ed. Exercise-Induced Asthma. Vol. 130. New York: Marcel Dekker, 1999:137–166.
60. Israel E, Drazen JM. Role of 5-lipoxygenase metabolites of arachidonic acid in exercise-induced asthma. In: McFadden ER Jr, ed. Exercise-Induced Asthma. Vol. 130. New York: Marcel Dekker Inc., 1999:167–180.
61. Pliss LB, Ingenito EP, Ingram RH Jr, Pichurko B. Assessment of broncho-alveolar cell and mediator response to isocapnic hyperpnea in asthma. Am Rev Respir Dis 1990; 142:73–78.

62. Kikawa Y, Miyanomae T, Inoue Y, Saito M, Nakai A, Shigematsu Y, Hosoi S, Sudo M. Urinary leukotriene E4 after exercise challenge in children with asthma. J Allergy Clin Immunol 1992; 89:1111–1119.
63. Yoshikawa T, Shoji S, Fujii T, Kanazawa H, Kudoh S, Hirata K, Yoshikawa J. Severity of exercise-induced broncho constriction is related to airway eosinophilic inflammation in patients with asthma. Eur Respir J 1998; 12:879–884.
64. Kivity S, Argaman A, Onn A, Shwartz Y, Man A, Greif J, Fireman E. Eosinophil influx into the airways in patients with exercise-induced asthma. Respir Med 2000; 94:1200–1205.
65. Ulrik CS, Backer V. Increased bronchial responsiveness to exercise as a risk factor for symptomatic asthma: findings from a longitudinal population study of children and adolescents. Eur Respir J 1996; 9:1696–1700.
66. Gauvreau GM, Ronnen GM, Watson RM, O'Byrne PM. Exercise-induced bronchoconstriction does not cause eosinophilic airway inflammation or airway hyperresponsiveness in subjects with asthma. Am J Respir Crit Care Med 2000; 162:1302–1307.
67. Freed AN, Davis MS. Hyperventilation with dry air increases airway surface fluid osmolality in canine peripheral airways. Am J Respir Crit Care Med 1999; 159:1101–1107.
68. Davis MS, McKiernan B, McCullough S, et al. Racing Alaskan sled dogs as a model of "ski asthma". Am J Respir Crit Care Med 2002; 166:878–882.
69. Bonsignore MR, Morici G, Vignola AM, et al. Increased airway inflammatory cells in endurance athletes: what do they mean? Clin Exp Allergy 2003; 33:14–21.
70. Helenius I, Rytila P, Sarna S, et al. Effect of continuing or finishing high-level sports on airway inflammation, bronchial hyperresponsiveness, and asthma: a 5-year prospective follow-up study of 42 highly trained swimmers. J Allergy Clin Immunol 2002; 109:962–968.
71. Parry DE, Lemanske RF Jr. Prevention and treatment of exercise-induced asthma. In: McFadden ER Jr, ed. Exercise-Induced Asthma. Vol. 130. New York: Marcel Dekker Inc., 1999:287–317.
72. Zawadski DK, Lenner KA, McFadden ER Jr. Effect of exercise on nonspecific airway reactivity in asthmatics. J Appl Physiol 1988; 64:812–816.
73. Smith BW, LaBotz M. Pharmacologic treatment of exercise-induced asthma. Clin Sports Med 1998; 17:343–363.
74. National Asthma Education and Prevention Program: Highlights of the Expert Panel Report 2: Guidelines for the Diagnosis and Management of Asthma. (Publication No. 97–4051A). Bethesda, MD: United States Department of Health and Human Services, Public Health Service, National Institutes of Health, National Heart, Lung, and Blood Institute; 1997.
75. Section on Allergy and Immunology, Section on Diseases of the Chest. Exercise and the asthmatic child. Pediatrics 1989; 84:392–393.
76. de Benedictis FM, Tuteri G, Bertotto A, Bruni L, Vaccaro R. Comparison of the protective effects of cromolyn sodium and nedocromil sodium in the treatment of exercise-induced asthma in children. J Allergy Clin Immunol 1994; 94:684–688.

77. Zimmermann T, Gulyas A, Bauer CP, Steinkamp G, Trautmann M. Salmeterol versus sodium cromoglycate for the protection of exercise induced asthma in children—a randomised cross-over study. Eur J Med Res 2003; 8:428–434.

78. Pearlman DS, Ostrom NK, Bronsky EA, Bonuccelli CM, Hanby LA. The leukotriene D_4-receptor antagonist zafirlukast attenuates exercise-induced bronchoconstriction in children. J Pediatr 1999; 134:273–279.

79. Melo RE, Sole D, Naspitz CK. Exercise-induced bronchoconstriction in children: montelukast attenuates the immediate-phase and late-phase responses. J Allergy Clin Immunol 2003; 111:301–307.

80. Helenius I, Lumme A, Ounap J, Obase Y, Rytila P, Sarna S, Alaranta A, Remes V, Haahtela T. No effect of montelukast on asthma-like symptoms in elite ice hockey players. Allergy 2004; 59:39–44.

81. Finnerty JP, Holgate ST. Evidence for the roles of histamine and prostaglandins as mediators in exercise-induced asthma: the inhibitory effect of terfenadine and flurbiprofen alone and in combination. Eur Respir J 1990; 3: 540–547.

82. Spooner C, Spooner G, Rowe B. Mast-cell stabilising agents to prevent exercise-induced bronchoconstriction. Cochrane Database Syst Rev 2003; 4: CD002307.

83. Anderson S, Brannan J. Long-acting beta2-agonists and exercise-induced asthma: lessons to guide us in the future. Pediatr Drugs 2004; 6:161–175.

84. Anderson SD, Rodwell LT, Du Toit J, Young IH. Duration of protection by inhaled salmeterol in exercise-induced asthma. Chest 1991; 100:1254–1260.

85. Ramage L, Lipworth BJ, Ingram CG, Cree IA, Dhillon DP. Reduced protection against exercise induced bronchoconstriction after chronic dosing with salmeterol. Respir Med 1994; 88:363–368.

86. Simons FE, Gerstner TV, Cheang MS. Tolerance to the bronchoprotective effect of salmeterol in adolescents with exercise-induced asthma using concurrent inhaled glucocorticoid treatment. Pediatrics 1997; 99:655–659.

87. Nelson HS, Bensch G, Pleskow WW, DiSantostefano R, DeGraw S, Reasner DS, Rollins TE, Rubin PD. Improved bronchodilation with levalbuterol compared with racemic albuterol in patients with asthma. J Allergy Clin Immunol 1998; 102:943–952.

88. Henriksen JM, Dahl R. Effects of inhaled budesonide alone and in combination with low-dose terbutaline in children with exercise-induced asthma. Am Rev Respir Dis 1983; 128:993–997.

89. Henriksen JM. Effect of inhalation of corticosteroids on exercise induced asthma: randomised double blind crossover study of budesonide in asthmatic children. Br Med J (Clin Res Ed) 1985; 291:248–249.

90. Jonasson G, Carlsen KH, Hultquist C. Low-dose budesonide improves exercise-induced bronchospasm in school children. Pediatr Allergy Immunol 2000; 11:120–125.

91. Pedersen S, Hansen OR. Budesonide treatment of moderate and severe asthma in children: a dose-response study. J Allergy Clin Immunol 1995; 95: 29–33.

92. Hofstra WB, Neijens HJ, Duiverman EJ, Kouwenberg JM, Mulder PG, Kuethe MC, Sterk PJ. Dose-responses over time to inhaled fluticasone

propionate treatment of exercise- and methacholine-induced bronchoconstriction in children with asthma. Pediatr Pulmonol 2000; 29:415–423.

93. Hancox RJ, Subbarao P, Kamada D, Watson RM, Hargreave FE, Inman MD. β2-agonist tolerance and exercise-induced bronchospasm. Am J Respir Crit Care Med 2002; 165:1068–1070.

94. Gibson PG, Simpson JL, Hankin R, Powell H, Henry RL. Relationship between induced sputum eosinophils and the clinical pattern of childhood asthma. Thorax 2003; 58:116–121.

95. Mickleborough TD, Murray RL, Ionescu AA, Lindley MR. Fish oil supplementation reduces severity of exercise-induced bronchoconstriction in elite athletes. Am J Respir Crit Care Med 2003; 168:1181–1189.

96. Shturman-Ellstein R, Zeballos RJ, Buckley JM, Souhrada JF. The beneficial effect of nasal breathing on exercise-induced bronchoconstriction. Am Rev Respir Dis 1978; 118:65–73.

97. Stewart EJ, Cinnamond MJ, Siddiqui R, Nicholls DP, Stanford CF. Effect of a heat and moisture retaining mask on exercise induced asthma. BMJ 1992; 304:479–480.

98. Godfrey S. Clinical and physiological features. In: McFadden ER Jr, ed. Exercise-Induced Asthma. Vol. 130. New York: Marcel Dekker Inc., 1999: 11–45.

99. Marchal F, Schweitzer C, Khallouf S. Respiratory conductance response to a deep inhalation in children with exercise-induced bronchoconstriction. Respir Med 2003; 97:921–927.

100. Carroll N, Sly P. Exercise training as an adjunct to asthma management. Thorax 1999; 54:190–191.

101. Counil FP, Varray A, Matecki S, Beurey A, Marchal P, Voisin M, Prefaut C. Training of aerobic and anaerobic fitness in children with asthma. J Pediatr 2003; 142:179–184.

102. Matsumoto I, Araki H, Tsuda K, Odajima H, Nishima S, Higaki Y, Tanaka H, Tanaka M, Shindo M. Effects of swimming training on aerobic capacity and exercise induced bronchoconstriction in children with bronchial asthma. Thorax 1999; 54:196–201.

103. Hallstrand TS, Bates PW, Schoene RB. Aerobic conditioning in mild asthma decreases the hyperpnea of exercise and improves exercise and ventilatory capacity. Chest 2000; 118:1460–1469.

22

Comorbid Illness Associated with Childhood Asthma

GAIL G. SHAPIRO

Northwest Asthma and Allergy Center, University of Washington Medical School
Seattle, Washington, U.S.A.

I. Asthma Comorbidities

Childhood asthma is a multidimensional inflammatory disease that is often found in association with other health problems. These associated conditions are known as comorbidities. They are not merely curious associations, but rather offer insight into disease prognosis and progression. Managing asthma comorbidity may be a critical element in disease control.

Children with asthma are often atopic individuals, producers of specific IgE after exposure to environmental and/or ingested allergens. The prevalence of allergy skin test positivity has been noted to be more than 80% among youngsters with asthma (1). Certain atopic conditions are particularly interesting in relationship to asthma: food allergy as a precursor of respiratory disease, atopic dermatitis as a marker for asthma, allergic rhinitis as a frequent cohabiter and modulator of airways reactivity.

Other common health problems travel with asthma. Sinus disease, which may stem from underlying allergic rhinitis, has features suggesting an upper airway equivalent of asthma (2). Inflammatory changes in the sinus mucosa have significant parallels to those in the pulmonary tree, including accumulation of inflammatory cells and destructive changes of the epithelium. Gastroesophageal reflux is a sometimes underappreciated cause of asthma instability, and it appears that reflux can directly or indirectly influence bronchoconstriction and inflammation.

Arguably more surprising than these atopic and respiratory conditions as asthma comorbidities is the association of obesity and asthma. Only in the last decade have observers connected the surge in asthma prevalence and morbidity with a similar increased prevalence of obesity-related issues.

This is clearly a relationship that is connected to lifestyle patterns that are different from exposure and sensitization but just as important.

A. Markers of Atopy as Asthma Comorbidities

Allergic rhinitis, atopic dermatitis, and food allergy are risk factors for the development of asthma as well as being comorbidities associated with asthma. Epidemiologic studies reveal that rising rates of atopic diseases—atopic dermatitis, food allergy, and allergic rhinitis— have increased in a similar manner to childhood asthma. In defining a profile to discern risk factors for developing asthma in the first years of life, atopic dermatitis and allergic rhinitis appear as major and minor risk factors, respectively (3) (Table 1). If a young child who wheezes possesses these risk factors, it is highly likely that he or she will develop persistent disease, and it is advisable to initiate preventive therapy to decrease the number and severity of exacerbations. While this profiling identifies patients at risk, this is not to say that the majority of children with asthma will come from this group.

Knowledge of these risk relationships is very valuable to the clinician who is assessing a young child who may have asthma and answering questions from parents about what to expect in the future. The child with recurrent wheezing in the first years of life who shows no signs of atopy is much more likely to have transient wheezing than the child with atopic dermatitis or rhinitis, who is more likely to have persistent disease. When these factors are combined with information about parental asthma, there may be some helpful information for the family regarding their child's future health care needs.

Table 1   A Clinical Index to Define Asthma Risk

Major criteria	Minor criteria
Parental asthma	Allergic rhinitis
Eczema	Wheezing apart from colds
	Eosinophilia (>3%)

Loose index for prediction of asthma: early wheezer plus at least one of two major criteria or two of three minor criteria. *Source*: From Ref. 3.

B. Atopic Dermatitis

Atopic dermatitis may be a harbinger of more allergic diseases to come, including asthma. An evaluation of the relationship between atopic dermatitis in infancy, allergic sensitization to aeroallergens, and allergic disease revealed that 50% of children with early atopic dermatitis and a strong family history of allergy had asthma by age five (4).

Estimates are that 15–30% of patients with atopic dermatitis have co-existent asthma (5). Atopic dermatitis, may be a severity marker for asthma. Atopic dermatitis, a more severe skin disease correlating with more difficult asthama, may be a severity marker for asthma a more severe skin disease correlating with more difficult asthma. In general, patients with atopic dermatitis may be more likely to have severe asthma (6).

Both atopic dermatitis (particularly in its acute form) and asthma appear to be manifestations of overactivity of the Th-2 lymphocyte population. This lymphocyte subset preferentially produces inflammatory mediators that support IgE production and mast cell and eosinophil maturation. In support of both asthma and atopic dermatitis being sequelae of a common systemic disorder, it has been demonstrated recently that epithelial Langerhans cell surface FcεR1–bound IgE can be found in the skin of subjects with active atopic dermatitis as well as those with active atopic respiratory disease (asthma and rhinitis). No surface FcεR1 was found in the skin of subjects with quiescent atopic dermatitis, asthma, or rhinitis (7). Also showing this cutaneous respiratory connection, animal models have shown that epicutaneous stimulation with allergen can lead to an asthmatic response when animals are later challenged with similar allergen in an aerosolized form (8,9). In spite of their clinical associations, genetic linkage studies for atopic dermatitis and asthma have not uniformly shown an association, though some common chromosomal linkages have been shown to occur (10,11).

C. Management of Atopic Dermatitis

There is no current evidence linking control of atopic dermatitis with degree of improvement in asthma. There are some interesting observations regarding prevention of asthma with antihistamine therapy for children with atopic dermatitis. A prospective, long-term study of cetirizine for therapy of atopic dermatitis showed a lower prevalence of asthma in a post hoc analysis of children with sensitization to two specific environmental allergens who were treated with cetirizine (12).

This effect was seen during the 18-month treatment phase and persisted in the 18-month observation phase ($p < 0.008$). A prospective trial of the antihistamine ketotifen in atopic dermatitis showed a decreased incidence of asthma in the ketotifen group (13.1%) compared to the placebo group (41.6%) $p < 0.001$ (13). It appears that antihistamine

Table 2 Overview of Atopic Dermatitis Control in Children with Asthma

Avoid pertinent environmental and food allergens
Anti-inflammatory therapy to areas of active rash
Topical corticosteroids—non-fluorinated for face and genital area
Calcineurin inhibitors as alternatives to topical corticosteroids
Emollients
Anti-pruritics—first- or second-generation antihistamines
Use of anti-inflammatory and bronchodilator asthma medications as indicated by
    disease severity

therapy represents an opportunity for primary prevention of airways disease that deserves further evaluation.

Recognition of atopic sensitization and the avoidance of environmental and ingested allergens is an important aspect of atopic dermatitis care that may be overlooked by dermatologists and primary care physicians who may not be considering the role of allergy. There is good evidence for worsening atopic dermatitis in connection with ingesting food allergens to which a person has become sensitized, most commonly wheat, egg, milk, soy, and peanut in young children and nuts, fish, and shellfish in older children and adults. Environmental allergen exposure by inhalation and direct contact are also capable of exacerbating atopic dermatitis (14).

Controlling cutaneous inflammation can usually be achieved with a program that includes topical anti-inflammatory agents, emollients, and systemic anti-pruritic agents, typically antihistamines. Topical corticosteroid therapy can be replaced or supplemented with the nonsteroidal antiinflammatories tacrolimus and pimecrolimus. These calcineurin inhibitors appear to have a favorable safety profile and avoid adverse effects of aggressive topical corticosteroid therapy such as dermal thinning and telangiectasia formation. First-generation antihistamines such as hydroxyzine and diphenhydramine, which are known to have sedative potential, can be very valuable in pruritus control and are often well tolerated when given at bedtime. There may be problems, however, with suboptimal functioning during daytime use, which may not always be appreciated by parents and teachers.

Second-generation antihistamines may provide pruritus control that is dissociated from sedation. The example of cetirizine as an effective intervention has been noted (Table 2).

D. Food Allergy

Food allergy and asthma may coexist as manifestations of atopic disease just as can atopic dermatitis and asthma. Those patients with food allergy and asthma certainly may also have atopic dermatitis. Asthma is a common component of food-induced anaphylaxis. It is less commonly a sole manifestation of food-induced allergies reactivity. The review by James (15) on respiratory manifestations of food allergies clearly illustrates studies to substantiate this. In one investigation of 300 consecutive patients with asthma, food-induced wheezing was documented in six (2%) (16). A trial of 140 children with asthma yielded eight (5.7%) with a specific asthmatic reaction after food challenge (17). Another trial reported food-induced bronchospasm in 8.5% of 284 children with asthma (18). Among a small sample of 42 children with atopic dermatitis and milk allergy, 11% or 27% developed asthma symptoms with challenge (19).

Long-term clinical experiences in centers devoted to allergy and asthma yield more striking correlations. During two decades of experience at the National Jewish Center for Immunology and Respiratory Medicine, 68% of children with a history of asthma also had a history of food-induced asthma (20). Positive food challenges occurred in 60% of the subgroup that were challenged. The most common foods causing reactions were peanut, cow's milk, egg, and tree nuts. It is important to appreciate that only 2% of patients had isolated wheezing after challenge. At the Johns Hopkins Hospital, 17% (34) of 205 children with positive food challenges developed wheezing as part of their reaction. Wheezing as the sole manifestation of respiratory reaction was rare. James (15) summarizes the correlation between food allergy and asthmatic reactions (Table 3). In addition to evaluation of acute wheezing with food ingestion, one specific study of blinded food challenges and effect on bronchial hyperresponsiveness suggests that food-induced reactions may increase bronchial reactivity in some patients with moderate to severe persistent asthma, even though acute symptoms are not elicited.

Food allergy in infancy appears to be a predictor for later respiratory tract disease. Among a cohort of 1218 children followed for four years, increased respiratory allergy was associated with egg allergy (odds ratio 5.0) with a positive predictive value of 55%. This rose to 80% with concomitant atopic dermatitis. Skin test sensitivity to egg and cow's milk

Table 3 Estimated Prevalence of Food Allergy–Induced Asthmatic Reactions

Clinical population	Estimated prevalence (%)
General population of children with asthma	5.7
Infants with cow's milk allergy	29
Food-induced wheezing during acute reactions	2–24
Food additive–induced wheezing	<5
Patients with atopic dermatitis	17–27

Source: From Ref. 15.

Table 4 Management of Food Allergy in Children with Asthma

Ascertain symptoms of food allergy that are more likely than respiratory disease
Perform skin tests or in vitro tests to clarify history of IgE-mediated disease
Avoid foods that appear to contribute to asthma comorbidity and perhaps asthma
Consider periodic challenge to determine clinically significant foods, if deemed safe
EpiPens® at hand for anaphylactic food allergy

in the first five years of life have been correlated with asthma (odds ratio 10.7).

Just as in the child with food allergies who does not have asthma, there should be a systematic approach to care that involves a thorough history, testing to clarify allergic sensitization, and avoidance of clinically significant food allergens. There may be change over time. Open or blinded challenges may be valuable and should be done only with supervision and emergency care available (Table 4).

E. Rhinitis and Asthma

There is growing evidence for a conceptual vision of the upper and lower airway as part of a continuum. The information to support this includes epidemiologic, histopathologic, physiologic, and clinical studies. The practical clinical outcome of this airway integration is that allergic rhinitis and asthma may be considered to be elements of a disease spectrum and that, in the individual, insults to one element actually influence the other.

Epidemiologic studies are sometimes plagued by problems of standardizing questions to address the prevalence of rhinitis among patients with asthma. There is probably a tendency of subjects to downplay or ignore their nasal disease if asthma is their focus of concern. Nevertheless, several studies confirm the almost ubiquitous nature of rhinitis among asthma subjects, as was nicely reviewed by Togias (21). A survey of public housing residents in Baltimore, Maryland, showed a rhinitis prevalence of 86% in the population with asthma (22).

A survey of Brown University alumni followed during their freshman year and again 23 years later found an 86% prevalence of rhinitis in the subgroup that had asthma at the time of the initial survey (23). The Copenhagen Allergy Study of the same population from 1990 to 1998 showed a strong relationship between rhinitis and asthma (24). The first European Community Respiratory Health Survey revealed that perennial rhinitis was a major risk factor for asthma in both the atopic and non-atopic population with odds ratios of 11 and 17, respectively (25).

Other studies have confirmed that rhinitis is a risk factor for asthma, including the Brown University and Copenhagen studies noted above. The Tucson Epidemiologic Study of Obstructive Lung Diseases is a longitudinal prospective study that showed an odds ratio for developing asthma if rhinitis was present of 2.59 over a period of 10 years. This number rose to 6.28 for patients with rhinitis and sinusitis (26). While most of the evaluations have involved adults, a similar pattern exists for children (21).

The common presence of inflammatory cells in rhinitis and asthma has been documented by studies that show increased numbers of eosinophils and mast cells as well as cytokines consistent with Th-2 lymphocyte expression (21). Allergen provocation trials show early- and late-phase reactions and increased hyperresponsiveness in both nasal and bronchial airways after allergen challenge exposure. It is interesting that subjects with allergic rhinitis and no asthma show immunopathologic findings of asthma, though often to a lesser degree than patients with clinical asthma (21). A recent trial of sensitization and local nasal provocation to antigen in mice showed marked eosinophilic infiltration in upper and lower airways as well as increased IL-5 in bronchoalveolar lavage fluid and increased PMN infiltrates (27). Segmental antigen bronchoprovocation in patients with allergic asthma and those with allergic rhinitis without asthma show a similar pattern of increases in inflammatory cells and soluble factors in both groups, but with a significantly lower antigen dose in asthma patients (28).

Laboratory and clinical evaluations substantiate what has been called communication between the upper and lower airways, and most specifically the modulation of lower airways disease by changes in the upper airway. An unsubstantiated but popular hypothesis is of a "nasobronchial reflex." This concept calls for irritating stimuli that originate in the upper airway to signal increased bronchoconstriction and inflammation through neurologic pathways and neurogenic mediators. An alternate theory supports the direct transfer of upper airway derivatives to the lower airway. Though there is no evidence of this sort of direct penetration in humans (29), Brugman et al. (30) showed direct penetration of upper airway secretions to the lower airway in a rabbit model.

More likely, on the basis of recent trials, is blood-born systemic communication between upper and lower airways. Braunstahl et al. (31) showed that nasal allergen provocation in patients with allergic rhinitis induced peripheral blood eosinophilia along with lower airway expression of inflammatory changes. This concept of systemic communication leaves a wide door open for research to examine the ingress and egress of informational molecules between the upper and lower airway and for observations connecting this movement to health and disease in animals and humans.

The clinical correlations of "the airway as a continuum" are important for the practitioner. Recent investigation shows that patients with allergic rhinitis who were being treated had lower risk of asthma-related events than those who were not treated (32). This agrees with findings of several clinical trials done in the 1990s that showed decreased bronchial hyperresponsiveness in patients with asthma who were treated with nasal corticosteroids (33–35). More recently, investigators have tried to define mechanisms for this connection and have noted a decrease in the lower airway inflammatory markers exhaled, nitric oxide and H_2O_2, in patients treated with nasal triamcinolone. The decrease in expiratory NO applied only to the subgroup of patients with both rhinitis and asthma who were treated with nasal corticosteroid, while the reduction in H_2O_2 applied to the rhinitis group as a whole, with or without concurrent asthma (36).

F. Medical Management of Rhinitis in Patients with Asthma

In children, atopy is a dominant factor in rhinitis and asthma. Measures to control environmental allergens can be valuable for decreasing airways reactivity. To accomplish appropriate avoidance, allergy skin testing or in vitro measures of specific IgE should be performed. Allergen avoidance measures can then be focused correctly. Evidence linking environmental exposure with asthma severity is reviewed elsewhere (Chapter 10) (Table 5).

First-line medical therapy generally involves the use of nasal steroids or second-generation (mainly non-sedating) antihistamines. Comparative studies favor the former both in terms of nasal symptom control and decreased bronchial hyperresponsiveness. Antihistamines are favored by those preferring oral medication and when parents harbor fear about corticosteroid-related adverse effects. Aside from a mild decrease in growth velocity with beclomethasone (37), clinical trials have not demonstrated adverse effects of nasal corticosteroids on growth and development. Another option for seasonal allergic rhinitis is the leukotriene antagonist montelukast. Using this monotherapy might be helpful to both upper and lower airway disease, though it is less potent than corticosteroid therapy.

More difficult rhinitis may require a combination of these medications. Pseudoephedrine-containing decongestants may be added for nasal vasoconstriction. Nasal cromolyn has value as a therapy that affects chloride channels and thereby blocks mast cell mediator release, though there is

Table 5 Management of Allergic Rhinitis in Patients with Asthma

---

Avoid pertinent environmental allergens based on history and skin testing or in vitro tests

Use nasal corticosteroids to decrease upper airway inflammation and decrease bronchial hyperresponsiveness

Use antihistamines ± decongestant if nasal corticosteroids are declined or if supplement is needed

Consider leukotriene modifier—generally not first choice but supplemental for asthma and rhinitis

Consider allergen immunotherapy—usually if medication need is escalating and response is inadequate where allergen(s) are a major factor in disease severity

---

controversy over whether nasal mucosal mast cells are actually responsive in this manner.

Allergen immunotherapy is well established as an effective modality for rhinitis control and is less well established for asthma control. In patients with bothersome persistent rhinitis and accompanying asthma, it may be that the likely benefits to the upper airway will translate into benefits for the lower airway through pathways that minimize inflammatory mechanisms.

G. Sinusitis and Asthma

Chronic rhinosinusitis and asthma frequently coexist in the same individual. A recent evaluation of sinus CT, pulmonary function, sputum eosinophilia, and nitric oxide in exhaled air in patients with severe asthma showed a direct relationship between sinonasal mucosal thickness and bronchial inflammation (38). Histologic samples from patients with rhinosinusitis and asthma demonstrate similar inflammatory cell infiltrate with biopsies of the upper and lower airway mucosa being almost interchangeable in appearance (2). During upper respiratory infection, patients with asthma experience selective increases in inflammatory cytokines and reduced T-cell responsiveness to steroids (39).

Sinus disease is a pronounced problem in children with asthma and is often underdiagnosed and undertreated. Twenty-years ago, Rachelefsky et al. (40) noted clinically apparent upper airway congestion and purulence in a large proportion of children with difficult-to-control wheezing. These patients had radiographic proof of sinusitis. When treated aggressively with antibiotics, most of these patients became clinically improved with normalized pulmonary function tests and sinus radiographs. Others confirmed this connection between bacterial sinusitis and asthma exacerbation (41).

H. Disease Characteristics Before and After Treatment of Sinus Disease in 48 Children

These observations have been reconfirmed more recently. Children with chronic sinusitis treated with amoxicillin-clavulanate for six weeks had improvement in bronchial hyperresponsiveness compared to treatment with nasal saline alone (42) (Table 6).

Children with chronic rhinosinusitis and asthma treated aggressively with a brief oral steroid course, steroid nasal spray, and amox-clavulanate showed a reduction in inflammatory cell numbers, decreased IL-4 levels, and increased interferon gamma levels (43).

I. Medical Management

Sinusitis in patients with asthma may be acute or chronic, infectious or not. Therapy will depend on the specific presentation. Acute disease usually

Table 6 Disease Characteristics Before and After Treatment for Sinus Disease in 48 Children

Characteristics	Before		After	
	Number	Percentage	Number	Percentage
Cough	48	100	14	29
Wheeze	48	100	7	15
Rhinorrhea	30	63	10	21
Bronchodilator treatment	48	100	10	21
Normal pulmonary function tests	0/30	0	20/30	67
Normal sinus radiograph	0	0	38	79

Source: From Ref. 40.

refers to symptoms of less than 3-weeks duration. Most common symptoms in children are cough and rhinorrhea, with headache, fever, and positional pressure being much more likely in adults. If upper respiratory infection symptoms persist for more than 7–10 days, or if there is fulminant rhinorrhea, acute bacterial sinusitis is reasonably likely and therapy should include antibiotics directed to typical pathogens as well as topical corticosteroids to reduce inflammation. Nasal saline may also be helpful for reducing symptoms. In situations where disease persists for many weeks or months, the likelihood of noninfectious inflammation increases, and the chance for resolution with antibiotics decreases (44–46). While a trial of antibiotic therapy is warranted, more attention must be paid to underlying structural problems and imaging studies (usually CT) to elucidate these. Therapy is more likely to include short-term oral corticosteroids, nasal saline lavage, and nasal corticosteroids. Adults are more likely than children to have chronic hyperplastic sinusitis with nasal polyps. There may be value in using leukotriene antagonists in this situation, considering cysteinyl leukotriene concentrations in sinus tissue from patients with this chronic situation (47). To date there are no published controlled trials of anti-leukotriene therapy in acute or chronic sinus disease.

II. Gastroesophageal Reflux Disease

Gastroesophageal reflux disease (GERD) is a common problem that appears to be more prevalent in the population with asthma than in normal subjects (Table 7). It appears that GERD can exacerbate asthma. Studies to corroborate this have appeared over many decades (48–50).

Table 7 Management of Sinus Disease in Children with Asthma

Appreciate presentation as chronic cough/rhinorrhea
Empiric treatment with antibiotics to cover common pathogens: *Haemophilus
 influenzae, Moraxella catarrhalis, Streptococcus pneumoniae*; Staphylococcus and
 anaerobes for more persistent disease
Ancillary measures: nasal corticosteroids, nasal saline irrigation (older children)
Consider imaging studies for persistent disease: screening CT or full coronal CT if
 ENT referral and/or surgery anticipated

Assessment is complicated by the fact that patients with asthma may have coexistent GERD and not have gastrointestinal symptoms. Another complexity is to ascertain when and to what degree asymptomatic GERD actually aggravates asthma versus simply existing as an associated condition. Most studies that explore this relationship have been carried out in adults, data in children being quite limited.

A questionnaire-based survey of more than 200 asthma patients and controls showed heartburn to be present in 77% of the asthma patients and 52% and 48% in two control groups (51). Patients with asthma have been noted to have more symptoms of regurgitation and dysphagia than controls. Physiologic studies show more esophageal dysmotility and lower esophageal sphincter hypotension than normal (52) as well as a high prevalence of esophagitis (53).

The most reliable test for diagnosing GERD is ambulatory 24-hour esophageal pH monitoring. A series of studies has documented higher esophageal acid contact times and more frequent reflux episodes in asthma patients compared to normal controls. Harding et al. showed that of 199 asthma patients referred for 24-hour esophageal pH testing, 72% with reflux symptoms had abnormal esophageal acid, contact times. Seventy-eight percent of respiratory symptoms were associated with esophageal acid, and 90% of coughs were associated with acid events (54). In addition 24% of asthma patients without reflux symptoms had abnormal esophageal acid contact times. Thus, it appears that GERD is highly prevalent in asthma patients. Symptomatic patients may or may not have asthma exacerbations due to GERD.

Several physiologic features related to asthma may promote GERD in patients with asthma (55): heightened vagal responsiveness due to autonomic dysregulation, increased pressure gradient from the abdomen to the esophagus, and defective crural diaphragm function contributing to inappropriate relaxation of the lower esophageal sphincter. Acid reflux may enhance vagal dysfunction and increase bronchial hyperresponsiveness. Tracheal microaspiration is also possible.

Numerous studies, many with small samples and no controls, suggest improvement in asthma symptoms with medical therapy of GERD. A review of all papers on the subject from 1966 to 1999 noted improved asthma symptoms in 69% of patients and reduction in asthma medication in 62%. Pulmonary function did not improve (56). While aggressive use of proton pump inhibitors is the current medical therapy of choice, there are no large-scale, double-blind, placebo-controlled trials of this intervention in relation to asthma outcome.

Many trials of surgical intervention have design shortcomings. Nevertheless, several reports on outcomes of hundreds of patients undergoing fundoplication show improvement in a substantial number of the subgroup of asthma patients, with symptoms improving in about 80% (57,58).

There are few trials of GERD focusing specifically on children. One randomized, double-blind, crossover, placebo-controlled trial of ranitidine showed little improvement in asthma symptoms (58). Two trials of surgical intervention in children have shown dramatic improvement in asthma symptoms (59,60). A recent trial evaluated proton pump inhibitor therapy in older children with persistent asthma (61). Patients were on a combination of ICS, LTRAs, and short- and long-acting bronchodilators. Those with documented GERD chose medical therapy with proton pump inhibitors, prokinetic medication, advice on diet, and positioning or surgical intervention with Nissen fundoplication. In both groups there was a significant reduction in bronchodilator use ($p < 0.05$). At the end of one year of follow-up, bronchodilator use was no longer required in 78% of the surgical group and 67% of the medical treatment group. Use of LTRAs and ICS also decreased in both groups. The probability of a significant decrease in asthma medication requirement following anti-GERD treatment was 100% in those who had abnormal pH study findings initially, compared to 25% with normal pH study findings. In certain cases a 6-month anti-GERD treatment period was needed in order to see a significant response.

A cost-effectiveness analysis in adults (62) concluded that for patients with moderate or severe asthma and typical reflux symptoms, the most efficient approach was the use of omeprazole 20 mg/day for three months, followed by pH testing while still on this treatment in non responders to clarify the role of GERD in asthma. Using a regimen of omeprazole 40 mg/day increased cost while adding relatively few responders.

III. Obesity as a Risk Factor for Asthma

Since the late 1990s, there has been considerable interest in the relationship between body mass index (BMI) and asthma in the pediatric and adult populations. Clearly, both obesity and asthma have had parallel ascendancies as issues of growing concern in the public health arena.

A number of trials have focused on the BMI–asthma association in children. Looking at black and Hispanic children, a controlled, prospective trial (63) found that the prevalence of being overweight was significantly higher in children with moderate to severe asthma than in their peers. The association was significant for number of school days missed per year, peak flow <60% of predicted, and number of asthma medications prescribed. Another evaluation of Hispanic children noted that those with asthma were significantly more overweight than controls, but measures of asthma severity were not related to obesity (64). An evaluation of British and Scottish children documented the association of obesity and asthma in mainly Caucasian children (65).

The results of the third national health and nutrition examination survey (NHANESIII) demonstrate that BMI and the prevalence of obesity is higher in children with asthma. Pediatric BMI is also related to the interaction of asthma and maternal BMI in white and African American youth (66). There was a lack of correlation with television viewing hours or amount of physical exercise, supporting the view that obesity rather than lack of exercise is the important issue (67).

There has been debate regarding whether having asthma leads to obesity or whether obesity leads to asthma. Proponents of the former relationship propose that poor lung function leads to inactivity, which then leads to obesity. This view has been challenged by prospective evaluations in women that show that increased BMI precedes development of asthma (67). It has further been challenged by studies in adults where severe obesity was treated surgically, with subsequent improvement in asthma symptoms and medication use (68).

Theories of how obesity might influence asthma are unproven but include several theses. One is the belief that obesity increases GERD, which then increases asthma severity. Another theory is that the diets of obese subjects may in some way potentiate asthma. There is interest in the possibility that obesity stimulates inflammatory mechanisms or mechanical properties of the respiratory system (66). Perhaps the obesity is actually an epiphenomenon in children who are less physically active because of asthma and therefore prone to gain weight, although trials in adults do not support this theory (67,68).

Studies differ regarding what segment of the population is most clearly involved in the BMI–asthma association. Questionnaire data from German children revealed a higher prevalence of being overweight and obese for girls but not boys (69). Gold et al. also found increased risk of asthma in girls with higher BMI at entry into their study and greater increase in BMI during follow-up (70). Among school-aged children, Gilliland and coworkers identified being overweight with increased risk of new-onset asthma in boys and in nonallergic children (71). These different findings hold true for adult studies as well. Gain in BMI predisposes to new asthma diagnosis in females (72,73), while Kim and Camargo cite a stronger association in women than men, but with strong positive associations among men from minority groups (74).

These observations regarding the BMI–asthma connection, along with observations that weight loss leads to improvement in asthma, support the importance of current public health initiatives to raise awareness regarding the surging increase in prevalence of obesity in much of the Western world. It remains to be seen whether efforts to change dietary patterns in children and adults will alter the current trend and, if so, whether asthma prevalence will decline in association with the weight of the population.

IV. Conclusions

Clearly, the relationship between asthma and its comorbidities is intriguing and much remains to be explored. Food allergy and atopic dermatitis are markers of atopic disease, and it is not difficult to accept that these would be common occurrences in children with asthma, a disease that is linked to atopy. Less obvious is the connection between upper airway disease, rhinitis and sinusitis, and asthma. While hypotheses regarding direct penetration of upper airway contents into the lower airway and neurological connections between the upper and lower airways have been worthy guesses, it is becoming increasingly likely that inflammatory changes are quite similar in upper and airway sites, and that blood-born transport of inflammatory mediators may create the continuum of upper and lower airway disease. New developments to clarify the details of this connection are certainly on the horizon.

The GERD–asthma connection has a substantial literature base, but, again, the mechanistic details are obscure. We surmise that pressure imbalances between stomach and esophagus and/or the insult of acid actually entering the esophagus trigger reflex bronchospasm. The blueprint of the molecular basis of these events is not yet available.

Similarly, the recently recognized connection between obesity and asthma connotes a true causal relationship, with the former adding risk for the latter. The biochemical basis of this association has not yet been established, so that current knowledge consists of observations and hypotheses.

No doubt future discussions of these fascinating topics and their interrelationships will contain the details that currently elude us. This foundation of observations should serve as the impetus for both bench and clinical discovery.

References

1. Childhood Asthma Management Program Research Group. Nelson HS, Szefler SJ, Jacobs J, Huss K, Shapiro G, Sternberg A. The relationships among environmental allergen sensitization, allergen exposure, pulmonary function,

and bronchial hyperresponsiveness in the childhood asthma management program (CAMP). J Allergy Clin Immunol 1999; 104:774–785.

2. Ponikau JU, Sherris DA, Kephart GM, Kern EB, Gaffey TA, Tarara JE, Kita H. Features of airway remodeling and eosinophilic inflammation in chronic rhinosinusitis: is the histopathology similar to asthma? J Allergy Clin Immunol 2003; 112:877.

3. Castro-Rodriguez JA, Holberg CJ, Wright AK, Martinez FD. A clinical index to define risk of asthma in young children with recurrent wheezing. Table 1, A Clinical Index to Define Asthma Risk. Am J Respir Crit Care Med 2000; 162:1404.

4. Bergmann RL, Edenharter G, Bergmann KE, Forster J, Bauer CP, Wahn V, Zepp F, Wahn U. Atopic dermatitis in early infancy predicts allergic airway disease at 5 years. Clin Exp Allergy 1998; 28:965–970.

5. Leung DY. Atopic dermatitis: new insights and opportunities for therapeutic intervention. J Allergy Clin Immunol 2000; 106:860–876.

6. Buffum WP, Settipane GA. Prognosis of asthma in childhood. Am J Dis Child 1966; 112:214–217.

7. Semper AE, Heron K, Woollard ACS, Kochan JP, Friedmann PS, Church MK, Reischl IG. Surface expression of FcεR1 on Langerhans' cells of clinically uninvolved skin is associated with disease activity in atopic dermatitis, allergic asthma, and rhinitis. J Allergy Clin Immunol 2003; 112:411–419.

8. Spergel JM, Mizoguchi E, Brewer JP, Martin TR, Bhan AK, Geha RS. Epicutaneous sensitization with protein antigen induces localized allergic dermatitis and hyperresponsiveness to methacholine after single exposure to aerosolized antigen in mice. J Clin Invest 1998; 101:1614–1622.

9. Herrick CA, MacLeon H, Glusac E, Tigelaar RE, Bottomly K. Th-2 responses induced by epicutaneous or inhalational protein exposure are differentially dependent on IL-4. J Clin Invest 2000; 105:765–775.

10. Folster-Holst R, Moises HW, Yang L, Fritsch W, Weissenbach J, Christophers E. Linkage between atopy and the IgE high-affinity receptor gene at 11q13 in atopic dermatitis families. Hum Genet 1998; 102(2):236–239.

11. Beyer K, Nickel R, Freidhoff L, Bjorksten B, Huang SK, Barnes KC, MacDonald S, Forster J, Zepp F, Wahn V, Beaty TH, Marsh DG, Wahn U. Association and linkage of atopic dermatitis with chromosome 13q12–14 and 6q31–33 markers. J Invest Dermatol 2000; 115:906–908.

12. Warner JO. A double-blinded, randomized, placebo-controlled trial of cetirizine in preventing the onset of asthma in children with atopic dermatitis: 18 months' treatment and 18 months' posttreatment follow-up. J Allergy Clin Immunol 2001; 108:929–937.

13. Iikura Y, Naspitz CK, Mikawa H, Talaricoficho S, Baba M, Sole D, Nishima S. Prevention of asthma by ketotifen in infants with atopic dermatitis. Ann Allergy 1992; 68:233–236.

14. Adinoff AD, Tellez P, Clark RA. Atopic dermatitis and aeroallergen contact sensitivity. J Allergy Clin Immunol 1988; 81:736–742.

15. James JM. Respiratory manifestations of food allergy. Pediatrics 2003; 111: 1625–1630.

16. Onorato J, Merland N, Terral C, Michel FB, Bousquet J. Placebo-controlled double-blind food challenges in asthma. J Allergy Clin Immunol 1986; 78:1139–1146.
17. Novembre E, deMartino M, Vierucci A. Foods and respiratory allergy. J Allergy Clin Immunol 1988; 81:1059–1065.
18. Oehling A, Baena Cagnani CE. Food allergy and child asthma. Allergol Immunopathol 1980; 8:7–14.
19. Businco L, Falconieri P, Giampietro P, Bellioni B. Food allergy and asthma. Pediatr Pulm Suppl 1995; 11:59–60.
20. Bock SA. Respiratory reactions induced by food challenges in children with pulmonary disease. Pediatr Allergy Immunol 1992; 3:188–194.
21. Togias A. Rhinitis and asthma: evidence for respiratory system integration. J Allergy Clin Immunol 2003; 111:1171–1183.
22. Horowitz E, Diemer FB, Poyser J, Rice V, Jean L-G, Britt V, Knight M, Togias A. Asthma and rhinosinusitis prevalence in Baltimore City public housing project (abstract #918). J Allergy Clin Immunol 2001; 107:S280.
23. Settipane RJ, Hagy GW, Settipane GA. Long-term risk factors for developing asthma and allergic rhinitis: a 23-year follow-up study of college students. Allergy Proc 1994; 15:21–25.
24. Linneberg A, Nielsen NH, Frølund L, Madsen F, Dirksen A, Jørgensen T. The link between allergic rhinitis and allergic asthma: a prospective population-based study. The copenhagen allergy study. Allergy 2002; 57:1048–1052.
25. Leynaert B, Bousquet J, Neukirch C, Liard R, Neukirch F. Perennial rhinitis: an independent risk factor for asthma in nonatopic subjects: results from the European Community Respiratory Health Survey. J Allergy Clin Immunol 1999; 104:301–304.
26. Guerra S, Sherrill DL, Martinez FD, Barbee RA. Rhinitis as an independent risk factor for adult-onset asthma. J Allergy Clin Immunol 2002; 109:419–425.
27. McCusker C, Chicoine M, Hamid Q, Mazer B. Site-specific sensitization in a murine model of allergic rhinitis: Role of the upper airway in lower airways disease. J Allergy Clin Immunol 2002; 110:891–898.
28. Becky Kelly EA, Busse WW, Jarjour NN. A comparison of the airway response to segmental antigen bronchoprovocation in atopic asthma and allergic rhinitis. J Allergy Clin Immunol 2003; 111:79–86.
29. Bardin PG, Van Heerden BB, Joubert JR. Absence of pulmonary aspirations of sinus contents in patients with asthma and sinusitis. J Allergy Clin Immunol 1990; 86:82–88.
30. Brugman SM, Larsen GL, Henson PM, Honor J, Irvin CG. Increased lower airways responsiveness associated with sinusitis in a rabbit model. AARD 1993; 147:314–320.
31. Braunstahl GJ, Fokkens WJ, Overbeek SE, KleinJan A, Hoogsteden HC, Prins J-B. Mucosal systemic inflammatory changes in allergic rhinitis and asthma: a comparison between upper and lower airways. Clin Exp Allergy 2003; 33:579–587.
32. Crystal-Peters J, Neslusan C, Crown WH, Torres A. Treating allergic rhinitis in patients with comorbid asthma: the risk of asthma-related hospitalizations and emergency department visits. J Allergy Clin Immunol 2002; 109:57–62.

33. Corren J, Adinoff AD, Buchmeier AD, Irvin CG. Nasal beclomethasone prevents the seasonal increase in bronchial responsiveness in patients with allergic rhinitis and asthma. J Allergy Clin Immunol 1992; 90:250–256.

34. Aubier M, Levy J, Clerici C, Neukirch F, Herman D. Different effects of nasal and bronchial glucocorticosteroid administration on bronchial hyperresponsiveness in patients with allergic rhinitis. Am Rev Respir Dis 1992; 146: 122–126.

35. Watson WT, Becker AB, Simons FE. Treatment of allergic rhinitis with intranasal corticosteroids in patients with mild asthma: effect on lower airway responsiveness. J Allergy Clin Immunol 1993; 91:97–101.

36. Sandrini A, Ferreira IM, Jardim JR, Zamel N, Chapman KR. Effect of nasal triamcinolone acetonide on lower airway inflammatory markers in patients with allergic rhinitis. J Allergy Clin Immunol 2003; 111:313–320.

37. Skoner DP, Rachelefsky GS, Meltzer EO, Chervinsky P, Morris RM, Seltzer JM, Storms WW, Wood RA. Detection of growth suppression in children during treatment with intranasal beclomethasone dipropionate. Pediatrics 2000; 105(2):E23.

38. ten Brinke A, Grootendorst DC, Schmidt JTh, de Bruüne FTvan Buchem MA, Sterk PJ, Rabe KF, Bel EH. Chronic sinusitis in severe asthma is related to sputum eosinophilia. J Allergy Clin Immunol 2002; 109:621–626.

39. Vianna EO, Westcott J, Martin RJ. The effects of upper respiratory infection on T-cell proliferation and steroid sensitivity of asthmatics. J Allergy Clin Immunol 1998; 102:592–597.

40. Rachelefsky GS, Katz RM, Siegel SC. Chronic sinus disease with associated reactive airway disease in children. Pediatrics 1984; 73(4):526–529.

41. Friedman R, Ackerman M, Wald E, Casselbrant M, Friday G, Fireman P. Asthma and bacterial sinusitis in children. J Allergy Clin Immunol 1984; 74: 185–189.

42. Oliveria CAA, Sole D, Naspitz CK, Rachelefsky GS. Improvement of bronchial hyperresponsiveness in asthmatic children treated for concomitant sinusitis. Ann Allergy 1997; 79:70–74.

43. Tsao CH, Chen LC, Yeh KW, Huang JL. Concomitant chronic sinusitis treatment in children with mild asthma, the effect on bronchial hyperresponsiveness. Chest 2003; 123:757–764.

44. Tosca MA, Cosentino C, Pallestrini E, Caligo G, Milanese M, Ciprandi G. Improvement of clinical and immunopathologic parameters in asthmatic children treated for concomitant chronic rhinosinusitis. Ann Allergy Asthma Immunol 2003; 91:71–78.

45. Dohlman AW, Hemstreet MP, Odrezin GT, Bartolucci AA. Subacute sinusitis: are antimicrobials necessary? J Allergy Clin Immunol 1993; 91:1015–1023.

46. Garbut JM, Goldstein M, Gellman E, Shannon W, Littenberg B. A randomized, placebo-controlled trial of antimicrobial treatment for children with clinically diagnosed acute sinusitis. Pediatrics 2001; 107:619–625.

47. Steinke JW, Bradley D, Arango P, Crouse CD, Frierson H, Kountakis SE, Kraft M, Borish L. Cysteinyl leukotriene expression in chronic hyperplastic sinusitis-nasal polyposis: Importance to eosinophilia and asthma. J Allergy Clin Immunol 2003; 111:342–349.

48. Overholt RH, Ashraff MM. Esophageal reflux as a trigger in asthma. NY State J Med 1966; 66:3030–3032.

49. Sontag S, O'Connell S, Greenlee H, Schnell T, Chintam R, Nemchausky B, Chejfec G, Van Drunen M, Wanner J. Is gastroesophageal reflux a factor in some asthmatics?. Am J Gastroenterol 1987; 82:119–126.

50. DeMeester TR, Bonavina L, Iascone C, Courtney JV, Skinner DB. Chronic respiratory symptoms and occult gastroesophageal reflux: a prospective clinical trial and results of surgical therapy. Ann Surg 1990; 211:337–345.

51. Field SK, Sutherland LR. Does medical antireflux therapy improve asthma in asthmatics with gastroesophageal reflux? A critical review of the literature. Chest 1998; 114:275–283.

52. Kjellen G, Tibbling L, Wranne B. Effect of conservative treatment of oesophageal dysfunction on bronchial asthma. Eur J Respir Dis 1981; 62:190–197.

53. Sontag SJ, O'Connell S, Khandelwal S, Greenlee H, Schnell T, Nemchausky B, Chejfec G, Miller T, Seidel J, Sonnenberg A. Asthmatics with gastroesophageal reflux: long term results of a randomized trial of medical and surgical antireflux therapies. Am J Gastroenterol 2003; 98:987–999.

54. Harding SM, Guzzo MR, Richter JE. 24-h esophageal pH testing in asthmatics: respiratory symptom correlation with esophageal acid events. Chest 1999; 115:654–659.

55. Harding SM. Gastroesophageal reflux and asthma: insight into the association. J Allergy Clin Immunol 1999; 104:251–259.

56. Hunter JG, Trus TL, Branum GD, Waring JP, Wood WC. A physiologic approach to laparoscopic fundoplication for gastroesophageal reflux disease. Ann Surg 1996; 223:673–687.

57. Johnson WE, Hagen JA, DeMeester TR, Kauer WKH, Ritter MP, Peters JH, Bremner CG. Outcome of respiratory symptoms after anti-reflux surgery on patients with gastroesophageal reflux disease. Arch Surg 1996; 131:489–492.

58. Gustafsson PM, Kjellman NIM, Tibbling L. Oesophageal function and symptoms in moderate and severe asthma. Acta Paediatr Scand 1986; 75:729–736.

59. Rothenberg SS, Bratton D, Larsen G, Deterding R, Milgrom H, Brugman S, Boguniewicz M Copenhaver S, White C, Wagener J, Fan L, Chang J, Stathos T. Laparoscopic fundoplication to enhance pulmonary function in children with severe reactive airway disease and gastroesophageal reflux disease. Surg Endosc 1997; 11:1088–1090.

60. Berquist WE, Rachelefsky GS, Kadden M, Siegel SC, Katz RM, Fonkalsrud EW, Ament ME. Gastroesophageal reflux-associated recurrent pneumonia and chronic asthma in children. Pediatrics 1981; 68:29–35.

61. Khoshoo V, Le T, Haydel RM Jr, Landry L, Nelson C. Role of Gastroesophageal reflux in older children with persistent asthma. Chest 2003; 123:1008–1013.

62. O'Conner JFB, Singer ME, Richter JE. The cost effectiveness of strategies to assess gastroesophageal reflux as an exacerbating factor in asthma. Am J Gastroenterol 1999; 94:1472–1480.

63. Luder E, Melnik TA, DiMaio M. Association of being overweight with greater asthma symptoms in inner city black and Hispanic children. J Pediatr 1998; 132:699–703.

64. Gennuso J, Epstein LH, Paluch RA, Cerny F. The relationship between asthma and obesity in urban minority children and adolescents. Arch Pediatr Adolesc Med 1998; 152:1197–1200.

65. Figueroa-Munoz JI, Chinn S, Rona RJ. Association between obesity and asthma in 4–11 year old children in the UK. Thorax 2001; 56:133–137.

66. Epstein LH, Wu YWB, Paluch RA, Cerny FJ, Dorn JP. Asthma and maternal body mass index are related to pediatric body mass index and obesity: results from the third national health and nutrition examination survey. Obes Res 2000; 8:575–581.

67. von Mutius E, Schwartz J, Neas LM, Dockery D, Weiss ST. Relation of body mass index to asthma and atopy in children: the national health and nutrition examination study III. Thorax 2001; 56:835–838.

68. Camargo CA Jr, Weiss ST, Zhang S, Willett WR, Speizer FE. Prospective study of body mass index, weight change, and risk of adult-onset asthma in women. Arch Intern Med 1999; 159:2582–2588.

69. von Kries R, Hermann M, Grunert VP, von Mutius E. Is obesity a risk factor for childhood asthma? Allergy 2001; 56:318–322.

70. Gold DR, Damokosh AI, Dockery DW, Berkey CS. Body-mass index as a predictor of incident asthma in a prospective cohort of children. Pediatr Pulmonol 2003; 36:514–521.

71. Gilliland FD, Berhane K, Islam T, McConnell R, Gauderman WJ, Gilliland SS, Avol E, Peters JB. Obesity and the risk of newly diagnosed asthma in school-aged children. Am J Epidemiol 2003; 158:406–415.

72. Beckett WS, Jacobs DR Jr, Yu X, Iribarren C, Williams OD. Asthma is associated with weight gain in females but not males, independent of physical activity. Am J Respir Crit Care Med 2001; 164:2045–2050.

73. Chen Y, Dales R, Krewski D, Tang M, Krewski D. Obesity may increase the incidence of asthma in women but not in men: longitudinal observations from the Canadian national population health surveys. Am J Epidemiol 2002; 155: 191–197.

74. Kim S, Camargo CA Jr. Sex-race differences in the relationship between obesity and asthma: the behavioral risk factor surveillance system, 2000. Ann Epidemiol 2003; 13:666–673.

23

Improving Asthma Medication Adherence

BRUCE G. BENDER

Department of Pediatrics, National Jewish
    Medical and Research Center
Denver, Colorado, U.S.A.

CYNTHIA RAND

Division of Pulmonary and Critical Care
    Medicine, Johns Hopkins University
    Medical Center
Baltimore, Maryland, U.S.A.

FREDERICK S. WAMBOLDT

Department of Medicine, National Jewish
    Medical and Research Center
Denver, Colorado, U.S.A.

I. Introduction

Much has been written about the high frequency with which patients do not adhere to a protocol for the treatment of a chronic illness. Non-adherence compromises patient quality of life and increases health care costs. The World Health Organization recently published a book addressing the world-wide problem of treatment adherence, which averages only 50% in developed countries and is even lower in developing countries, and concluded that increasing adherence may have a more beneficial impact on the health of the population than improving specific treatments (1).

Despite this apparent broad recognition of the problem, there is little evidence to indicate that adherence rates have improved in the past two decades. Newer, more effective drugs may be somewhat forgiving in the face of partial adherence, but too often non-adherence is so pervasive and extreme that many patients are receiving minimal benefit. Numerous studies have introduced adherence interventions, but few have delivered cost-effectiveness or easy distribution across a large population. The national trend toward shifting increasing drug costs to patients will almost certainly serve to further decrease adherence. In short, the problem of non-adherence may be getting worse and is driving up the cost of health care.

II. Non-adherence and Health Care Cost

The United States is the largest consumer of health care in the world, with total health costs reaching 1.6 trillion in 2002, representing 14.9% of the GDP (2). The average cost of health care expenses for each person in the United States in 2002 was $5440, with an average of 3.1 physician office visits per person (2), resulting in a total of over 880 million physician office visits. Yet, adherence research suggests that a significant portion of the health care advice and prescriptions dispensed at these 880 million medical encounters was wasted. DiMatteo (3) has estimated that over 188 million medical visits result with patients failing to adhere with physician advice. While acknowledging that it is impossible to precisely estimate the waste and excess cost associated with non-adherence, DiMatteo's meta-analysis of the prevalence of non-adherence suggests that the costs may be as high as $300 billion a year.

Even more troubling are the health care costs resulting from non-adherence–related disease exacerbations. For example, when a non-adherent asthma patient presents with continuing symptoms, the physician may unnecessarily step up therapy because the physician believes the patient is nonresponsive to the original less intensive, and less costly, therapy. In addition, when a patient fails to respond to an apparently appropriate therapy, the physician may feel compelled to order expensive diagnostic tests to try to better understand the patient's poor response to treatment. While not all non-adherence results in dangerous or costly complications, research across a range of chronic diseases, including asthma, suggests that non-adherence results in excess urgent care and hospitalizations. For example, Milgrom et al. have demonstrated that pediatric asthma patients who were the least adherent were more likely to have asthma exacerbations requiring a prednisone burst (4). On a national level, Iskedjian et al. estimated the economic burden of hospitalization attributable to patient non-adherence with controller therapy in Canada. Using national health statistics and an average admission rate due to non-adherence of 5.2% (based on literature review) they concluded that Canadian hospital expenditures due to non-adherence exceeded $1.6 billion (5).

Finally, even when patients follow physician advice as far as filling prescriptions and initiating therapy, research suggests that a portion of all prescribed medication is wasted or discarded. For example, a study by Morgan used home-based pill counts and surveys to examine the economic impact of wasted prescriptions among older outpatients (>65 years).

Morgan found that waste (i.e., no intention of using remaining medication) represented 2.3% of total medication costs and that the average annual cost of the wasted medication was \$30.47 (range = \$0–131.56) per person. The study estimated that this modest per person cost of waste would translate into national cost for adults older than 65 years of age over \$1 billion per year (6).

The overall implications of these analyses are clear and compelling. As health care costs spiral upward and national health policy debates consider severe limitations on health care benefits, strategies to reduce non-adherence–related costs offer a promising (and cost-effective) avenue for intervention.

III. Why Do Patients Not Take Their Medication as Prescribed?

Most non-adherence is not the result of patients' forgetfulness, and hence significant behavior change is unlikely to result exclusively from attempts to help patients remember. Underlying beliefs about the prescribed medication have a large impact on adherence (7). Patients make a decision, actively or passively, as to whether they are going to take their medicine. In this "cost–benefit" analysis, the patient's conviction about taking a medication will depend upon the balance between concerns about the medicine, and the necessity of taking the medicine to control their disease (7). If patient's concerns, including questions about potential side effects or financial costs, are strong enough, they may outweigh the perceived necessity of the medicine. In this case, the patient's perception of the concern/necessity balance may lead them to decide not to take the medicine, or to take it less often. The patient's concern/necessity analysis may be based on inaccurate or incomplete information about the risks and benefits associated with medication. Patients with asthma often do not accurately understand why a controller medication must be taken daily, particularly when the patient feels asymptomatic, in order to control underlying inflammation. They may "test" their medicine by taking it for a short period of time to determine whether it is beneficial to them without understanding that a short interval is insufficient to appreciate benefit. Alternatively, the patient who is using a controller medication may cease using it and, seeing no change over one or two weeks, decide that they do not need the medication. Such experimentation can lead to faulty conclusions and cement the patient's belief that daily use of the medication is not a necessity. The attitude of a patient towards any individual medication may reflect their general perception about medications (8). Some patients are skeptical about prescription drugs, do not have faith in medical research, do not trust pharmaceutical companies, and may adopt the attitude that "the less medicine taken the better." Patients may use their controller medication sparingly,

Table 1 Factors Affecting Patient Adherence

1. Agreement with the physician's diagnosis
2. Perception of disease severity
3. Characteristics of the treatment regimen
4. Practical asthma knowledge
5. Personal habits, routines, and organization
6. Health beliefs
7. Provider–patient communication
8. Family competence

only taking it when symptoms are present, to avoid potential side effects or to extend the interval between pharmacy refills in order to save money.

Several key factors affect patients' perceptions about medicine, their concern/necessity analysis, and their willingness to faithfully follow a treatment regimen requiring daily behavior (Table 1).

A. Perception of Disease Severity

Patients' estimates of the severity of their asthma often differ from those of their health care provider. Patients who misjudge their asthma severity may inappropriately decrease or discontinue therapy. This discrepancy was illustrated in a study by Nguyen et al. that compared adult patients' perceptions of their asthma severity with that obtained by using the guidelines published by the National Asthma Education and Prevention Program's Expert Panel and with functional impairment measured by spirometry. When compared with a severity composite based on National Asthma Education Program criteria, only 54% of patients accurately estimated their own asthma severity, while 27% overestimated, and 20% underestimated their asthma severity (9). Similar discrepancies have been described by Wolfenden et al. (10) and Osborne et al. (11).

Many factors can contribute to this discrepancy in severity assessment. Asthma is an episodic disease with frequent periods of quiescence. Patients may prefer to consider asthma as a temporary acute illness that will eventually resolve, rather than accept a diagnosis of a chronic illness. In a qualitative study of asthma beliefs, Adams et al. (12) identified a subset of adult asthma patients who denied persistent asthma or claimed that they had "slight" or "not proper" asthma. These patients reported that asthma had no effect on their lives. However, with probing, these patients often described complex avoidance behaviors that they had developed to avoid physical symptoms (e.g., not running and staying indoors in certain seasons). Consistent with their denial of a chronic illness, none of these patients were using their daily prophylactic asthma medications (12). Patients who have adapted their lifestyles to the restrictions of asthma may underestimate their asthma severity or may ascribe asthma symptoms such as cough or sleep disturbances to other factors. Finally, some patients may have poor symptom perception and be relatively insensitive to changes in airway obstruction. This lack of sensitivity to airway obstruction may cause patients to dangerously underestimate their asthma severity, resulting in non-adherence and delays in treatment. For example, Magadle et al. (13) found that patients with blunted perception of dyspnea (POD) had statistically significantly emergency department visits, hospitalizations, near-fatal asthma attacks, and deaths during the 24-month follow-up period than patients with normal POD (13).

B. Characteristics of the Treatment Regimen

Consistent with common sense, the lengthier and more complicated the treatment regimen, the greater the likelihood of patient non-adherence (14,15). This observation has led to the expectation that simpler, once-daily asthma therapies will inevitably lead to improved patient adherence. Non-randomized pharmacy review-based studies do suggest some adherence advantage for once-daily asthma therapies compared to therapies with twice-daily dosing (16–18). However, while once-daily therapy may simplify daily regimens and decrease inadvertent missed doses due to forgetting, simplifying therapy is unlikely to promote adherence in the patient who is intentionally decreasing or discontinuing therapy because they believe that they no longer need to use it (19) or because they are concerned about side effects (20). Apart from adherence considerations, however, once-daily asthma therapy appears to be preferred by most patients (21). Venables et al. (21) examined patients' preference in asthma therapy and found that 61% of patients expressed a preference for once-a-day treatment, 12% preferred twice-a-day treatment, and 27% expressed no preference. While selecting therapies based on patients' preference may not necessarily lead to improved adherence, it may well reduce the burden of therapy and enhance patients' quality of life.

Other characteristics of the regimen can also impair or enhance adherence. For example, adherence with asthma therapies may be compromised by poor device technique (e.g., MDI, peak flow monitoring) (22). Actual or perceived treatment side effects or risks can also reduce adherence levels. Patients concerned by real or imagined risks of inhaled steroids may deliberately reduce dosing in an effort to decrease exposure (23). The high cost of many asthma drugs or rising pharmacy co-pays may contribute to non-adherence when patients fail to fill prescriptions, delay refills, or reduce dosing frequency to reduce costs (24). A study by Alexander et al. suggests that even though the cost of prescribed therapies may be important to a patient's ability to adhere, patients and physicians rarely discuss the patient's out-of-pocket costs related to heath care expenditures (25).

C. Health Knowledge and Beliefs

Patients' understanding and beliefs about asthma and asthma therapy are strongly associated with adherence to preventive treatment (7). Asthma patients frequently misunderstand the purpose of daily controller therapy and confuse the side effects of inhaled steroids with anabolic steroids (20). The most frequent reason that patients report not using their controller therapy is a belief that they do not need it any more (19). This confusion about therapies may occur even when physicians provide appropriate information and education during the clinical encounter. Studies of patient retention of health information suggest that immediately after an office visit, patients recall less than 50% of the information conveyed by the physician (26). In addition to general limitations in patients' abilities to recall, some patients may inherently have more difficulty recalling and comprehending medical information. Individuals with lower health literacy may be at particular risk of non-adherence resulting from misunderstanding of the therapeutic regimen (27).

Cultural and lay beliefs about asthma within minority or ethnic communities may differ from those of conventional medical models. Individuals from ethnic minorities may have different health belief systems or health practices than those of the medical practitioner. Divergent beliefs may impair adherence through competing therapies, fear of the health care system, or distrust of prescribed therapies (23,28,29). In one study, the level of cultural acculturation of inner-city Puerto Rican families attending an asthma clinic was positively associated with greater adherence with prescribed asthma therapies (28). Several studies within inner-city African American communities have reported parent concerns about their child becoming "addicted" to asthma drugs, or fears that medications will become less effective if used too frequently (30,31). In one study, inner-city caregivers of children with asthma who have negative health beliefs about the benefits of inhaled corticosteroid therapy were found to be more likely to deny having been prescribed inhaled corticosteroid therapy, despite their primary care provider's positive report (32).

D. Provider–Patient Communication

The content and quality of doctor–patient communication are important contributing factors to patient adherence (33). Clearly, the patient who is not sure about the difference between one's controller and one's rescue medication, who has unexpressed fears about using inhaled steroids, or who finds the therapy burdensome will be less likely to be adherent with therapy. Therefore, effective doctor–patient communication not only needs to provide information, but assess understanding, discuss concerns, and consider patient preference and abilities.

Physicians who use closed-ended questioning and who do not directly ask patients about their adherence level are no better than chance in assessing their patients' adherence (34). Conversely, physicians who use an information-intensive style of interacting have been found to be better able to assess patients' true adherence level (34). One study found that diabetic patients with low health literacy whose physicians actively assessed patient understanding and recall (interactive communication) had better adherence and lower hemoglobin A_{1c} levels. Effective provider–patient communication is not didactic, but rather interactive (27). Active listening not only educates patients about asthma, but also recognizes and respects the personal validity of patient beliefs and personal goals.

Without effective communication, the physician's goals for treatment may be markedly discordant with those of the patient's. For example, the physician following NAEPP guidelines might prescribe daily controller therapy to completely control mild persistent asthma symptoms. The patient, however, might prefer to treat symptoms with their rescue medication or live with occasional symptoms rather than take a daily medication. Shared decision making may be one communication approach that providers and patients can use to find "common ground" (35). Shared decision making attempts to increase concordance about treatment choices and goals by promoting greater involvement of the individual patient in deliberations about treatment options. This promising communication strategy may have significant potential for improving patient adherence (36–38). DiMatteo (39) has suggested, " . . . for the therapeutic relationship to be successful and for the physician's advice to improve the patient's life, doctors and patients must communicate and agree on treatment goals. Patients must be given the opportunity to assess the potential risks or drawbacks in a proposed treatment and its potential effect on the quality of their lives" (Ref. 39, p. 79).

E. Family Factors

The special case of pediatric asthma requires a careful look at the child's entire family. Successful asthma management is a family affair. Although this is most obvious in pediatric asthma where parents unconditionally need to aid infants and young children with virtually all aspects of asthma care, even for adults the care of asthma involves multiple family members. A handful of asthma-related activities that ultimately involve the entire family include ensuring that medications are taken on time, prescription refills are anticipated and filled in a timely fashion, and environmental irritants and triggers are controlled or eliminated. Hence, just as the partnership between patient and provider is a major determinant of treatment adherence, evidence has accumulated that various aspects of the relational partnership(s) within the family also are important determinants of adherence.

Family Confidence and Competence

One key dimension of the family partnership is the degree to which family members have the knowledge, competence, and confidence to handle asthma-related tasks and situations. A number of studies have offered family-based interventions to families who were having limited success managing asthma. Although these interventions attempted to alter various family processes [including those posited by the poorly supported Psychosomatic Family model of Minuchin et al. (40,41)] they all consistently provided practical instruction in the use of effective asthma management techniques, and a strong case can be made that this was the basis of their success (42). In a similar vein, Fiese and Wamboldt (43) recently reported that parents whose "stories" of the impact of their child's asthma on themselves and their family contained more elements of anxiety and uncertainty and had lower medication adherence and higher rates of urgent health care utilization than parents whose stories were rated as more confident and coordinated.

For this reason, health care providers are advised to ascertain, especially in the context of hard-to-manage asthma, the family's competence and confidence in practical asthma management. Although lack of competence, at times, is due to the family simply needing to be taught what to do, clinicians should be especially careful to look for excessive anxiety, depression, or traumatic experience. Such psychological problems may cause individuals who have the knowledge of what to do to fail to recognize important asthma symptoms or cues, or minimize and/or avoid putting their knowledge into action (42). In recent years, it has become increasingly apparent that medical interventions cause or aggravate anxiety disorders up to and including post-traumatic stress disorders (44–47). Emergency intubations while the patient remains conscious or awakening in the middle of the night to see the infant blue and in respiratory distress are examples of relatively common situations that can traumatize patients and family members. Furthermore, given the genetic predisposition for asthma and allergy, there is some evidence that the parents' traumatic experience with respiratory illness can influence their management of their child's asthma (47). Similarly, patient and/or parental depression increasingly is being recognized as a risk factor for poorer asthma treatment adherence and outcomes (48–50).

Family Organization and Routines

A second important determinant is the degree to which a family is organized and has routines that promote successful asthma management (51,52). In some families, life has a clear and consistent pattern with regular wake-up times, shared meals, and organized bedtime habits. The regular taking of asthma medications can be relatively easily facilitated by pairing medication taking with an already well-established routine, such as using the inhaler before tooth brushing or taking a nebulized treatment while a bedtime story is read (53). Additionally, while together for meals or other shared events, family members are more likely to have the opportunity to monitor, evaluate, and even discuss each other's health status.

In other families, every day is a new and different challenge, with little to no consistency across days or weeks. Once the clinician recognizes this, the opportunity exists to discuss other strategies to promote adherence, ranging from increasing the ease of being regularly "cued" to remember medication taking to discussing the "creation" of a new medication taking routine (53,54).

Family Conflict and Dysfunction

The presence of overt family conflict or more limited and subtle disruption of the family's "teamwork" with the member with asthma has been related to poor asthma adherence and outcomes (55–59). Indeed, even with infants and toddlers, "parenting difficulties," including problems with the marital and parent–child relationship, have been associated with both the onset and persistence of asthma into young childhood (60–63). Given the importance of family partnership and teamwork in the successful management of asthma, these are not surprising findings, but nonetheless warrant greater attention during routine clinical contacts, again, especially once a particular case of asthma has become "hard to manage" (42).

A seemingly important variant of family conflict affecting pediatric asthma management, which has received virtually no prior research attention, is the relatively frequently encountered clinical situation where parents disagree about the presence and/or appropriate management of asthma in their child. Typically, this involves the father taking the position that the mother "overemphasizes" the importance of the child's asthma and/or associated prescribed treatments, with the father advocating for greater physical conditioning or exertion as the "cure" for the child's breathing problems. Similarly, adolescence has been consistently shown to be a time when asthma adherence suffers, in part due to the difficulties involved in the passing of asthma management responsibilities from parent to growing child (64–66). Recognition and monitoring of such potential "asthma-related belief" and "role transition" problems among family members is recommended in all clinical contacts with children and adolescents.

Finally, it is important to remember that family conflict, at times, merges with other risk factors, such as social disadvantage, deficient nurturing, and intrafamilial aggression, that negatively impact children's mental and physical health in many ways (for a detailed discussion see the excellent recent review on "risky families" by Repetti and colleagues) (67). In such cases, improving asthma management may require, first and foremost, a multidisciplinary effort to improve the family's management of life in general.

IV. Who Is Responsible for Changing Patient Behavior?

Despite a large published literature addressing how to change patient behavior in order to improve medication adherence, remarkably little success has been recorded. Patients in adherence-intervention studies may achieve higher scores on a test of asthma knowledge and report increased medication use, but most frequently an objectively established change in medication adherence or disease status is not achieved (1,68). Because many factors can contribute to treatment non-adherence, no single intervention will affect change in every individual. Patient understanding of the disease and its treatment is essential to treatment adherence and improved outcomes, yet studies employing comprehensive asthma education programs often do not result in significant change (1,68). Patient education remains an important component in the comprehensive care of asthma, but it is likely to affect change only in that group of patients for whom lack of information is the primary reason for non-adherence.

Changing adherence behavior is a difficult but not impossible task. Smoking, which is both physiologically and psychologically addictive, is a behavior very resistant to change. Nonetheless, comprehensive efforts to reduce smoking frequency have resulted in a decrease over the past 25 years in the proportion of Americans who smoke. Further, the Surgeon General's Report in 2000 outlined a plan for cutting U.S. smoking rates in half that included (1) implementation of school-based anti-tobacco programs, (2) a media campaign including anti-tobacco messages from popular celebrities, (3) encouragement of inclusion of state-of-the art smoking cessation programs in health insurance plans, (4) training of physicians to more effectively address tobacco cessation, (5) passage of legislation that would include stricter indoor air regulations, and (6) increased funding to develop more effective smoking-cessation interventions. The application of a broad spectrum of strategies that influence behavior may similarly help to improve self-management of chronic medical conditions, including asthma, diabetes, and hypertension. While the health care provider has the most direct contact with patients, and hence the greatest opportunity to affect behavior change, the caregiver cannot alone improve patient management of chronic illness, relieve the patient of disease burden, and reduce health care cost.

In a recent report, the World Health Organization cited the worldwide problem of treatment non-adherence in both developed and developing countries and across all chronic conditions, including communicable diseases such as tuberculosis and human immunodeficiency virus/acquired immunodeficiency syndrome; mental and neurological conditions such as depression and epilepsy; substance dependence; and a range of other conditions, including asthma, hypertension, and cancer. The international panel of writers of the World Health Organization report took this position

Table 2 Who Is Responsible for Helping to Make Sure That Patients Adhere to Their Treatment Plan?

1. The patient
2. The health care provider
3. The health care industry, including health maintenance organizations and insurance carriers
4. The pharmaceutical companies

with regard to which elements of the health care system must assume responsibility for improving disease management:

> Over the past few decades, we have witnessed several phases in the development of approaches aimed at ensuring that patients continue therapy for chronic conditions for long periods of time. Initially the patient was thought to be the source of the "problem of compliance." Later, the role of the providers was also addressed. Now we acknowledge that a systems approach is required. The idea of compliance is associated too closely with blame, be it of providers or patients, and the concept of adherence is a better way of capturing the dynamic and complex changes required of many players over long periods to maintain optimal health in people with chronic diseases (1).

Widespread change in patient medication adherence, as well as other aspects of the self-management of chronic illness, will occur when, as with the campaign to lower smoking rates, the problem is approached from multiple avenues using multiple strategies. To accomplish this, neither the patient nor the health care provider can be expected to assume sole responsibility for effective disease self-management. The health care provider, health care industry, and pharmaceutical industry must all accept responsibility for helping enable patients to better care for their asthma (Table 2).

A. Health Care Provider

The relationship between the health caregiver and the patient has a large influence on whether the patient will engage in health care behaviors sufficient to insure successful treatment of the disease. The *Expert Panel Report: Guidelines for the Diagnosis and Management of Asthma* (69) emphasizes that patient education must occur within this caregiver–patient "partnership." This relationship has a more powerful influence on adherence than almost any other factor (70,71). The strength of the physician–patient treatment alliance, as rated by the physician, predicted treatment adherence and non-routine office visits in the year after hospitalization of 60 adolescents with severe, chronic asthma (72). In psychotherapy for emotional disorders, stronger therapeutic alliance has similarly been positively related to better outcomes (73). In some cases, the behavior and attitude of the patient prevents the health caregiver from developing an optimal working relationship. However, there is considerable evidence that the behavior of the physician plays a significant role in defining the strength of the treatment alliance. Patients are more adherent to their treatment regimen when their physician has answered all their questions (74) and communicated clearly (75) and positively (76). The physician's interest in spending time with a patient, attempting to understand the patient's beliefs and perceptions about the illness, communicates the desire to developing a partnership that will result in treatment success (76).

In a masterfully written book, published in 1987 and now out of print, Meichenbaum and Turk (77) described the caregiver behaviors that improve treatment adherence. These behavioral scientists used established behavior-change techniques to promote strategies for health care providers to improve patients' adherence to their treatment (Table 3). In the 15 years following the publication of this book, numerous studies of patients with chronic illness have demonstrated the effectiveness of each of these strategies, and underlying concepts have been further refined. For example, Meichenbaum and Turk urged that the health care provider must foster a collaborative relationship with the patient that includes a willingness to share control of treatment decisions with the patient. This concept is embraced in recent promotions of a shared decision-making model in which patient and physician exchange information, deliberate about treatment options, and collaboratively decide upon which treatment to initiate (78). It is also included in the recommendation of the NHLBI guidelines that caregivers establish a "partnership" with patients within which goals and treatments are negotiated (69).

B. Health Care Industry

The health care industry includes insurance companies, health maintenance organizations, and the hospitals, clinics, and medical centers that provide clinical care. The needs and objectives of these organizations are sometimes in conflict. For example, the amount and type of health care that medical facilities may wish to offer is restricted by patients' health care insurance policies. Further, the need for insurance providers and health maintenance organizations to remain profitable may at times conflict with the patient's wish to receive quality health care in a rapid and unrestricted manner. Nonetheless, the objectives of increased patient adherence and consequent improved disease control are in the best interests of both the health care industry and the patient. Patients who are adherent to their treatment plan and able to effectively self manage a chronic illness are less burdensome to health care providers. Such patients are less frustrating to their providers and less likely to require emergent medical services, in turn saving money for the insurer.

Table 3 Health Caregiver Behaviors That Promote Adherence

Health caregiver behavior	Explanation	Recent evidence
Anticipate non-adherence	Caregivers should expect that most patients will take less than 100% and many will take less than half of their medication	Bender (78)
Consider the treatment from the patient's perspective	Patient's health care experiences, health beliefs, expectations, fears, and goals all influence commitment to the treatment regimen	Apter et al. (76)
Foster a collaborative relationship based on negotiation	An acceptable, negotiated regimen that is carried out appropriately is better than an ideal one that is ignored	Charles et al. (79)
Customize treatment	Adherence can improve when the treatment regimen is adjusted, modified, and simplified to improve convenience to the patient	Jones et al. (80)
Enlist family support	When family members or other people significant to the patient understand the treatment plan and are called upon to support the patient, adherence improves	Fiese and Wamboldt (43)
Make use of other health care resources	Nurses, health educators, pharmacists, and any member of the health care team can be enlisted to ensure understanding of the treatment and encourage adherence to it	Levy et al. (81)
Provide continuity and accessibility	Follow-up phone calls and office visits enhance continuity and adherence	McDonald et al. (82)
Repeat everything	Patients frequently remember less than half of what health care providers tell them during office visits; oral repetition and provision of a written plan can enhance adherence	Schillinger et al. (27)

Source: From Ref. 77.

Because many emergency room visits and hospitalizations for asthma can be traced to treatment non-adherence (83), increased adherence can be cost-saving for insurance and health maintenance organizations. Inadequate disease management frequently underlies the largest health care costs related to asthma, including on average more than $500 per emergency room visit and $2000 per hospitalization (84). Urgent care, including hospital stays and visits to the emergency room or urgent care clinic, amount to almost $2 billion; (85) when indirect costs such as work absenteeism are taken into account, the total cost of poorly controlled asthma is much higher (86). The potential cost-savings achieved by promoting adherence must be weighed against the apparent cost-savings of restricting access to care, shortening office visits, and passing increasing medication costs to patients. Physicians and other care providers who experience pressure to see more patients in shorter office visits often report that they are allowed insufficient time to address patient adherence (87). If increased emergency room and hospital visits by patients who are not well motivated or informed about caring for their illness are at least partially the result of shortened office visits, then the apparent cost savings resulting from seeing more patients in less time is not real. Similarly, the apparent cost savings anticipated when insurance companies shift increasing medication cost to patients must be calculated against the cost resulting when patients stop taking medication for their disease (88).

Following are recommendations for the health care industry to help promote patient adherence to their treatment for chronic health conditions:

Do Not Blame the Patient

It is easy to view non-adherence as the fault of patients who fail to use health care resources appropriately and whose behavior is a nuisance, which drives up health care costs. In certain circumstances, health care may be denied to non-adherent patients, as occurs when organ transplant candidates are screened and only those who provide evidence of adherence sufficient to assure the viability of the transplanted organ become recipients. For most medical conditions, however, a more productive view is to see non-adherence not as a behavior to be punished, but as a problem that the health care industry must help to solve.

Provide Education and Support to the Providers Who Prescribe Treatment

There is evidence that physicians provided with training in communication and motivation skills can improve patient adherence to their treatment. One study demonstrated change in physician behavior by randomizing 69 primary-care physicians to either a communication-skill training group or a control group. Patients of physicians who received the intervention, consisting of training in recognizing and addressing patient distress, demonstrated a greater reduction in psychological distress and a short-term reduction in health care utilization (89). A program aimed at physicians who treat diabetes reported that patients of residents who were randomized to an intervention (which included focused seminars conducted by specialists, small group discussions, and emphasis toward patient attitudes, beliefs, skills, and clinical support systems) had improved fasting plasma glucose relative to control patients. The disease control improvements were even greater when physician education was combined with programmatic patient education (90).

Studies of patients with asthma have revealed significantly improved outcomes when teaching and communication skills were taught to physicians (91–93). Seventy-four general practitioners in Ann Arbor, Michigan, and New York City were randomized to an intervention or control condition (91). Those in the intervention condition received training to improve their ability to communicate effectively, understand patient behavior, create a supportive atmosphere, and educate patients in problem solving and asthma management. In contrast to the control group, patients of physicians in the intervention group received more oral and written information directing them in modifying their therapy, even though the average amount of time spent per patient was no greater than in the control group. Patients in this group were also more likely to receive a prescription for inhaled anti-inflammatory medication, which resulted in a significant decrease in office visits, ED visits, and hospitalizations during the two-year follow up (91).

Involve All Members of the Health Care Team

When patients' education and motivation are viewed as the responsibility of the entire health care team, and not just the physician, the possibility of affecting behavior change is dramatically improved. Physician assistants, nurses, medical assistants, and pharmacists can all help patients to understand their disease and its treatment, and to encourage greater adherence (81). The 1997 NHLBI guidelines captured this concept in their recommendations for interactions with patients, which included (1) patient education beginning at the time of diagnosis and integrated into every step of asthma care; (2) patient education provided by all members of the team, including mental health practitioners; and (3) teaching and reinforcing at every opportunity such behavioral skills as inhaler use, self-monitoring, and environmental control (69).

Establish a Communication Loop

Establishing communication systems that extend outside of the exam room can facilitate better adherence. Contacting patients to remind them of a scheduled office visit (94), asking patients to restate information or instructions to ensure that they were understood and remembered (95), following an office visit with an automated telephone call to assess health status (96), and providing home asthma telemonitoring (97) have helped to improve visit attendance, adherence, and treatment outcome. Similarly, clinically relevant information from pharmacy databases (e.g., repeat refills of rescue but not controller medications) can be fed back to providers who then can engage in non-judgmental, collaborative, problem-finding, and problem-solving discussions with their patients during subsequent clinic visits.

Recognize That Passing the Burden of Drug Costs to the Patient Will Likely Decrease Adherence

Shifting medication cost to patients is a rapidly growing national trend that may be short sighted. Incentive-based drug formularies, which allow patients a smaller co-payment when choosing generic or alternative medications, reduce drug utilization and cost (98,99). However, the savings may come at a yet undetermined price. Data from two large employer-sponsored health plans revealed a reduction in medication use when patients were switched from a one-tiered medication reimbursement plan to a three-tiered plan. A significant number of patients chose not simply to change drugs within the class of medications required for their illness, but to stop taking all drugs in the same class, including 16% of those on ACE inhibitors, 32% of those on proton-pump inhibitors, and 21% of those on statins (88). A potential consequence of this phenomenon, therefore, is to discourage patients from taking medication for their chronic illness.

C. Pharmaceutical Industry

Drug development, manufacturing, marketing, and pricing all have potential impact on patient acceptance and adherence. The fact that patients are more adherent to medications that are easily taken has been understood for many years (80,100–102). Recognizing this phenomenon, pharmaceutical firms have increasingly attempted to develop once-daily treatments, to obtain FDA approval to convert multiple-dosing regimens to once daily, and to produce asthma medications with tablet rather than inhaler delivery systems. Longer-acting and "depot" preparations of medications are not currently available for asthma, but such preparations have been useful in other chronic illnesses, especially in contexts when risk factors for very poor adherence are high and/or the consequences of poor adherence are especially dangerous.

Developing medications with higher patient acceptance helps adherence, but the pharmaceutical industry could do more to assist in the pursuit of improved self-management. Much of the research in adherence to asthma metered-dose inhalers has advanced because of the availability of electronic devices, which allows researchers to collect information about patterns of medication use. The most recent generation of dry-powder inhaled medications include a variety of delivery systems that do not accept electronic adherence-tracking equipment. As new asthma medications are developed, the inclusion of technology that can permit objective monitoring of adherence in clinical and research contexts would represent an important contribution to increasing patient adherence.

Finally, pharmaceutical firms may benefit from consideration of the growing phenomena of patient rejection of new, expensive drugs for which they are expected to shoulder a large portion of cost in their insurance plan. Management of high medication cost must be the responsibility of the pharmaceutical industry as well as the health insurance industry, the care provider, and the patient.

V. Conclusions

Many factors combine to determine patient adherence to their asthma treatment regimen. Some important factors include patient perception of illness severity that is at variance from that of the health caregiver, misunderstanding of the disease or its treatment, excessive demands of the treatment regimen, high medication costs, and inadequate communication with the health caregiver. For children, family confidence and competence, emotional health, positive relationships, absence of conflict, and the presence of established routines promote better adherence. The responsibility for improving adherence must be shared by various elements of the health care system, including the physician, insurance providers, and the pharmaceutical industry. Collaborative efforts to improve adherence to treatments for chronic illness, recently promoted by the World Health Organization (1), may follow the success of anti-tobacco efforts, including adherence promoting messages conveyed in the popular media, communication training for physicians, and increased funding to test new adherence intervention strategies. Research efforts to improve patient adherence to treatments should include development of interventions that are simple and easily applicable to the clinical setting, target vulnerable populations of patients at particular risk for non-adherence, address prevention of decay of adherence over time, and determine effective methods to train health caregivers in communication skills (103).

References

1. Adherence to Long-Term Therapies: Evidence for Action. World Health Organization, 2003.
2. National Ambulatory Medical Care Survey 2001, http://cms.hhs.gov/statistics/nhe/historical/highlights.asp.

3. DiMatteo MR. Variations in patients' adherence to medical recommendations: a quantitative review of 50 years of research. Med Care. In press.
4. Milgrom H, Bender B, Ackerson L, Bowry P, Smith B, Rand C. Noncompliance and treatment failure in children with asthma. J Allergy Clin Immunol 1996; 98:1051–1057.
5. Iskedjian M, Addis A, Einarson TR. Estimating the economic burden of hospitalization due to patient nonadherence in Canada. Value Health 2002; 5:470.
6. Morgan TM. The economic impact of wasted prescription medication in an outpatient population of older adults. J Fam Pract 2001; 50:779–781.
7. Horne R, Weinman J. Patients' beliefs about prescribed medicines and their role in adherence to treatment in chronic physical illness. J Psychosom Res 1999; 47:555–567.
8. Conrad P. The meaning of medications: another look at compliance. Soc Sci Med 1985; 20:29–37.
9. Nguyen BP, Wilson SR, German DF. Patients' perceptions compared with objective ratings of asthma severity. Ann Allergy Asthma Immunol 1996; 77:209–215.
10. Wolfenden LL, Diette GB, Krishnan JA, Skinner EA, Steinwachs DM, Wu AW. Lower physician estimate of underlying asthma severity leads to undertreatment. Arch Intern Med 2003; 163:231–236.
11. Osborne ML, Vollmer WM, Pedula KL, Wilkins J, Buist AS, O'Hollaren M. Lack of correlation of symptoms with specialist-assessed long-term asthma severity. Chest 1999; 115:85–91.
12. Adams S, Pill R, Jones A. Medication, chronic illness and identity: the perspective of people with asthma. Soc Sci Med 1997; 45:189–201.
13. Magadle R, Berar-Yanay N, Weiner P. The risk of hospitalization and near-fatal and fatal asthma in relation to the perception of dyspnea. Chest 2002; 121:329–333.
14. Sackett DL, Haynes RB. Compliance with therapeutic regimens. Baltimore: Johns Hopkins University Press, 1976.
15. Bender BG. Overcoming barriers to nonadherence in asthma treatment. J Allergy Clin Immunol 2002; 109(suppl 6):S554–S559.
16. Sherman J, Patel P, Hutson A, Chesrown S, Hendeles L. Adherence to oral montelukast and inhaled fluticasone in children with persistent asthma. Pharmacotherapy 2001; 21:1464–1467.
17. Bukstein DA, Henk HJ, Luskin AT. A comparison of asthma-related expenditures for patients started on montelukast versus fluticasone propionate as monotherapy. Clin Ther 2001; 23:1589–1600.
18. Bukstein DA, Luskin AT, Bernstein A. "Real-world" effectiveness of daily controller medicine in children with mild persistent asthma. Ann Allergy Asthma Immunol 2003; 90:543–549.
19. Chambers CV, Markson L, Diamond JJ, Lasch L, Berger M. Health beliefs and compliance with inhaled corticosteroids by asthmatic patients in primary care practices. Respir Med 1999; 93:88–94.
20. Boulet LP. Perception of the role and potential side effects of inhaled corticosteroids among asthmatic patients. Chest 1998; 113:587–592.

21. Venables TL, Addlestone MB, Smithers AJ. A comparison of the efficacy and patient acceptability of once-daily budesonide via Turbuhaler and twice-daily fluticasone propionate via a disc-inhaler at an equal dose of 400 mcg in adult asthmatics. Br J Clin Res 1996; 7:15–32.

22. Shrestha M, Parupia H, Andrews B, Kim SW, Martin MS, Park DI, Gee E. Metered-dose inhaler technique of patients in an urban ED: prevalence of incorrect technique and attempt at education. Am J Emerg Med 1996; 14: 380–384.

23. Apter AJ, Reisine ST, Affleck G, Barrows E, ZuWallack RL. Adherence with twice-daily dosing of inhaled steroids. Socioeconomic and health-belief differences. Am J Respir Crit Care Med 1998; 157:1810–1817.

24. Steinman MA, Sands LP, Covinsky KE. Self-restriction of medications due to cost in seniors without prescription coverage. J Gen Intern Med 2001; 16:793–799.

25. Alexander GC, Casalino LP, Meltzer DO. Patient–physician communication about out-of-pocket costs. JAMA 2003; 290:953–958.

26. DiMatteo MR. The Psychology of Health, Illness and Medical Care: an Individual Perspective. Pacific Grove: 1991.

27. Schillinger D, Piette J, Grumbach K, Wang F, Wilson C, Daher C, Leong-Grotz K, Castro C, Bindman AB. Closing the loop: physician communication with diabetic patients who have low health literacy. Arch Intern Med 2003; 163:83–90.

28. Pachter LM, Weller SC. Acculturation and compliance with medical therapy. J Dev Behav Pediatr 1993; 14:163–168.

29. Pachter LM. Culture and clinical care. Folk illness beliefs and behaviors and their implications for health care delivery. JAMA 1994; 271:690–694.

30. Bauman LJ, Wright E, Leickly FE, Crain E, Kruszon-Moran D, Wade SL, Visness CM. Relationship of adherence to pediatric asthma morbidity among inner-city children. Pediatrics 2002; 110:1–7.

31. Butz AM, Malveaux FJ, Eggleston P, Thompson L, Schneider S, Weeks K, Huss K, Murigande C, Rand CS. Use of community health workers with inner-city children who have asthma. Clin Pediatr (Phila) 1994; 33: 135–141.

32. Riekert KA, Bartlett S, Kolodner K, Malveaux F, Rand CS. Inner-city caregiver's reports of their physicians' asthma management practices. Am J Respir Crit Care Med 2001; 163.

33. Roter D, Hall J, Katz N. Patient–physician communication: a descriptive summary of the literature. Patient Educ Counsel 1988; 12:99–119.

34. Steele DJ, Jackson TC, Gutmann MC. Have you been taking your pill? The adherence-monitoring sequence in the medical interview. J Fam Pract 1990; 30:294–299.

35. Wensing M, Elwyn G, Edwards A, Vingerhoets E, Grol R. Deconstructing patient centered communication and uncovering shared decision making: an observational study. BMC Med Inform Decis Making 2002; 2:2.

36. Moumjid N, Bremond A, Carrere MO. From information to shared decision-making in medicine. Health Expect 2003; 6:187–188.

37. Ruland CM, Bakken S. Developing, implementing, and evaluating decision support systems for shared decision making in patient care: a conceptual model and case illustration. J Biomed Inform 2002; 35:313–321.

38. Fenton WS. Shared decision-making: a model for the physician–patient relationship in the 21st century? Acta Psychiatr Scand 2003; 107:401–402.

39. DiMatteo MR. Enhancing patient adherence to medical recommendations. JAMA 1994; 271:79–83.

40. Minuchin S, Baker L, Rosman BL, Liebman R, Milman L, Todd TC. A conceptual model of psychosomatic illness in children. Family organization and family therapy. Arch Gen Psychiatry 1975; 32:1031–1038.

41. Minuchin S, Rosman BL, Baker L. Psychosomatic Families. Cambridge: Harvard University Press, 1978.

42. Wamboldt MZ, Wamboldt FS. Psychosocial aspects of severe asthma in children. In: Szefler SJ, Leung DYM, eds. Severe Asthma: Pathogenesis and Clinical Management, 2d ed. New York: Marcel Dekker, 2001:471–503.

43. Fiese BH, Wamboldt FS. Tales of pediatric asthma management: family-based strategies related to medical adherence and health care utilization. J Pediatr 2003; 143:457–462.

44. Gavin LA, Roesler TA. Post-traumatic distress in children and families after intubation. Pediatr Emerg Care 1997; 13:222–224.

45. Kazak AE. Post-traumatic distress in childhood cancer survivors and their parents. Med Pediatr Oncol 1998; Suppl 1:60–68.

46. Stuber ML, Shemesh E, Saxe GN. Post-traumatic stress responses in children with life-threatening illnesses. Child Adolesc Psychiatr Clin N Am 2003; 12:195–209.

47. Wamboldt FS, Wamboldt MZ, Gavin LA, Roesler TA, Brugman SM. Parental criticism and treatment outcome in adolescents hospitalized for severe, chronic asthma. J Psychosom Res 1995; 39:995–1005.

48. Bartlett SJ, Kolodner K, Butz AM, Eggleston P, Malveaux FJ, Rand CS. Maternal depressive symptoms and emergency department use among inner-city children with asthma. Arch Pediatr Adolesc Med 2001; 155: 347–353.

49. DiMatteo MR, Lepper HS, Croghan TW. Depression is a risk factor for noncompliance with medical treatment: meta-analysis of the effects of anxiety and depression on patient adherence. Arch Intern Med 2000; 160: 2101–2107.

50. Weil CM, Wade SL, Bauman LJ, Lynn H, Mitchell H, Lavigne J. The relationship between psychosocial factors and asthma morbidity in inner-city children with asthma. Pediatrics 1999; 104:1274–1280.

51. Markson S, Fiese BH. Family rituals as a protective factor for children with asthma. J Pediatr Psychol 2000; 25:471–480.

52. Fiese BH, Tomcho TJ, Douglas M, Josephs K, Poltrock S, Baker T. A review of 50 years of research on naturally occurring family routines and rituals: cause for celebration? J Fam Psychol 2002; 164:381–390.

53. Fiese B, Wamboldt F. Family routines and asthma management: a proposal for family-based strategies to increase treatment adherence. Fam Syst Health 2000; 18:405–418.

54. Cramer JA. Optimizing long-term patient compliance. Neurology 1995; 45(suppl 1):S25–S28.
55. Chen E, Bloomberg GR, Fisher EB Jr, Strunk RC. Predictors of repeat hospitalizations in children with asthma: the role of psychosocial and socio-environmental factors. Health Psychol 2003; 22:12–18.
56. Christiaanse ME, Lavigne JV, Lerner CV. Psychosocial aspects of compliance in children and adolescents with asthma. Dev Behav Pediatr 1989; 10:75–80.
57. Hermanns J, Florin I, Dietrich M, Rieger C, Hahlweg K. Maternal criticism, mother–child interaction, and bronchial asthma. J Psychosom Res 1989; 33:469–476.
58. Schobinger R, Florin I, Reichbauer M, Lindemann H, Zimmer C. Childhood asthma: mothers' affective attitude, mother–child interaction and children's compliance with medical requirements. J Psychosom Res 1993; 37:697–707.
59. Wamboldt MZ, Weintraub P, Krafchick D, Berce N, Wamboldt FS. Links between past parental trauma and the medical and psychological outcome of asthmatic children: a theoretical model. Fam Syst Med 1995; 13:129–149.
60. Gustafsson PA, Kjellman NI, Bjorksten B. Family interaction and a supportive social network as salutogenic factors in childhood atopic illness. Pediatr Allergy Immunol 2002; 13:51–57.
61. Klinnert MD, Mrazek PJ, Mrazek DA. Early asthma onset: the interaction between family stressors and adaptive parenting. Psychiatry 1994; 57:51–61.
62. Klinnert MD, Nelson HS, Price MR, Adinoff AD, Leung DY, Mrazek DA. Onset and persistence of childhood asthma: predictors from infancy. Pediatrics 2001; 108:E69.
63. Mrazek DA, Klinnert M, Mrazek PJ, Brower A, McCormick D, Rubin B, Ikle D, Kastner W, Larsen G, Harbeck R, Jones J. Prediction of early-onset asthma in genetically at-risk children. Pediatr Pulmonol 1999; 27:85–94.
64. Bender B, Wamboldt FS, O'Connor SL, Rand C, Szefler S, Milgrom H, Wamboldt MZ. Measurement of children's asthma medication adherence by self-report, mother report, canister weight, and Doser CT. Ann Allergy Asthma Immunol 2000; 85:416–421.
65. McQuaid EL, Kopel SJ, Klein RB, Fritz GK. Medication adherence in pediatric asthma: reasoning, responsibility, and behavior. J Pediatr Psychol 2003; 28:323–333.
66. Wasilewski Y, Clark N, Evans D, Feldman CH, Kaplan D, Rips J, Mellins RB. The effect of paternal social support on maternal disruption caused by childhood asthma. J Community Health 1988; 13:33–42.
67. Repetti RL, Taylor SE, Seeman TE. Risky families: family social environments and the mental and physical health of offspring. Psychol Bull 2002; 128:330–366.
68. Bernard-Bonnin A-C, Stachenko S, Bonin D, Charette C, Rousseau E. Self-management teaching programs and morbidity of pediatric asthma: a meta-analysis. J Allergy Clin Immunol 1995; 95:23–41.
69. NHLBI. Expert Panel Report 2. Guidelines for the diagnosis and management of asthma. U.S. Department of Health and Human Services 1997.

70. Cromer BA. Behavioral strategies to increase compliance in adolescents. In: Cramer JA, Spilker B, eds. Patient Compliance in Medical Practice and Clinical Trials. New York: Raven Press, 1991:99–105.

71. Stewart MA. Effective physician–patient communication and health outcomes: a review. Can Med Assoc J 1995; 152:1423–1433.

72. Gavin LA, Wamboldt MZ, Sorokin N, Levy SY, Wamboldt FS. Treatment alliance and its association with family functioning, adherence, and medical outcome in adolescents with severe, chronic asthma. J Pediatr Psychol 1999; 24:355–365.

73. Krupnick JL, Sotsky SM, Simmens S. The role of the therapeutic alliance in psychotherapy and pharmocotherapy outcome: findings in the National Institute of Mental Health treatment of depression collaborative research program. J Consult Clin Psychol 1996; 64:532.

74. DiMatteo MR, Sherbourne CD, Hays RD. Physicians' characteristics influence patients' adherence to medical treatment: results from the medical outcomes study. Health Psychol 1993; 12:93–102.

75. Armstrong D, Glanville T, Bailey E, O'Keefe G. Doctor-initiated consultations: a study of communication between general practitioners and patients about the need for reattendance. Brit J Gen Pract 1990; 40:241–242.

76. Apter AJ, Boston RC, George M, Norfleet AL, Tenhave T, Coyne JC, Birck K, Reisine ST, Cucchiara AJ, Feldman HI. Modifiable barriers to adherence to inhaled steroids among adults with asthma: it's not just black and white. J Allergy Clin Immunol 2003; 111:1219–1226.

77. Meichenbaum D, Turk DC. Facilitating Treatment Adherence. A Practitioner's Guidebook. New York: Plenum Press, 1987.

78. Bender BG. Strategies that improve adherence to asthma therapy. Contemp Pediatr 2003; 4–11.

79. Charles C, Gafni A, Whelan T. Decision-making in the physician–patient encounter: revisiting the shared treatment decision-making model. Soc Sci Med 1999; 49:651–661.

80. Jones C, Santanello NC, Boccuzzi SJ, Wogen J, Strub P, Nelsen LM. Adherence to prescribed treatment for asthma: evidence from pharmacy benefits data. J Asthma. In press.

81. Levy ML, Robb M, Allen J, Doherty C, Bland JM, Winter RJD. A randomized controlled evaluation of specialist nurse education following accident and emergency department attendance for acute asthma. Respir Med 2000; 94:900–908.

82. McDonald HP, Garg AX, Haynes RB. Interventions to enhance patient adherence to medication prescriptions. JAMA 2002; 288:2868–2879.

83. Bauman LJ, Wright E, Leickly FE, Crain E, Kruszon-Moran D, Wade SL. Visness CM. Relationship of adherence to pediatric asthma morbidity among inner-city children. Pediatrics 2002; 110:1–7.

84. Weiss KB, Sullivan SD. The health economics of asthma and rhinitis. I. Assessing the economic impact. J Allergy Clin Immunol 2001; 107:3–8.

85. Cisternas MG, Blanc PD, Yen IH, Katz PP, Earnest G, Eisner MD, Shiboski S, Yelin EH. A comprehensive study of the direct and indirect costs of adult asthma. J Allergy Clin Immunol 2003; 111:1212–1218.

86. Birnbaum HG, Berger WE, Greenberg PE, Holland M, Auerbach R, Atkins KM, Wanke LA. Direct and indirect costs of asthma to an employer. J Allergy Clin Immunol 2002; 109:264–270.

87. Ammerman AS, DeVellis RF, Carey TS, Keyserling TC, Strogatz DS, Haines PS, Simpson RJ Jr, Siscovick DS. Physician-based diet counseling for cholesterol reduction: current practices, determinants, and strategies for improvement. Prev Med 1993; 22:96–109.

88. Huskamp HA, Deverka PA, Epstein AM, Epstein RS, McGuigan KA, Frank RG. The effect of incentive-based formularies on prescription-drug utilization and spending. New Eng J Med 2003; 349:2224–2232.

89. Roter D, Hall J, Dern D. Improving physicians' interviewing skills and reducing patients' emotional distress: a randomized clinical trial. Arch Intern Med 1995; 155:1877–1884.

90. Vinicor F, Cohen SJ, Mazzuca SA. DIABEDS: a randomized trial of the effects of physician and/or patient education on diabetes patient outcomes. J Chronic Dis 1987; 40:345–356.

91. Clark NM, Gong M, Schork MA, Evans D, Roloff D, Hurwitz M, Maiman L, Mellins RB. Impact of education for physicians on patient outcomes. Pediatrics 1998; 101:831–836.

92. Clark NM, Gong M, Schork MA, Kaciroti N, Evans D, Roloff D, Hurwitz M, Maiman LA, Mellins RB. Long-term effects of asthma education for physicians on patient satisfaction and use of health services. Eur Respir J 2000; 16:15–21.

93. Evans D, Mellins R, Lobach K, Ramos-Bonoan C, Pinkett-Heller M, Wiesemann S, Klein I, Donahue C, Burke D, Levison M, Levin B, Zimmerman B, Clark N. Improving care for minority children with asthma: professional education in public health clinics. Pediatrics 1997; 99:157–164.

94. Macharia WM, Leon G, Rowe BH. An overview of interventions to improve compliance with appointments for medical services. JAMA 1992; 267: 374–378.

95. Schillinger D, Piette J, Grumback K, Wang F, Wilson C, Daher C, Leong-Grotz K, Castro C, Bindman AB. Closing the loop. Physician communication with diabetic patients who have low health literacy. Arch Intern Med 2003; 163:83–90.

96. Piette JD, Weinberger M, McPhee SJ, Mah CA, Kraemer FB, Crapo LM. Do automated calls with nurse follow-up improve self-care nand glycemic control among vulnerable patients with diabetes? Am J Med 2000; 108:20–27.

97. Finkelstein J, O'Connor G, Friedman RH. In: Patel V, ed. Development and Implementation of the Home Asthma Telemonitoring (HAT) System to Facilitate Asthma Self-Care. Amsterdam: IOS Press, 2001:810–814.

98. Motheral BR, Fairman KA. Effect of a three-tier prescription copay on pharmaceutical and other medical utilization. Med Care 2001; 39:1293–1304.

99. Joyce GF, Escarce JJ, Solomon MD, Goldman DP. Employer drug benefit plans and spending on prescription drugs. JAMA 2002; 288:1733–1739.

100. Becker MH, Matman LA. Sociobehavioral determinants of compliance with health and medical care recommendations. Med Care 1975; 13:10–24.

101. Cramer J, Mattson R, Prevey M, Scheyer R, Oullette V. How often is medication taken as prescribed? A novel assessment technique. JAMA 1989; 261:3273–3277.

102. Kelloway JS, Wyatt RA, Adlis SA. Comparison of patients' compliance with prescribed oral and inhaled asthma medications. Arch Intern Med 1994; 154:1349–1359.

103. Bender BG, Berning S, Dudden R, Milgrom H, vu Tran Z. Sedation and performance impairment of diphenhydramine and second generation antihistamines: a meta-analysis. J Allergy Clin Immunol 2003; 111:770–776.

24

Potential Applications of New Drugs in the Management of Childhood Asthma

PETER J. BARNES

Department of Thoracic Medicine, National Heart and Lung Institute, Imperial College London, U.K.

I. Introduction

Development of new treatments for childhood asthma poses particular problems in view of safety concerns and the difficulty of accurately measuring clinical outcomes. There are several novel drugs in development for the management of asthma, but these are always studied initially in adults, and studies in children generally follow when the drug is in advanced clinical development. This chapter reviews some of the new drugs in development for asthma, some of which are currently in clinical trials for asthma in adults. A few drugs that are improvements in existing classes of drugs, such as corticosteroids, are testable at an earlier stage in children and adverse effects are more predictable.

Currently available therapy for asthma is highly effective and, if used appropriately, usually has no problems in terms of adverse effects. However, some patients (~5% of asthmatic adults and children) remain poorly controlled, despite what appears to be optimal therapy. There are also continuing concerns about the safety of asthma therapy, particularly in the treatment of childhood asthma, as this treatment has to be given over very long periods. Compliance with inhaled therapy, particularly with inhaled corticosteroid therapy, is very poor and might be improved with oral therapy (once-daily calendar pack). Yet oral therapy presents a problem of side effects, since the drug exerts effects throughout the body, whereas asthma is localized to the airways. This will necessitate the development of drugs that are specific for asthma and do not have effects on other systems or on normal physiological mechanisms (unlike β-agonists and corticosteroids). None of the currently available therapy is curative nor has it so far been shown to alter the natural history of the disease. Perhaps it is difficult to seek a cure for asthma until more about the molecular causes is known.

Despite considerable efforts by the pharmaceutical industry, it has proved very difficult to develop new classes of therapeutic agents. This is partly because existing drugs are effective and safe, and partly because animal models of asthma are poor and do not appear to predict clinical efficacy. Asthma is one of the most rapidly growing therapeutic markets in the world, reflecting the enormous worldwide increase in prevalence of asthma and the increasing recognition that chronic anti-inflammatory treatment is needed for many patients. In addition, despite the availability of effective and relatively cheap treatments, there is still a considerable degree of undertreatment of asthma. For example, a European survey showed that only ~25% of patients of all ages with severe asthma were receiving inhaled corticosteroids (1). The current worldwide asthma market exceeds US $4 billion and is increasing rapidly (2,3).

It is clearly important to understand more about the underlying mechanisms of asthma (4) and also about how the currently used drugs work before rational improvements in therapy can be expected. Better understanding of the cellular and molecular mechanisms of asthma has identified new molecular targets for the development of novel classes of drug, and there are several opportunities for new drug development in asthma (5–7).

There are three major approaches to the development of new anti-asthma treatments:

- improvements in existing classes of effective drugs—e.g., development of long-acting inhaled β2-agonists (LABA) (salmeterol and formoterol) or long-acting anticholinergics (tiotropium bromide);
- development of novel compounds, based on rational developments and improved understanding of asthma—e.g., anti-leukotrienes, anti-IgE, and IL-5 inhibitors;
- development of novel compounds based on serendipity, often arising from other disease areas—e.g., furosemide.

II. Problems of Drug Development in Children

Although the pathophysiological mechanisms and the inflammatory process are similar in childhood asthma to those in adult asthma, there may be important differences in the handling and response to drugs. This means that specific clinical trials need to be conducted in asthmatic children. For new drugs, this is usually only possible once the drug has been tested in adults, so that clinical trials in children are planned late in the clinical development program.

Assessment of the response to anti-asthma therapy is more difficult in children because of the difficulties of measuring lung function, particularly in young children. Invasive investigations, such as bronchial biopsies, are more difficult in children because of ethical concerns. This has led to a search for less invasive approaches. Induced sputum is widely used to measure anti-inflammatory effects of drugs in adults, but is less successful in children, with less than 50% of patients able to provide satisfactory samples (8). Noninvasive techniques, such as exhaled nitric oxide (NO) and exhaled breath condensate, are now being applied to investigating anti-inflammatory treatments in children (9–12).

There are particular problems in studying new treatments in very young children. Yet, this is a very important age group as there may be a greater potential to switch off the disease process before it becomes fully established and possibly less reversible. This is an impetus for developing noninvasive methods for assessing drug effects in young children. This may be of particular importance in approaches that might result in a cure such as vaccination.

There are also, problems in delivering inhaled drugs to children, but the use of large-volume spacers with valves has greatly increased the efficiency of inhaled drug delivery, even in young children. However, oral therapy is much easier to deliver in children, so there has been an intense search for effective oral anti-asthma therapies.

III. New Bronchodilators

Bronchodilators are presumed to act by reversing the contraction of airway smooth muscle, although some may have additional effects on mucosal edema or inflammatory cells. The biochemical basis of airway smooth muscle relaxation has been studied extensively, yet no new types of bronchodilator have so far had any clinical impact. The molecular basis of bronchodilatation involves an increase in intracellular cyclic adenosine $3',5'$ monophosphate (cAMP) and a reduction in cytosolic calcium ion concentration ($[Ca^{2+}]$). The rise in cAMP is linked to the opening of Ca^{2+}-activated K^+ channels (maxi-K channels) in animal and human airway smooth muscle (13,14). However, β-agonists may open maxi-K channels via a direct G-protein (G_s) coupling to the channel, and this may occur at low concentrations of β-agonist that do not involve any increase in cAMP concentration (15). The molecular mechanisms underlying bronchodilatation may be exploited in the development of new broncho-dilators, several of which are under development (Fig. 1).

A. β2-Agonists

Many selective β2-agonists are now available and there has been a search for β-agonists that have even greater selectivity for β2-receptors. However, it is unlikely that any greater selectivity would be an advantage clinically, since when the drugs are given by inhalation, a high degree of functional β2-receptor selectivity is obtained. Furthermore, many of the side effects of β-agonists (tremor, tachycardia, and hypokalemia) are mediated via β2-receptors. The recent concern that inhaled β2-agonists might be associated with increased asthma morbidity and mortality is controversial, and there is little evidence that the normally used doses of inhaled β2-agonists are a problem, particularly when these drugs are used as required for symptom relief rather than on a regular basis (16,17). The most important recent advance

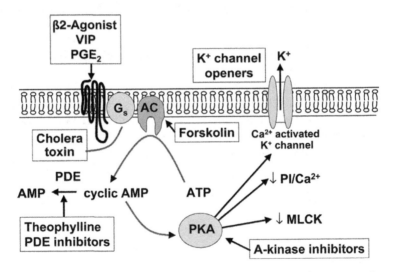

Figure 1 Molecular mechanism of action of β2-agonists on airway smooth muscle cells. Activation of β2AR, VIP, and PGE$_2$ receptors results in activation of AC via a stimulatory G$_s$ and increase in cyclic AMP. This activates protein kinase A which then phosphorylates several target proteins which result in opening of K$_{Ca}$ or maxi-K channels, decreased PI hydrolysis, increased Na$^+$/Ca^{2+} exchange, increased Na$^+$/K$^+$ ATPase, and decreased MLCK activity. In addition, β2-receptors may be coupled directly via G$_s$ to K$_{Ca}$. *Abbreviations:* β2AR, β2-receptors; VIP, vasoactive intestinal peptide; PGE$_2$, prostaglandin E$_2$; AC, adenylyl cyclase; G$_s$, G-protein; AMP, 3′,5′ adenosine monophosphate; K$_{Ca}$, calcium-activated potassium channels; PI, phosphoinositide; Na$^+$/Ca^{2+}, sodium/calcium ion; ATP, adenosine triphosphate; MLCK, myosin light chain kinase.

in bronchodilator therapy has been the introduction of the LABA, salmeterol and formoterol, that give bronchodilatation and protection against bronchoconstriction for over 12 hours (18). These drugs have proved to be very useful clinically and provide additional control of asthma when added to inhaled corticosteroids, and they are safe. This has made development of new bronchodilators that would have any advantage extremely difficult. The recent introduction of fixed combination inhalers of a corticosteroid and a LABA (fluticasone propionate/salmeterol and budesonide/formoterol) is having a major impact on asthma treatment in children with more severe asthma, as this provides increased control, reduced risk of side effects, and greater convenience (19). It is likely that several other LABA/corticosteroid inhalers will be introduced, including generic versions, and that this will be the mainstay of treatment for most patients with asthma over the next 10–15 years.

Several β2-agonists with an even longer duration of action have now been developed and will be suitable for once-daily administration. These once-daily inhaled β2-agonists are now in clinical trials.

B. Drugs That Increase Cyclic AMP

Understanding the molecular mechanism of β-agonists has prompted a search for other drugs that increase intracellular cyclic AMP concentrations in airway smooth muscle cells. Several other receptors on airway smooth muscle, other than β-receptors, may activate adenylyl cyclase via a stimulatory G_s.

Vasoactive intestinal peptide (VIP) is a potent bronchodilator of human airways in vitro, but is ineffective in asthmatic patients in vivo (20), reflecting degradation of the peptide by airway epithelial cells. A more stable cyclic analogue of VIP (Ro-25–1553) has a more prolonged effect in vitro and in vivo (21), and has been shown to have a useful bronchodilator effect when given by inhalation to adult asthmatics (22). However, there is no advantage over a β2-agonist and its duration of action is less than formoterol.

Prostaglandin E_2 (PGE$_2$) stimulates adenylyl cyclase and relaxes airways in vitro. However PGE has not proved to be as effective as a bronchodilator in vivo, and may even lead to constriction and coughing in asthmatics since PGE also stimulates afferent nerve endings in airways. There are at least four subtypes of PGE (EP) receptor and it is likely that the EP-receptor subtype on sensory nerves differs from the receptor subtype on airway smooth muscle (EP$_2$), so that a selective agonist may be developed (23). In addition, there is evidence that PGE$_2$ has an inhibitory action on eosinophils, monocytes, and T lymphocytes (24), and might therefore have anti-inflammatory potential. Inhaled PGE$_2$ inhibits the early and late response to allergen and is involved in the refractory response to exercise in the airways, suggesting that PGE$_2$ may have some therapeutic potential (25). Receptor subtype–selective PGE-agonists may avoid the problem of coughing and may be worthy of further exploration as bronchodilator/anti-inflammatory drugs.

Forskolin directly activates the catalytic subunit of adenylyl cyclase, and produces large increases in cyclic AMP concentration in airway smooth muscle cells, but has not proved to be effective as a bronchodilator in vitro (26). This may be because $\beta2$-agonists are effective as bronchodilators via direct coupling to maxi-K channels via G_s in addition to a rise in cyclic AMP that is seen with high concentrations of β-agonists (15).

C. Drugs That Increase Cyclic GMP

Atrial natriuretic peptide (ANP), when given by intravenous infusion, produces a significant bronchodilator response and protects against bronchoconstrictor challenges (27,28). It is likely that the effects of ANP on airways are mediated by stimulation of particulate guanylyl cyclase and subsequent generation of cyclic $3',5'$ guanosine monophosphate (GMP) (29). While ANP itself may be difficult to use, it is possible that non-peptide agonists of ANP receptors may be developed in the future for inhaled use. A related peptide urodilatin (ularitide) has a longer duration of action than ANP as it is less susceptible to enzymatic breakdown and is as potent as albuterol when given by intravenous infusion in asthmatic subjects (30,31).

Nitrovasodilators, such as isosorbide dinitrate and glyceryl trinitrate (GTN), activate soluble guanylyl cyclase (29). The endogenous neural bronchodilator in human airways is NO (32). However, previous studies with nitrovasodilators in asthma have not been promising as the dose may be limited by vasodilator effects.

D. Selective Anticholinergics

There are several distinct subtypes of muscarinic receptor, which have differing physiological roles in the airway, and there is a rationale for the development of selective anti-muscarinics that block M_3-(and possibly M_1-) receptors, but avoiding blockade of prejunctional M_2-receptors that would lead to an increase in the release of acetylcholine. Tiotropium bromide is a new anticholinergic with a duration of action of > 24 hours and kinetic selectivity for M_1- and M_3-receptors (33). It has recently been introduced for the treatment of chronic obstructive pulmonary disease, but it is likely that it will also be useful as an additional bronchodilator in children with severe asthma, particularly when there is an element of fixed airflow obstruction.

E. K$^+$ Channel Openers

Potassium (K^+) channels play an important role in the recovery of excitable cells after activation and in maintaining cell stability. K^+ channels openers relax airway smooth muscle and act as bronchodilators. Drugs that selectively activate an adenosine $5'$-triphosphate-dependent K^+ channel (K_{ATP}), such as levcromakalim, are effective bronchodilators of human airways in vitro, but are ineffective in vivo at maximally tolerated oral doses (34).

Several K^+ channel openers have been in phase-I/II studies but their development for asthma was halted because of dose-limiting vasodilator side effects (headaches and postural hypotension). The bronchodilator response to β2-agonists is mediated in part by opening of a large conductance calcium-dependent K^+ channel (K_{Ca}). Benzimidazole compounds, such as NS 1619, are K_{Ca} openers and bronchodilators (35). K_{Ca} openers may also be effective as inhibitors of sensory nerve activation. This class of drug may, therefore, be useful in inhibiting cough and airway hyperresponsiveness (36).

IV. Mediator Antagonists

Many inflammatory mediators have been implicated in asthma, and several specific receptor antagonists and synthesis inhibitors have been developed that have proved to be useful in working out the contribution of each mediator (37). As over 100 mediators probably contribute to the pathophysiology of asthma and many mediators have similar effects, it is unlikely that a single antagonist could have a major clinical effect compared with nonspecific agents such as β-agonists and corticosteroids. Antihistamines, platelet-activating factor antagonists, thromboxane inhibitors, and bradykinin antagonists have all proved to have little or no clinical benefit in asthma (Fig. 2).

A. Leukotriene Modifiers

Leukotriene modifiers, including anti-leukotrienes (cys-LT_1-receptor antagonists: montelukast, pranlukast, and zafirlukast) and $5'$-lipoxygenase inhibitors (zileuton), were the first new class of anti-asthma treatment to be introduced in over 30 years of intense research. Although anti-leukotrienes have some clinical effects in asthma, they are considerably less effective and more expensive than inhaled corticosteroids (38). They may be useful in patients with aspirin-sensitive asthma (39) and when exercise-induced asthma is a particular problem (40), but cannot be considered as a substitute for inhaled corticosteroids. Some patients respond better than others, but it is not possible to predict good responders on any clinical parameters, and even genetic polymorphisms in the $5'$-LO pathway do not help to select responders. Anti-leukotrienes have been particularly popular in the treatment of childhood asthma because of their oral delivery. This has prompted a search for new drugs that interact with leukotriene pathways.

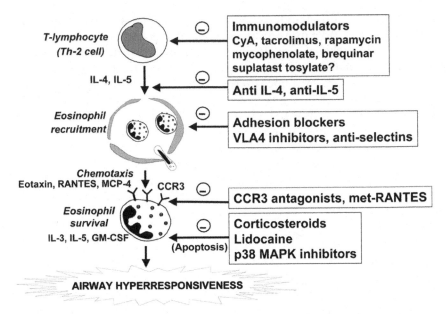

Figure 2   Inhibition of eosinophilic inflammation. Several strategies are possible to inhibit eosinophil inflammation in tissues, including immunomodulators, inhibitors of driving cytokines (IL-4 and IL-5), inhibition of critical adhesion molecules (VLA4, selectins, and ICAM-1), blockade of chemokine receptors on eosinophils (CCR3), and induction of apoptosis.

Currently available anti-leukotrienes (montelukast, pranlukast, and zafirlukast) are potent competitive antagonists of cys-LT$_1$ receptors and it is unlikely that any increase in potency would increase their efficacy, although a more prolonged duration of action might be beneficial. These anti-leukotrienes are selective inhibitors of cys-LT$_1$ receptors, which mediate bronchoconstriction, plasma exudation, and mucous secretion, but a second receptor termed cys-LT$_2$ may be important in mediating some responses to cys-LTs, such as airway smooth muscle proliferation (41). Drugs that inhibit both cys-LT$_1$ and cys-LT$_2$ receptors may therefore have some theoretical advantage.

Zileuton is a relatively poor 5′-LO inhibitor; it is weak, has a short duration of action, and frequently causes disturbed liver function tests. However, in terms of clinical efficacy, it is similar to the more potent anti-leukotrienes, perhaps indicating that better 5′-LO inhibitors may be more effective clinically. The 5′-LO inhibitors block the generation of cys-LTs, but also of LTB$_4$, which might play a role particularly in more severe asthma and in exacerbations where neutrophilic inflammation may become more prominent. The concentration of LTB$_4$ is increased in exhaled breath condensate of children with asthma, particularly in severe asthma (11). It has proved difficult to develop 5'-LO inhibitors as many of these drugs have redox effects and are limited by toxicity. Inhibitors of 5'-lipoxygenase activating protein (FLAP) appear to be less toxic, but in clinical studies lacked efficacy (42). More potent 5'-LO inhibitors may therefore be useful, particularly in severe asthma. LTB$_4$-receptor antagonists (BLT$_1$-antagonists) do not inhibit allergen-induced responses in asthmatic patients (43), but might have a role in more severe asthma and during exacerbations where neutrophil recruitment is evident.

B. Prostaglandin Inhibitors

Prostaglandins have potent effects on airway function and there is increased expression of the inducible form of cyclo-oxygenase-2 (COX-2) in asthmatic airways (44). COX inhibitors, such as aspirin or ibuprofen, and COX-2 inhibitors do not have any beneficial effects.

Prostaglandin D$_2$ is a bronchoconstrictor prostaglandin that is produced predominantly by mast cells. Deletion of the PGD$_2$ receptors in mice significantly inhibits inflammatory responses to allergen and AHR, suggesting that this mediator may be important in asthma (45). PGD$_2$ activates a novel receptor termed chemoattractant receptor of Th-2 cells (CRTH2), which is expressed on Th-2 cells, eosinophils, and basophils and mediates chemotaxis of these cell types, providing a possible link between mast cell activation and allergic inflammation (46). There is a search for inhibitors of CRTH2, but the observation that blocking the production of PGD$_2$ with COX inhibitors is not beneficial in asthma makes this approach unpromising.

C. Endothelin Antagonists

Endothelins are potent vasoconstrictor and bronchoconstrictor peptide mediators (47). Endothelin-1 levels are increased in the sputum of patients with asthma; they are further increased by allergen exposure and reduced by corticosteroid treatment (48,49). Endothelins induce airway smooth muscle cell proliferation and promote a profibrotic phenotype and may, therefore, play a role in the chronic inflammation and airway remodeling in asthma. Several relatively potent antagonists of endothelin receptors have been developed (50). In asthma, both ET$_A$ and ET$_B$ receptors may be involved in bronchoconstriction and structural changes, so that non-selective antagonists are preferable. It is uncertain whether ET antagonists will be beneficial in asthma, as many growth factors are involved in the structural changes in the airways and it would also be difficult to detect any effect of a drug on these processes, which proceed very slowly and for which there are no validated biomarkers yet developed.

D. Antioxidants

As in all inflammatory diseases, there is increased oxidative stress in asthmatic inflammation, as activated inflammatory cells, such as macrophages and eosinophils, produce reactive oxygen species. Evidence for increased oxidative stress in childhood asthma is provided by the increased concentrations of 8-isoprostane (a product of oxidized arachidonic acid) in exhaled breath condensates (51). Increased oxidative stress is related to disease severity and may amplify the inflammatory response and reduce responsiveness to corticosteroids, particularly in severe disease and during exacerbations. Oxidative stress impairs responsiveness to corticosteroids by inhibition of histone deacetylase activity (probably through the formation of peroxynitrite) (52), which is the major mechanism whereby corticosteroids switch off inflammatory genes. Antioxidants are therefore a logical approach in asthma therapy, particularly in severe disease. However, existing antioxidants are weak and are not able to neutralize the high level of oxidative stress in the airways, so that more potent antioxidants are needed in the future (53).

E. Purine Receptor Modulators

Adenosine is a potent bronchoconstrictor in patients with asthma and appears to activate mast cells via adenosine A_{2B} receptors (54). The effects of adenosine are markedly potentiated by prior exposure to allergen (55). A_{2B} receptor antagonists may therefore be of value in inhibiting mast cell activation in asthma, although it has been difficult to identify selective compounds (56). On the other hand, adenosine has an inhibitory effect on granulocytes, including eosinophils, and this action is mediated via adenosine A_{2A} receptors (57). This has led to the development of A_{2A} agonists and several selective drugs are in development, such as CGS 21680, which inhibits allergic inflammation in rats (58).

ATP may also be a mediator of asthma acting through P_2 receptors. ATP enhances the release of mediators from sensitized human mast cells via P_{2Y2} receptors, which are also expressed on eosinophils (59), suggesting that P_{2Y2} antagonists may be beneficial (60).

F. Inducible NO Synthase Inhibitors

NO is produced by several cells in the airway by NO synthases (61). The concentration of NO in the exhaled air of children with asthma is higher than in normal subjects (10,62), and this is likely to be derived from inducible NO synthase (iNOS), which shows increased expression in asthmatic patients, particularly in airway epithelial cells and infiltrating inflammatory cells (63,64). The combination of increased oxidative stress and NO derived from iNOS leads to the formation of the potent radical peroxynitrite that may result in nitration of proteins in the airways (63). Peroxynitrite may nitrate certain histone deacetylases, thus impairing responsiveness to corticosteroids. This suggests that an inhibitor of iNOS might be useful in the treatment of asthma, particularly in patients with severe disease in whom it may restore steroid responsiveness and make asthma control easier to achieve. Several potent and long-lasting iNOS inhibitors are now in development. The prodrug L-N^6-(1-iminoethyl) lysine 5-tetrazole amide (SC-51) is rapidly converted in vivo to the active metabolite L-N^6-(1-iminoethyl) lysine (L-NIL) and when given orally markedly reduces the levels of exhaled NO in asthmatic patients for several days (65).

G. Tryptase Inhibitors

Mast cell tryptase has several effects on airways, including increasing responsiveness of airway smooth muscle to constrictors, increasing plasma exudation, potentiating eosinophil recruitment, and stimulating fibroblast and airway smooth muscle proliferation (66). Some of these effects are mediated by activation of the proteinase-activated receptor PAR2, which is widely expressed in the airways of asthmatic patients (67). A tryptase inhibitor, APC366, is effective in a sheep model of allergen-induced asthma (68), but is only poorly effective in asthmatic patients (69). More potent tryptase inhibitors and PAR2 antagonists are in development (70).

V. Cytokine Inhibitors

Multiple cytokines and chemokines have been implicated in the pathophysiology of asthma (71), and cytokine inhibitors figure prominently among novel therapeutic approaches to asthma (72–74).

A. Anti-interleukin-5

IL-5 plays an essential role in orchestrating the eosinophilic inflammation of asthma (75) (Fig. 2). In IL-5 gene knockout mice the eosinophilic response to allergen and the subsequent AHR are markedly suppressed, and yet animals have a normal survival, validating the strategy to inhibit IL-5. This has also been achieved using blocking antibodies to IL-5. Blocking antibodies to IL-5 inhibit eosinophilic inflammation and AHR in animal models of asthma, including primates (75). This blocking effect may last for up to three months after a single intravenous injection of antibody in primates, making treatment of chronic asthma with such a therapy a feasible proposition. Humanized monoclonal antibodies to IL-5 have been developed and a single intravenous infusion of one of these antibodies (mepolizulab) markedly reduces blood eosinophils for over three months and prevents eosinophil recruitment into the airways after allergen challenge in patients with mild asthma (76). However, this treatment has no significant effect on the early or late response to allergen challenge or on baseline AHR, suggesting that eosinophils may not be of critical importance for these responses in humans. A clinical study in patients with moderate to severe asthma not controlled on inhaled corticosteroids therapy confirmed a profound reduction in circulating eosinophils, but no significant improvement in either asthma symptoms or lung function (77). In both of these studies, it would be expected that high doses of corticosteroids would improve these functional parameters. These surprising results question the critical role of eosinophils in asthma and indicate that other strategies aimed at inhibiting eosinophilic inflammation might not be effective. However, mepolizumab, while profoundly reducing eosinophils in the circulation (by over 95%), is less effective at reducing eosinophils in bronchial biopsies (by ~50%), which may explain why this treatment is not clinically effective (78). Nevertheless, this suggests that blocking IL-5 is unlikely to be useful as an asthma therapy.

Non-peptidic IL-5 receptor antagonists would be an alternative strategy and there is a search for such compounds using molecular modeling of the IL-5 receptor α-chain and through large-scale throughput screening. One such molecule YM-90709 appears to be a relatively selective inhibitor of IL-5-receptors (79). However, the lack of clinical benefit of anti-IL-5 antibodies has made this a less attractive approach.

B. Anti-interleukin-4

IL-4 is critical for the synthesis of IgE by B lymphocytes and is also involved in eosinophil recruitment to the airways (80). A unique function of IL-4 is to promote differentiation of Th-2 cells and therefore act at a proximal and critical site in the allergic response, making IL-4 an attractive target for inhibition. IL-4 blocking antibodies inhibit allergen-induced AHR, goblet cell metaplasia, and pulmonary eosinophilia in a murine model (81). Inhibition of IL-4 may, therefore, be effective in inhibiting allergic diseases, and soluble humanized IL-4 receptors (sIL-4r) have been tested in clinical trials. A single nebulized dose of sIL-4r prevents the fall in lung function induced by withdrawal of inhaled corticosteroids in patients with moderately severe asthma (82), and weekly nebulization of sIL-4R improves asthma control over a 12-week period (83). Subsequent studies in patients with milder asthma proved disappointing, however, and this treatment has now been withdrawn. One reason soluble receptors to IL-4 may not be very effective is that monomeric receptors have a relatively low binding affinity. Recently, a heterodimeric soluble receptor containing each component of the IL-4R (cytokine trap) has been shown to have a much higher affinity and may, therefore, be more useful (84). Another approach is blockade of IL-4 receptors with a mutated form of

IL-4 (BAY 36–1677), which binds to and blocks IL-4Rα and IL-13Rα1, thus blocking both IL-4 and IL-13 (85). This treatment has a short duration of action and has also been withdrawn.

IL-4 and the closely related cytokine IL-13 signal through a shared surface receptor, IL-4Ra, which activates a specific transcription factor STAT-6 (86). Deletion of the STAT-6 gene has a similar effect to IL-4 gene knockout (87). This has led to a search for inhibitors of STAT-6, and although peptide inhibitors that interfere with the interaction between STAT-6 and JAKs linked to IL-4Rα have been discovered, it will be difficult to deliver these intracellularly, so that small molecule inhibitors are being sought through screening.

C. Anti-interleukin-13

There is increasing evidence that IL-13 mimics many of the features of asthma, including AHR, mucous hypersecretion and airway fibrosis, independently of eosinophilic inflammation (88). It potently induces the secretion of eotaxin from airway epithelial cells and transforms airway epithelium into a secretory phenotype. Knocking out the IL-13, but not the IL-4, gene in mice prevents the development of AHR after allergen, despite a vigorous eosinophilic response (89), and the increase in AHR induced by IL-13 is only seen when the expression of STAT6 is lost in airway epithelial cells (90). IL-13 signals through the IL-4Rα, but may also activate different intracellular pathways via activation of IL-13Rα1 (86), so that it may be an important target for the development of new therapies. A second specific IL-13 receptor, IL-13Rα2, exists in soluble form and has a high affinity for IL-13, thus acting as a decoy receptor for secreted IL-13. Soluble IL-13Rα2 is effective in blocking the actions of IL-13, including IgE generation, pulmonary eosinophilia, and AHR in mice (91). In the murine model IL-13Rα2 is more effective than IL-4-blocking antibodies, highlighting the potential importance of IL-13 as a mediator of allergic inflammation. Blocking IL-13 may be more important in established asthma where concentrations of IL-13 are much higher than those of IL-4. Humanized IL-13Rα2 and anti-IL-13 antibodies are now in clinical development as a therapeutic approach for asthma.

D. Anti-interleukin-1

Pro-inflammatory cytokines, particularly IL-1β and tumor necrosis factor-α (TNF-α), may amplify the inflammatory response in asthma and COPD and may be linked to disease severity. This suggests that blocking IL-1β or TNF-α may have beneficial effects, particularly in severe airway disease. IL-1 expression is increased in asthmatic airways (92) and activates many inflammatory genes that are expressed in asthma. There are no small molecule inhibitors of IL-1, but the endogenous cytokine IL-1 receptor antagonist (IL-1Ra), binds to IL-1 receptors to block the effects of IL-1 (93). In experimental animals IL-1Ra reduces AHR induced by allergen. Human recombinant IL-1Ra (anakinra) does not appear to be effective in the treatment of asthma, however (94).

E. Anti-TNF

TNF-α is expressed in asthmatic airways and may play a key role in amplifying asthmatic inflammation through the activation of transcription factors nuclear factor-κB (NF-κB), activator protein-1 (AP-1), and other transcription factors (95). In rheumatoid arthritis and inflammatory bowel disease a blocking humanized monoclonal antibody to TNF-α (infliximab) and soluble TNF receptors (etanercept) have produced remarkable clinical responses, even in patients who are relatively unresponsive to steroids (96). Such TNF inhibitors are a logical approach to asthma therapy, particularly in patients with severe disease, and several clinical trials are now underway. Because of the problems associated with antibody-based therapies that have to be given by injection, there is a search for small molecule inhibitors of TNF. TNF-α-converting enzyme (TACE) is a matrix metalloproteinase-related enzyme critical for the release of TNF from the cell surface. Small molecule TACE inhibitors are in development as oral TNF inhibitors (97), but the concern is that while preventing the release of TNF-α, it may remain tethered to its cells of origin and still exert proinflammatory effects.

VI. Anti-inflammatory Cytokines

Some cytokines have anti-inflammatory effects in inflammation and therefore have therapeutic potential (98,99). While it may not be feasible or cost-effective to administer these proteins as long-term therapy, it may be possible to develop drugs in the future that increase the release of these endogenous cytokines or activate their receptors and specific signal transduction pathways.

A. Interleukin-10

IL-10 is a potent anti-inflammatory cytokine that inhibits the synthesis of many inflammatory proteins, including cytokines (TNF-α, GM-CSF, IL-5, and chemokines) and inflammatory enzymes (iNOS and COX2) that are over-expressed in asthma (Fig. 3) (100). Indeed, there may be a defect in IL-10 transcription and secretion from macrophages in asthma, suggesting that IL-10 might be defective in atopic diseases (101,102). In sensitized animals, IL-10 is effective in suppressing the inflammatory response to allergen (103) and CD4$^+$ cells engineered to secrete IL-10 suppress airway inflammation in a murine model of asthma (104). Specific allergen

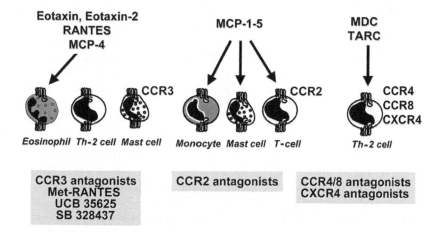

Figure 3 Chemokine receptor antagonists in asthma. Several chemokines are likely to be involved in the pathophysiology of asthma. There are three major chemokine receptor targets in asthma: CCR3, which is most advanced in terms of small molecule inhibitor development, but also CCR2 and CCR4, for which small molecule inhibitors are now in development.

immunotherapy results in increased production of IL-10 by a subpopulation of regulatory Th cells that may mediate the beneficial effects of immunotherapy (105). Recombinant human IL-10 has proved to be effective in controlling inflammatory bowel disease and psoriasis, where similar cytokines are expressed, and may be given as a weekly injection (106). Although IL-10 is reasonably well tolerated, there are hematological side effects. In the future, drugs that activate the unique signal transduction pathways activated by the IL-10 receptor or drugs that increase endogenous production of IL-10 may be developed. In mice, drugs that elevate cyclic AMP increase IL-10 production, but this does not appear to be the case in human cells (107).

B. Interferons

IFN-γ inhibits Th-2 cells and should, therefore, reduce atopic inflammation. In sensitized animals nebulized IFN-γ inhibits eosinophilic inflammation induced by allergen exposure (108). However, administration of IFN-γ by nebulization to asthmatic patients does not significantly reduce eosinophilic inflammation, possibly due to the difficulty in obtaining a high enough concentration locally in the airways (109). Specific immunotherapy increases IFN-γ production by circulating T cells in patients with clinical benefit (110) and increased numbers of IFN-γ expressing cells in nasal biopsies of patients with allergic rhinitis (111). A preliminary report suggests that IFN-α may be useful in the treatment of patients with severe asthma who have reduced responsiveness to corticosteroids (112).

C. Interleukin-12

IL-12 is the endogenous regulator of Th-1 cell development and determines the balance between Th-1 and Th-2 cells (113). IL-12 administration to rats inhibits allergen-induced inflammation (114) and sensitization to allergens. IL-12 releases IFN-γ, but has additional effects on T-cell differentiation. IL-12 levels released from whole blood cells are lower in asthmatic patients, indicating a possible reduction in IL-12 secretion (115). Recombinant IL-12 has several toxic effects in clinical studies that are diminished by slow escalation of the dose (116). In patients with mild asthma, weekly infusions of human recombinant IL-12 in escalating doses over four weeks caused a progressive fall in circulating eosinophils and a reduction in the normal rise in circulating eosinophils after allergen challenge (117). There was a concomitant reduction in eosinophils in induced sputum. However, there was no reduction in either early or late response to inhaled allergen challenge or any reduction in AHR (as with anti-IL-5 therapy). Furthermore, most of the patients suffered from malaise and one out of the 12 subjects had an episode of cardiac arrhythmia. This suggests that IL-12 is not a suitable treatment for asthma. In mice, administration of an IL-12-allergen fusion protein results in the development of a specific Th-1 response to the allergen, with increased production of an allergen-specific IgG2, rather than the normal Th-2 response with IgE formation (118). This indicates the possibility of using local IL-12 together with specific allergens to provide a more specific immunotherapy, which might even be curative if applied early in the course of the atopic disease.

VII. Chemokine Inhibitors

Many chemokines are involved in the recruitment of inflammatory cells in asthma. Over 50 different chemokines are now recognized and they activate more than 20 different surface receptors (119). Chemokine receptors belong to the 7 transmembrane receptor superfamily of G-protein-coupled receptors and this makes it possible to find small molecule inhibitors, which has not yet proved feasible for classical cytokine receptors (120). Another approach is to use antibodies, which may give a long duration of blockade and avoid some of the toxicity issues associated with many small molecule inhibitors. Some chemokines appear to be selective for single chemokines, whereas others are promiscuous and mediate the effects of several related chemokines (Fig. 3).

A. CCR3 Inhibitors

Several chemokines, including eotaxin, eotaxin-2, eotaxin-3, RANTES, and macrophage chemoattractant protein-4 (MCP-4) activate a common receptor on eosinophils designated CCR3 (121). A neutralizing antibody against eotaxin reduces eosinophil recruitment into the lung after allergen and the associated AHR in mice (122). There is increased expression of eotaxin, eotaxin-2, MCP-3, MCP-4, and CCR3 in the airways of asthmatic patients and this is correlated with increased AHR (123). Several small molecule inhibitors of CCR3, including UCB35625, SB-297006, and SB-328437, are effective in inhibiting eosinophil recruitment in allergen models of asthma and drugs in this class are currently undergoing clinical trials in asthma (124). Although it was thought that CCR3 were restricted to cosinophils, there is some evidence for their expression on Th-2 cells and mast cells, so that these inhibitors may have a more widespread effect than on eosinophils alone, making them potentially more valuable in asthma treatment. RANTES, which shows increased expression in asthmatic airways (125), also activates CCR3, but also has effects on CCR1 and CCR5, which may play a role in T-cell recruitment. Modification of the N-terminal of RANTES, met-RANTES, has a blocking effect on RANTES by inhibiting these receptors (126).

B. CCR2 Inhibitors

Monocyte chemoattractant protein-1 (MCP-1) activates CCR2 on monocytes and T lymphocytes. Blocking MCP-1 with ncutralizing antibodies reduces recruitment of both T cells and eosinophils in a murine model of ovalbumin-induced airway inflammation, with a marked reduction in AHR (122). MCP-1 also recruits and activates mast cells, an effect that is mediated via CCR2 (127). MCP-1 instilled into the airways induces marked and prolonged AHR in mice, which is associated with mast cell degranulation. A neutralizing antibody to MCP-1 blocks the development of AHR in response to allergen (127). Several small molecule inhibitors of CCR2 are now in clinical development.

C. Other CCR Inhibitors

CCR4 and CCR8 are selectively expressed on Th-2 cells and are activated by the chemokines monocyte-derived chemokine (MDC) and thymus-and activation-dependent chemokine (TARC), both of which are expressed in asthmatic airways (128). Inhibitors of CCR4 and CCR8 may, therefore, inhibit the recruitment of Th-2 cells and thus persistent eosinophilic inflammation in the airways. CCR8 gene deletion does not have any effects on allergic inflammation in mice, suggesting that this receptor may not be an effective target (129). CXCR4 are also selectively expressed on Th-2 cells and a small molecule inhibitor AMD3100 inhibits allergen-induced inflammation in a murine model of asthma (130). CCR7 plays a role in the migration of immature dendritic cells to regional lymph nodes and therefore blocking this receptor might suppress antigen presentation (131).

VIII. New Corticosteroids

There has been an intensive search for anti-inflammatory treatments that
are as effective in children as corticosteroids but with fewer side effects.
One approach is to seek corticosteroids with a greater therapeutic ratio.
Corticosteroids are by far the most effective treatments for childhood
asthma but cannot routinely be given systemically because of side effects.
This led to the development of inhaled corticosteroids with topically active
molecules, which suppress local airway inflammation with a marked
reduction in systemic exposure. However, currently available inhaled corticosteroids (including beclomethasone dipropionate, budesonide, fluticasone, mometasone, triamcinolone, and flunisolide) are all absorbed from
the lungs into the systemic circulation and therefore have the potential for
systemic side effects at high doses (132,133). There has, therefore, been
a search for new topical corticosteroids that have fewer tendencies to
produce systemic (and local) side effects.

A. Soft Steroids

One approach was the development of corticosteroids that are inactivated
by esterases in the airways, with the idea that any corticosteroids not taken
into airway cells would be inactivated so that systemic absorption from the
lungs would be avoided. Such "soft" steroids as butixocort and tipredane
were developed, but turned out to be ineffective in clinical studies in asthma
(134). This may be because they were inactivated before they were able to
enter target cells in the airways.

B. Ciclesonide

A novel corticosteroid, ciclesonide, appears to have an improved therapeutic ratio. Ciclesonide is an inactive prodrug that liberates the active des-
ciclesonide in response to esterases in the airways (135). This steroid is
associated with fewer local side effects, as presumably these esterases are
less expressed in the oropharynx. Ciclesonide is effective after inhalation
in asthmatic patients and has anti-inflammatory effects (136). It is effective
in controlling asthma when given as a once-daily inhalation as it has a long lung
retention time (137). Ciclesonide has a favorable therapeutic ratio because it is
highly bound to plasma proteins (>99%) so it is not available for systemic side
effects. Several large clinical trials in children are now underway.

C. Dissociated Corticosteroids

All currently available inhaled corticosteroids are absorbed from the
lungs into the systemic circulation and, therefore, inevitably have some
systemic component. Understanding the molecular mechanisms of action

of corticosteroids has led to the development of a new generation of corticosteroids. A major mechanism of the anti-inflammatory effect of corticosteroids appears to be inhibition of the effects of proinflammatory transcription factors, such as NF-κB and AP-1, which are activated by pro-inflammatory cytokines (transrepression) via an inhibitory action on histone acetylation and stimulation of histone deacetylation (138). By contrast, the endocrine and metabolic effects of steroids that are responsible for the systemic side effects of corticosteroids are likely to be mediated predominantly via DNA binding (transactivation). This has led to a search for novel corticosteroids that selectively transrepress without significant transactivation, thus reducing the potential risk of systemic side effects. Since corticosteroids bind to the same GR, this seems at first to be an unlikely possibility, but while DNA binding involved a GR homodimer, interaction with transcription factors AP-1 and NF-κB and coactivators involves only a single GR (139). A separation of transactivation and transrepression has been demonstrated using reporter gene constructs in transfected cells using selective mutations of the glucocorticoid receptor (140). In addition, in mice with GR that do not dimerize there is no transactivation, but transrepression appears to be normal (141,142). Furthermore, some steroids, such as the antagonist RU486, have a greater transrepression than transactivation effect. Indeed, the topical steroids used in asthma therapy today, such as fluticasone propionate and budesonide, appear to have more potent transrepression than transactivation effects, which may account for their selection as potent anti-inflammatory agents (143). Recently, a novel class of steroids has been described in which there is potent transrepression with relatively little transactivation. These "dissociated" steroids, including RU24858 and RU40066, have anti-inflammatory effects in vitro (144), although there is little separation of anti-inflammatory effects and systemic side effects in vivo (145). Several dissociated corticosteroids are now in clinical development and show good separation between transrepression and transactivation actions. Selective estrogen receptor modulators (SERM), such as raloxifene, are now well established in the treatment of osteoporosis, and the equivalent type of selective agonist is now needed for glucocorticoid receptors. The development of steroids with a greater margin of safety is possible and may even lead to the development of oral steroids that do not have significant adverse effects. The crystal structure of the ligand-binding domain of GR reveals a distinct binding pocket that may be important for selectivity and the better design of dissociated steroids (146).

IX. Phosphodiesterase-4 Inhibitors

Phosphodiesterases (PDEs) break down cyclic nucleotides that inhibit cell activation, and at least 10 families of enzymes have now been discovered (147). Theophylline, long used as an asthma treatment, is a weak but non-selective PDE inhibitor. PDE4 is the predominant family of PDEs in inflammatory cells, including mast cells, eosinophils, T lymphocytes, macrophages, and structural cells such as sensory nerves and epithelial cells (148,149). This has suggested that PDE4 inhibitors would be useful as an anti-inflammatory treatment in asthma, particularly as there is some evidence for over-expression of PDE4 in cells of atopic patients (Fig. 4). In animal models of asthma, PDE4 inhibitors reduce eosinophil infiltration and AHR responses to allergen. Several PDE4 inhibitors have been tested in asthma, but with disappointing results (150). One PDE4 inhibitor, CDP840, had a marginal inhibitory effect on the late response to allergen, but is not being further developed (151). Another PDE4 inhibitor, roflumilast, appears to be better tolerated and has a long duration of action so that it is suitable for once-daily oral administration (152). It appears to be clinically effective in reducing exercise-induced asthma and has a similar effect to BDP 200 mg twice daily (153). At these doses roflumilast inhibits LPS-induced TNF-α release from whole blood by $\sim$20% (153). However, most of the PDE4 inhibitors so far tested clinically have had unacceptable side effects, particularly nausea and vomiting; these are the very side effects that have limited the use of theophylline.

Several steps may be possible to overcome the limitation of side effects. It is possible that vomiting is due to the inhibition of a particular subtype of PDE4. At least four human PDE4 genes have been identified and each has several splice variants (149). This raises the possibility that subtype-selective inhibitors may be developed that may preserve the anti-inflammatory effect, while having less propensity to side effects.

PDE4D appears to be of particular importance in nausea and vomiting and is expressed in the chemosensitive trigger zone in the brain stem

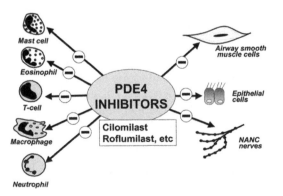

Figure 4 Phosphodiesterase 4 inhibitors have a broad spectrum of anti-inflammatory effects.

(154), and in mice deletion of the gene for PDE4D prevents a behavioral equivalent of emesis (155). This isoenzyme appears to be less important in anti-inflammatory effects, and knockout studies indicate that PDE4B is more important than PDE4D in inflammatory cells (156). PDE4B selective inhibitors may therefore have a greater therapeutic margin and theoretically might be effective anti-inflammatory drugs. Cilomilast is the PDE4 inhibitor that has been most fully tested in clinical studies, particularly in COPD (157), but this drug is selective for PDE4D and therefore has a propensity to cause emesis. Roflumilast, which is non-selective, looks more promising, as it has a more favorable therapeutic ratio (152).

X. Transcription Factor Inhibitors

Several transcription factors are involved in the expression of inflammatory genes in asthmatic airways and are, therefore, possible targets for anti-inflammatory drugs. Indeed, many of the anti-inflammatory actions of corticosteroids in asthma may be ascribed to inhibition of NF-κB- and AP-1-regulated gene expression (138). However, inhibition of transcription factors is difficult and it is necessary to target the specific activating enzymes (kinases).

A. NF-κB Inhibitors

NF-κB is naturally inhibited by the inhibitory protein IκB, which is degraded after activation by specific kinases (IKK). IKK2 is the isoenzyme that is important for activation of NF-κB by inflammatory stimuli (158). Inhibitors of IKK2 or the proteasome, the multifunctional enzyme that degrades IκB, would thus inhibit NF-κB and selective inhibitors are now in development (159). One concern about long-term inhibition of NF-κB is that effective inhibitors may result in immune suppression and impair host defenses, since mice that lack NF-κB genes succumb to septicemia. However, there are alternative pathways of NF-κB activation that might be more important in inflammatory disease (160).

B. NF-AT/Calcineurin Inhibitors

Ciclosporin A, tacrolimus, and pimecrolimus inhibit T-lymphocyte function by inhibiting the transcription factor NF-AT (nuclear factor of activated T cells) by blocking activation of calcineurin. This results in suppression if IL-2, IL-4, IL-5, IL-13, and GM-CSF and, therefore, these drugs have therapeutic potential in asthma. However, ciclosporin A is of little value in chronic asthma as the dose is probably limited by toxicity (161). These drugs have serious side effects, particularly nephrotoxicity, and this limits their usefulness in a common disease such as asthma. Inhaled formulations of ciclosporin and tacrolimus are being tested for efficacy in asthma, but it remains to be determined whether this would give a favorable therapeutic ratio, as the drugs may be absorbed into the systemic circulation from the lungs. Rapamycin (sirolimus) has a similar action to calcineurin inhibitors, but acts more distally and has a different toxicity.

XI. Kinase Inhibitors

Multiple kinases are involved in the activation of inflammatory pathways, and selective kinase inhibitors represent a novel approach to controlling inflammation (162).

A. MAP Kinase Inhibitors

Mitogen-activated protein (MAP) kinases play a key role in inflammatory and remodelling responses (163). There has been particular interest in the p38 MAP kinase pathway, which is involved in expression of multiple inflammatory proteins that are relevant to asthma (164). The p38 MAP kinase is blocked by a novel class of drugs, the cytokine suppressant anti-inflammatory drugs (CSAIDs), such as SB203580, SB 239063, and RWJ67657. These drugs inhibit the synthesis of many inflammatory cytokines, chemokines, and inflammatory enzymes. Interestingly, they appear to have a preferential inhibitory effect on the synthesis of Th-2 compared to Th-1 cytokines, indicating their potential application in the treatment of atopic diseases (165).

Furthermore, p38 MAPK inhibitors have also been shown to decrease eosinophil survival by activating apoptotic pathways (166) and are involved in corticosteroid resistance in asthma (167). The p38 MAP kinase inhibitors are now in phase-II development. Whether this new class of anti-inflammatory drugs will be safe in long-term studies remains to be established; it is likely that such a broad-spectrum anti-inflammatory drug will have some toxicity, but inhalation may be a feasible therapeutic approach.

Jun-N-terminal kinases (JNK) may be involved in activation of the transcription factor AP-1, and small molecule inhibitors have now been developed that have anti-inflammation effects in animal models (168). Steroid resistance in asthma is associated with increased activation of JNK (169).

B. Protein Tyrosine Kinase Inhibitors

Several protein tyrosine kinases have been implicated in allergic inflammation. Syk (p72syk) kinase is a protein tyrosine kinase that plays a pivotal role in the signaling of the high affinity IgE receptor (FcεRI) in mast cells, and in syk-deficient mice mast cell degranulation is inhibited, suggesting that this might be an important potential target for the development of mast cell stabilizing drugs (170). Syk is also involved in antigen receptor signaling of B and T lymphocytes and in eosinophil survival in response to IL-5 and GM-CSF (171), so that syk inhibitors might have several useful beneficial effects in atopic diseases. Aerosolized syk anti-sense oligodeoxynucleotide inhibits allergen-induced inflammation in a rat model, indicating that this may be a target for drug development (172).

Another tyrosine kinase, lyn, is upstream of syk and an inhibitor of lyn kinase, PP1, has an inhibitory effect on inflammatory and mast cell activation (173). Lyn is also involved in eosinophil activation and IL-5 signaling (174,175) and a lyn-blocking peptide inhibits eosinophilic inflammation in a murine model (175). Since lyn and syk are widely distributed in the immune system, there are doubts about the long-term safety of selective inhibitors.

C. EGF Receptor Kinase

Epidermal growth factor receptors (EGFR) may play a critical role in the regulation of mucous secretion from airways in response to multiple stimuli (176). An orally active small-molecule inhibitor of EGFR, tyrosine kinase gifitinib, has now been developed for the treatment of epidermal cancers, but may also suppress mucous secretion (177). However, treatment of the underlying inflammation that drives mucous hypersecretion in asthma, via release of IL-13 and other cytokines, is more likely to be useful as mucous hypersecretion is not an isolated problem.

XII. Immunomodulators

T lymphocytes may play a critical role in initiating and maintaining the inflammatory process in allergy via the release of cytokines that result in eosinophilic inflammation, suggesting that T-cell inhibitors may be useful in controlling asthmatic inflammation.

A. Nonspecific Immunomodulators

The nonspecific immunomodulator ciclosporine A has limited efficacy as discussed above, as side effects limit the oral dose (161). Delivery of cyclosporine and the related calcineurin inhibitor tacrolimus via the inhaled route is now being explored. Novel immunomodulators that inhibit purine or pyrimidine pathways, such as mycophenolate mofetil, leflunomide, and brequinar sodium, may be less toxic and therefore of greater potential value in asthma therapy. Mycophenolate inhibits IL-5 production from a peripheral blood mononuclear cell preparation from patients with asthma, indicating that it might be useful (178,179), but no clinical studies of this drug have been reported in asthma.

B. Anti-CD4

CD4$^+$ T cells have been implicated in asthma and a chimeric antibody directed against CD4$^+$ (keliximab), which reduces circulating CD4$^+$ cells, appears to have some beneficial effect in asthma (180), although long-term safety of such a treatment might be a problem. Furthermore, there is increasing evidence that CD8$^+$ cells (Tc2 cells), through release of IL-5 and other cytokines, might also be involved in allergic diseases, particularly in response to infections with certain viruses (181).

C. Th-2 Cell Inhibitors

One problem with these nonspecific immunomodulators is that they inhibit both Th-1 and Th-2 cells, and therefore do not restore the imbalance between these Th-1 and Th-2 cells in atopy. They also inhibit suppresser T-cells (Tc cells) that may modulate the inflammatory response. Selective inhibition of Th-2 cells may be more effective and better tolerated and there is now a search for such drugs. One approach is to block the chemoattractant receptors expressed on Th-2 cells that recruit these cells to the airways, namely CCR4, CCR8, CXCR4, and CRTH2, as discussed above. Suplatast tosilate (IPD-1151T) is a dimethylsulphonium compound that inhibits the release of cytokines (IL-4 and IL-5) from Th-2 cells without effects on IFN-γ from Th-1 cells in vitro (182). In clinical studies this drug has some clinical benefit in symptomatic asthmatic patients (183) and reduces markers of inflammation and AHR (184). However, it has a short duration of action and it has not been compared to inhaled corticosteroids. The drug is only available in Japan and its mechanism of action is uncertain.

XIII. Cell Adhesion Blockers

Infiltration of inflammatory cells into tissues is dependent on adhesion of blood born inflammatory cells to endothelial cells prior to migration to the inflammatory site (185). This depends upon specific glycoprotein adhesion molecules, including integrins and selectins, on both leukocytes and on endothelial cells, which may be upregulated or show increased binding affinity in response to various inflammatory stimuli such as cytokines or lipid mediators. Monoclonal antibodies, which inhibit these adhesion molecules, therefore may prevent inflammatory cell infiltration. A monoclonal antibody to ICAM-1 on endothelial cells prevents the eosinophil infiltration into airways and the increase in bronchial reactivity after allergen exposure in sensitized primates (186), although this has not been found in other species (187).

A. VLA4 Inhibitors

The interaction between VLA4 and VCAM-1 is important for eosinophil inflammation and humanized antibodies to VLA4 ($\alpha4\beta1$) have been developed (188). Small molecule peptide inhibitors of VLA4 have subsequently been developed that are effective in inhibiting allergen-induced responses in sensitized sheep (189). Natalizumab, a monoclonal antibody to $\alpha4$ integrin, which is a component of VLA4, has recently been shown to be effective in Crohn's disease indicating its anti-inflammatory potential in humans (190). Small molecule inhibitors of VLA4 are now in clinical development for asthma.

B. Selectin Inhibitors

Inhibitors of selectins, particularly L-selectin, based on the structure of sialyl-Lewis[x], inhibit the influx of inflammatory cells in response to inhaled allergen in sensitized sheep (191) and inhibit adhesion of human eosinophils in vitro (192). While blocking adhesion molecules is an attractive new approach to the treatment of inflammatory disease, there may be potential dangers in inhibiting immune responses, as a result of inhibiting T-cell trafficking, leading to increased infections and increased risks of neoplasia.

XIV. Anti-allergic Drugs

Although corticosteroids are very effective in controlling atopic diseases, there are continuing concerns in children about systemic side effects when high doses are needed. This has prompted a search for anti-inflammatory agents that would more selectively target the atopic disease process. There are several approaches to inhibiting allergen-induced responses.

A. Cromones

Cromolyn sodium and nedocromil sodium are the most specific anti-allergic drugs so far discovered, but their effectiveness is considerably less than low doses of inhaled corticosteroids, probably due to their very short duration of action. Indeed, the clinical value of cromoglycate has been questioned in a meta-analysis of results (193). Cromones appear to have a specific action on allergic inflammation, yet their molecular mechanism of action remains obscure. Although it was believed that the primary mode of action of cromones involves inhibiting mast-cell mediator release, they also inhibit other inflammatory cells and sensory nerves. Cromones may act on certain types of chloride channels that are expressed in mast cells and sensory nerves (194). Cromolyn phosphorylates a specific cytoskeletal protein moesin in mast cells, indicating a possible mechanism that may inhibit degranulation (195). Identification of the molecular mechanism of action is important, as it may be possible to develop more potent and long-lasting drugs in the future. Both cromolyn and nedocromil must be given topically and all attempts to develop orally active drugs of this type have been unsuccessful, possibly suggesting that topical administration is critical to their efficacy.

B. Furosemide

The diuretic furosemide shares many of the actions of cromones in inhibiting indirect bronchoconstrictor challenges (allergen, exercise, cold air, adenosine, and metabisulfite) but not direct bronchoconstriction (histamine and methacholine) when given by inhalation (196). The mechanism of action of furosemide is not shared by the more potent loop diuretic bumetanide, indicating that some other mechanism than the inhibition of the $Na^+/K^+/Cl^-$ co-transporter (which accounts for their diuretic action) must be involved. This is most likely to involve inhibition of the same chloride channel that is inhibited by cromones. Furosemide itself does not appear to be very effective when given regularly by metered dose inhaler in asthma (197), but it is possible that more potent and long-lasting chloride channel blockers might be developed in the future.

C. Co-stimulation Inhibitors

Co-stimulatory molecules may play a critical role in augmenting the interaction between antigen-presenting cells (predominantly dendritic cells) and $CD4^+$ cells (198). The interaction between B7 and CD28 may determine whether a Th-2-type cell response develops, and there is some evidence that B7.2 (CD86) skews towards a Th-2 response. Blocking antibodies to B7.2 inhibit the development of specific IgE, pulmonary eosinophilia, and AHR in mice, whereas antibodies to B7.1 (CD80) are ineffective (199).

A molecule on activated T cells, CTL4, appears to act as an endogenous inhibitor of T-cell activation and a soluble fusion protein construct, CTLA4-Ig, blocks the development of AHR in a murine model of asthma (200), although it appears to be less effective when the allergic inflammation is severe (201). Anti-CD28, anti-B7.2, and CTLA4-Ig also block the proliferative response of T cells to allergen (202), indicating that these are potential targets for novel therapies that should be effective in all atopic diseases.

Inducible co-stimulator (ICOS) is a costimulatory molecule related to CD28 and binds to a B7-like molecule B7RP-1. ICOS appears to be important in polarizing the immune response and an antibody to ICOS blocks Th-2 cell development, whereas CD28 plays a role in priming T cells (203). The ICOS pathway is also critical for the development of regulatory T cells that secrete IL-10 and suppress the allergic inflammatory response (204), so that stimulating rather than blocking its action may be beneficial.

D. Anti-IgE

Since release of mediators from mast cells in asthma is IgE dependent, an attractive approach is to block the activation of IgE using blocking antibodies that do not result in cell activation (Fig. 5). A humanized monoclonal antibody directed to the high affinity IgE-receptor (FcεRI) binding domain of human IgE (omalizumab) has beneficial effects in the treatment of patients with asthma when given by subcutaneous injection every two to four weeks, particularly those with severe steroid-dependent disease (205). Omalizumab has been shown to be equally effective in children and is well tolerated (206). Omalizumab is now approved for asthma therapy in some countries, but its high cost means that it is only likely to be used in patients with very severe disease not controlled by low doses of oral corticosteroids. The success of omalizumab has now prompted a search for small molecule inhibitors of IgE.

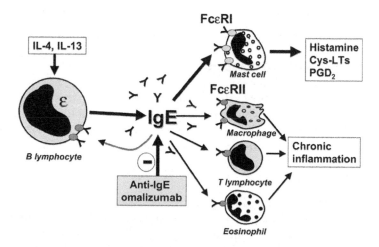

Figure 5 IgE plays a central role in allergic diseases and blocking IgE using an antibody, such as omalizumab, is a logical approach. IgE may activate high affinity receptors (FcεRI) on mast cells as well as low affinity receptors (FcεRII and CD23) on other inflammatory cells. *Abbreviations*: IL, interleukin; cys-LT, cysteinyl-leukotriene; PG, prostaglandin.

E. Specific Immunotherapy

Subcutaneous injection of small amounts of purified allergen has been used for many years in the treatment of allergy, but is not very effective in asthma and has a risk of serious side effects (207). The molecular mechanism of desensitization is unknown, but may be related to stimulation of IL-10 and transforming growth factor-β release from a subset of regulatory T cells (105). Cloning of several common allergen genes has made it possible to prepare recombinant allergens for injection, although this purity may detract from their allergenicity, as most natural allergens contain several proteins. Intramuscular injection of rats with plasmid DNA expressing house dust mite allergen results in its long-term expression and prevents the development of IgE responses to inhaled allergen (208). This suggests that allergen gene immunization with a DNA vaccine might be a therapeutic strategy in the future.

F. Peptide Immunotherapy

T-cell derived peptides from cat allergen (*fel* d1) appear to be effective in blocking allergen responses to cat dander, but may induce an isolated late response to allergen by direct T-cell activation followed by prolonged hyporesponsiveness (209). *Fel* d1 peptides inhibit the cutaneous response to cat allergens, but whether this will be a useful strategy in asthma is not yet certain. One problem of this approach is that there are differences between individuals in recognizing T-cell peptides epitopes, so this approach may not be effective in all patients and many patients are sensitized to more than one allergen.

XV. Preventive Therapies

Atopy, which underlies most asthma, appears to be due to immune deviation from Th-1 to Th-2 cells, which may arise because of a failure to inhibit the normal Th-2 preponderance at birth as a result of lack of environmental factors (infections and endotoxins) that stimulate a normal Th-1 response.

A. Vaccination

A relative lack of infections may be a factor predisposing to the development of atopy in genetically predisposed individuals, leading to the concept of vaccination to induce protective Th-1 responses to prevent sensitization and thus prevent the development of atopic diseases. BCG inoculation in mice 14 days before allergen sensitization reduced the formation of specific IgE in response to allergen and the eosinophilic response and AHR responses to allergen, with an increase in production of IFN-γ (210). This has prompted several clinical trials of BCG to prevent the development of atopy. In one study BCG vaccination has been shown to improve asthma control and reduce markers of Th-2 activation (211). Similar results have been obtained in mice with a single injection of heat-killed *Mycobacterium vaccae*, another potent inducer of Th-1 responses (212). In a clinical study, *M. vaccae* had no effect on clinical parameters of asthma, IgE, or cytokine profile, however (213).

B. CpG Oligonucleotides

Immunostimulatory DNA sequences, such as unmethylated cytosine-guanosine dinucleotide-containing oligonucleotides (CpG ODN), are also potent inducers of Th-1 cytokines through stimulation of IL-12 release (214) and in mice administration of CpG ODN increases the ratio of Th-1 to Th-2 cells, decreases formation of specific IgE, and reduces the eosinophilic response to allergen, an effect that lasts for over six weeks (215). CpG ODN treatment is also able to reverse established allergen-driven eosinophilic inflammation in mice (216) and reverse AHR in mice sensitized to ragweed pollen antigen (217). These promising animal studies encourage the possibility that CpG ODN and DNA vaccines might prevent or cure atopic diseases in the future and clinical trials are currently underway (218).

Although these approaches aimed at tipping the balance back in favor of Th-1 responses are promising in terms of disease modification, there are concerns that a therapeutic shift might increase the chance of developing Th-1-mediated diseases, such as autoimmune diseases, multiple sclerosis, inflammatory bowel disease, rheumatoid arthritis, and diabetes. These concerns particularly apply to infants.

XVI. Gene Therapy

Since atopic diseases are polygenic, it is unlikely that gene therapy will be of value in long-term therapy. However, understanding the genes involved in atopic diseases and in disease severity may identify new molecular targets (219) and may also predict the response to different forms of therapy (pharmacogenetics) (220). Several novel genes have recently been linked to asthma, providing new therapeutic opportunities (221–223).

A. Gene Transfer

Transfer of anti-inflammatory genes may provide specific anti-inflammatory or inhibitory proteins in a convenient manner, and gene transfer has been shown to be feasible in animals using viral vectors (224). Anti-inflammatory proteins relevant to asthma include IL-10, IL-12, IL-18, and IκB.

B. Anti-sense Oligonucleotides

Anti-sense oligonucleotides may switch off specific genes, but there are considerable problems in getting these molecules into cells. An inhaled anti-sense oligonucleotide directed against the adenosine A_1-receptor reduces AHR in a rabbit model of asthma, demonstrating the potential of this approach in treating asthma (225). Respirable anti-sense oligonucleotides (RASONS) are a novel approach to asthma therapy, and clinical trials with the A_1-receptor oligonucleotide (EPI-2010) have shown that this therapy is well tolerated (226). Suitable target genes may be IL-13 or CCR3, as well as novel genes discovered through the human genome project (227).

C. Interference RNA

Interference RNA (RNAi) is sequence-specific gene silencing induced by double-stranded RNA, which knocks down specific genes. This has proved invaluable in determining the role of specific genes in human cells, but also has the potential for therapy (228). This technique appears to be more effective than anti-sense oligonucleotides in switching off genes, although there is still a problem in getting these small interfering RNA (siRNA) sequences into cells. Recent studies suggest that nasal application of siRNA sequences may inhibit gene expression in the lungs even without the need for viral vectors (229).

XVII. Conclusions

Many different therapeutic approaches to the treatment of asthma may be possible, yet there have been few new drugs that have reached the clinic. Inhaled corticosteroids are very effective as chronic treatment in childhood asthma and suppress the underlying inflammatory process. An advance in therapy would be the development of more specific antiasthma drugs that lack side effects. If these treatments can be taken orally this would also treat atopic diseases, such as rhinitis and eczema, which often coincide. The possibility of developing a "cure" for asthma is remote, but strategies to inhibit the development of sensitization in early childhood offer such a prospect in the future.

References

1. Rabe KF, Vermeire PA, Soriano JB, Maier WC. Clinical management of asthma in 1999: the Asthma Insights and Reality in Europe (AIRE) study. Eur Respir J 2000; 16:802–807.
2. Barnes PJ, Jonsson B, Klim J. The costs of asthma. Eur Respir J 1996; 9: 636–642.

3. Weiss KB, Sullivan SD. The health economics of asthma and rhinitis. I. Assessing the economic impact. J Allergy Clin Immunol 2001; 107:3–8.
4. Barnes PJ. Pathophysiology of asthma. Eur Respir Mon 2003; 8:84–113.
5. Barnes PJ. Therapeutic strategies for allergic diseases. Nature 1999; 402: B31–B38.
6. Barnes PJ. New directions in allergic disease: mechanism-based anti-inflammatory therapies. J Allergy Clin Immunol 2000; 106:5–16.
7. Barnes PJ. New treatments for asthma. Eur J Int Med 2000; 11:9–20.
8. Jones PD, Hankin R, Simpson J, Gibson PG, Henry RL. The tolerability, safety, and success of sputum induction and combined hypertonic saline challenge in children. Am J Respir Crit Care Med 2001; 164:1146–1149.
9. Baraldi E, Azzolin NM, Zanconato S, Dario C, Zacchello F. Corticosteroids decrease exhaled nitric oxide in children with acute asthma [see comments]. J Pediatr 1997; 131:381–385.
10. Byrnes CA, Dinarevic S, Shinebourne EA, Barnes PJ, Bush A. Exhaled nitric oxide measurements in normal and asthmatic children. Pediatr Pulmonol 1997; 24:312–318.
11. Csoma Z, Kharitonov SA, Balint B, Bush A, Wilson NM, Barnes PJ. Increased leukotrienes in exhaled breath condensate in childhood asthma. Am J Respir Crit Care Med 2002; 166:1345–1349.
12. Shahid SK, Kharitonov SA, Wilson NM, Bush A, Barnes PJ. Increased interleukin-4 and decreased interferon-g in exhaled breath condensate of asthmatic children. Am J Respir Crit Care Med 2002; 165:1290–1293.
13. Jones TR, Charette L, Garcia ML, Kaczorowski GJ. Interaction of iberiotoxin with β-adrenoceptor agonists and sodium nitroprusside on guinea pig trachea. J Appl Physiol 1993; 74:1879–1884.
14. Miura M, Belvisi MG, Stretton CD, Yacoub MH, Barnes PJ. Role of potassium channels in bronchodilator responses in human airways. Am Rev Respir Dis 1992; 146:132–136.
15. Kume H, Hall IP, Washabau RJ, Takagi K, Kotlikoff MI. Adrenergic agonists regulate K_{Ca} channels in airway smooth muscle by cAMP-dependent and -independent mechanisms. J Clin Invest 1994; 93:371–379.
16. Drazen JM, Israel E, Boushey HA, Chinchilli VM, Fahy JV, Fish JE, Lazarus SC, Lemanske RF, Martin RJ, Peters SP, Sorkness C, Szefler SJ. Comparison of regularly scheduled with as needed use of albuterol in mild asthma. New Engl J Med 1996; 335:841–847.
17. Dennis SM, Sharp SJ, Vickers MR, Frost CD, Crompton GK, Barnes PJ, Lee TH. Regular inhaled salbutamol and asthma control: the TRUST randomized trial. Lancet 2000; 355:1675–1679.
18. Kips JC, Pauwels RA. Long-acting inhaled β2-agonist therapy in asthma. Am J Respir Crit Care Med 2001; 164:923–932.
19. Barnes PJ. Scientific rationale for combination inhalers with a long-acting β2-agonists and corticosteroids. Eur Respir J 2002; 19:182–191.
20. Barnes PJ, Dixon CMS. The effect of inhaled vasoactive intestinal peptide on bronchial hyperreactivity in man. Am Rev Respir Dis 1984; 130: 162–166.

21. O'Donnel M, Garippa RJ, Rinaldi N, Selig WM, Smiko B, Renzetti L, Tanno SA, Wasserman MA, Welton A, Bolin DR. Ro25–1553: a novel long-acting vasoactive intestinal peptide agonist. Part 1: in vitro and in vivo bronchodilator studies. J Pharmacol Exp Ther 1994; 270:1282–1288.

22. Linden A, Hansson L, Andersson A, Palmqvist M, Arvidsson P, Lofdahl CG, Larsson P, Lotvall J. Bronchodilation by an inhaled VPAC(2) receptor agonist in patients with stable asthma. Thorax 2003; 58:217–221.

23. Coleman RA, Smith WL, Narumiya S. International Union of Pharmacology classification of prostanoid receptors: properties, distribution, and structure of the receptors and their subtypes. Pharmacol Rev 1994; 46:205–229.

24. Meja KK, Barnes PJ, Giembycz MA. Characterization of the prostanoid receptor(s) on human blood monocytes at which prostaglandin E_2 inhibits lipopolysaccharride-induced tumour necrosis factor-a. Br J Pharmacol 1997; 122:149–157.

25. Pavord ID, Tattersfield AE. Bronchoprotective role for endogenous prostaglandin E2. Lancet 1995; 344:436–438.

26. Waldeck B, Widmark E. Comparison of the effects of forskolin and isoprenaline on tracheal, cardiac and skeletal muscles from guinea pig. Eur J Pharmacol 1985; 112:349–353.

27. Angus RM, Mecallaum MJA, Hulks G, Thomson NC. Bronchodilator, cardiovascular and cyclic guanylyl monophosphate response to high dose infused atrial natriuretic peptide in asthma. Am Rev Respir Dis 1993; 147: 1122–1125.

28. Angus RM, Millar EA, Chalmers GW, Thomson NC. Effect of inhaled atrial natriuretic peptide and a neutral endopeptidase inhibitor on histamine-induced bronchoconstriction. Am J Respir Crit Care Med 1995; 151: 2003–2005.

29. Hamad AM, Range S, Holland E, Knox AJ. Regulation of cGMP by soluble and particulate guanylyl cyclases in cultured human airway smooth muscle. Am J Physiol 1997; 273:L807–L813.

30. Fluge T, Fabel H, Wagner TO, Schneider B, Forssmann WG. Bronchodilating effects of natriuretic and vasorelaxant peptides compared to salbutamol in asthmatics. Regul Pept 1995; 59:357–370.

31. Fluge T, Forssmann WG, Kunkel G, Schneider B, Mentz P, Forssmann K, Barnes PJ, Meyer M. Bronchodilation using combined urodilatin—albuterol administration in asthma: a randomized, double-blind, placebo-controlled trial. Eur J Med Res 1999; 4:411–415.

32. Belvisi MG, Stretton CD, Barnes PJ. Nitric oxide is the endogenous neurotransmitter of bronchodilator nerves in human airways. Eur J Pharmacol 1992; 210:221–222.

33. Hansel TT, Barnes PJ. Tiotropium bromide: a novel once-daily anticholinergic bronchodilator for the treatment of COPD. Drugs Today 2002; 38: 585–600.

34. Kidney JC, Fuller RW, Worsdell Y-M, Lavender EA, Chung KF, Barnes PJ. Effect of an oral potassium channel activator BRL 38227 on airway function and responsiveness in asthmatic patients: comparison with oral salbutamol. Thorax 1993; 48:130–134.

35. Macmillan S, Sheridan RD, Chilvers ER, Patmore L. A comparison of the effects of SCA40, NS 004 and NS 1619 on large conductance Ca^{2+}-activated K^+ channels in bovine tracheal smooth muscle cells in culture. Br J Pharmacol 1995; 116:1656–1660.

36. Fox AJ, Barnes PJ, Venkatesan P, Belvisi MG. Activation of large conductance potassium channels inhibits the afferent and efferent function of airway sensory nerves. J Clin Invest 1997; 99:513–519.

37. Barnes PJ, Chung KF, Page CP. Inflammatory mediators of asthma: an update. Pharmacol Rev 1998; 50:515–596.

38. Barncs PJ. Anti-leukotrienes: here to stay? Curr Opin Pharmacol 2003; 3: 257–263.

39. Dahlen SE, Malmstrom K, Nizankowska E, Dahlen B, Kuna P, Kowalski M, Lumry WR, Picado C, Stevenson DD, Bousquet J, Pauwels R, Holgate ST, Shahane A, Zhang J, Reiss TF, Szczeklik A. Improvement of aspirin-intolerant asthma by montelukast, a leukotriene antagonist: a randomized, double-blind, placebo-controlled trial. Am J Respir Crit Care Med 2002; 165:9–14.

40. Leff JA, Busse WW, Pearlman D, Bronsky EA, Kemp J, Hendeles L, Dockhorn R, Kundu S, Zhang J, Seidenberg BC, Reiss TF. Montelukast, a leukotriene-receptor antagonist, for the treatment of mild asthma and exercise-induced bronchoconstriction [see comments]. N Engl J Med 1998; 339: 147–152.

41. Back M. Functional characteristics of cysteinyl-leukotriene receptor subtypes. Life Sci 2002; 71:611–622.

42. Nasser SMS, Bell GS, Hawksworth RJ, Spruce KE, MacMillan R, Williams AJ, Lee TH, Arm JP. Effect of the 5-lipoxygenase inhibitor ZD2138 on allergen-induced early and late responses. Thorax 1994; 49:743–748.

43. Evans DJ, Barnes PJ, Coulby LJ, Spaethe SM, van Alstyne EC, Pcchous PA, Mitchell MI, O'Connor BJ. The effect of a leukotriene B_4 antagonist LY293111 on allergen- induced responses in asthma. Thorax 1996; 51: 1178–1184.

44. Taha R, Olivenstein R, Utsumi T, Ernst P, Barnes PJ, Rodger IW, Giaid A. Prostaglandin H synthase 2 expression in airway cells from patients with asthma and chronic obstructive pulmonary disease. Am J Respir Crit Care Med 2000; 161:636–640.

45. Matsuoka T, Hirata M, Tanaka H, Takahashi Y, Murata T, Kabashima K, Sugimoto Y, Kobayashi T, Ushikubi F, Aze Y, Eguchi N, Urade Y, Yoshida N, Kimura K, Mizoguchi A, Honda Y, Nagai H, Narumiya S. Prostaglandin D2 as a mediator of allergic asthma. Science 2000; 287:2013–2017.

46. Hirai H, Tanaka K, Yoshie O, Ogawa K, Kenmotsu K, Takamori Y, Ichimasa M, Sugamura K, Nakamura M, Takano S, Nagata K. Prostaglandin D2 selectively induces chemotaxis in T helper type 2 cells, eosinophils, and basophils via seven-transmembrane receptor CRTH2. J Exp Med 2001; 193:255–261.

47. Goldie RG, Henry PJ. Endothelins and asthma. Life Sci 1999; 65:1–15.

48. Chalmers GW, Little SA, Patel KR, Thomson NC. Endothelin-1-induced bronchoconstriction in asthma. Am J Respir Crit Care Med 1997; 156: 382–388.

49. Redington AE, Springall DR, Ghatei MA, Madden J, Bloom SR, Frew AJ, Polak JM, Holgate ST, Howarth PH. Airway endothelin levels in asthma: influence of endobronchial allergen challenge and maintenance corticosteroid therapy. Eur Respir J 1997; 10:1026–1032..

50. Benigni A, Remuzzi G. Endothelin antagonists. Lancet 1999; 353:133–138.

51. Baraldi E, Ghiro L, Piovan V, Carraro S, Ciabattoni G, Barnes PJ, Montuschi P. Increased exhaled 8-isoprostane in childhood asthma. Chest 2003; 124:25–31.

52. Barnes PJ, Ito K, Adcock IM. A mechanism of corticosteroid resistance in COPD: inactivation of histone deacetylase. Lancet 2004; 363:731–733.

53. Cuzzocrea S, Riley DP, Caputi AP, Salvemini D. Antioxidant therapy: a new pharmacological approach in shock, inflammation, and ischemia/reperfusion injury. Pharmacol Rev 2001; 53:135–159.

54. Feoktistov I, Biaggioni I. Pharmacological characterization of adenosine A2B receptors: studies in human mast cells co-expressing A2A and A2B adenosine receptor subtypes. Biochem Pharmacol 1998; 55:627–633.

55. Hannon JP, Tigani B, Williams I, Mazzoni L, Fozard JR. Mechanism of airway hyperresponsiveness to adenosine induced by allergen challenge in actively sensitized Brown Norway rats. Br J Pharmacol 2001; 132:1509–1523.

56. Fozard JR, McCarthy C. Adenosine receptor ligands as potential therapeutics in asthma. Curr Opin Invest Drugs 2002; 3:69–77.

57. Yukawa T, Kroegel C, Dent G, Chanez P, Ukena D, Barnes PJ. Effect of theophylline and adenosine on eosinophil function. Am Rev Respir Dis 1989; 140:327–333.

58. Fozard JR, Ellis KM, Villela Dantas MF, Tigani B, Mazzoni L. Effects of CGS 21680, a selective adenosine A2A receptor agonist, on allergic airways inflammation in the rat. Eur J Pharmacol 2002; 438:183–188.

59. Mohanty JG, Raible DG, McDermott LJ, Pelleg A, Schulman ES. Effects of purine and pyrimidine nucleotides on intracellular Ca^{2+} in human eosinophils: activation of purinergic P2Y receptors. J Allergy Clin Immunol 2001; 107:849–855.

60. Schulman ES, Glaum MC, Post T, Wang Y, Raible DG, Mohanty J, Butterfield JH, Pelleg A. ATP modulates anti-IgE-induced release of histamine from human lung mast cells. Am J Respir Cell Mol Biol 1999; 20:530–537.

61. Barnes PJ, Liew FY. Nitric oxide and asthmatic inflammation. Immunol Today 1995; 16:128–130.

62. Baraldi E, Dario C, Ongaro R, Scollo M, Azzolin NM, Panza N, Paganini N, Zacchello F. Exhaled nitric oxide concentrations during treatment of wheezing exacerbation in infants and young children. Am J Respir Crit Care Med 1999; 159:1284–1288..

63. Saleh D, Ernst P, Lim S, Barnes PJ, Giaid A. Increased formation of the potent oxidant peroxynitrite in the airways of asthmatic patients is associated with induction of nitric oxide synthase: effect of inhaled glucocorticoid. FASEB J 1998; 12:929–937.

64. Guo FH, Comhair SA, Zheng S, Dweik RA, Eissa NT, Thomassen MJ, Calhoun W, Erzurum SC. Molecular mechanisms of increased nitric oxide (NO) in asthma: evidence for transcriptional and post-translational regulation of NO synthesis. J Immunol 2000; 164:5970–5980.
65. Hansel TT, Kharitonov SA, Donnelly LE, Erin EM, Currie MG, Moore WM, Manning PT, Recker DP, Barnes PJ. A selective inhibitor of inducible nitric oxide synthase inhibits exhaled breath nitric oxide in healthy volunteers and asthmatics. FASEB J 2003; 17:1298–1300.
66. He S, Walls AF. Human mast cell tryptase: a stimulus of microvascular leakage and mast cell activation. Eur J Pharmacol 1997; 328:89–97.
67. Knight DA, Lim S, Scaffidi AK, Roche N, Chung KF, Stewart GA, Thompson PJ. Protease-activated receptors in human airways: upregulation of PAR-2 in respiratory epithelium from patients with asthma. J Allergy Clin Immunol 2001; 108: 797–803.
68. Clark JM, Abraham WM, Fishman CE, Forteza R, Ahmed A, Cortes A, Warne RL, Moore WR, Tanaka RD. Tryptase inhibitors block allergen-induced airway and inflammatory responses in allergic sheep. Am J Respir Crit Care Med 1995; 152:2076–2083.
69. Krishna MT, Chauhan A, Little L, Sampson K, Hawksworth R, Mant T, Djukanovic R, Lee T, Holgate S. Inhibition of mast cell tryptase by inhaled APC 366 attenuates allergen-induced late-phase airway obstruction in asthma. J Allergy Clin Immunol 2001; 107:1039–1045.
70. Slusarchyk WA, Bolton SA, Hartl KS, Huang MH, Jacobs G, Meng W, Ogletree ML, Pi Z, Schumacher WA, Seiler SM, Sutton JC, Treuner U, Zahler R, Zhao G, Bisacchi GS. Synthesis of potent and highly selective inhibitors of human tryptase. Bioorg Med Chem Lett 2002; 12:3235–3238.
71. Chung KF, Barnes PJ. Cytokines in asthma. Thorax 1999; 54:825–857.
72. Barnes PJ. Cytokine modulators as novel therapies for asthma. Ann Rev Pharmacol Toxicol 2002; 42:81–98.
73. Barnes PJ. New treatments for COPD. Nat Rev Drug Discov 2002; 1: 437–445.
74. Barnes PJ. Cytokine modulators as novel therapies for airway disease. Eur Respir J Suppl 2001; 34:67s–77s.
75. Greenfeder S, Umland SP, Cuss FM, Chapman RW, Egan RW. The role of interleukin-5 in allergic eosinophilic disease. Respir Res 2001; 2:71–79.
76. Leckie MJ, ten Brincke A, Khan J, Diamant Z, O'Connor BJ, Walls CM, Mathur M, Cowley H, Chung KF, Djukanovic RJ, Hansel TT, Holgate ST, Sterk PJ, Barnes PJ. Effects of an interleukin-5 blocking monoclonal antibody on eosinophils, airway hyperresponsiveness and the late asthmatic response. Lancet 2000; 356:2144–2148.
77. Kips JC, O'Connor BJ, Langley SJ, Woodcock A, Kerstjens HA, Postma DS, Danzig M, Cuss F, Pauwels RA. Effect of SCH55700, a humanized anti-human interleukin-5 antibody, in severe persistent asthma: a pilot study. Am J Respir Crit Care Med 2003; 167:1655–1659..
78. Flood-Page PT, Menzies-Gow AN, Kay AB, Robinson DS. Eosinophil's role remains uncertain as anti-interleukin-5 only partially depletes numbers in asthmatic airways. Am J Respir Crit Care Med 2003; 167:199–204.

79. Morokata T, Ida K, Yamada T. Characterization of YM-90709 as a novel antagonist, which inhibits the binding of interleukin-5 to interleukin-5 receptor. Int Immunopharmacol 2002; 2:1693–1702.

80. Steinke JW, Borish L. Interleukin-4: its role in the pathogenesis of asthma, and targeting it for asthma treatment with interleukin-4 receptor antagonists. Respir Res 2001; 2:66–70.

81. Gavett SH, O'Hearn DJ, Karp CL, Patel EA, Schofield BH, Finkelman FD, Wills-Karp M. Interleukin-4 receptor blockade prevents airway responses induced by antigen challenge in mice. Am J Physiol 1997; 272:L253–61..

82. Borish LC, Nelson HS, Lanz MJ, Claussen L, Whitmore JB, Agosti JM, Garrison L. Interleukin-4 Receptor in Moderate Atopic Asthma. A phase I/II randomized, placebo-controlled trial. Am J Respir Crit Care Med 1999; 160:1816–1823..

83. Borish LC, Nelson HS, Corren J, Bensch G, Busse WW, Whitmore JB, Agosti JM. Efficacy of soluble IL-4 receptor for the treatment of adults with asthma. J Allergy Clin Immunol 2001; 107:963–970.

84. Economides AN, Carpenter LR, Rudge JS, Wong V, Koehler-Stec EM, Hartnett C, Pyles EA, Xu X, Daly TJ, Young MR, Fandl JP, Lee F, Carver S, McNay J, Bailey K, Ramakanth S, Hutabarat R, Huang TT, Radziejewski C, Yancopoulos GD, Stahl N. Cytokine traps: multi-component, high-affinity blockers of cytokine action. Nat Med 2003; 9:47–52.

85. Shanafelt AB, Forte CP, Kasper JJ, Sanchez-Pescador L, Wetzel M, Gundel R, Greve JM. An immune cell-selective interleukin 4 agonist. Proc Natl Acad Sci U S A 1998; 95:9454–9458.

86. Jiang H, Harris MB, Rothman P. IL-4/IL-13 signalling beyond JAK/STAT. J Allergy Clin Immunol 2000; 105:1063–1070.

87. Foster PS. STAT6: an intracellular target for the inhibition of allergic disease. Clin Exp Allergy 1999; 29:12–16.

88. Wills-Karp M, Chiaramonte M. Interleukin-13 in asthma. Curr Opin Pulm Med 2003; 9:21–27.

89. Walter DM, McIntire JJ, Berry G, McKenzie AN, Donaldson DD, DeKruyff RH, et al. Critical role for IL-13 in the development of allergen-induced airway hyperreactivity. J Immunol 2001; 167:4668–4675.

90. Kuperman DA, Huang X, Koth LL, Chang GH, Dolganov GM, Zhu Z, Elias JA, Sheppard D, Erle DJ. Direct effects of interleukin-13 on epithelial cells cause airway hyperreactivity and mucus overproduction in asthma. Nat Med 2002; 8:885–889.

91. Wills-Karp M, Luyimbazi J, Xu X, Schofield B, Neben TY, Karp CL, Donaldson DD. Interleukin-13: central mediator of allergic asthma. Science 1998; 282:2258–2261.

92. Sousa AR, Lane SJ, Nakhosteen JA, Lee TH, Poston RN. Expression of interleukin-1 beta (IL-1b) and interleukin-1 receptor antagonist (IL-1Ra) on asthmatic bronchial epithelium. Am J Respir Crit Care Med 1996; 154: 1061–1066.

93. Arend WP, Malyak M, Guthridge CJ, Gabay C. Interleukin-1 receptor antagonist: role in biology. Annu Rev Immunol 1998; 16:27–55.

94. Rosenwasser LJ. Biologic activities of IL-1 and its role in human disease. J Allergy Clin Immunol 1998; 102:344–350.
95. Kips JC, Tavernier JH, Joos GF, Peleman RA, Pauwels RA. The potential role of tumor necrosis factor a in asthma. Clin Exp Allergy 1993; 23: 247–250.
96. Palladino MA, Bahjat FR, Theodorakis EA, Moldawer LL. Anti-TNF-alpha therapies: the next generation. Nat Rev Drug Discov 2003; 2:736–746.
97. Rabinowitz MH, Andrews RC, Becherer JD, Bickett DM, Bubacz DG, Conway JG, Cowan DJ, Gaul M, Glennon K, Lambert MH, Leesnitzer MA, McDougald DL, Moss ML, Musso DL, Rizzolio MC. Design of selective and soluble inhibitors of tumor necrosis factor-α converting enzyme (TACE). J Med Chem 2001; 44:4252–4267.
98. Barnes PJ, Lim S. Inhibitory cytokines in asthma. Mol Med Today 1998; 4: 452–458.
99. Barnes PJ. Endogenous inhibitory mechanisms in asthma. Am J Respir Crit Care Med 2000; 161:S176–S181.
100. Barnes PJ. IL-10: a key regulator of allergic disease. Clin Exp Allergy 2001; 31:667–669.
101. Borish L, Aarons A, Rumbyrt J, Cvietusa P, Negri J, Wenzel S. Interleukin-10 regulation in normal subjects and patients with asthma. J Allergy Clin Immunol 1996; 97:1288–1296.
102. John M, Lim S, Seybold J, Robichaud A, O'Connor B, Barnes PJ, Chung KF. Inhaled corticosteroids increase IL-10 but reduce MIP-1α, GM-CSF and IFN-g release from alveolar macrophages in asthma. Am J Respir Crit Care Med 1998; 157:256–262.
103. Zuany-Amorim C, Haile S, Leduc D, Dumarey C, Huerre M, Vargaftig BB, Pretolani M. Interleukin-10 inhibits antigen-induced cellular recruitment into the airways of sensitized mice. J Clin Invest 1995; 95:2644–2651.
104. Oh JW, Seroogy CM, Meyer EH, Akbari O, Berry G, Fathman CG, DeKruyff RH, Umetsu DT. CD4 T-helper cells engineered to produce IL-10 prevent allergen-induced airway hyperreactivity and inflammation. J Allergy Clin Immunol 2002; 110:460–468.
105. Jutel M, Akdis M, Budak F, Aebischer-Casaulta C, Wrzyszcz M, Blaser K, Akdis CA. IL-10 and TGF-β cooperate in the regulatory T cell response to mucosal allergens in normal immunity and specific immunotherapy. Eur J Immunol 2003; 33:1205–1214.
106. Fedorak RN, Gangl A, Elson CO, Rutgeerts P, Schreiber S, Wild G, Hanauer SB, Kilian A, Cohard M, LeBEAUT A, Feagan B. Recombinant human interleukin 10 in the treatment of patients with mild to moderately active Crohn's disease. Gastroenterology 2000; 119:1473–1482.
107. Seldon PM, Giembycz MA. Suppression of granulocyte/macrophage colony-stimulating factor release from human monocytes by cyclic AMP-elevating drugs: role of interleukin-10. Br J Pharmacol 2001; 134:58–67.
108. Lack G, Bradley KL, Hamelmann E, Renz H, Loader J, Leung DY, Larsen G, Gelfand EW. Nebulized IFN-gamma inhibits the development of secondary allergic responses in mice. J Immunol 1996; 157:1432–1439.

109. Boguniewicz M, Martin RJ, Martin D, Gibson U, Celniker A. The effects of nebulized recombinant interferon-y in asthmatic airways. J Allergy Clin Immunol 1995; 95:133–135.
110. Benjaponpitak S, Oro A, Maguire P, Marinkovich V, DeKruyff RH, Umetsu DT. The kinetics of change in cytokine production by CD4 T cells during conventional allergen immunotherapy. J Allergy Clin Immunol 1999; 103: 468–475.
111. Durham SR, Ying S, Varney VA, Jacobson MR, Sudderick RM, Mackay IS, Kay AB, Hamid QA. Grass pollen immunotherapy inhibits allergen-induced infiltration of CD4+ T lymphocytes and eosinophils in the nasal mucosa and increases the number of cells expressing messenger RNA for interferon-gamma. J Allergy Clin Immunol 1996; 97:1356–1365.
112. Simon HU, Seelbach H, Ehmann R, Schmitz M. Clinical and immunological effects of low-dose IFN-alpha treatment in patients with corticosteroid-resistant asthma. Allergy 2003; 58:1250–1255.
113. Trinchieri G, Pflanz S, Kastelein RA. The IL-12 family of heterodimeric cytokines: new players in the regulation of T-cell responses. Immunity 2003; 19: 641–644.
114. Gavett SH, O'Hearn DJ, Li X, Huang SK, Finkelman FD, Wills-Karp M. Interleukin 12 inhibits antigen-induced airway hyperresponsivness, inflammation and Th-2 cytokine expression in mice. J Exp Med 1995; 182:1527–1536.
115. van der Pouw Kraan TC, Boeije LC, de Groot ER, Stapel SO, Snijders A, Kapsenberg ML, van der Zee JS, Aarden LA. Reduced production of IL-12 and IL-12-dependent IFN-gamma release in patients with allergic asthma. J Immunol 1997; 158:5560–5565.
116. Leonard JP, Sherman ML, Fisher GL, Buchanan LJ, Larsen G, Atkins MB, Sosman JA, Dutcher JP, Vogelzang NJ, Ryan JL. Effects of single-dose interleukin-12 exposure on interleukin-12- associated toxicity and interferon-gamma production. Blood 1997; 90:2541–2548.
117. Bryan S, O'Connor BJ, Matti S, Leckie MJ, Kanabar V, Khan J, Warrington S, Renzetti L, Rames A, Bock JA, Boyce M, Hansel TT, Holgate ST, Sterk PJ, Barnes PJ. Effects of recombinant human interleukin-12 on eosinophils, airway hyperreactivity and the late asthmatic response. Lancet 2000; 356: 2149–2153.
118. Kim TS, DeKruyff RH, Rupper R, Maecker HT, Levy S, Umetsu DT. An ovalbumin-IL-12 fusion protein is more effective than ovalbumin plus free recombinant IL-12 in inducing a T helper cell type 1-dominated immune response and inhibiting antigen-specific IgE production. J Immunol 1997; 158:4137–4144.
119. Rossi D, Zlotnik A. The biology of chemokines and their receptors. Annu Rev Immunol 2000; 18:217–242.
120. Proudfoot AE. Chemokine receptors: multifaceted therapeutic targets. Nat Rev Immunol 2002; 2:106–115.
121. Gutierrez-Ramos JC, Lloyd C, Gonzalo JA. Eotaxin: from an eosinophilic chemokine to a major regulator of allergic reactions. Immunol Today 1999; 20:500–504.

122. Gonzalo JA, Lloyd CM, Kremer L, Finger E, Martinez A, Siegelman MH, Cybulsky M, Gutierrez-Ramos JC. Eosinophil recruitment to the lung in a murine model of allergic inflammation. The role of T cells, chemokines, and adhesion receptors. J Clin Invest 1996; 98:2332–2345.

123. Ying S, Meng Q, Zeibecoglou K, Robinson DS, Macfarlane A, Humbert M, Kay AB. Eosinophil chemotactic chemokines (eotaxin, eotaxin-2, RANTES, monocyte chemoattractant protein-3 (MCP-3), and MCP-4), and C-C chemokine receptor 3 expression in bronchial biopsies from atopic and nonatopic (Intrinsic) asthmatics. J Immunol 1999; 163:6321–6329.

124. Erin EM, Williams TJ, Barnes PJ, Hansel TT. Eotaxin receptor (CCR3) antagonism in asthma and allergic disease. Curr Drug Targets Inflamm Allergy 2002; 1:201–214.

125. Berkman N, Krishnan VL, Gilbey T, O'Connor BJ, Barnes PJ. Expression of RANTES mRNA and protein in airways of patients with mild asthma. Am J Respir Crit Care Med 1996; 15:382–389.

126. Elsner J, Petering H, Hochstetter R, Kimmig D, Wells TN, Kapp A, Proudfoot AE. The CC chemokine antagonist Met-RANTES inhibits eosinophil effector functions through the chemokine receptors CCR1 and CCR3. Eur J Immunol 1997; 27:2892–2898.

127. Campbell EM, Charo IF, Kunkel SL, Strieter RM, Boring L, Gosling J, Lukacs NW. Monocyte chemoattractant protein-1 mediates cockroach allergen-induced bronchial hyperreactivity in normal but not CCR2-/- mice: the role of mast cells. J Immunol 1999; 163:2160–2167.

128. Lloyd CM, Delaney T, Nguyen T, Tian J, Martinez A, Coyle AJ, Gutierrez-Ramos JC. CC chemokine receptor (CCR)3/eotaxin is followed by CCR4/monocyte-derived chemokine in mediating pulmonary T helper lymphocyte type 2 recruitment after serial antigen challenge in vivo. J Exp Med 2000; 191:265–274.

129. Chung CD, Kuo F, Kumer J, Motani AS, Lawrence CE, Henderson WR, Jr., Venkataraman C. CCR8 is not essential for the development of inflammation in a mouse model of allergic airway disease. J Immunol 2003; 170:581–587.

130. Lukacs NW, Berlin A, Schols D, Skerlj RT, Bridger GJ. AMD3100, a CxCR4 antagonist, attenuates allergic lung inflammation and airway hyperreactivity. Am J Pathol 2002; 160:1353–1360.

131. Sallusto F, Lanzavecchia A. Understanding dendritic cell and T-lymphocyte traffic through the analysis of chemokine receptor expression. Immunol Rev 2000; 177:134–140.

132. Barnes PJ, Pedersen S, Busse WW. Efficacy and safety of inhaled corticosteroids: an update. Am J Respir Crit Care Med 1998; 157:S1–S53.

133. Lipworth BJ. Systemic adverse effects of inhaled corticosteroid therapy: a systematic review and meta-analysis [see comments]. Arch Intern Med 1999; 159:941–955.

134. Brattsand R, Axelsson B. New inhaled glucocorticosteroids. In: Barnes PJ, ed. New Drugs for Asthma. Vol 2. London: IBC Technical Services Ltd, 1992:192–207.

135. Dent G. Ciclesonide. Curr Opin Invest Drugs 2002; 3:78–83.

136. Taylor DA, Jensen MW, Kanabar V, Englestatter R, Steinjans VW, Barnes PJ, O'Connor BJ. A dose-dependent effect of the novel inhaled corticosteroid ciclesonide on airway responsiveness to adenosine-5'-monophosphate in asthmatic patients. Am J Respir Crit Care Med 1999; 160:237–243.

137. Postma DS, Sevette C, Martinat Y, Schlosser N, Aumann J, Kafe H. Treatment of asthma by the inhaled corticosteroid ciclesonide given either in the morning or evening. Eur Respir J 2001; 17:1083–1088.

138. Barnes PJ, Adcock IM. How do corticosteroids work in asthma? Ann Intern Med 2003; 139:359–370.

139. Ito K, Jazrawi E, Cosio B, Barnes PJ, Adcock IM. p65-Activated histone acetyltransferase activity is repressed by glucocorticoids: Mifepristone fails to recruit HDAC2 to the p65/HAT complex. J Biol Chem 2001; 276: 30208–30215.

140. Heck S, Kullmann M, Grast A, Ponta H, Rahmsdorf HJ, Herrlich P, Cato ACB. A distinct modulating domain in glucocorticoid receptor monomers in the repression of activity of the transcription factor AP-1. EMBO J 1994; 13:4087–4095.

141. Reichardt HM, Kaestner KH, Tuckermann J, Kretz O, Wessely O, Bock R, Gass P, Schmid W, Herrlich P, Angel P, Schutz G. DNA binding of the glucocorticoid receptor is not essential for survival. Cell 1998; 93:531–541.

142. Reichardt HM, Tuckermann JP, Gottlicher M, Vujic M, Weih F, Angel P, Herrlich P, Schutz G. Repression of inflammatory responses in the absence of DNA binding by the glucocorticoid receptor. EMBO J 2001; 20:7168–7173.

143. Adcock IM, Nasuhara Y, Stevens DA, Barnes PJ. Ligand-induced differentiation of glucocorticoid receptor trans-repression and transactivation: preferential targetting of NF-κB and lack of I-κB involvement. Br J Pharmacol 1999; 127:1003–1011.

144. Vayssiere BM, Dupont S, Choquart A, Petit F, Garcia T, Marchandeau C, Gronemeyer H, Resche-Rigon M. Synthetic glucocorticoids that dissociate transactivation and AP-1 transrepression exhibit antiinflammatory activity in vivo. Mol Endocrinol 1997; 11:1245–1255.

145. Belvisi MG, Wicks SL, Battram CH, Bottoms SE, Redford JE, Woodman P, Brown TJ, Webber SE, Foster ML. Therapeutic benefit of a dissociated glucocorticoid and the relevance of in vitro separation of transrepression from transactivation activity. J Immunol 2001; 166:1975–1982.

146. Bledsoe RK, Montana VG, Stanley TB, Delves CJ, Apolito CJ, McKee DD, Consler TG, Parks DJ, Stewart EL, Willson TM, Lambert MH, Moore JT, Pearce KH, Xu HE. Crystal structure of the glucocorticoid receptor ligand binding domain reveals a novel mode of receptor dimerization and coactivator recognition. Cell 2002; 110:93–105.

147. Essayan DM. Cyclic nucleotide phosphodiesterases. J Allergy Clin Immunol 2001; 108:671–680.

148. Torphy TJ. Phosphodiesterase isoenzymes. Am J Respir Crit Care Med 1998; 157:351–370.

149. Houslay MD, Adams DR. PDE4 cAMP phosphodiesterases: modular enzymes that orchestrate signalling cross talk, desensitization and compartmentalization. Biochem J 2003; 370:1–18.
150. Giembycz MA. Cilomilast: a breath of relief? Trends Mol Med 2001; 7: 433–434.
151. Harbison PL, MacLeod D, Hawksworth R, O'Toole S, Sullivan PJ, Heath P, Kilfeather S, Page CP, Costello J, Holgate ST, Lee TH. The effect of a novel orally active selective PDE4 isoenzyme inhibitor (CD840) on allergen-induced responses in asthmatic subjects. Eur Respir J 1997; 10:1008–1014.
152. Reid P. Roflumilast. Curr Opin Invest Drugs 2002; 3:1165–1170.
153. Timmer W, Leclerc V, Birraux G, Neuhauser M, Hatzelmann A, Bethke T, Wurst W. The new phosphodiesterase 4 inhibitor roflumilast is efficacious in exercise-induced asthma and leads to suppression of LPS-stimulated TNF-alpha ex vivo. J Clin Pharmacol 2002; 42:297–303.
154. Lamontagne S, Meadows E, Luk P, Normandin D, Muise E, Boulet L, Pon DJ, Robichaud A, Robertson GS, Metters KM, Nantel F. Localization of phosphodiesterase-4 isoforms in the medulla and nodose ganglion of the squirrel monkey. Brain Res 2001; 920:84–96.
155. Robichaud A, Stamatiou PB, Jin SL, Lachance N, MacDonald D, Laliberte F, Liu S, Huang Z, Conti M, Chan CC. Deletion of phosphodicstcrasc 4D in mice shortens alpha(2)-adrenoceptor-mediated anesthesia, a behavioral correlate of emesis. J Clin Invest 2002; 110:1045–1052.
156. Jin SL, Conti M. Induction of the cyclic nucleotide phosphodiesterase PDE4B is essential for LPS-activated TNF-alpha responses. Proc Natl Acad Sci USA 2002; 99:7628–7633.
157. Compton CH, Gubb J, Nieman R, Edelson J, Amit O, Bakst A, Ayres JG, Creemers JP, Schultzc-Wcrninghaus G, Brambilla C, Barnes NC. Cilomilast, a selective phosphodiesterase-4 inhibitor for treatment of patients with chronic obstructive pulmonary disease: a randomised, dose-ranging study. Lancet 2001; 358:265–270.
158. Delhase M, Li N, Karin M. Kinase regulation in inflammatory response. Nature 2000; 406:367–368.
159. Roshak AK, Callahan JF, Blake SM. Small-molecule inhibitors of NF-κB for the treatment of inflammatory joint disease. Curr Opin Pharmacol 2002; 2: 316–321.
160. Nasuhara Y, Adcock IM, Catley M, Barnes PJ, Newton R. Differential IKK activation and IkBa degradation by interleukin-1b and tumor necrosis factor-a in human U937 monocytic cells: evidence for additional regulatory steps in kB-dependent transcription. J Biol Chem 1999; 274:19965–19972.
161. Evans DJ, Cullinan P, Geddes DM. Cyclosporin as an oral corticosteroid sparing agent in stable asthma (Cochrane Review). Cochrane Database Syst Rev 2001; 2:CD002993.
162. Cohen P. Protein kinases—the major drug targets of the twenty-first century? Nat Rev Drug Discov 2002; 1:309–315.
163. Johnson GL, Lapadat R. Mitogen-activated protein kinase pathways mediated by ERK, JNK, and p38 protein kinases. Science 2002; 298:1911–1912.

164. Kumar S, Boehm J, Lee JC. p38 MAP kinases: key signalling molecules as therapeutic targets for inflammatory diseases. Nat Rev Drug Discov 2003; 2: 717–726.

165. Schafer PH, Wadsworth SA, Wang L, Siekierka JJ. p38a Mitogen-activated protein kinase is activated by CD28-mediated signaling is required for IL-4 production by human CD4$^+$CD45RO$^+$ T cells Th-2 effector cells. J Immunol 1999; 162:7110–7119.

166. Kankaanranta H, Giembycz MA, Barnes PJ, Lindsay DA. SB203580, an inhibitor of p38 mitogen-activated protein kinase, enhances constitutive apoptosis of cytokine-deprived human eosinophils. J Pharmacol Exp Ther 1999; 290: 621–628.

167. Irusen E, Matthews JG, Takahashi A, Barnes PJ, Chung KF, Adcock IM. p38 Mitogen-activated protein kinase-induced glucocorticoid receptor phosphorylation reduces its activity: role in steroid-insensitive asthma. J Allergy Clin Immunol 2002; 109:649–657.

168. Huang TJ, Adcock IM, Chung KF. A novel transcription factor inhibitor, SP100030, inhibits cytokine gene expression, but not airway eosinophilia or hyperresponsiveness in sensitized and allergen-exposed rat. Br J Pharmacol 2001; 134:1029–1036.

169. Sousa AR, Lane SJ, Soh C, Lee TH. In vivo resistance to corticosteroids in bronchial asthma is associated with enhanced phosyphorylation of JUN N-terminal kinase and failure of prednisolone to inhibit JUN N-terminal kinase phosphorylation. J Allergy Clin Immunol 1999; 104:565–574.

170. Costello PS, Turner M, Walters AE, Cunningham CN, Bauer PH, Downward J, Tybulewicz VL. Critical role for the tyrosine kinase Syk in signalling through the high affinity IgE receptor of mast cells. Oncogene 1996; 13:2595–2605.

171. Yousefi S, Hoessli DC, Blaser K, Mills GB, Simon HU. Requirement of lyn and syk tyrosine kinases for the prevention of apoptosis by cytokines in human eosinophils. J Exp Med 1996; 183:1407–1414.

172. Stenton GR, Ulanova M, Dery RE, Merani S, Kim MK, Gilchrist M, Puttagunta L, Musat-Marcu S, James D, Schreiber AD, Befus AD. Inhibition of allergic inflammation in the airways using aerosolized antisense to Syk kinase. J Immunol 2002; 169:1028–1036.

173. Amoui M, Draber P, Draberova L. Src family-selective tyrosine kinase inhibitor, PP1, inhibits both Fc epsilonRI- and Thy-1-mediated activation of rat basophilic leukemia cells. Eur J Immunol 1997; 27:1881–1886.

174. Lynch OT, Giembycz MA, Daniels I, Barnes PJ, Lindsay MA. Pleiotropic role of *lyn* kinase in leukotriene B$_4$-induced eosinophil activation. Blood 2000; 95:3541–3547.

175. Adachi T, Stafford S, Sur S, Alam R. A novel Lyn-binding peptide inhibitor blocks eosinophil differentiation, survival, and airway eosinophilic inflammation. J Immunol 1999; 163:939–946.

176. Takeyama K, Dabbagh K, Lee HM, Agusti C, Lausier JA, Ueki IF, Grattan KM, Nadel JA. Epidermal growth factor system regulates mucin production in airways. Proc Natl Acad Sci U S A 1999; 96:3081–3086.

177. Wakeling AE. Epidermal growth factor receptor tyrosine kinase inhibitors. Curr Opin Pharmacol 2002; 2:382–387.

178. Powell N, Till S, Bungre J, Corrigan C. The immunomodulatory drugs cyclosporin A, mycophenolate mofetil, and sirolimus (rapamycin) inhibit allergen-induced proliferation and IL-5 production by PBMCs from atopic asthmatic patients. J Allergy Clin Immunol 2001; 108:915–917.

179. Moder KG. Mycophenolate mofetil: new applications for this immunosuppressant. Ann Allergy Asthma Immunol 2003; 90:15–19.

180. Kon OM, Sihra BS, Compton CH, Leonard TB, Kay AB, Barnes NC. Randomized dose-ranging placebo-controlled study of chimeric anribody to CD4 (keliximab) in chronic severe asthma. Lancet 1998; 352:1109–1113.

181. Schwarze J, Cieslewicz G, Joetham A, Ikemura T, Hamelmann E, Gelfand EW. CD8 T cells are essential in the development of respiratory syncytial virus-induced lung eosinophilia and airway hyperresponsiveness. J Immunol 1999; 162:4207–4211.

182. Oda N, Minoguchi K, Yokoe T, Hashimoto T, Wada K, Miyamoto M, Tanaka A, Kohno Y, Adachi M. Effect of suplatast tosilate (IPD-1151T) on cytokine production by allergen-specific human Th1 and Th2 cell lines. Life Sci 1999; 65:763–770.

183. Tamaoki J, Kondo M, Sakai N, Aoshiba K, Tagaya E, Nakata J, Isono K, Nagai A. Effect of suplatast tosilate, a Th2 cytokine inhibitor, on steroid-dependent asthma: a double-blind randomised study. Lancet 2000; 356: 273–278.

184. Yoshida M, Aizawa H, Inoue H, Matsumoto K, Koto H, Komori M, Fukuyama S, Okamoto M, Hara N. Effect of suplatast tosilate on airway hyperresponsiveness and inflammation in asthma patients. J Asthma 2002; 39:545–552.

185. Schleimer RP, Bochner BS. The role of adhesion molecules in allergic inflammation and their suitability as targets of antiallergic therapy. Clin Exp Allergy 1998; 28(suppl 3):15–23.

186. Wegner CD, Gundel L, Reilly P, Haynes N, Letts LG, Rothlein R. Intracellular adhesion molecule-1 (ICAM-1) in the pathogenesis of asthma. Science 1990; 247:456–459.

187. Sun J, Elwood W, Haczku A, Barnes PJ, Hellewell PG, Chung KF. Contribution of intracellular adhesion molecule-1 in allergen-induced airway hyperesponsiveness and inflammation in sensitised Brown-Norway rats. Int Arch Allergy Immunol 1994; 104:291–295.

188. Yuan Q, Strauch KL, Lobb RR, Hemler ME. Intracellular single-chain antibody inhibits integrin VLA-4 maturation and function. Biochem J 1996; 318:591–596.

189. Lin Kc, Ateeq HS, Hsiung SH, Chong LT, Zimmerman CN, Castro A, Lee WC, Hammond CE, Kalkunte S, Chen LL, Pepinsky RB, Leone DR, Sprague AG, Abraham WM, Gill A, Lobb RR, Adams SP. Selective, tight-binding inhibitors of integrin alpha4beta1 that inhibit allergic airway responses. J Med Chem 1999; 42:920–934.

190. Ghosh S, Goldin E, Gordon FH, Malchow HA, Rask-Madsen J, Rutgeerts P, et al. Natalizumab for active Crohn's disease. N Engl J Med 2003; 348:24–32.

191. Abraham WM, Ahmed A, Sabater JR, Lauredo IT, Botvinnikova Y, Bjercke RJ, Hu X, Revelle BM, Kogan TP, Scott IL, Dixon RA, Yeh ET, Beck PJ.

Selectin blockade prevents antigen-induced late bronchial responses and airway hyperresponsiveness in allergic sheep. Am J Respir Crit Care Med 1999; 159:1205–1214.

192. Kim MK, Brandley BK, Anderson MB, Bochner BS. Antagonism of selectin-dependent adhesion of human eosinophils and neutrophils by glycomimetics and oligosaccharide compounds. Am J Respir Cell Mol Biol 1998; 19:836–841.

193. Wouden JC, Tasche MJ, Bernsen RM, Uijen JH, Jongste JC, Ducharme FM. Inhaled sodium cromoglycate for asthma in children. Cochrane Database Syst Rev 2003;CD002173.

194. Heinke S, Szucs G, Norris A, Droogmans G, Nilius B. Inhibition of volume-activated chloride currents in endothelial cells by chromones. Br J Pharmacol 1995; 115:1393–1398.

195. Wang L, Correia I, Basu S, Theoharides TC. Ca^{2+} and phorbol ester effect on the mast cell phosphoprotein induced by cromolyn [In Process Citation]. Eur J Pharmacol 1999; 371:241–249.

196. Bianco S, Pieroni MG, Refini RM, Robuschi M, Vaghi A, Sestini P. Inhaled loop diuretics as potential new anti-asthmatic drugs. Eur Respir J 1993; 6:130–134.

197. Yates DH, O'Connor BJ, Yilmaz G, Aikman S, Chen-Worsdell M, Barnes PJ, Chung KF. Effect of acute and chronic inhaled furosemide on bronchial hyperresponsiveness in mild asthma. Am J Respir Crit Care Med 1995; 152:892–896.

198. Djukanovic R. The role of co-stimulation in airway inflammation. Clin Exp Allergy 2000; 30(suppl 1):46–50.

199. Haczku A, Takeda K, Redai I, Hamelmann E, Cieslewicz G, Joetham A, Loader J, Lee JJ, Irvin C, Gelfand EW. Anti-CD86 (B7.2) treatment abolishes allergic airway hyperresponsiveness in mice [In Process Citation]. Am J Respir Crit Care Med 1999; 159:1638–1643.

200. Van Oosterhout AJ, Hofstra CL, Shields R, Chan B, van Ark I, Jardieu PM, Nijkamp FP. Murine CTLA4-IgG treatment inhibits airway eosinophilia and hyperresponsiveness and attenuates IgE upregulation in a murine model of allergic asthma. Am J Respir Cell Mol Biol 1997; 17:386–392.

201. Deurloo DT, van Esch BC, Hofstra CL, Nijkamp FP, Van Oosterhout AJ. CTLA4-IgG reverses asthma manifestations in a mild but not in a more "severe" ongoing murine model. Am J Respir Cell Mol Biol 2001; 25: 751–760.

202. van Neerven RJ, Van de Pol MM, van der Zee JS, Stiekema FE, De Boer M, Kapsenberg ML. Requirement of CD28–CD86 costimulation for allergen-specific T cell proliferation and cytokine expression [see comments]. Clin Exp Allergy 1998; 28:808–816.

203. Gonzalo JA, Tian J, Delaney T, Corcoran J, Rottman JB, Lora J, Al garawi A, Kroczek R, Gutierrez-Ramos JC, Coyle AJ. ICOS is critical for T helper cell-mediated lung mucosal inflammatory responses. Nat Immunol 2001; 2: 597–604.

204. Akbari O, Freeman GJ, Meyer EH, Greenfield EA, Chang TT, Sharpe AH, Berry G, DeKruyff RH, Umetsu DT. Antigen-specific regulatory T cells

develop via the ICOS-ICOS-ligand pathway and inhibit allergen-induced airway hyperreactivity. Nat Med 2002; 8:1024–1032.

205. Walker S, Monteil M, Phelan K, Lasserson TJ, Walters EH. Anti-IgE for chronic asthma. Cochrane Database Syst Rev 2003; CD003559.

206. Lemanske RF Jr, Nayak A, McAlary M, Everhard F, Fowler-Taylor A, Gupta N. Omalizumab improves asthma-related quality of life in children with allergic asthma. Pediatrics 2002; 110:e55.

207. Creticos PS, Reed CE, Norman PS, Khoury J, Adkinson NF, Buncher R, Busse WW, Bush RK, Gaddie J, Li JT, Richerson HB, Rosenthal RR, Solomon WR, Steinberg P, Yunginger JW. Ragweed immunotherapy in adult asthma. New Engl J Med 1996; 334:501–506.

208. Hsu CH, Chua KY, Tao MH, Lai YL, Wu HD, Huang SK, Hsieh KH. Immunoprophylaxis of allergen-induced immunoglobulin E synthesis and airway hyperresponsiveness in vivo by genetic immunization [see comments]. Nat Med 1996; 2:540–544.

209. Oldfield WL, Larche M, Kay AB. Effect of T-cell peptides derived from Fel d 1 on allergic reactions and cytokine production in patients sensitive to cats: a randomised controlled trial. Lancet 2002; 360:47–53.

210. Herz U, Gerhold K, Gruber C, Braun A, Wahn U, Renz H, Paul K. BCG infection suppresses allergic sensitization and development of increased airway reactivity in an animal model. J Allergy Clin Immunol 1998; 102: 867–874.

211. Choi IS, Koh YI. Therapeutic effects of BCG vaccination in adult asthmatic patients: a randomized, controlled trial. Ann Allergy Asthma Immunol 2002; 88:584–591.

212. Wang CC, Rook GA. Inhibition of an established allergic response to ovalbumin in BALB/c mice by killed Mycobacterium vaccae. Immunology 1998; 93:307–313.

213. Shirtcliffe PM, Easthope SE, Cheng S, Weatherall M, Tan PL, Le Gros G, Beasley R. The effect of delipidated deglycolipidated (DDMV) and heat-killed Mycobacterium vaccae in asthma. Am J Respir Crit Care Med 2001; 163:1410–1414.

214. Horner AA, Van Uden JH, Zubeldia JM, Broide D, Raz E. DNA-based immunotherapeutics for the treatment of allergic disease. Immunol Rev 2001; 179:102–118.

215. Sur S, Wild JS, Choudhury BK, Sur N, Alam R, Klinman DM. Long term prevention of allergic lung inflammation in a mouse model of asthma by CpG oligodeoxynucleotides [In Process Citation]. J Immunol 1999; 162: 6284–6293.

216. Kline JN, Kitagaki K, Businga TR, Jain VV. Treatment of established asthma in a murine model using CpG oligodeoxynucleotides. Am J Physiol Lung Cell Mol Physiol 2002; 283:L170–L179.

217. Santeliz JV, Van Nest G, Traquina P, Larsen E, Wills-Karp M. Amb a 1-linked CpG oligodeoxynucleotides reverse established airway hyperresponsiveness in a murine model of asthma. J Allergy Clin Immunol 2002; 109: 455–462.

218. Agrawal S, Kandimalla ER. Medicinal chemistry and therapeutic potential of CpG DNA. Trends Mol Med 2002; 8:114–121.
219. Cookson WO. Asthma genetics. Chest 2002; 121:7S–13S.
220. Hall IP. Pharmacogenetics of asthma. Eur Respir J 2000; 15:449–451.
221. Powell RM, Hamilton LM, Holgate ST, Davies DE, Holloway JW. ADAM33: a novel therapeutic target for asthma. Expert Opin Ther Targets 2003; 7: 485–494.
222. Allen M, Heinzmann A, Noguchi E, Abecasis G, Broxholme J, Ponting CP, et al. Positional cloning of a novel gene influencing asthma from Chromosome 2q14. Nat Genet 2003; 35:258–263.
223. Zhang Y, Leaves NI, Anderson GG, Ponting CP, Broxholme J, Holt R, Edser P, Bhattacharyya S, Dunham A, Adcock IM, Pulleyn L, Barnes PJ, Harper JI, Abecasis G, Cardon L, White M, Burton J, Matthews L, Mott R, Ross M, Cox R, Moffatt MF, Cookson WO. Positional cloning of a quantitative trait locus on chromosome 13q14 that influences immunoglobulin E levels and asthma. Nat Genet 2003; 34:184–186.
224. Xing Z, Ohkawara Y, Jordana M, Grahern FL, Gauldie J. Transfer of granulocyte-macrophage colony-stimulating factor gene to rat induces eosinophilia, monocytosis and fibrotic lesions. J Clin Invest 1996; 97:1102–1110.
225. Nyce JW, Metzger WJ. DNA antisense therapy for asthma in an animal model. Nature 1997; 385:721–725.
226. Sandrasagra A, Leonard SA, Tang L, Teng K, Li Y, Ball HA, Mannion JC, Nyce JW. Discovery and development of respirable antisense therapeutics for asthma. Antisense Nucleic Acid Drug Dev 2002; 12:177–181.
227. Ball HA, Sandrasagra A, Tang L, Van Scott M, Wild J, Nyce JW. Clinical potential of respirable antisense oligonucleotides (RASONs) in asthma. Am J Pharmacogenomics 2003; 3:97–106.
228. Wall NR, Shi Y. Small RNA: can RNA interference be exploited for therapy? Lancet 2003; 362:1401–1403.
229. Zhang X, Shan P, Jiang D, Noble PW, Abraham NG, Kappas A, Lee PJ. Small interfering RNA targeting heme oxygenase-1 enhances ischemia-reperfusion-induced lung apoptosis. J Biol Chem 2004; 279:10677–10684.

25

Difficult-to-Control Asthma

JOHN F. PRICE

Guy's, King's and St. Thomas School of Medicine, King's College Hospital
Denmark Hill, London, U.K.

I. Introduction

Good asthma control can be achieved in most children with a short-acting beta-agonist and with low doses of inhaled steroid given alone or in combination with a long-acting beta-agonist or a leukotriene recepter antagonist. Inhaled steroids have a flat dose–response curve for efficacy, the top of the dose–response curve being reached at approximately 400–800 mcg beclomethasone equivalent in children (1). Children who have asthma that is difficult to control, despite being prescribed high doses (800 mcg or more of beclomethasone equivalent) of inhaled steroids combined with other asthma medication, should be reviewed by a pediatrician specializing in respiratory disease. The first consideration will be whether the diagnosis of asthma is correct. There may be environmental or psychosocial factors affecting the asthma that have not been recognized or the prescribed treatment may not be being taken. A small proportion of children with severe asthma remain symptomatic despite appropriate environmental measures and treatment that includes high doses of an inhaled steroid and beta-agonists. The care of these children requires considerable skill and sometimes a therapeutic approach that may involve a delicate balance of risk against benefit. They comprise no more than 5% of the childhood asthma population but, because asthma is so common, there will be 5000 to 10,000 such children in the United Kingom. They are a heterogeneous group in whom the pathophysiology is poorly understood. They require frequent consultations, complex treatment regimes, and are often admitted to the hospital. As a result, they consume the bulk of the £250 million spent on childhood asthma care in the United Kingdom.

II. Poor Control Unrelated to Asthma Severity

A. Diagnosis—Is It Asthma?

Wheezing in Early Childhood

Wheezing illness is more common in infancy and early childhood than at any other age and has the widest differential diagnosis. Congenital malformations are suggested by very early onset of wheezing, associated stridor, difficulty swallowing, choking with feeds, and recurrent vomiting. Wheezing associated with frequent lower respiratory tract infection may indicate cystic fibrosis or immune deficiency. In addition to immunoglobulin and common variable immune deficiency, functional antibody deficiencies to *Pneumococcus* and *Haemophilus influenzae* capsular polysaccharide antigens are increasingly recognized in children with recurrent lower respiratory tract symptoms, including wheezing (2). If there is also a history of unexplained dyspnea and nasal obstruction from birth, consider primary ciliary dyskinesia (Table 1). Although persistent nocturnal cough may precede the onset of wheezing in a preschool child with asthma, it has been estimated that less than 10% of asthma presents with cough alone (3,4). Cough without bronchial hyperreactivity is unlikely to be asthma (5).

Table 1 Some Non-asthmatic Causes of Cough and Wheezing

Diagnostic indicators	Consider
Wheeze after feeding/vomiting	Gastrooesophageal reflux/aspiration
Inspiratory/expiratory stridor	Tracheal stenosis/mediastinal mass
With dysphagia	Vascular ring
Frequent severe infections	Immune deficiency/immotile cilia syndrome
Poor weight gain/fatty stools	Cystic fibrosis
Hilar lymphadenopathy	TB/lymphoma
Persistent symptoms/hypoxia after a severe lower respiratory illness	Obliterative bronchiolitis

Gastroesophageal Reflux and Inhalation

Reflux resulting in inhalation causes coughing and wheezing that may be mistaken for asthma or may make asthma worse. The relationship between reflux and problematic asthma is controversial. A Swedish study found no relationship between episodes of reflux and either wheezing or changes in peak flow (6). A U.K. study, on the other hand, observed an increase in bronchial reactivity to histamine after an acid drink in children with asthma and reflux and suggested this could be a mechanism for exacerbation of nocturnal symptoms (7). The degree of reflux does not correlate well with the severity of wheezing, suggesting that host responsiveness such as underlying bronchial hyperreactivity may be more relevant than the amount of reflux (8).

Vocal Cord Dysfunction

In this condition there is paradoxical adduction of the vocal cords sufficient to cause airflow limitation at the level of the larynx. The obstruction is predominantly in inspiration, but there may be paradoxical vocal cord motion in early expiration as well. The predominant symptom is stridor, with dyspnea, chest tightness, cough, and sometimes wheezing. The symptoms of vocal cord dysfunction can mimic asthma but do not respond to bronchodilator or anti-inflammatory therapy. Children may receive high doses of corticosteroid treatment before the correct diagnosis is made. It can present with dyspnea on exertion and be mistaken for exercise-induced asthma (9). Vocal cord dysfunction can coexist with asthma and this makes the diagnosis particularly difficult. A review of 95 cases found that 53 had asthma as well, and at the time of correct diagnosis those without asthma were receiving similar treatment to those with asthma (10). Lung function tests may show attenuation of the inspiratory flow volume loop. The definitive diagnosis is made by observing paradoxical vocal cord adduction during visualization of the vocal cords with flexible laryngoscopy. Supraglottic anteroposterior constriction and false vocal cord approximation have been described in some cases (11). Treatment is often unsatisfactory. Careful explanation, speech therapy, and psychological counseling are sometimes successful (12).

B. Adverse Environment

The presence of unrecognized allergens to which the child is sensitized, outdoor and indoor air pollution, and psychosocial stress may, individually or in combination, make asthma difficult to control.

Allergen Exposure

An allergic precipitant of asthma often causes acute symptoms and is easy to identify. Studies using repeated low-dose allergen challenge, however, suggest that persistent allergen exposure in sensitized subjects increases bronchial reactivity and eosinophilic inflammation (13). It also decreases glucocorticoid receptor binding affinity and so could affect the response to steroid treatment (14). Less obvious low-dose allergen exposure may therefore cause symptoms that are difficult to control or increased vulnerability to asthma attacks provoked by other factors such as viral infection or exercise. Improvement in asthma when children go on holiday without any other change in their management strongly suggests an environmental trigger in the home. Children in temperate countries commonly become sensitized to the house dust mite *Dermatophagoides pteronissinus*. Unfortunately, no particular pattern of symptoms characterizes house dust mite allergy. Exposure to mite allergens is highest at night, but asthma symptoms in children generally tend to be worse at night. Severe nasal symptoms in the early morning are sometimes an indicator of dust mite allergy. When families have pets, one must be as sure as possible that the pet is contributing to difficult asthma before advising its removal. The resulting emotional upset could make things worse. It can also take months after the animal is removed before the relevant allergens disappear completely from the home (15).

Air Pollution and Smoking

Air pollutants may influence the severity of asthma by a direct irritant action provoking bronchoconstriction by causing airway inflammation and increased bronchial reactivity, or by altering the immune response to environmental allergens. Children living in polluted areas have more frequent asthma attacks than those living in non-polluted areas (16). Certain climatic conditions may combine with environmental pollutants to cause asthma symptoms, for example, ground level ozone accumulates in cities during sunny periods with little wind.

Children exposed to adults who smoke have elevated salivary cotinine concentrations (17) and there is good evidence that children with asthma have more severe symptoms if their parents smoke (18). Both passive and active smoking influence attainment of maximal lung function. Active smoking impairs the efficacy of both oral (19) and inhaled (20) corticosteroid treatment. Unfortunately, intervention informing parents about the harmful effects of smoking on their children with asthma generally does not encourage them to stop smoking (21). Behavior associated with smoking may also impact indirectly on asthma control in children. For example, parental smoking is an important factor in non-attendance at education programs about asthma (22).

Psychosocial Issues

Individual or family psychopathology can contribute to difficult asthma directly by its association with deteriorating symptoms, or indirectly by acting as a barrier to asthma education and adherence to treatment. Stressful events in children's lives have been linked with decreased school performance (23), a requirement for increased doses of steroids (24), and prolonged admissions to the hospital (25). Several mechanisms have been proposed to explain the association between psychopathology and deterioration in asthma control. The pathophysiology and clinical manifestations of asthma depend on complex neural mechanisms and changes in the autonomic nervous system. β-Adrenergic hyporesponsiveness has been demonstrated in subjects who are depressed. Certain neuropeptides thought to regulate airway inflammation and responsiveness are released during stress. Alterations in immune responses observed during stress may have implications for the exacerbation of asthma particularly by increasing the risk of respiratory infections (26). Family support naturally has an important influence on a child's asthma. Many of the psychosocial factors implicated in poor asthma control—childhood anxiety, depression, non-adherence, and family conflict—are dependent on family structure and function. There is some evidence that exposure to violence is associated with deterioration in asthma among inner-city children (27).

Psychosocial factors may affect perception of asthma control and can have an adverse influence on attitudes to treatment and self-management. Adherence to prescribed treatment is poorer in families with psychological problems, although very few studies have examined this specifically in children with asthma. One study, however, found that the level of family conflict predicted adherence with theophylline treatment (28). Psychosocial barriers to asthma education include economic status, literacy level, and ethnicity. Socioeconomic status has a significant effect on patterns of asthma symptoms. A study in the United Kingdom has shown that socioeconomic status does not influence asthma diagnosis or prescribed treatment, but children in less privileged social classes have more frequent asthma attacks, especially at night (29).

In the past, there has been a tendency for polarization of views about the role of psychosocial issues in asthma. Collaborative research between respiratory physicians and psychologists is needed to advance our knowledge in this complex area.

C. Non-adherence with Treatment

The Scale of the Problem

It is unusual for a child with asthma and their parents to adhere precisely to the prescribed treatment and unrealistic to expect that medication will be taken if the doctor simply describes asthma and demonstrates the treatment recommendations (30). Estimates of overall adherence rates vary according to the methodology used. As one might expect, the most objective and "blinded" assessments produce the lowest figures for adherence (31). Diary card records generally overestimate the frequency with which treatment is taken. In one study of children aged 8–12 years with asthma the median use of inhaled steroid recorded on diary cards was 95%. Electronic monitoring with MDI chronologs indicated the true adherence was a median of 58% (32). Both overall non-adherence and an imbalance of adherence may influence asthma control. Non-adherence may result in an increase in symptoms. However, underuse of regular anti-inflammatory medication plus overuse of bronchodilator relief medication may result in relatively good symptom control but increased vulnerability to asthma attacks. For example, in the study described above adherence to inhaled steroid in children who had exacerbations during the 13 weeks of observation was a median of 14% compared with 68% in those who had no exacerbations (33). Over 100 children aged 7–16 years took part in a 27-month randomized trial of inhaled budesonide given by Turbohaler. During the first 12 weeks of the study, mean adherence according to the diary cards was 93%, but estimated mean adherence derived from counting the remaining doses in the Turbohalers was 77%. Adherence steadily declined over the 27 months of the study and by the end had fallen to less than 50%. While this information is useful and warns us that non-adherence may be a cause of difficult-to-control asthma, it does not help us in the individual case. It is therefore important to consider the underlying child and family characteristics that lead to non-adherence even in the presence of persisting symptoms and/or impaired quality of life.

Patterns of Non-adherence

Intelligence, education, and the ability to understand information about the nature of asthma bears little relationship to adherence (34). Non-adherence may occur because of misunderstanding or because other life events take priority. Misunderstanding arises if the wrong language is used to describe the treatment or, for example, because it has not been explained that inhaled steroids have no immediate benefit. Highly complicated regimes also cause confusion. Difficult social circumstances or the tasks of adolescence may impose more pressing demands and asthma treatment gets low priority. When prescribed medication twice a day young people often have routines for one of the doses but not the other (35). When symptoms improve regular treatment is easily forgotten. Deliberate rather than accidental omission of treatment may arise from anxiety about side effects. The most commonly described concern among parents of children taking inhaled steroids is the possible adverse effect on growth. A survey of teenage students in Australia revealed that nearly 60% of them believed asthma drugs were addictive (36). Many people feel a powerful disincentive to take any form of regular medication (37). Conrad described three patterns of personal style that result in non-adherence to prescribed treatment regimes. With each pattern of behavior treatment is self-regulated, but for different reasons. The first is testing "do I really need it?"—treatment is stopped to find out. The second is pragmatic practice "stop and start"—start when I feel ill and stop when I feel better. The third is de-stigmatization—taking treatment regularly confirms I have a chronic illness (38).

Groups identified as at risk of non-adherence include the socially disadvantaged, the very young, and adolescents. In the preschool age group where treatment is normally supervised by adult carer-givers, adherence overall is no better than in older children (39).

Oral therapy has a potential advantage in preschool children who may have difficulty with inhalers. It is also less visible to take—an important factor, especially for adolescents. Compliance assessments made after studying medical records and pharmacy claims data suggest that adherence is better than with inhaled medication (40), but this is a comparatively crude assessment of adherence.

III. Poor Control Due to Severe Asthma

A. Clinical Features

The European Respiratory Society Task Force on Difficult/Therapy Resistant Asthma defines poor control in difficult asthma as the need for a bronchodilator more than three times a week, school absence of more than five days a term, or one episode or more of wheezing each month (41). In practice many children with difficult asthma experience far more symptoms than this and may be using a bronchodilator several times a day. A child and their family are severely disrupted by hospital visits, admissions and limitation of normal daily activities. Deaths are rare but many parents live in fear that their child may die. Characteristically, a child with severe asthma will have unremitting symptoms of cough, wheeze, and dyspnea, usually most troublesome at night, and severe impairment of exercise tolerance. Such children show clinical and physiological evidence of airways obstruction and hyperinflation even between asthma attacks. Although this is typical, the pattern may occasionally be one in which the child has periods when they are relatively free of symptoms, with only mild impairment of lung function punctuated by sudden and apparently unexpected severe episodes of asthma resulting in hospital admission. Although not well defined in children, this pattern is sometimes seen in adolescents, particularly girls, and may correspond to what has been described as "brittle asthma" in adults (42). There are also some preschool children who appear to show a similar pattern but in whom the sudden severe attacks are usually associated with viral upper respiratory tract infection. Virtually nothing is known about the pathophysiology of this difficult-to-manage group of very young children. Overall, severe childhood asthma is twice as common in boys as it is in girls and is associated with a personal or family history of atopic illness. Early manifestation of symptoms and abnormal lung function are features of persistent or relapsing symptoms in adolescence (43) and of severe asthma unremitting into adult life (44).

Several recent reports have indicated differences between severe childhood asthma and severe adult asthma. The ENFUMOSA study carried out in 12 European centers found that severe adult asthma is more common in females than males (ratio 4.4:1) and shows a lower prevalence of atopy than mild or moderate adult asthma (45). The female predominance and lower prevalence of atopy in severe adult asthma has been confirmed in another cross-sectional study (46). There are also differences between children and adults with severe asthma in the nature and degree of lung function abnormality. Two cross-sectional studies have examined the relationship between lung function abnormality and age of onset and duration of symptoms. In the first, children classified as having severe asthma on the basis of their requirement for oral or high-dose inhaled corticosteroid showed less airflow limitation and lower airway resistance but larger lung volumes than adults classified as severe by the same criteria. In both the children with asthma and the adults with severe asthma of childhood onset there was a relationship between duration of asthma and lung function impairment. However, the rate of decline in lung function was more rapid in childhood, calculated as being 1.8% of predicted per year, compared with the rate of lung function loss in adulthood, calculated to be 0.4% of predicted per year. In adults with severe asthma that had its onset in adult life there appeared to be no relationship between severity of airflow obstruction and duration of symptoms (47). The second study compared adults with severe asthma whose onset of symptoms had been either before or after the age of 12 years. Lung function was more abnormal in subjects with adult-onset asthma compared with those who had an onset of asthma in childhood, despite a shorter duration of symptoms (48). This observation is compatible with a previous report that had noted rapid decline in lung function in adult-onset asthma soon after diagnosis (49). There are a few non-atopic children who develop difficult asthma and it would be interesting to know whether they show a pattern of lung function decline similar to that seen in adult-onset severe asthma. Children of comparable severity in terms of inhaled and oral steroid requirement show greater steroid responsiveness than adults. The underlying mechanism for this greater sensitivity to the anti-inflammatory effects of steroids is at present unknown (Table 2).

B. Pathology

Relatively little is known about the pathology of severe asthma and less is known in children than in adults. The limited information available strongly suggests that severe asthma is not a single condition but represents a variety of different phenotypes. There are different patterns of inflammation seen in adults with severe asthma, differences between adults with childhood

Table 2 Comparison of Severe Asthma of Childhood and Adult Onset

Characteristic	Childhood onset	Adult onset
Male:female	2:1	1:4
Atopy	+	−
Lung function abnormality related to duration of symptoms	+	−
Airways obstruction	++	+++
Lung hyperinflation	+++	++
Eosinophilic inflammation	+	+
Neutrophilic inflammation	+	+
Lymphocyte/mast cell inflammation	+	−

and adult onset of asthma, and probably several different pathologies in children with difficult asthma. Although the presence of eosinophils is generally associated with severe symptoms and poor lung function (48), a neutrophilic inflammation has been observed in broncho-alveolar lavage (BAL) from adults and older children with severe asthma (50). Non-eosinophilic corticosteroid unresponsive asthma is also described in adults (51), and there may be a distinct phenotype of severe adult asthma that is not associated with airway eosinophilia (52). Early- but not late-onset adult asthma is associated with a lymphocyte and mast cell inflammation (48).

Our knowledge of the pathology of severe asthma in children is derived from post-mortem studies, measurement of inflammatory markers in induced sputum and exhaled breath, BAL, and a few endobronchial biopsies. Information has been obtained from BAL in children with and without asthma undergoing a general anesthetic for reasons unrelated to asthma. Krawiec et al. investigated mainly atopic children under the age of two years with frequent wheezing and compared them with young children of the same age who had never wheezed. They found that the wheezy children had a significantly higher number of inflammatory cells in samples of BAL. The highest cell counts were of lymphocytes and neutrophils rather than eosinophils (53). Because the children were so young this study may give us some insight into the initiation rather than the sustaining of airway inflammation. It may also be directing our attention towards the role of neutrophils. Studies in adults suggest that in some phenotypes of severe asthma there may be a predominantly neutrophilic type of inflammation in the bronchi (54). In young children with asthma there is an association between the presence of eosinophils in BAL and allergic sensitization, but not an association between the presence of neutrophils and persistence of asthma (55).

Exhaled nitric oxide (eNO) is an indirect measure of airway inflammation. In adults with mild or moderate asthma it is usually elevated and falls rapidly in response to steroid treatment. However, in adults with difficult asthma the highest levels are found in those taking oral steroids and perhaps therefore in these patients it is a marker for steroid insensitivity (56). Grouped data suggest the level of eNO is raised in children with difficult asthma and reduced by steroid treatment. However, in some the level remains high after treatment with prednisolone, and in others it is not raised at all. This suggests that some children with difficult asthma have a type of inflammation that is not responsive to corticosteroids and others may not have the airway inflammation normally associated with asthma (57). There is an association between levels of eNO and eosinophils in induced sputum in school-age children with mild or moderate asthma who are not taking inhaled steroids (58,59). In children with difficult asthma a high eNO after two weeks treatment with oral prednisolone is associated with a high eosinophil score in endobronchial biopsies. The relationship was strongest in children who showed a poor therapeutic response to prednisolone. This may indicate that a persistent elevation of eNO after prednisolone is a non-invasive way to identify children with difficult asthma in whom the inflammatory pattern in the airways is predominantly eosinophilic (60). In children with asthma that is difficult to control despite high doses of inhaled steroid, an association has been demonstrated between the presence of current symptoms and high eosinophil and neutrophil counts in bronchial biopsies. In this particular study both symptomatic and relatively asymptomatic children had previously shown some resistance to the effects of prednisolone. Levels of IFNγ in the BAL supernatants obtained from relatively asymptomatic children were higher than in those obtained from symptomatic children. This is an indication that IFNγ and perhaps other Th-1 related cytokines may modulate the local inflammatory response in severe asthma. The authors of this study proposed that eosinophils and a Th-2 cytokine profile could be contributing to symptoms and deterioration in lung function in children with difficult asthma (61).

Although changes in the structure of the airway wall, with epithelial reticular basement membrane (RBM) thickening, is a characteristic finding in adults with asthma (62), little is known about the rate of development of RBM thickening or its relationship to airway inflammation in children. RBM thickening has been described qualitatively in school-age children with moderate asthma (63). When the degree of thickening was assessed quantitatively in children with difficult asthma there appeared to be no relationship with age, duration of symptoms, lung function, or eosinophilic inflammation in the bronchial mucosa. The thickness of RBM in these children was similar to that seen in adults with either mild or life-threatening asthma (64). RBM thickening is also similar in symptomatic and relatively asymptomatic children with difficult asthma (61).

Our understanding of the pathology of severe childhood asthma is still rudimentary. We are hampered by the absence of longitudinal studies, and there are issues to be resolved concerning the ethics of performing longitudinal studies that involve invasive tests. Children with severe and difficult symptoms that are unresponsive to standard asthma treatment show several different types of airway pathology. Whether this represents different conditions or different phases of the same condition remains to be determined. If there are different patterns of inflammation and indeed phenotypes of severe childhood asthma that are associated with minimal airway inflammation, this has important implications for the choice of treatment in individual cases.

IV. Management of Difficult Asthma

A. Assessment and Algorithm

A possible algorithm to guide management of difficult asthma is suggested in Figure 1. Unfortunately, the therapeutic components of this algorithm can only be based on indirect and anecdotal evidence. It is important to obtain as much information as possible because treatment "beyond the guidelines" inevitably involves a fine balance between benefit and adverse effects. Detailed measurement of lung function is essential. Assessment of bronchial responsiveness is valuable but may be very difficult in the child with severe asthma. Some attempt should be made to document by noninvasive methods the presence of airway inflammation before and after steroid treatment. Some centers are now advocating BAL and bronchial biopsy as part of the assessment process, particularly in children who do not show a therapeutic response to a course of high-dose prednisolone. In experienced hands bronchoscopy in children with difficult asthma is safe, yields information that may contribute to therapeutic decision making, and adds to our understanding of the condition (65). It has been suggested by the group at the Royal Brompton Hospital in London that the histology seen on bronchial biopsy could be used to help direct therapy in children with severe asthma. An eosinophilic type of inflammation might point to the use of a combination of a corticosteroid and an immunosuppressive agent; a neutrophil type of inflammation might suggest the addition of a macrolide antibiotic such as azithromycin (66); and minimal inflammation but a bronchodilator response might suggest a trial of subcutaneous terbutaline.

B. Corticosteroids

Prednisolone

Regular oral prednisolone is recommended as the final step in asthma guidelines.

A survey in the United Kingdom of almost 4000 asthmatic children under 16 years of age found only 27 children who were taking regular oral steroids (67). The use of regular prednisolone involves a balance between the benefits and the side effects. Both excessive doses of prednisolone and poorly controlled asthma may suppress growth in childhood. The use

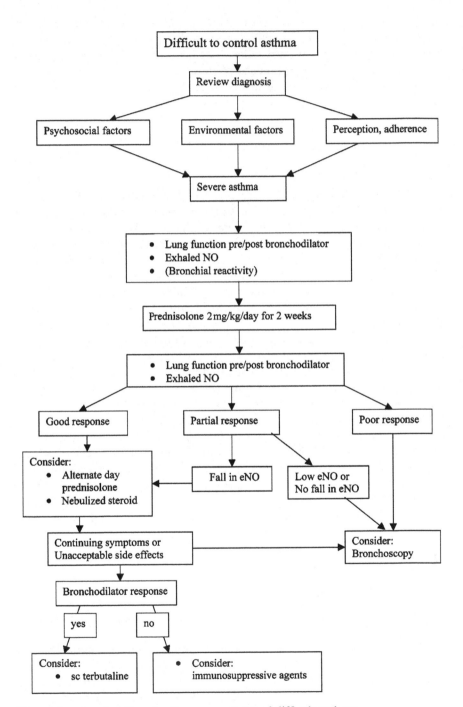

Figure 1 An algorithm for the management of difficult asthma.

of prednisolone to control asthma may therefore actually accelerate rather than retard growth. Oral prednisolone suppresses the hypothalamo-pituitary-adrenal axis, but this may be lessened by taking the dose in the morning and, if possible, on alternate days. The drug should never be stopped suddenly, and additional doses may be required for patients undergoing surgery. In addition, children on regular oral prednisolone should not have live vaccines and are at increased risk of severe chickenpox. Assays of serum prednisolone are available and can help with the assessment of treatment adherence.

Nebulized Corticosteroids

The use of nebulized steroids in very severe childhood asthma is controversial. In a small open study in adults, 55% were able to reduce their oral steroid intake when treated with nebulized budesonide 2 mg/day (68). A small reduction in daily prednisolone was also seen in adults with steroid-dependent asthma when they were given nebulized fluticasone 4 mg/day (69). One randomized, controlled trial has been done in preschool children with oral steroid–dependent asthma. There was a reduction in oral steroid dose and subjective improvement in symptoms in those children treated with nebulized budesonide 2 mg/day (70). However, it is not clear whether high-dose inhaled steroid given by spacer device would have been equally effective. There is little evidence to support the use of high-dose nebulized corticosteroid in older children with steroid-dependent asthma. There may occasionally be a place for nebulized steroid in very young children with severe asthma when inhaled steroid by spacer has failed, but in older children who can use a spacer device efficiently it seems unlikely that switching to a nebulized steroid will confer additional benefit.

C. "Add On" Compounds

These include long-acting beta-agonists, leukotriene receptor antagonists, and theophyllines. All these compounds have some beneficial effect on symptoms and lung function in school-age children with asthma that is not controlled by low doses of inhaled steroid (step 3). There is less convincing evidence that they are of benefit or reduce the requirement for oral steroids in children with severe asthma, and it is likely that they will already have been tried at an earlier stage in the child's management. If this is not the case then the child could have a therapeutic trial over about six weeks with careful monitoring of symptoms and lung function (71).

D. Subcutaneous Terbutaline

Continuous subcutaneous terbutaline and salbutamol have been shown to be useful in adults with severe chronic or brittle asthma (72,73). This form of treatment has been reported in acute severe infantile asthma (74). There are no controlled trials of the long-term use of subcutaneous short-acting beta-agonists in children with severe asthma. However, a retrospective review has been published of eight children aged 8–14 years with severe symptoms despite regular predisolone, who were treated with subcutaneous terbutaline for at least two months. Five of the children experienced an improvement in symptoms and reduction in the dose of prednisolone. In three children there was no benefit. All the children had some side effects from the treatment that included tremor, agitation, tachycardia, and discomfort at the injection site (75). The intravenous preparation (0.5 mg/mL) is administered by a pump, (Graseby Medical Ltd., Watford, UK; MiniMed Inc., Sylmar, California, USA), at a starting dose of 2.5–5 mg/day. In addition to tremor, hyperactivity, tachycardia, palpitations, headache, and muscle cramps, hypokalemia is a theoretical possibility. Local problems include tender subcutaneous nodules and hematomas at the site of injection. It is advisable to start this treatment in the hospital for safety reasons, and to allow adequate time for educating the child and family. It is often useful to start with saline for 48–72 hours and perform an $n = 1$ single blind therapeutic trial; this ensures that any symptom improvement is not simply a placebo effect.

E. Immunosuppressive Agents

Cyclosporin

Cyclosporin is an immunosuppressive agent used after organ transplantation that works by inhibiting T lymphocyte activation. Small trials in adults with severe asthma, in which oral cyclosporin has been given for 12 weeks (76) and 36 weeks (77), have shown improvement in lung function, reduction in exacerbations, and reduced prednisolone use compared to placebo. No controlled trials have been carried out on children. However, there is a case report of its use in five children on regular oral steroids, three of whom experienced a definite benefit (78). The adverse effects in adults include hirsutism, paraesthesia, mild hypertension, headaches, and tremor. Of these side effects the only one so far reported in children is hirsutism, but this led to one girl stopping its use even though her steroid dose had been greatly reduced (78). There is concern about renal impairment with long-term use of cyclosporin, so renal function must be carefully monitored, and blood concentrations maintained at 80–150 mg/L. A randomized, controlled trial in children is needed as this drug has considerable potential in very severe asthma. Nebulized cyclosporin, which has been used in some adults after heart-lung transplant, unfortunately causes marked bronchospasm and has no place in the treatment of asthma.

Methotrexate

This compound has both immunosuppressive and anti-inflammatory properties. It has been shown to reduce steroid use in adults with asthma. Two meta-analyses (79,80) concluded that methotrexate allowed a modest reduction in daily prednisone dosage (4.3 and 3.3 mg) compared to placebo. Three small open-label studies have shown that steroid doses could be reduced in some children while lung function was maintained or improved (81–83). The doses of methotrexate used were between 7.5 and 17 mg/week for up to two years (81,82), and 0.6 mg/kg/week for three months (83). Side effects in the children were gastrointestinal upset and transiently raised liver enzymes. There are many potentially serious adverse effects associated with the drug (pulmonary fibrosis, pneumonitis, hepatic cirrhosis, and myelosuppression), particularly when given in high doses. However, low doses seem to be relatively safe, and its use may be considered in carefully selected children.

F. Intravenous Immunoglobulin

Three small open-label studies have found that infusions of intravenous immunoglobulin (IVIG) led to a reduction in oral steroid use in children aged over six years (84–86). Two proposed mechanisms of action are in vitro inhibition of IgE production from human B cells and, acting synergistically with corticosteroid, suppression of lymphocyte proliferation (86,87). There have also been reports of improvement in glucocorticoid receptor binding affinity in peripheral blood mononuclear cells and a reduction in numbers of all cell types (especially CD3+, CD4+, and activated CD25+ T lymphocytes) in bronchial biopsy (86,88). The results of randomized, placebo-controlled trials are conflicting. One study of 31 children and adolescents given 4 g/kg over eight weeks showed no improvement in lung function, bronchial hyper-reactivity, or symptom scores (89). A more recent trial involving 28 children and adults, given 2 g/kg at the start of treatment followed by 400 mg/kg every three weeks for nine months, demonstrated a significant steroid-sparing effect in a subgroup of patients taking more than 5.5 mg/day of prednisolone (90). Another trial demonstrated no difference between two different doses of immunoglobulin (2 and 1 g/kg) and placebo given monthly for seven months. This last study reported three cases of aseptic meningitis in the high-dose treatment group (91). Other reported side effects of intravenous immunoglobulin include rash and hypertension. As it is a blood product, there is also the theoretical risk of transmission of viral infections. Although the open studies offer some encouragement, the controlled trials have failed to provide conclusive evidence to support the use of intravenous immunoglobulin in severe childhood asthma.

G. Future Therapies

Several other compounds have been shown to have steroid-sparing effects in adults with asthma, but trials have not been done in children. These include parenteral gold salts, the macrolide antibiotic troleandomycin, dapsone, and hydroxychloroquine. As the mechanisms involved in the initiation and progression of asthma become clearer, new therapies are being developed. These include antibodies directed against specific components of the inflammatory cascade, such as T cells, IgE, interleukin-5, and adhesion molecules. A recent trial of monoclonal anti-IgE antibody demonstrated a steroid-sparing effect in a subgroup of patients taking regular oral prednisolone (92). There is also renewed interest in the anti-inflammatory effects of theophylline (93,94). Selective phosphodiesterase inhibitors targeting the isoenzymes III and IV have been developed, which should maximize these anti-inflammatory effects with potentially fewer side effects than theophylline. New corticosteroids are in preparation that are designed to have greater anti-inflammatory potency and fewer unwanted systemic effects.

V. Conclusions

If a child or adolescent has wheezing illness that does not respond to asthma treatment it is important to review the diagnosis, seek out unrecognized provoking factors, and improve adherence. Very early onset of symptoms, stridor, feeding difficulties, and failure to thrive are some of the features that will cast doubt on the diagnosis. Environmental allergens and air pollution are causes of poor asthma control. There is a need for good collaborative studies of the impact of psychosocial factors on asthma. Many patients wish to have some control over the medication they or their children are prescribed. Adherence to asthma treatment can be improved by using simple, clearly explained, written management plans. Adolescents with difficult or severe asthma present a special challenge and we are unlikely to make progress unless we recognize the impact of their asthma on their psychosocial development.

For the small number of children with very severe asthma, a greater understanding of the pathological basis of persistent symptoms is needed. It is becoming increasingly clear that very severe childhood asthma comprises more than one phenotype. The way to define the different phenotypes is by combining careful documentation of symptoms and measurement of lung function with examination of material obtained by bronchoscopic BAL and endobronchial biopsy. This will lead to more rational prescribing in difficult-to-control asthma and inform the design of trials with new therapeutic agents.

References

1. Pedersen S, Hansen OR. Budesonide treatment of moderate and severe asthma in children: a dose response study. J Allergy Clin Immunol 1995; 95:29–33.
2. Sanders LA, Rijkers GT, Kuis W, Tenbergen-meeks AJ, de Graeff-Meeder BR, Hiemstra I, Zegers BJ. Defective anti-pneumococcal polysaccharide antibody response in children with recurrent respiratory tract infections. J Allergy Clin Immunol 1993; 91:110–119.

3. Kelly YJ, Brabin BJ, Milligan PJM, Reif JA, Heaf D, Pearson MG. The clinical significance of cough in the diagnosis of asthma in the community. Arch Dis Child 1996; 75:489–493.

4. Ninan TK, MacDonald L, Russell G. Persistent nocturnal cough in childhood: a population base study. Arch Dis Child 1995; 73:403–407.

5. De Benedictus FM, Canny GJ, Levison H. Methacholine inhalational challenge in the evaluation of chronic cough in children. J Asthma 1986; 23:303–308.

6. Ekstrom T, Tibbling L. Gastro-oesophageal reflux and triggering of bronchial asthma: a negative report. Eur J Respir Dis 1987; 71:177–180.

7. Wilson NM, Charette L, Thomson AH, Silverman M. Gastro-oesophageal reflux and childhood asthma: the acid test. Thorax 1985; 40:592–597.

8. Hampton FJ, MacFayden UM, Beardsmore CS, Simpson H. Gastro-oesophageal reflux and respiratory function in infants with respiratory symptoms. Arch Dis Child 1991; 66:848–853.

9. Mc Fadden ER Jr, Zawadski DK. Vocal cord dysfunction masquerading as exercise-induced asthma. Am J Resp Crit Care Med 1996; 153:942–947.

10. Newman KB, Mason UG, Schmaling KB. Clinical features of vocal cord dysfunction. Am J Resp Crit Care Med 1995; 152:1382–1386.

11. Powell DM, Karanfilov BI, Beechler KB, Yreole K, Trudeau MD, Forrest LA. Paradoxical vocal cord dysfunction in juveniles. Arch Otolaryngol 2000; 126:29–34.

12. Bahrainwala AH, Simon MR. Wheezing and vocal cord dysfunction mimicking asthma. Curr Opin Pulm Med 2001; 7:8–13.

13. Sulakvelidze I, Inman MD, Rerecich T, O'Byrne PM. Increases in airway eosino-phils and interleukin-5 with minimal bronchoconstriction during repeated low dose allergen challenge in atopic asthmatics. Eur Respir J 1998; 11:821–827.

14. Nimmagadda SR, Szefler SJ, Spahn JD, Surs W, Leung DY. Allergen exposure decreases glucocorticoid receptor binding affinity and steroid responsiveness in atopic asthmatics. Am J Respir Crit Care Med 1997; 155:87–93.

15. Van de Brempt X, Charpin D, Haddi E, da Mata P, Vervoe D. Cat removal and Fel d1 levels in mattresses. J Allergy Clin Immunol 1991; 87:595–596.

16. Berciano FA, Dominguez J, Alvarez FV. Influence of air pollution on extrinsic asthma in childhood. Ann Allergy 1989; 5:201–207.

17. Cook DG, Whincup PH, Papacosta O, Strachan DP, Jarvis MJ, Bryant A. Relation of passive smoking as assessed by salivary cotinine concentration and questionnaire to spirometric indices in children. Thorax 1993; 48:14–20.

18. Strachan DP. Parental smoking and childhood asthma: longitudinal and case control studies. Thorax 1998; 53:204–212.

19. Chaudhuri R, Livingstone E, McMahon AD, Thomson L, Borland W, Thomson NC. Cigarette smoking impairs the therapeutic response to oral corticosteroids in chronic asthma. Am J Respir Crit Care Med 2003; 168:1308–1311.

20. Chamers GW, MacLeod KJ, Little SA, Thomson LJ, McSharry CP, Thomson NC. Influence of cigarette smoking on inhaled corticosteroid treatment in mild asthma. Thorax 2002; 57:226–230.

21. Irvine L, Crombie IK, Clark RA, Slane PW, Feyerbend C, Goodman KE, Cater JI. Advising parents of asthmatic children on passive smoking: rando-mised controlled trial. BMJ 1999; 318:1456–1459.

22. Fish L, Wilson SR, Latini DM, Starr NJ. An education program for parents of children with asthma: differences in attendance between smoking and non-smoking parents. Am J Public Health 1996; 86:246–248.

23. Gutstadt LB, Gillette JW, Mrazek DA, Fukuhara JT, LaBrecque JF, Strunk RC. Determinants of school performance in children with chronic asthma. Am J Dis Child 1989; 143:471–475.

24. Fritz GK, Overholser JC. Patterns of response to childhood asthma. Psychosom Med 1989; 51:347–355.

25. Kaptein AA. Psychological correlates of length of hospitalisation and re-hospitalisation in patients with severe acute asthma. Soc Sci Med 1982; 16: 725–729.

26. Wright RJ, Rodriguez M, Cohen S. Review of psychosocial stress and asthma: an integrated biopsychosocial approach. Thorax 1998; 53:1066–1074.

27. Wright RJ, Steinbach SF. Violence: an unrecognized environmental exposure that may contribute to greater asthma morbidity in a high risk inner city population. Environmental Health Perspectives 2001; 109:1085–1089.

28. Christiaanse ME, Labigne JV, Lerner CV. Psychosocial aspects of compliance in children and adolescents with asthma. J Dev Behav Pediatr 1989; 10: 75–80.

29. Strachan DP, Anderson HR, Limb ES, O'Neill A, Wells N. A national survey of asthma prevalence, severity and treatment in Great Britian. Arch Dis Child 1994; 70:174–178.

30. Ley P. Communicating with patients: improving communication, satisfaction and compliance. New York: Chapman & Hall 1988:53–71.

31. Bender B, Wamboldt FS, O'Connor SL, Rand C, Szefler S, Milgrom H, Wamboldt MZ. Measurement of children's asthma medication adherence by self report, mother report, canister weight and doser CT. Ann Allergy Asthma Immunol 2000; 85:416–421.

32. Milgrom H, Bender B, AckersonL, Bowry P, Smith B, Rand C. Non-compliance and treatment failure in children with asthma. J Allergy Clin Immunol 1996; 98: 1051–1057.

33. Jonasson G, Carlsen K-H, Sodal A, Jonasson C, Mowinckel P. Patient compliance in a clinical trial with inhaled budesonide in children with mild asthma. Eur Respir J 1999; 14:150–154.

34. Rand CS, Wise RA. Measuring adherence to asthma medication regimes. Am J Respir Crit Care Med 1994; 149:869–876.

35. Swyer SM, Dakin V. Adherence in adolescents with asthma: comparison of self report with parental report and objective measurement (abstr). Respirology 2000; 5:25.

36. Gibson PG, Henry RL, Vimpani GV, Halliday J. Asthma knowledge, attitudes and quality of life in adolescents. Arch Dis Child 1995; 73:321–326.

37. Osman LM, Russell IT, Friend JA, Legge JS, Douglas JG. Predicting patient attitudes to asthma medication. Thorax 1993; 48:827–830.

38. Conrad P. The meaning of medications: another look at compliance. Soc Sci Med 1985; 20:29–37.

39. Gibson NA, Ferguson AE, Aitchison TC, Paton JY. Compliance with inhaled asthma medication in preschool children. Thorax 1995; 50:1274–1279.

40. Kelloway JS, Wyatt RA, Adlis SA. Comparison of patient's compliance with prescribed oral and inhaled asthma medications. Arch Intern Med 1994; 154:1349–1352.
41. Chung KF, Godard P, Adelroth E, Ayres J, Barnes N, Bel E, Chanez P, Connett G, Corrigan C, de Blic J, Fabbri L, Holgate ST, Ind P, Joos G, Kerstjens H, Leuenberger P, Lofdhal CG, MsKensie S, Magnussen H, Postma D, Saetta M, Salmeron S, Sterk P. Difficult/Therapy resistant asthma: the need for an integrated approach to define clinical phenotypes, evaluate risk factors, understand pathophysiology and find novel therapies. ERS Task Force on Difficult/Therapy Resistant asthma. Eur Respir J 1999; 13:1198–1208.
42. Ayres JG, Miles JF, Barnes PJ. Brittle asthma. Thorax 1998; 53:315–321.
43. Sears MR, Greene JM, Willan AR, Wiecek EM, Taylor DR, Flannery EM, Cowan JO, Herbison GP, Silva PA, Poulton R. A longitudinal, population-based, cohort study of childhood asthma followed to adulthood. New Eng J Med 2003; 349:1414–1422.
44. Oswald H, Phelan PD, Lanigan A, Hibbert M, Carlin JB, Bowes G, Olinski A. Childhood asthma and lung function in mid adult life. Pediatr Pulmonol 1997; 23:14–20.
45. The ENFUMOSA cross-sectional European multicentre study of the clinical phenotype of chronic severe asthma. Eur Respir J 2003; 22:470–477.
46. ten Brinke A, Zwinderman AH, Sterk PJ, Rabe KF, Bel EH. Factors associated with persistent airflow limitation in severe asthma. Am J Respir Crit Care Med 2002; 164:744–748.
47. Jenkins HA, Cherniak R, Szefler SJ, Covar R, Gefland EW, Spahn JD. A comparison of the clinical characteristics of children and adults with severe asthma. Chest 2003; 124:1318–1324.
48. Miranda C, Busacker A, Balzar S, Trudeau J, Wenzel S. Distinguishing severe asthma phenotypes: role of age of onset and eosinophilic inflammation. J Allergy Clin Immunol 2004; 113:101–108.
49. Burrows B, Lebowitz MD, Barbee RA, Cline MG. Findings before diagnosis of asthma among the elderly in a longitudinal study of a general population sample. J Allergy Clin Immunol 1991; 88:870–877.
50. Wenzel SE, Szefler SJ, Leung DYM, Sloan SI, Rex MD, Martin RJ. Bronchoscopic evaluation of severe asthma. Persistent inflammation associated with high dose glucocorticoids. Am J Respir Crit Care Med 1997; 156:737–743.
51. Pavord ID, Brightling G, Woltman G, Wardlaw AJ. Non-eosinophilic corticosteroid unresponsive asthma. Lancet 1999; 353:2213–2214.
52. Wenzel SE, Schwartz LB, Langmack EL, Halliday JL, Trudeau JB, Gibbs RL, Chu HW. Evidence that severe asthma can be divided pathologically into two inflammatory subtypes with distinct physiologic and clinical characteristics. Am J Respir Crit Care Med 1999; 160:1001–1008.
53. Krawiec ME, Wescott JY, Chu HW, Balzar S, Trudeau JB, Schwartz LB, Wenzel SE. Persistent wheezing in very young children is associated with lower respiratory inflammation. Am L Respir Crit Care Med 2001; 163:1338–1343.
54. Jatakanon A, Uasuf C, Maziak W, Lim S, Chung KF, Barnes PJ. Neutrophilic inflammation in severe persistent asthma. Am J Respir Crit Care Med 1999; 160:1532–1539.

55. Just J, Fournier L, Momas I, Zambetti C, Sahraoui F, Grimfeld A. Clinical significance of bronchoalveolar eosinophils in childhood asthma. J Allergy Clin Immunol 2002; 110:42–44.

56. Stirling RG, Kharitonov SA, Campbell D, Robinson DS, Durham SR, Chung KF, Barnes PJ. Increase in exhaled nitric oxide levels in patients with difficult asthma and correlation with symptoms and disease severity despite treatment with oral and inhaled corticosteroids. Thorax 1998; 53:1030–1034.

57. Payne DNR, Wilson NM, James A, Hablas H, Agrafioti C, Bush A. Evidence for different subgroups of difficult asthma in children. Thorax 2001; 56:345–350.

58. Piacentini GL, Bodini A, Costella S, Vicentini L, Mazzi P, Sperandio S, Boner AL. Exhaled nitric oxide and sputum eosinophil markers of inflammation in asthmatic children. Eur Respir J 1999; 13:1386–1390.

59. Mattes J, Storm van's Gravesande K, Reining U, Alving K, Ihorst G, Henschen M, Kuehr J. Nitric oxide in exhaled air is correlated with markers of eosinophilic airway inflammation in corticosteroid-dependent childhood asthma. Eur Respir J 1999; 13:1391–1395.

60. Payne DNR, Adcock IM, Wilson NM, Oates T, Scallon M, Bush A. Relationship between exhaled nitric oxide and mucosal eosinophilic inflammation in children with difficult asthma, after treatment with oral prednisolone. Am J Respir Crit Care Med 2001; 164:1376–1381.

61. de Blic J, Tillie-Leblond I, Bernard Tonnel A, Jaubert F, Scheinmann P, Gosset P. Difficult asthma in children: an analysis of airway inflammation. J Allergy Clin Immunol 2004; 113:94–100.

62. Bousquet J, Jeffery PK, Busse WW, Johnson M, Vignola AM. Asthma: from bronchoconstriction to airways inflammation and remodelling. Am J Respir Crit care Med 2000; 161:1720–1745.

63. Cokugras H, Akcakaya N, Seckin, Camcioglu Y, Sarimurat N, Aksoy F. Ultrastructural examination of bronchial biopsy specimens from children with moderate asthma. Thorax 2001; 56:25–29.

64. Payne DNR, Rogers AV, Adelroth E, Bandi V, Guntupalli KK, Bush A, Jeffery PK. Early thickening of the reticular basement membrane in children with difficult asthma. Am J Respir Crit Care Med 2003; 167:78–82.

65. Payne DNR, McKenzie SA, Stacey S, Misra D, Haxby E, Bush A. Safety and ethics of bronchoscopy and endobronchial biopsy in difficult asthma. Arch Dis Child 2001; 84:422–425.

66. Jaffe A, Bush A. Anti-inflammatory effects of macrolides in lung disease. Pediatr Pulmonol 2001; 31:464–473.

67. Hoskins G, McCowan C, Neville RG, Thomas GE, Smith B, Silverman S. Risk factors and costs associated with an asthma attack. Thorax 2000; 55:19–24.

68. Higenbottam TW, Clark RA, Luksza AR. The role of nebulised budesonide in permitting a reduction in the dose of oral steroid in persistent severe asthma. Eur J Clin Res 1994; 5:1–10.

69. Westbroek J, Saarelainen S, Laher M, O'Brien J, Barnacle H, Efthimiou J. Oral steroid-sparing effect of two doses of nebulised fluticasone propionate and placebo in patients with severe chronic asthma. Respir Med 1999; 93:689–699.

70. Llangovan P, Pedersen S, Godfrey S, Nikander K, Noviski N, Warner JO. Treatment of severe steroid dependent preschool asthma with nebulised budesonide suspension. Arch Dis Child 1993; 68:356–359.
71. British Guideline on the Management of Asthma. Thorax 2003; 58(suppl 1): I20–I23.
72. O'Driscoll BRC, Ruffles SP, Ayres JG, Cochrane GM. Long term treatment of severe asthma with subcutaneous terbutaline. Br J Dis Chest 1988; 82:360–367.
73. Cluzel M, Bousquet J, Daures JP, Renon D, Clauzel AM, Godard PH, Michel FB. Ambulatory long-term subcutaneous salbutamol infusion in chronic severe asthma. J Allergy Clin Immunol 1990; 85:599–605.
74. Brémont F, Moisan V, Dutau G. Continuous subcutaneous infusion of beta2-agonists in infantile asthma. Pediatr Pulmonol 1992; 12:81–83.
75. Payne DNR, Balfour-Lynn IM, Biggart EA, Bush A. Subcutaneous terbutaline in children with chronic severe asthma. Pediatr Pulmonol 2002; 33:356–361.
76. Alexander AG, Barnes NC, Kay AB. Trial of cyclosporin in corticosteroid-dependent chronic severe asthma. Lancet 1992; 339:324–328.
77. Lock SH, Kay AB, Barnes NC. Double blind placebo controlled study of cyclosporin A as a corticosteroid-sparing agent in corticosteroid-dependent asthma. Am J Resp Crit Care Med 1996; 153:509–514.
78. Coren ME, Rosenthal M, Bush A. The use of cyclosporin in corticosteroid dependent asthma. Arch Dis Child 1997; 77:522–523.
79. Marin MG. Low-dose methotrexate spares steroid usage in steroid-dependent asthmatic patients: a meta-analysis. Chest 1997; 112:29–33.
80. Aaron SD, Dales RE, Pham B. Management of steroid-dependent asthma with methotrexate: a meta-analysis of randomised clinical trials. Respir Med 1998; 92:1059–1065.
81. Stempel DA, Lammert J, Mullarkey MF. Use of methotrexate in the treatment of steroid-dependent adolescent asthmatics. Ann Allergy 1991; 67:346–348.
82. Guss S, Portnoy J. Methotrexate treatment of severe asthma in children. Pediatrics 1992; 89:635–639.
83. Sole D, Costa-Carvalho BT, Soares FJ, Rullo VV, Naspitz CK. Methotrexate in the treatment of corticodependent asthmatic children. J Invest Allergol Clin Immunol 1996; 6:126–130.
84. Mazer BD, Gelfand EW. An open-label study of high-dose intravenous immunoglobulin in severe childhood asthma. J Allergy Clin Immunol 1991; 87:976–983.
85. Jakobsson T, Croner S, Kjellman NI, Pettersson A, Vassella C, Bjorksten B. Slight steroid-sparing effect of intravenous immunoglobulin in children and adolescents with moderately severe bronchial asthma. Allergy 1994; 49:413–420.
86. Spahn JD, Leung DY, Chan MT, Szrfler SJ, Gelfand EW. Mechanisms of glucocorticoid reduction in asthmatic subjects treated with intravenous immunoglobulin. J Allergy Clin Immunol 1999; 103:421–426.
87. Sigman K, Ghibu F, Sommerville W, Toledano BJ, Bastein Y, Cameron L, Hamid QA, Mazer B. Intravenous immunoglobulin inhibits IgE production in human B lymphocytes. J Allergy Clin Immunol 1998; 102(3):421–427.
88. Vrugt B, Wilson S, van Velzen E, Bron A, Shute JK, Holgate ST, Djukanovic R, Aalbers R. Effects of high dose intravenous immunoglobulin in two severe corticosteroid insensitive asthmatic children. Thorax 1997; 52:662–664.

89. Niggemann B, Leupold W, Schuster A, Schuster R, v Berg A, Grubl A, v d Hardt H, Eibl MM, Wahn U. Prospective, double-blind, placebo-controlled, multicentre study on the effect of high-dose, intravenous immuno-globulin in children and adolescents with severe bronchial asthma. Clin Exp Allergy 1998; 28:205–210.

90. Salmun LM, Barlau I, Wolf HM, Eibl M, Twarog FJ, Geha RS, Scheider LC. Effect of intravenous immunoglobulin on steroid consumption in patients with severe asthma: a double-blind, placebo-controlled, randomised trial. J Allergy Clin Immunol 1999; 103:810–815.

91. Kishimaya JL, Valacer D, Cunningham-Rundles C, Sperber K, Richmond GW, Abramson S, Glovsky AI, Stiehm R, Stocks J, Rosenberg I, Shames RS, Corn B, Shearer WT, Bacot B, DiMaio M, Tonetta S, Adelman DC. A multicenter, ran-domised, double-blind, placebo-controlled trial of intravenous immunoglobulin for oral corticosteroid-dependent asthma. Clin Immunol 1999; 91(2):126–133.

92. Milgrom H, Fick RB, Su JQ, Reimann JD, Bush RK, Watrous ML, Metzger WJ. Treatment of allergic asthma with monoclonal anti-IgE antibody. N Engl J Med 1999; 341:1966–1973.

93. Hatzelmann A, Tenor H, Schudt C. Differential effects of non-selective and selective phosphodiesterase inhibitors on human eosinophil functions. Br J Pharmacol 1995; 114:821–831.

94. Sullivan P, Bekir S, Jaffar Z, Page C, Jeffrey P, Costello J. Anti-inflammatory effects of low-dose oral theophylline in atopic asthma. Lancet 1994; 343: 1006–1008.

26

Childhood Asthma Management in the Next 10 Years

STANLEY J. SZEFLER

Department of Pediatrics and Pharmacology
  Divisions of Clinical Pharmacology and
Allergy and Immunology,
Helen Wohlberg and Herman
Lambert Chair in Pharmacokinetics,
National Jewish Medical and
Research Center, University of Colorado
Health Sciences Center,
Denver, Colorado, U.S.A.

SØREN PEDERSEN

Department of Pediatrics,
  University of Southern Denmark,
Kolding Hospital
Kolding, Denmark

I. Introduction

We can feel some comfort that recent statistics indicate that the concerted effort to halt the trend of increasing asthma mortality and morbidity has been successful (1). However, as indicated in our opening chapter by Dr. David Stempel, there is still considerable room for improvement. An effort must now be made to achieve a decline in morbidity and mortality. This may be possible by developing a system to recognize patients at risk for persistent asthma and to intervene early, as indicated in Dr. Søren Pedersen's chapter on early intervention. This summary will highlight the

This chapter supported in part by Public Health Services Research Grants 1NO1-HR-16048, HL36577, HL51834, General Clinical Research Center Grant 5 MO1 RR00051 from the Division of Research Resources, and the NICHHD Pediatric Pharmacology Research Unit Network Grant 1-U01-HD37237.

673

current status of asthma management and also indicate where advances are possible if new principles identified in this book are applied judiciously.

New knowledge regarding the origins of asthma was comprehensively summarized in chapters by Prescott and Holt and Warner et al. As a consequence of this change in direction regarding asthma pathogenesis and the chronic inflammatory nature of the disease, inhaled glucocorticoids, the most potent anti-inflammatory asthma medication, are recognized as the cornerstone for the management of persistent asthma for all age groups. As summarized by Hamid and Minshall, we have witnessed extraordinary gains in understanding the pathogenesis of asthma through the application of bronchoscopy, bronchoalveolar lavage and biopsy (2). This effort, combined with advances in molecular biology and identification of key inflammatory mediators, has resulted in the introduction of new medications, new delivery systems, and also new initiatives to improve medication labeling for young children. Consequently, new opportunities have emerged to improve the overall management of childhood asthma through early intervention with dosing strategies that ensure the safe use of available medications. As indicated in the chapter by Spahn and Covar, there are significant differences between asthma in children and adults and much of this is probably related to the duration of the disease and its consequent effect on airway structure.

New directions in the management of childhood asthma now include early recognition, early intervention, more effective environmental control, and new principles in applying long-term control therapy. The high interest in the natural history of childhood asthma should lead to even better methods to diagnose asthma and a continuing assessment of the efficacy of early intervention in altering the natural history of asthma. The use of inhaled glucocorticoid therapy has appeared to play a major role in stabilizing the rise in asthma morbidity and mortality, but questions still remain about whether it is effective in preventing progression of asthma and thus altering the natural history of asthma (3). Although the current information around the safety of inhaled glucocorticoids is reassuring, there is still a hesitancy to intervene early with inhaled glucocorticoids and to maintain continuous treatment with high doses. Dr. Allen indicated in his chapter that the benefit-to-risk ratio remains high for inhaled glucocorticoid therapy as long as we focus on the use of low to medium doses and limit the duration of treatment with high-dose, high-potency inhaled glucocorticoids.

We will begin with a brief summary of the recommended principles of asthma management. This will be followed by a discussion of methods that could strengthen current areas of weakness. To achieve a "cure" for asthma, or at least to be able to induce remission, we must be able to take a more proactive approach and recognize the disease early and intervene appropriately.

II. Evolving Changes in Asthma Management

Approximately 50 years ago, the treatment of asthma was directed toward the relief of bronchospasm, with an emphasis on bronchodilator therapy. Theophylline, primarily a bronchodilator with some recently recognized anti-inflammatory effects, was the preferred maintenance therapy for asthma during the 1970s and for almost 15 years. The 1980s marked the shift to preventative therapy, initially with cromolyn and subsequently inhaled glucocorticoids. One feature of inhaled cromolyn viewed as advantageous is the ability to block the early and late pulmonary response to an allergen challenge in a sensitized patient as well as the resultant airways hyperresponsiveness that often follows an allergen challenge in a sensitized patient. However, several studies have now found that the efficacy of cromolyn and the next generation mast cell inhibitor medication, nedocromil, is rather limited.

Principles of inhaled glucocorticoid therapy dosing emerged with their recognized efficacy in the management of asthma for both adults and children (4). Over the last 10 years, several new classes of medications have been approved for use in the treatment of asthma. The long-acting β2-adrenergic agonists, salmeterol and formoterol, with a 12-hour duration of action were introduced as long-term control therapies and the stereoisomer of albuterol, levalbuterol, was introduced to limit the adverse effects of short-acting β-agonists for acute asthma episodes. Another new class of medications are the leukotriene modifiers. Although a few have been lost in the short time span of five years, the oral leukotriene receptor antagonist, montelukast, has become a popular first-line long-term control therapy, especially for children in some countries, because some perceive oral administration as more convenient.

Renewed interest has developed for combination therapy, such as the combination of an inhaled steroid and a long-acting β-adrenergic agonist in one delivery device and combined treatment with inhaled corticosteroids and oral leukotriene modifiers. The success of the inhaled steroid and a long-acting β-adrenergic agonist in one delivery device is based on evidence of additive effects, convenience for the patient, and the potential to further reduce the risk for significant exacerbations (5). Each new medication results in the reorganization of treatment guidelines for the management of asthma. Introduction of new medications always engenders considerable debate and this discussion was summarized by Dr. Alan Becker.

III. Childhood Asthma—Current Management Approach

Our current management approach for asthma emphasizes environmental control, objective monitoring, cooperative management, and pharmacotherapy. Asthma is currently classified as intermittent, mild persistent, moderate persistent, and severe persistent based on the number of symptoms and nighttime episodes, along with measures of pulmonary function (6–8). The GINA guidelines also attempted to factor the level of treatment along with measures of asthma control to determine the severity level of asthma (6).

The recently revised NAEPP guidelines attempted to address the needs of childhood asthma with evidence-based reviews (8). The available evidence for various steps in asthma management for children less than five years of age is very limited. Therefore, many recommendations regarding the management of young children are based on studies conducted in older children and adults. To fill some of the gaps in information, investigators and the pharmaceutical industry are conducting additional studies and developing new medications.

The revised NAEPP guidelines recommend inhaled glucocorticoids as the preferred first-line treatment in adults and children of all ages (8). For inadequate control, the preferred additive therapy to low to medium dose inhaled glucocorticoid is a long-acting β-adrenergic agonist. However, the documentation for efficacy in children is less than for adults, and there are no head-to-head comparisons with add-on therapy in children. Leukotriene antagonists are also alternative additive therapy once inhaled glucocorticoids are started. Five major areas of need for additional research include defining the benefits of early intervention with long-term control therapy, new approaches for the management of severe persistent asthma, the best alternative to inhaled corticosteroids in patients who are not given this treatment as first-line therapy, the best add-on treatment to inhaled corticosteroids in children, and studies assessing various treatment modalities in children with intermittent asthma as defined in the guidelines. Recent additions to the therapeutic armamentarium include anti-IgE, but it is currently only approved for use in children 12 years of age and older and only in a few countries.

IV. Asthma in Young Children—New Opportunities to Make Significant Strides in Asthma Management

As previously discussed, the current approach to asthma management focuses on chronic inflammation as a major feature of asthma. Since the time of onset of inflammation is unknown but must begin early in life, attention is now directed toward identifying better methods to recognize the disease early and to develop new approaches to early intervention. It is assumed that early intervention with anti-inflammatory therapy could potentially modify the disease process and the natural history of asthma but this has not been verified in a prospective study (8,9). Therefore, well designed, randomized, controlled studies are needed to determine whether early intervention can alter long-term outcomes as it seems to be able to in animal models (10).

Although the core approach to asthma management in young children is similar to the approach developed for older children and adults, there are special challenges posed in managing asthma in young children. The assessment of asthma control in young children is primarily based on symptoms as reported by a caretaker and thus subject to interpretation. As indicated in the chapter by Morgan et al., pulmonary function cannot be measured reliably in young children; however, new techniques are being developed to help gauge this important feature of the disease. If allergen sensitivity is defined and exposure confirmed, environmental control measures can be applied. Also, as indicated in the chapter by Gern et al., limiting exposure to viral respiratory infections could potentially reduce the frequency of significant acute exacerbations; however, this is very difficult to achieve in the high exposure areas such as day care settings and schools, as well as carrier exposure from other family members and siblings, especially with household crowding. Choosing appropriate medications for management can also be a challenge. The route of administration for inhaled medication administration must be adjusted to facilitate patient cooperation as summarized by Dr. Myrna Dolovich in this book. Until recently, another problem has been the limited information on the appropriate dose of medications for children less than five years of age.

A nebulized budesonide preparation has been recently approved in the United States for use in children as young as one year of age with dosage guidelines for this age group. This medication and delivery device have been available for quite a while in many other countries and the benefits have been well recognized. First-line therapy may begin with low-dose inhaled glucocorticoid via nebulizer or a spacer/holding chamber and face mask (8). An alternative to inhaled glucocorticoids is montelukast, an oral leukotriene receptor antagonist that is now available in a formulation that can be administered in children as young as one year of age. Of note, current global guidelines and recent revisions to the U.S. guidelines recommend an inhaled glucocorticoid by face mask or nebulized administration as first-line therapy in young children (8). Outside of the United States, studies have been conducted to show that inhaled glucocorticoids delivered with a metered dose inhaler and large-volume spacer can provide effective therapy in young children (11). Comparative studies are now needed to determine whether the inhaled glucocorticoid by spacer/face mask and nebulized administration do indeed provide equivalent efficacy.

No inhaled glucocorticoid in the dry powder or metered dose inhaler formulation is approved for use in children less than four years of age. This is largely based on the inability of young children to consistently generate the necessary inspiratory flow rate to deliver adequate amounts of drug to the lungs. Since it is anticipated that available hydrochlorofluorocarbon-based metered dose inhalers will be removed from the market in the next several years, the new hydrofluoroalkane-based preparations should be evaluated for use in young children.

For moderate persistent levels of asthma severity, it is now recommended that a medium dose of inhaled glucocorticoid be administered or that a long-acting β-adrenergic agonist or a leukotriene modifier be added to low-dose inhaled glucocorticoid (6,8). The addition of a long-acting β-adrenergic agonist approach is based on observations that were derived from adult studies with no specific studies of comparative efficacy in young children. Furthermore, there is currently no long-acting β-adrenergic agonist formulation approved for use in children less than four years of age. Therefore, utilization of a long-acting β-adrenergic agonist is a non-approved use of an approved medication if administered. Also, there is no longer a metered dose inhaler preparation of a long-acting β-adrenergic agonist available. It would therefore be useful to develop a nebulized form of a long-acting β-adrenergic agonist for those patients unable to cooperate with the metered dose inhaler and spacer. Currently, the combination of inhaled fluticasone and salmeterol is approved, with labeling down to four years of age, but adequate inspiration technique must be ensured before relying on this device for management of asthma in young children, especially those four and five years of age.

Since the leukotriene receptor antagonist montelukast is approved for use in children down to one year of age with an age-appropriate formulation, this long-term controller could be added to an inhaled glucocorticoid as an alternative non-steroid supplemental control therapy. For young children with more severe asthma, high-dose inhaled glucocorticoids are recommended. If needed, systemic glucocorticoid with adjustment to the lowest dose either daily or on alternate days can be added to stabilize symptoms. This approach will obviously be refined as we obtain more information on the efficacy of the available approved medications for young children. For example, anti-IgE is a logical consideration for severe asthma in young children thought to be related to allergic airway inflammation but it is currently only approved for use in children 12 years of age and older, and it is only available in a limited number of countries.

V. Potential New Directions for the Management of Childhood Asthma

Recent advances in asthma research provide new insight for the management of asthma. While these studies have fortified the role of inhaled glucocorticoids as first-line therapy in the management of persistent asthma for all age groups, several studies identify some limitations in the overall efficacy of inhaled glucocorticoids, for example, loss of pulmonary function in early asthma, especially in young children. These concepts should now be applied in designing individualized asthma management plans for children.

A. Long-Term Outcomes

Results of recent studies focused on asthma management in children, such as the series of publications from the Childhood Asthma Management Program (CAMP) Research Group and the START study, provide supportive information for the safety and efficacy of long-term inhaled glucocorticoid therapy as compared to a symptom-based treatment plan (12–19). While the major outcome report in CAMP resolved a number of questions regarding the approach to asthma management, it generated a number of questions that form the base of ongoing studies (16). This long-term study was started in 1991 with the main goal being to determine whether continuous long-term treatment with either an inhaled glucocorticoid (budesonide) or an inhaled non-steroid (nedocromil) control medication could improve lung growth safely over a four- to six-year-treatment period compared to a symptom-based treatment plan (albuterol as needed).

The results of the CAMP trial showed that budesonide treatment increased postbronchodilator $FEV_1\%$ predicted from a mean of 103.2% predicted to 106.8% predicted within several months, but this measurement gradually diminished to 103.8% predicted by the end of the four- to six-year-study period. At the end of this study period, the postbronchodilator $FEV_1\%$ predicted in the budesonide group was similar to that in the placebo group. The nedocromil group was identical to the placebo group in postbronchodilator $FEV_1\%$ predicted throughout the treatment period. The CAMP study results thus raised questions about whether airway remodeling occurs in the population of mild to moderate persistent asthma and whether inhaled glucocorticoids have any effect on preventing this change in airway pathology. The START study indicated that declines in pulmonary function compared to predicted levels occur in younger children and adults but not as significantly in adolescence. Furthermore, inhaled glucocorticoids at best attenuate but do not prevent the decline in pulmonary function (19).

Based on this absence of decline in postbronchodilator $FEV_1\%$ predicted in adolescence, it is possible that one or more factors may be playing a role in the pathogenesis of asthma. First, $FEV_1\%$ predicted may be an insensitive marker for airway remodeling. Second, patients susceptible to airway remodeling or a progressive loss in $FEV_1\%$ predicted may have been screened out since only mild to moderate persistent asthmatics fit the entry criteria. Third, it is possible that the most significant effect on FEV_1 or airway remodeling occurred prior to entering the study since the mean duration of asthma at the time of randomization was five years (20,21). This latter observation would support the concept of evaluating the role of early recognition and early intervention on altering the natural history of asthma.

However, further analysis of the CAMP data by Covar et al. (18) has indicated that a decline in pulmonary function is actually occurring in a subset, approximately 20% of patients irrespective of the treatment arm. The etiology of this decline in percent predicted pulmonary function, whether structural or indicative of persistent inflammation, is under investigation.

The most distinct effect observed on a measure of pulmonary function in the CAMP study was the significant and consistent effect of inhaled budesonide on reducing airway hyperresponsiveness (16). Also, the most consistent effects on the clinical outcomes measures were observed with the inhaled glucocorticoid treatment arm as compared to the symptom-based treatment group. Hospitalizations, urgent care visits, and prednisone courses were significantly lower for the inhaled budesonide group (by approximately 45%) as compared to the placebo arm. The latter observation was also documented in the START study (19). Other clinical indicators showing a difference with inhaled budesonide as compared to placebo included lower symptom score, higher number of episode-free days per month, and less albuterol inhalations per week. However, the medications used in CAMP and START did not completely eliminate the morbidity associated with asthma (16,19).

The CAMP study helped alleviate concerns regarding the long-term effect of inhaled glucocorticoid therapy on body development by showing that the only detectable adverse effect was a transient reduction in growth velocity that was limited to one centimenter in the first year of treatment. Agertoft and Pedersen, in a long-term follow-up study, reported that final height is not reduced in young adults who received inhaled glucocorticoid therapy during childhood (22).

The rich CAMP database will continue to be evaluated as the ongoing 10-year post-treatment CAMP Continuation Study progresses. The CAMP participants are being followed into early adulthood in an attempt to define maximal lung and body growth parameters. The START study will also report on outcomes once the two-year-treatment period has ended. Both should yield useful information on the effect of early intervention in mild to moderate persistent asthma.

B.   Clinical Indicators for Early Diagnosis of Asthma

Having reliable indicators that would help identify the young child with wheezing episodes who was most likely to develop persistent asthma would be very useful. This type of information was derived from the Tucson Children's Respiratory Study (23). An Asthma Predictive Index was established from this study that suggests that frequent wheezing during the first three years of life and either one major risk factor (parental history of asthma or eczema) or two of three minor risk factors [eosinophilia (>4%), wheezing without colds, and allergic rhinitis] could predict the persistence of asthma (24).

Reports from this study also show that children who wheezed during lower respiratory tract illnesses in the first three years of life and were still wheezing at age six ("persistent wheezers") had slightly but not significantly lower levels of lung function than children who never wheezed before age six. At the age of six, however, persistent wheezers had significant deficits in lung function. The lowest levels of infant lung function were observed among children who wheezed before age three and were not current wheezers at age six ("transient wheezers") (20,23).

Therefore, the potential consequence of under-treatment may be a loss of pulmonary function over time that is greater than that observed in patients without asthma. This decline in pulmonary function could have an overall effect on long-term outcomes. Patients differ markedly in their clinical presentation and their susceptibility to this decline in lung function as demonstrated in the follow-up study of CAMP and START participants even in the presence of inhaled glucocorticoid therapy (18,19).

It has been proposed that early intervention with inhaled glucocorticoid therapy can be effective in preventing the progression of the disease and the risk for irreversible changes in the airways that could contribute to the persistence of symptoms. The Prevention of early Asthma in Kids (PEAK) study that is currently in progress as part of the NHLBI Childhood Asthma Research and Education Network utilized a positive Asthma Predictive Index as an entry criteria for the study. If this study yields positive results, the combination of the Asthma Predictive Index and effective inhaled glucocorticoid therapy could lead the way to improved long-term management through early recognition and early intervention. If the response is incomplete, it will generate new questions regarding the limitation of inhaled glucocorticoids, optimal doses of inhaled corticosteroids, how the results can be applied to low-risk groups of children, or perhaps the use of combination therapy with inhaled glucocortiocids and other long-term controllers or immunomodulators. Long-term early asthma prevention study (LEAP) is a four to five year study on both high- and low-risk groups of children younger than three. This placebo-controlled study was initiated in 1996. It uses initially high and later disease severity tailored doses of inhaled corticosteroids and follows the children until their sixth birthday (25). Although none of these studies will answer all questions, they are supplementary and will provide valuable information about the early use of inhaled corticosteroids in young children.

C. Interpatient and Intrapatient Variability in Response to Asthma Therapy

A study conducted by the NHLBI Asthma Clinical Research Network reported significant variability in response to inhaled glucocorticoids in adults with persistent asthma and reduced pulmonary function (26). This study examined pulmonary response to inhaled glucocorticoid therapy in 30 adult subjects with persistent asthma with FEV_1 between 55% and 85% predicted. Several observations were reported on this study population. First, near maximal FEV_1 and methacholine PC_{20} effects occurred with low to medium dose for inhaled fluticasone propionate and inhaled beclomethasone dipropionate administered via metered dose inhaler with a spacer device. Subsequently, the high dose of each inhaled glucocorticoid did not significantly increase either measure of efficacy; however, there was a measurable increase in systemic effect, overnight plasma cortisol. Second, there was significant inter-subject variability in both response measures noted with these two inhaled glucocorticoids. The investigators provided a note of caution that perhaps high doses of inhaled glucocorticoids may still be necessary to manage severe asthma or to prevent severe asthma exacerbations.

Approximately one-third of the subjects had a good response, defined as greater than 15% improvement in FEV_1 over the baseline, while another one-third had a marginal response, defined as 5% to 15% improvement in FEV_1 over the baseline, and yet another one-third had no response (defined as <5% improvement in FEV_1 over the baseline). This same distribution of responses was observed with methacholine PC_{20} improvement. Of interest, the FEV_1 improvement did not correlate to the PC_{20} improvement in this group of subjects, indicating that patients vary individually in their response to inhaled glucocorticoids. It was helpful to observe that certain biomarkers, such as exhaled nitric oxide and sputum eosinophils, and asthma characteristics, such as duration of asthma and bronchodilator response, were associated with differentiating the two types of response (26). The NHLBI Asthma Clinical Research Network is currently conducting studies to understand the reasons for poor response to inhaled glucocorticoid therapy as well as the association of a poor response to inhaled glucocorticoids to the possibility of an increased frequency of significant asthma exacerbations.

In addition, studies are also being completed in the NHLBI Childhood Asthma Research and Education Network to examine variable response to two classes of medications, inhaled glucocorticoids and oral leukotriene receptor antagonists (LTRA). This study was designed to determine if the refractoriness to inhaled glucocorticoid therapy reported in studies with adult participants is also present in children and whether the high proportion of poor responders identified in the adult population is of a similar proportion in children. This study will also characterize the response to an LTRA in these patients to determine if the response to an LTRA is proportional to the response to an inhaled glucocorticoid, or whether there are patients who respond to one of these two medications but not to the other medication, or who fail to respond to both of these medications. This careful assessment of response to two medications combined with careful phenotypic and genotypic analysis promises to provide insight into the identification of predictors of response to these two medications in children with mild to moderate persistent asthma. This would aid the clinician in choosing a medication most likely to achieve the desired response in an individual patient—so-called "personalized medicine." At present, our understanding of how to best assess and characterize individual responses is at an early stage. Asthma is a fluctuating disease and treatment effects on individual outcomes may not only depend on dose but also time of treatment. Maximum effects on some outcomes may take days while it may take years for others. Furthermore, the finding that the same person may be a "responder" with respect to one outcome and not to another further complicates the interpretation with respect to clinical conclusions. However, even if we still have a long way to go, each new study and design will add a new piece to the jigsaw puzzle.

D. Refractory Asthma

This area was addressed in detail by John Price in the chapter on difficult-to-control asthma. In addition, chapters in this book review special features of education (Patton), adolescence (Bacharier and Strunk), controlling the environment (Apter and Eggleston), special considerations in inner-city asthma (Kattan), adherence to medications (Bender), exercise management (Milgrom), and comorbid illness (Shapiro) that must be attended to in these patients. A provocative review by Payne and Balfour-Lynn also provides a summary of our understanding of difficult-to-control asthma in children, a very concerning group of patients (27). They presented an approach to the evaluation of children. They propose that once this type of patient is recognized, behavior and environmental control should be addressed, along with the appropriate use of medications, including medication delivery technique for inhaled therapy. Decisions must be made regarding the appropriate combination of bronchodilator and anti-inflammatory therapy, including dose, delivery device for inhaled medications, and timing of the treatment to take account of variability in symptom presentation. Interestingly, they propose that certain tools that are used to measure airway inflammation such as exhaled nitric oxide, induced sputum, bronchoalveolar lavage, and biopsy should be applied to assist in decisions centered around pursuing more aggressive forms of anti-inflammatory and immunomodulator therapy (methotrexate, cyclosporine, intravenous gamma globulin, etc.) or a course of bronchodilator therapy (subcutaneous terbutaline). Unfortunately, there is very little evidence in either children or adults, for that matter, that these measures can be reliably applied for clinical management decisions. In addition, Peter Gibson in his chapter on inflammatory markers discussed the application and limitation of these measures in children.

Two recent reports provide evidence that such a treatment approach, i.e., involving additional indicators of response, could be helpful in the overall management of asthma. The first is a report by Sont et al. (28). This group provided evidence indicating that a treatment approach for anti-inflammatory medication adjustment that is guided by measures of airway hyperresponsiveness leads to better overall asthma control, as indicated by improved pulmonary function and reduced symptoms, including significant exacerbations. They also provided data on an additional benefit on reduction in airway collagen deposition, perhaps an indicator of resolving airway remodeling. However, the previously discussed report by Szefler et al. (26) adds a note of caution for this approach. Since certain patients may be refractory to improvements in FEV_1 or reduction in airway hyperresponsiveness despite escalation of treatment to high-dose inhaled glucocorticoid therapy, an aggressive approach to treatment should be approached cautiously; if, indeed, high doses of inhaled glucocortiocids are needed to control asthma, then the current inhaled glucocorticoids have limitations of safety when administered at high doses for long periods of time. Perhaps new inhaled glucocortiocids, such as ciclesonide and mometasone, could provide a safety benefit at these high-dose ranges. Both medications are awaiting approval.

Those patients who are refractory to additional improvement with high-dose glucocorticoid therapy may have structural airway changes that are refractory to treatment, and thus failure to respond may not be indicative of persistent inflammation. These patients may be candidates for alternative forms of treatment. There is limited information on guiding the direction of treatment to reverse losses in pulmonary function that are poorly responsive to conventional therapy, except that cessation of smoking will both increase the effect of inhaled corticosteroids and reduce the time-dependent loss of lung function.

Another interesting observation in this patient population of severe asthma that deserves further investigation is the variable pattern of pulmonary function that can persist despite optimal management. Chan et al. (29) documented that there were two different patterns of pulmonary function in the population of patients classified as steroid-resistant asthma, specifically those who failed to see an improvement in pulmonary function despite a trial of high dose daily oral and inhaled glucocorticoid therapy. One group of patients maintains an FEV_1 below 70% and fail to improve (fixed or non-chaotic) while another group has a pattern characterized by variable pulmonary function throughout the day (brittle or chaotic) with periodic measurements below an FEV_1 of 70% predicted. Of additional importance is the observation that African Americans had a 38% prevalence of steroid-resistant asthma as compared to 12% in Caucasians. Further investigation is needed to identify the differing mechanisms for these two different patterns of steroid resistance as well as the high prevalence rate of steroid resistance in the African American population. This type of information should lead to new approaches to the management of refractory asthma.

E. Promising New Therapies

The new insight obtained through research reporting on observations from bronchoscopy, bronchoalveolar lavage, biopsy, molecular biology, and non-invasive measures of airway inflammation has stimulated thoughts around the new use of available medications and ideas for new medications. Identification of specific mediators associated with airway inflammation, such as IL-4, IL-5, IL-13, and interferon gamma, has stimulated the development of pharmaceutical agents to counteract the activity of these inflammatory mediators (30). To date, these approaches have not been very successful, likely due to the cascade of mediators involved or the failure to hit the key pathway for persistence of inflammation. The role of immunotherapy in the management of childhood asthma was reviewed in this book by Liu and Nelson. Another approach to immunomodulation of allergen sensitivity has been an attempt to develop DNA vaccine therapy with anti-sense oligonucleotides that theoretically could be applied to blocking the inflammatory response through a variety of pathways (31).

Although most of these early attempts at selective therapy have been disappointing, research should be designed to identify the population that does show a response to the treatment. Recent experience with anti-IgE should lead the way for the application of biologic response modifiers to asthma management (32,33). Experience with these medications should shed light on responders and non-responders and reason for treatment failure. In addition, inhibitors of phosphodiesterase 4 are undergoing early clinical trials. Other agents are at the phase 1 level of testing and are summarized in the chapter by Dr. Peter Barnes.

F. Pharmacogenetics

The area of genetics should provide insight related to the predisposition for asthma as well as response to medications (34–36). Available information is summarized in chapters by Weiss et al. and Szefler and Whelan in this review. It is important to define features of patients likely to develop persistent asthma, patients predisposed to severe exacerbations, patients predisposed to developing decline in lung function and irreversible airway obstruction, and patients with refractory asthma. It is the hope that advances in genetic associations could help define patients likely to follow these different pathways of disease presentation and also to identify features associated with response to available medications. This insight should pave the way for an individualized or "personalized" approach to treatment.

Genetic analysis is now being directed to genes related to the response to β-adrenergic agonists, to enzymes controlling leukotriene synthesis pathways and the leukotriene receptor, and to genes that control response to glucocorticoids (36).

Genes related to the origins and persistence of asthma are also likely associated with the response to available medications. For example, a predominant feature of asthma is allergic inflammation, considered to be an IgE-mediated response. IgE synthesis is regulated via IL-4 stimulation of B lymphocytes. Therefore, it is assumed that IL-4 has a disease-modifying role. Genetic features of IL-4-mediated IgE synthesis have been correlated to two mechanisms associated with genetic polymorphisms, increased IL-4 synthesis (C589T), or increased sensitivity to IL-4 at the IL-4 receptor level (R576 IL-4 receptor α) (37–42). An association of a sequence variant in the IL-4 gene promoter region at the C589T locus has also been correlated to asthma severity (40). The R576 IL-4 receptor α polymorphism has been linked to the severity of asthma (41). Since IL-13 also acts at the IL-4 receptor level, polymorphisms at the IL-13 level are also of interest (43,44).

Therefore, it is likely that further research will be successful in linking the benefit of a medication to an active disease pathway influenced, for example, leukotriene synthesis and leukotriene receptor antagonists as well as cytokine synthesis and a variability in response at the level of the glucocorticoid receptor (36,45,46). Failure to respond to treatment could therefore be related to excessive activity of a mediator synthesis pathway or an alternative pathway associated with disease activity. It is possible that response to one treatment may mask other features of the disease that are refractory to this treatment. For example, a bronchodilator medication may be very successful in improving overall pulmonary function but may not be successful in preventing progression of the disease that leads to long-term deterioration in pulmonary function. This area of investigation is in its infancy but holds promising opportunities to understand the variability in response to treatment as well as to provide unique insights into developing new medications, defining the best treatment combinations and an individualized approach to treatment.

VI. Summary and Conclusions

The understanding of asthma and the consequent approach to treatment has evolved considerably over the last 50 years. It is possible that the correct assembly of early indicators of asthma, such as a symptom pattern, patient features, biomarkers, and genetics, could further refine the approach to early intervention. With the right intervention, it is possible that the disease could be induced into remission and thus, in a sense, maintain a relative "cure"; however, there are a number of issues that must be addressed, including access to health care by all who have asthma (47). Current interest regarding early pharmacologic intervention options centers around the comparative effects of inhaled glucocorticoids and leukotriene antagonists; however, neither of these agents may be sufficient to control asthma progression, and new approaches, such as combination therapy, or new treatments with modest clinical effects but marked effects on airway remodeling could evolve as a result of careful investigation. We can also learn from the experience gained by the research into other modes of treatment, as well as overall experience with appropriate introduction of immunomodulator therapy, for example, in diseases such as rheumatoid arthritis and psoriasis (48,49).

Prevention of asthma at an early stage could therefore have an effect on preventing the development of severe asthma. Patients with severe asthma are characterized by low and irreversible pulmonary function. Their disease often has its origins in early childhood. It is therefore important to recognize patients at risk for developing severe asthma and to provide more effective interventions at critical stages of their disease progression. Consequently, it is important to develop good measures of persistent inflammation and to use this technology as a gauge to adjusting and individualizing therapy.

Once asthma is established, it is necessary to measure the response to treatment by evaluating all of the individual parameters of response, for example, symptoms, pulmonary function, and long-term features of progression. Recent studies have demonstrated that over a certain treatment period, certain patients may clearly respond to conventional treatment in one category, for example, improvement in FEV_1, but not in another category, such as reduction in airways hyperresponsiveness (26). Recognizing this deficiency in selective areas of responses should prompt direction of treatment to improve individual response categories. The new tools, such as exhaled nitric oxide, measurement of mediators in exhaled breath condensates and blood markers of inflammation, should be useful in tailoring response or treatment in order to optimize response and prevent significant exacerbations and even disease progression.

This review has focused on our understanding of the current therapeutic interventions and the possibilities for improving asthma management and potentially inducing a remission or cure for the disease. However, all of the benefits of science will not be achieved unless there is a concomitant integrated approach to patient care. There are currently serious deficiencies in the present health care system that influence access to health care worldwide. The recent observation of an arrest in the rise in asthma mortality and morbidity in certain countries is very encouraging but offers a challenge to determine whether a further reduction in morbidity and mortality is achievable (1). There are obviously discrepancies within populations, for example, asthma in inner-city children, that remain to be addressed. Concerted efforts are now being directed toward understanding this phenomenon and recommendations have been made to integrate the various resources available to improve outcomes of asthma care for children (47).

Acknowledgments

The authors would like to thank Gretchen Hugen for assistance in the manuscript preparation.

References

1. Mannino DM, Homa DM, Akinbami LJ, Moorman JE, Gwynn C, Redd SC. Surveillance for asthma—United States, 1980–1999. MMWR 2002; 51:1–13.
2. Hamid QA, Minshall EM. Molecular pathology of allergic disease: I: lower airway disease. J Allergy Clin Immunol 2000; 105:20–36.
3. Suissa S, Ernst P. Inhaled corticosteroids: impact on asthma morbidity and mortality. J Allergy Clin Immunol 2001; 107:937–944.
4. Spahn JD, Szefler SJ. Inhaled glucocorticoids from combination therapy for asthma and COPD. In: Martin RJ, Kraft M, eds. Lung biology in health and diseases series. New York: Marcel Dekker, 2000; 145:1–52.
5. Matz J, Emmett A, Rickard K, Kalberg C. Addition of salmeterol to low-dose fluticasone versus higher-dose fluticasone: an analysis of asthma exacerbations. J Allergy Clin Immunol 2001; 107:783–789.
6. National Institutes of Health, National Heart, Lung, and Blood Institute. Global Initiative for Asthma. Global strategy for asthma management and prevention, NHLBI/NIH workshop report. 2002.
7. National Asthma Education and Prevention Program Expert Panel Report 2: Guidelines for the Diagnosis and Management of Asthma. National Institutes of Health, National Heart, Lung, and Blood Institute, Publ. No. 97-4051,1997.
8. National Asthma Education and Prevention Program Report: Guidelines for the Diagnosis and Management of Asthma Update on Selected Topics— 2002. J Allergy Clin Immunol 2002; 110:S141–S219.
9. Agertoft L, Pedersen S. Effects of long-term treatment with an inhaled corti-costeroid on growth and pulmonary function in asthmatic children. Respir Med 1994; 88:373–381.
10. Inman M. Is there a place for anti-remodeling drugs in asthma which may not display immediate clinical efficacy? Eur Respir J 2004; 24:1–2.
11. Bisgaard H, Price MJ, Maden C, Olsen NA. Cost-effectiveness of fluticasone propionate administered via metered-dose inhaler plus babyhaler spacer in the treatment of asthma in pre-school aged children. Chest 2001; 120:1835–1842.
12. Zeiger RS, Dawson C, Weiss S. Relationships between duration of asthma and asthma severity among children in the childhood asthma management program (CAMP). J Allergy Clin Immunol 1999; 103:376–387.
13. Nelson HS, Szefler SJ, Jacobs J, Huss K, Shapiro G, Sternberg AL. The relationships among environmental allergen sensitization, allergen exposure,

pulmonary function, and bronchial hyperresponsiveness in the Childhood Asthma Management Program. J Allergy Clin Immunol 1999; 104:775–785.

14. Bender BG, Annett RD, Iklé D, DuHamel TR, Rand C, Strunk RC. Relationship between disease and psychological adaptation in children in the Childhood Asthma Management Program and their families. CAMP Research Group. Arch Pediatr Adolesc Med 2000; 154:706–713.

15. Annett RD, Aylward EH, Lapidus J, Bender BG, DuHamel T. Neurocognitive functioning in children with mild and moderate asthma in the childhood asthma management program. The childhood asthma management program (CAMP) Research Group. J Allergy Clin Immunol 2000; 105:717–724.

16. The Childhood Asthma Management Program Research Group. Long-term effects of budesonide or nedocromil in children with asthma. N Engl J Med 2000; 343:1054–1063.

17. Covar RA, Szefler SJ, Martin RJ, Sundstrom DA, Silkoff PE, Murphy J, Young DA, Spahn JD. Relationships between exhaled nitric oxide and measures of disease activity among children with mild to moderate asthma. J Pediatr 2003; 142: 469–475.

18. Covar RA, Spahn JD, Murphy JR, Szefler SJ, for the Childhood Asthma Management Program Research Group. Progression of asthma measured by lung function in the Childhood Asthma Management Program. Am J Respir Crit Care Med 2004; 170:235–241.

19. Pauwels RA, Pedersen S, Busse WW, Tan WC, Chen YZ, Ohlsson SV, Ullman A, Lamm CJ, O'Byrne PM, on behalf of the START Investigators Group. Early intervention with budesonide in mild persistent asthma: a randomized, double-blind trial. Lancet 2003; 361:1071–1076.

20. Martinez FD, Wright AL, Taussig LM, Holberg CJ, Halonen M, Morgan WJ. Associates TGHM. Asthma and wheezing in the first six years of life. N Engl J Med 1995; 332:133–138.

21. Phelan PD, Robertson CF, Olinsky A. The Melbourne Asthma Study: 1964–1999. J Allergy Clin Immunol 2002; 109:189–194.

22. Agertoft L, Pedersen S. Effect of long-term treatment with inhaled budesonide on adult height in children with asthma. N Engl J Med 2000; 343:1064–1069.

23. Martinez FD. Development of wheezing disorders and asthma in preschool children. Pediatrics 2002; 109:362–367.

24. Castro-Rodriguez JA, Holberg CJ, Wright AL, Martinez FD. A clinical index to define risk of asthma in young children with recurrent wheezing. Am J Respir Crit Care Med 2000; 162:1403–1406.

25. Agertoft L, Pedersen S. Inhaled steroid treatment in early wheeze in children younger than three years. Long-term Early Asthma Prevention (LEAP) study. Rationale and design. Control Clin Trials 2004, in press.

26. Szefler SJ, Martin RJ, Sharp-King T, Boushey HA, Cherniack RM, Chinchilli VM, Craig TJ, Dolovich M, Drazen JM, Fagan JK, Fahy JV, Fish JE, Ford JG, Israel E, Kiley J, Kraft M, Lazarus SC, Lemanske RF, Mauger E, Peters SP, Sorkness CA, for the Asthma Clinical Research Network of the National Heart, Lung, and Blood Institute. Significant variability in response to inhaled corticosteroids for persistent asthma. J Allergy Clin Immunol 2002; 109:410–418.

27. Payne DNR, Balfour-Lynn IM. Children with difficult asthma: A practical approach. J Asthma 2001; 38:189–203.
28. Sont JK, Willems LNA, Bel EH, van Krieken JHJM, Vendenbroucke JP, Sterk PJ, the AMPUL Study group. Clinical control and histopathologic outcome of asthma when using airway hyperresponsiveness as an additional guide to long-term treatment. Am J Respir Crit Care Med 1999; 159:1043–1051.
29. Chan MT, Leung DYM, Szefler SJ, Spahn JD. Difficult-to-control asthma: clinical characteristics of steroid- insensitive asthma. J Allergy Clin Immunol 1998; 101(5):594–601.
30. Barnes P. New targets for future asthma therapy. In: Yeadon M, Diamont Z, eds. New and exploratory therapeutic agents for asthma, lung biology in health and disease. Vol. 139. New York: Marcel Dekker, 2000:361–389.
31. Kline JN. DNA therapy for asthma. Curr Opin Allergy Immunol 2002; 2:69–73.
32. Corren J, Casale T, Deniz Y, Ashby M. Omalizumab, a recombinant humanized anti-IgE antibody, reduces asthma-related emergency room visits and hospitalizations in patients with allergic asthma. J Allergy Clin Immunol 2003; 111:87–90.
33. Finn A, Gross G, van Bavel J, Lee T, Windom H, Everhard F, Fowler-Taylor A, Liu J, Gupta N. Omalizumab improves asthma-related quality of life in patients with severe allergic asthma. J Allergy Clin Immunol 2003; 111:278–284.
34. Ober C, Moffatt ME. Contributing factors to the pathobiology: the genetics of asthma. Clin Chest Med 2000; 21:245–261.
35. Fenech A, Hall IP. Pharmacogenetics of asthma. Br J Clin Pharmacol 2002; 53:2–15.
36. Palmer LJ, Silverman ES, Weiss ST, Drazen JM. Pharmacogenetics of asthma. Am J Respir Crit Care Med 2002; 165:861–866.
37. Marsh DG, Neely JD, Breazeale DR, Ghosh B, Freidhoff LR, Ehrlich-Kautzky E, Schou C, Krishnaswamy G, Beaty TH. Linkage analysis of IL4 and other chromosome 5q31.1 markers and total serum immunoglobulin E concentrations. Science 1994; 264:1152–1156.
38. Borish L, Mascali JJ, Klinnert M, Leppert M, Rosenwasser LJ. SSC polymorphisms in interleukin genes. Hum Mol Genet 1995; 4:974.
39. Rosenwasser LJ, Klemm DJ, Dresback JK, Inamura H, Mascali JJ, Klinnert M, Borish L. Promoter polymorphisms in the chromosome 5 gene cluster in asthma and atopy. Clin Exp Allergy 1995; 25(Suppl 2):74–78; discussion 95–96.
40. Burchard EG, Silverman EK, Rosenwasser LJ, Borish L, Yandava C, Pillari A, Weiss ST, Hasday J, Lilly CM, Ford JG, Drazen JM. Association between a sequence variant in the IL-4 gene promoter and FEV(l) in asthma. Am J Respir Crit Care Med 1999; 160:919–922.
41. Hershey GK, Friedrich MF, Esswein LA, Thomas ML, Chatila TA. The association of atopy with a gain-of-function mutation in the alpha subunit of the interleukin-4 receptor. N Engl J Med 1997; 337:1720–1725.
42. Rosa-Rosa L, Zimmermann N, Bernstein JA, Rothenberg ME, Khurana Hershey GK. The R576 IL-4 receptor alpha allele correlates with asthma severity. J Allergy Clin Immunol 1999; 104:1008–1014.

43. Martinez FD. Maturation of immune responses at the beginning of asthma. J Allergy Clin Immunol 1999; 103:355–361.
44. Spahn JD, Szefler SJ, Surs W, Doherty DE, Nimmagadda SR, Leung DYM. A novel action of IL-13: induction of diminished monocyte glucocorticoid receptor-binding affinity. J Immunol 1996; 157:2654–2659.
45. Kam JC, Szefler SJ, Surs W, Sher ER, Leung DYM. Combination IL-2 and IL-4 reduces glucocorticoid receptor binding affinity and T cell response to glucocorticoids. J Immunol 1993; 151:3460–3466.
46. Sher ER, Leung DYM, Surs W, Kam JC, Zieg, G, Kamada AK, Szefler SJ. Steroid resistant asthma: cellular mechanisms contributing to inadequate response to glucocorticoid therapy. J Clin Invest 1994; 93:33–39.
47. Lara M, Rosenbaum S, Rachelefsky G, Nicholas W, Morton SC, Emont S, Branch M, Genovese B, Vaiana ME, Smith V, Wheeler L, Platts-Mills T, Clark N, Lurie N, Weiss KV. Improving childhood asthma outcomes in the United States: a blueprint for policy action. Pediatrics 2002; 109:919–930.
48. O'Dell JR. Therapeutic strategies for rheumatoid arthritis. New Engl J Med 2004; 350:2591–2602.
49. Nickoloff BJ, Nestle FO. Recent insights into the immunopathogenesis of psoriasis provide new therapeutic opportunities. J Clin Invest 2004; 113: 1664–1675.

Index